264 – 275

× 281

16
8
128

4 16

8
1286
136.6

2.54
72
508
1778 0
182.88

72
×2.54
183

Inches to CM

× 2.54

BONTRAGER and ANTHONY

Textbook of
RADIOGRAPHIC POSITIONING
and
Related
Anatomy

About the Authors

Barry T. Anthony, R.T. (R) has used his considerable teaching experience to best advantage in writing educational media for radiologic technologists. His reputation as a leading educator and as an authority in the subjects of anatomy and positioning, including special procedures and radiographic pathology, have brought invitations to present workshops and symposia on these subjects at state and national conventions.

Mr. Anthony majored in zoology at the University of Denver and received his training in radiologic technology at the University of Colorado Medical Center. He has served as an instructor and technical director of a hospital school of radiologic technology, an administrative technologist of a large Denver area hospital and as an instructor at an associate degree program in radiologic technology.

He has been employed as an author/editor by Multi-Media Publishing, Inc. since 1978. Mr. Anthony has authored and co-authored with Mr. Kenneth L. Bontrager numerous audiovisual programs in radiologic technology, including the 21-unit Radiographic Anatomy and Positioning series.

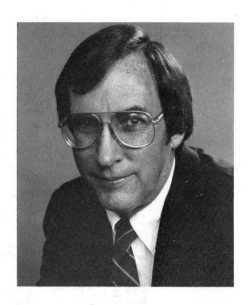

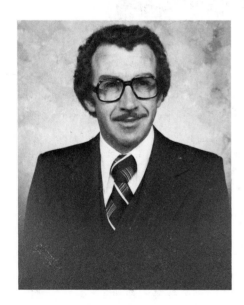

Kenneth L. Bontrager, M.A., R.T. (R), who was trained in radiologic technology at St. Luke's Hospital in Denver, received B.A. and M.A. degrees from the University of Colorado and the University of Northern Colorado, respectively. He has served as technical director of a hospital school of radiologic technology, administrative technologist in a large hospital and director of an associate degree college program in radiologic technology. His extensive teaching experience includes presentations of numerous workshops and symposia on teaching methods and instructional media at state and national conventions.

Mr. Bontrager founded Multi-Media Publishing, Inc. in 1971 for the express purpose of developing educational resources for radiologic technology and other health care professions. Mr. Bontrager has mastered the techniques involved in the challenging field of writing and developing successful self-instructional audiovisual programs. He has authored, co-authored and/or edited over 100 such programs since 1970. Among his best known radiologic technology programs are an x-ray physics and technique series, a dental radiography series and the 21-unit Radiographic Anatomy and Positioning series, co-authored with Barry T. Anthony. These self-instructional programs are being used by literally thousands of students each year in the U.S., Canada and many countries throughout the world.

Mr. Bontrager lives with his wife and two sons in a mountain setting west of Denver where he enjoys such hobbies as woodworking, hiking, photography, horseback riding and snowmobiling. He is active in his local church as a teacher and Christian Education Director. He has studied theology at Denver Seminary where he received the M.A. degree in Christian Education.

Radiographic Anatomy and Positioning
A Self-Paced Multimedia Learning Series
by Kenneth L. Bontrager, M.A., R.T. (R)
Barry T. Anthony, R.T. (R)

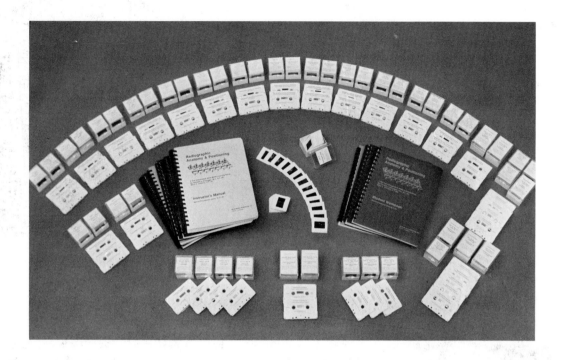

Content of Audiovisual Series

The anatomy and positioning audiovisual series covers all of the routine procedures and the common procedures presented in this text. The audiovisual units on cerebral pneumography, cerebral angiography and computed tomography are directed toward advanced, second-year students and practicing technologists. This knowledge is presented in less depth for the student users of the textbook.

Each audiovisual unit contains a series of visuals accompanied by an audio tape narration. The student workbook contains review exercises and a self-administered test on the material presented in the unit. The instructor's manual that accompanies each unit contains a lesson evaluation to measure each student's mastery of the material.

The complete 21-unit series contains **1,536 slides, 48 audio tapes,** a **three-volume student workbook** and a **five-volume set of instructor's manuals.**

Relationship of Audiovisual Series to Textbook

The textbook covers the anatomy and positioning information needed by students and can be used by itself, without the A-V series. But the A-V series provides an excellent adjunct to the text. The series presents the subject matter in the multi-media format of seeing, hearing and doing. Each year thousands of students use the audiovisual series. It has a proven history of increasing comprehension and retention, resulting in improved Registry and Certification scores.

The A-V series can be used as either an individualized, self-paced learning program or as a teaching aid in classroom instruction. Either way, it enhances the use of the text. A student could read a chapter of the text, then take the corresponding A-V unit to reinforce and expand knowledge in that area; or an instructor could use the audiovisual presentation as a classroom aid while teaching a chapter in the textbook.

Availability of Audiovisual Series

This series is only available from the publisher. For ordering and pricing information, please write to Multi-Media Publishing, Inc., 1393 S. Inca, Denver, CO 80223, or call (303) 778-1404.

BONTRAGER and ANTHONY

Textbook of
RADIOGRAPHIC POSITIONING
and Related Anatomy

Kenneth L. Bontrager
M.A., R.T. (R)

Barry T. Anthony
R.T. (R)

Multi·Media Publishing, inc.
1393 South Inca Street, Denver, Colorado 80223

© 1982 by Multi-Media Publishing, Inc., Denver Colorado
First Edition — Fifth Printing 1985

Printed in the United States of America

MULTI-MEDIA PUBLISHING, INC., BOOK DIVISION
1393 S. INCA STREET, DENVER, COLORADO 80223

Library of Congress Cataloging in Publication Data

Bontrager, 1937-
    Textbook of radiographic positioning and related anatomy.

    Bibliography: p.
    Includes index.
    1. Radiography, Medical— Positioning.
2. Anatomy, Human. I. Anthony, 1937-
II. Title. [DNLM: 1. Technology, Radiologic.
WN 160 B722t]
RC78.4.B66   1982   616.07′572   81-82006
ISBN 0-940122-01-4

MMP/M/M   9 8 7 6 5

Acknowledgments

Determination of the appropriate acknowledgments for this project is very difficult because of the many persons who contributed in such significant ways. Contributors include professional models and the dedicated radiology staff at Swedish Medical Center, Englewood, Colorado. Also included are the staff photographers, editors, typists, typesetters, artists, graphic designers and layout personnel here at Multi-Media Publishing, Inc. who have worked so many, many hours on this project. These persons are specifically recognized at the end of this book.

K.L.B. and B.T.A.

Personal Acknowledgments

I want to especially acknowledge and thank my longtime personal secretary and friend, Vi Fast, for her many contributions both to this project and to the audiovisual series from which came much of the basic information for this textbook. In addition to Vi, Jo Spilver and Freda Friesen also aided and supported me personally with their patience in typing and retyping drafts and revisions, and with the final typesetting. Phil Christie, as the principal editor and Project Manager for this project, aided both Barry and myself in so many ways. I personally thank him for his dedication, his belief in this project and his willingness to work with two authors with somewhat different writing styles, combining these writings into a unified entity. Dave Spilver, as Chief Editor of the Health Science Division, also gave me advice and encouragement.

I thank you, Barry, for your willingness to work with me these past years and to lend your expertise in special procedures and your extensive knowledge of anatomy to this project.

Last, and most important, I want to thank my wife, Mary Lou, and our two teenage sons, Neil and Troy, for their love and encouragement, and their willingness to "give up" their husband and father to this project for the past year, during which time the majority of evenings were spent at the office writing.

K.L.B.

Personal Acknowledgments

My deepest appreciation goes to Kenneth Bontrager for his support, interaction and understanding throughout the arduous writing, rewriting and compilation of this textbook. Indeed, my gratitude extends back to our earliest association and endeavors in the early 1970's. I wish to thank the entire radiology department at Swedish Medical Center in Englewood, Colorado, and especially Drs. William Jobe and Charles Seibert, and department administrator, Mrs. Vonnie Molgaard. I sincerely appreciate the technical expertise and excellent cooperation of the extraordinary staff of Multi-Media Publishing, Inc. of Denver, Colorado. Thanks, Phil, Vi, Mary Lou, Jo, Freda, Steve, Julie, Bob, Dick, Barb, CaroLee, Lois, Greg and Dave.

My biggest and best thank-you goes to my wife, Cecilia Holland, and my son, Jeffrey, for their support, encouragement and love.

B.T.A.

Preface

Purpose

This book is designed to meet the need for a thorough, clearly illustrated, simply written anatomy and positioning textbook for student radiographers. This textbook is **not** another comprehensive reference atlas. Instead it encompasses in one volume explanations and illustrations of the anatomy and positioning that all practicing radiographers must master. All of the basic or routine projections or positions for all body parts and systems are described and illustrated. Some of the more common optional projections and/or positions are also covered.

Uniqueness of Book

What is unique about this book is the way that it incorporates the techniques of self-paced, multimedia instruction into a textbook format. The writing is concise and visually oriented. The content is programmed to build from known to unknown, simple to difficult. All anatomy and positioning descriptions are accompanied by extensive visuals. These visuals and the written descriptions are grouped together to enable the student to quickly comprehend the relationship between body parts and systems, between patient and part positioning, and between the correct central ray direction and location.

The authors developed this writing style through many years of writing self-paced audiovisual programs for student radiographers. The testimony from literally hundreds of instructors has shown that self-paced, visually oriented instruction dramatically increases student retention and comprehension. A major purpose of this book is to provide the students with proven benefits of this method presented in textbook form.

Combining Anatomy & Positioning

The authors firmly believe in the importance of learning anatomy and positioning concurrently. Unless they are studied together, positioning is often learned by simply memorizing body positions and central ray locations. A thorough understanding of body structures and anatomical relationships helps develop highly competent, "thinking" radiographers who can conceptually visualize what is being radiographed and change or adapt positioning routines as needed.

This instructional approach and the combining of anatomy and positioning has also been used by the authors in their audiovisual series. According to instructors from around the U.S. and Canada, this approach has resulted in dramatic improvements in anatomy and positioning scores on certification and registry exams.

Contents

BONTRAGER and ANTHONY

Textbook of
RADIOGRAPHIC POSITIONING
and
Related
Anatomy

CHAPTER 1

General, Systemic and Skeletal Anatomy, Arthrology, and Basic Principles and Terminology of Radiographic Positioning

Part I. General, Systemic and Skeletal Anatomy

A. General Anatomy

Anatomy is the science of the structure of the human body, while **physiology** deals with functions of the body, or how the body parts work. In the living subject, it is almost impossible to study **anatomy** without also studying physiology. Radiographic study of the human body is primarily a study of the anatomy of the various systems with lesser emphasis on the physiology. Consequently, anatomy of the human system will be emphasized in this radiographic anatomy and positioning text.

Structural Organization

Several levels of structural organization compose the human body. The lowest level of organization is the **chemical level.** All of the chemicals necessary for maintaining life are composed of **atoms,** joined in various ways to form **molecules.** Various chemicals in the form of molecules are organized to form **cells.**

Cells: The cell is the basic structural and functional unit of the entire human being. Every single part of the body, whether muscle, bone, cartilage, fat, nerve, skin or blood, is composed of cells.

Tissues: Tissues, groups of similar cells together with their intercellular material, perform a specific function. The four basic types of tissues are: (1) epithelial, (2) connective, (3) muscular, and (4) nervous.

Organs: When various tissues are joined together to perform a specific function, the result is an organ. Organs usually have a specific shape. Some of the organs of the human body are the heart, liver, lungs, stomach and brain.

System: A system consists of a group or association of organs that has a similar or a common function. The digestive system is an example of several organs that combine to function in the breakdown of food for the total being.

Organism: All of the systems of the body functioning together constitute the total organism — one living being.

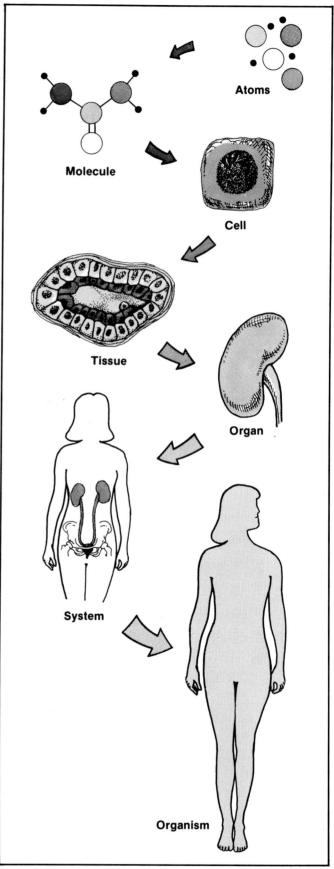

Fig. 1-1

Levels of Human Structural Organization

B. Systemic Anatomy

Body Systems

The human body is a structural and functional unit made up of ten lesser units termed systems. These ten systems are: (1) skeletal, (2) circulatory, (3) digestive, (4) respiratory, (5) urinary, (6) reproductive, (7) nervous, (8) muscular, (9) endocrine, and (10) integumentary.

1. Skeletal System: The skeletal system is the most important system to be studied by the radiographer. The skeletal system includes the 206 separate bones of the body and their associated cartilages and joints. The study of bones is termed **osteology,** while the study of joints is termed **arthrology.**

Four functions of the skeletal system are: (1) to support and protect the body, (2) to allow movement by interacting with the muscles to form levers, (3) to produce blood cells, and (4) to store calcium.

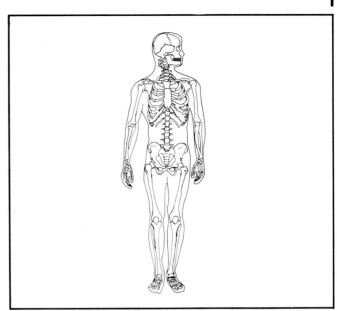

Skeletal System   Fig. 1-2

2. Circulatory System: The circulatory system is composed of the cardiovascular organs — heart, blood and blood vessels, as well as the lymphatic organs — lymph nodes, lymph and lymph vessels.

Six functions of the circulatory system are: (1) to distribute oxygen and nutrients to the cells of the body; (2) to carry cell waste and carbon dioxide from the cells; (3) to transport water, electrolytes, hormones and enzymes; (4) to protect against disease; (5) to prevent hemorrhage by forming blood clots; and (6) to help regulate body temperature.

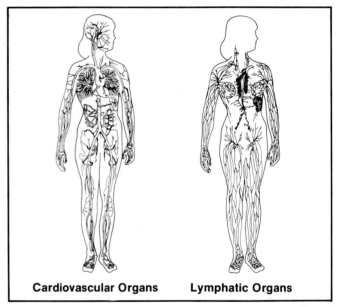

Cardiovascular Organs   **Lymphatic Organs**

Circulatory System   Fig. 1-3

3. Digestive System: The digestive system includes the alimentary canal and certain accessory organs. The alimentary canal is made up of the mouth, pharynx, esophagus, stomach, small intestine, large intestine and anus. Accessory organs of digestion include the salivary glands, liver, gallbladder and pancreas.

The twofold function of the digestive system is (1) to prepare food for absorption by the cells through numerous physical and chemical breakdown processes and (2) to eliminate solid wastes from the body.

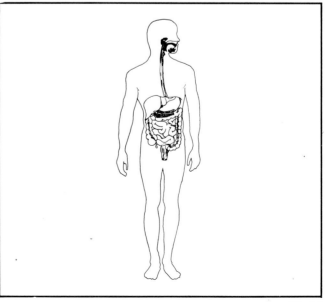

Digestive System   Fig. 1-4

4. Respiratory System: The respiratory system is composed of two lungs and a series of passages connecting the lungs to the outside atmosphere. The structures making up the passageway from the exterior to the alveoli of the lung interior are the nose, mouth, pharynx, larynx, trachea and bronchial tree.

Three functions of the respiratory system are: (1) to supply oxygen to the blood and eventually to the cells, (2) to eliminate carbon dioxide from the blood, and (3) to assist in regulating the acid-base balance of the blood.

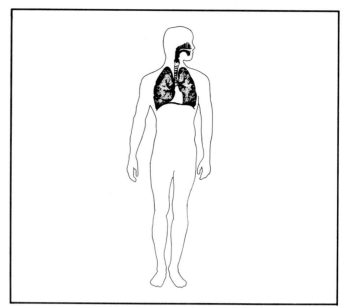

Respiratory System   Fig. 1-5

5. Urinary System: The urinary system includes those organs that produce, collect and eliminate urine. The organs of the urinary system are the kidneys, ureters, bladder and urethra.

The urinary system functions (1) to regulate the chemical composition of the blood, (2) to eliminate many waste products, (3) to regulate fluid and electrolyte balance and volume, and (4) to maintain the acid-base balance of the body.

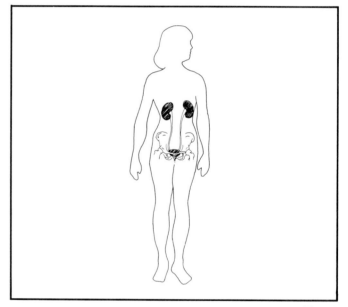

Urinary System   Fig. 1-6

6. Reproductive System: The reproductive or genital system includes those organs that produce, transport and store the germ cells. The testes in the male and the ovaries in the female produce mature germ cells. Transport and storage organs of the male include the vas deferens, prostate gland and penis. Additional organs of reproduction in the female are the uterine tubes, uterus and vagina.

The function of the reproductive system is to reproduce the organism.

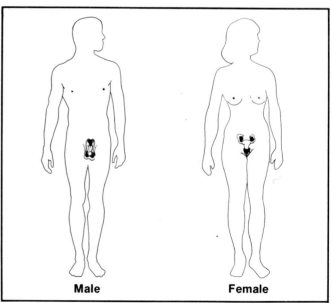

Male   **Female**

Reproductive System   Fig. 1-7

7. Nervous System: The nervous system is composed of the brain, spinal cord, nerves, ganglia and special sense organs such as the eyes and ears.

The function of the nervous system is to regulate body activities with electrical impulses traveling along various nerves.

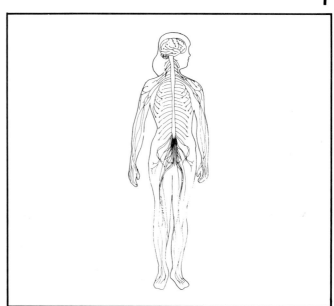

Nervous System   Fig. 1-8

8. Muscular System: The muscular system includes all muscle tissues of the body and is subdivided into three types: (1) skeletal, (2) visceral, and (3) cardiac. Most of the muscle mass of the body is skeletal muscle, which is striated and under voluntary control. The voluntary muscles act in conjunction with the skeleton to allow body movement. About 43 percent of the weight of the human body is composed of voluntary or striated skeletal muscle. Visceral muscle, which is smooth and involuntary, is located in the walls of hollow internal organs such as blood vessels, stomach and intestines. These muscles are termed involuntary because their contraction is usually not under voluntary or conscious control. Cardiac muscle is found only in the walls of the heart and is involuntary, but striated.

Three functions of muscle tissue are: (1) to allow movement, such as locomotion of the body or movement of substances through the alimentary canal, (2) to maintain posture, and (3) to produce heat.

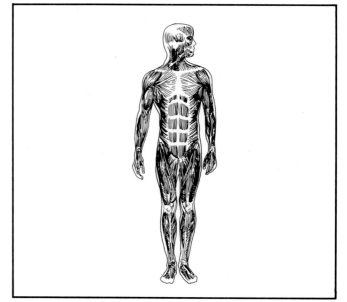

Muscular System   Fig. 1-9

9. Endocrine System: The endocrine system includes all of the ductless glands of the body. These glands include the testes, ovaries, pancreas, adrenals, thymus, thyroid, parathyroids, pineal and pituitary. The placenta acts as a temporary endocrine gland.

Hormones, which are the secretions of the endocrine glands, are released directly into the bloodstream.

The function of the endocrine system is to regulate bodily activities through the various hormones carried by the cardiovascular system.

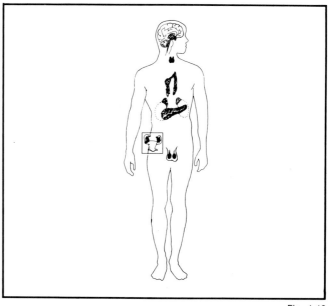

Endocrine System   Fig. 1-10

10. Integumentary System: The integumentary system is composed of the skin and all structures derived from the skin. These derived structures include hair, nails, and sweat and oil glands. The skin is an organ that is essential to life. In fact, the skin is the largest organ of the body, covering a surface area of approximately 7,620 square centimeters in the average adult.

Four functions of the integumentary system are: (1) to regulate body temperature, (2) to protect the body, (3) to eliminate waste products through perspiration, and (4) to receive certain stimuli such as temperature, pressure and pain.

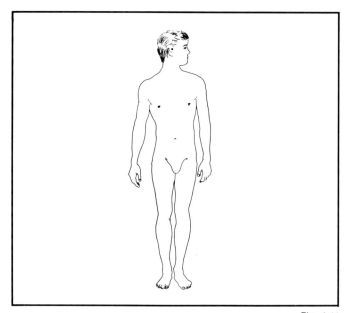

Integumentary System   Fig. 1-11

C. Skeletal Anatomy

Since a large part of general diagnostic radiography involves examinations of the bones and joints, **osteology** (the study of bones) and **arthrology** (the study of joints) are important subjects for the radiographer.

Osteology

The adult skeletal system is composed of 206 separate bones, forming the framework of the entire body. Certain cartilages, such as the costal cartilages and cartilage at the ends of long bones, are included in the skeletal system. These bones and cartilages are united by ligaments and provide surfaces to which the muscles attach. Since muscles and bones must combine to allow body movement, these two systems are sometimes collectively referred to as the loco-motor system.

Axial Skeleton: The adult human skeleton is divided into either the axial skeleton or the appendicular skeleton. The **axial skeleton** includes all bones that lie on or near the central axis of the body. The axial skeleton consists of 80 bones and includes the skull, vertebral column, ribs and sternum.

Axial Skeleton

Skull		
Cranium	—	8
Facial Bones	—	14
Hyoid	—	1
Auditory Ossicles	—	6
(Small bones in each ear)		
Vertebral column		
Cervical	—	7
Thoracic	—	12
Lumbar	—	5
Sacrum	—	1
Coccyx	—	1
Thorax		
Sternum	—	1
Ribs	—	24
Total		80

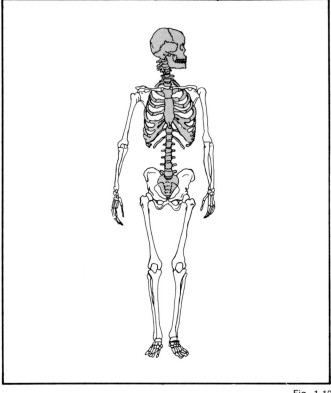

Axial Skeleton   Fig. 1-12

Appendicular Skeleton: The second division of the skeleton is the **appendicular** portion. This division consists of all bones of the upper and lower extremities, as well as the shoulder and pelvic girdles. There are 126 separate bones in the appendicular skeleton.

Appendicular Skeleton

Shoulder Girdles		
Clavicle	—	2
Scapula	—	2
Upper Extremities		
Humerus	—	2
Ulna	—	2
Radius	—	2
Carpals	—	16
Metacarpals	—	10
Phalanges	—	28
Pelvic Girdle		
Hip bone	—	2
Lower Extremities		
Femur	—	2
Tibia	—	2
Fibula	—	2
Patella	—	2
Tarsals	—	14
Metatarsals	—	10
Phalanges	—	28
Total		126

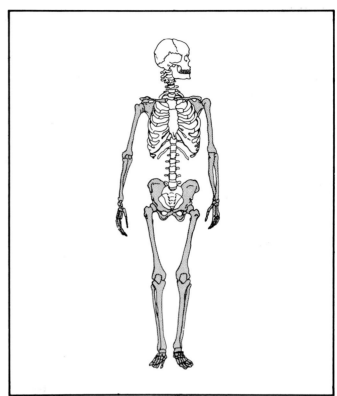

Appendicular Skeleton   Fig. 1-13

Classification of Bones

Each of the 206 bones of the body can be classified according to shape as a (1) long bone, (2) short bone, (3) flat bone, or (4) irregular bone.

1. Long Bones: Long bones consist of a shaft or diaphysis and two ends or extremities. The ends of long bones articulate with other bones; thus the ends are enlarged, smooth and covered with hyaline cartilage. Long bones are found only in the appendicular skeleton and are usually curved for strength. *Figure 1-14* is a radiograph of a humerus, a typical long bone.

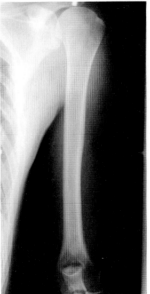

Long Bone Fig. 1-14
(Humerus)

The outer shell of most bones is composed of hard or dense bone tissue known as **compact bone.** Compact bone has few intercellular empty spaces and serves to protect and support the entire bone. The **diaphysis** or **shaft** contains a thicker layer of compact bone than the ends to help resist the stress of the weight placed on them.

Inside the shell of compact bone, and especially at both ends of each long bone, is found **spongy** or **cancellous bone.** Cancellous bone is highly porous and usually contains red bone marrow, which is responsible for production of red blood cells.

The shaft of a long bone is hollow. This hollow portion is known as the **medullary cavity.** In the adult the medullary cavity usually contains fatty yellow marrow. A dense fibrous membrane, the **periosteum,** covers bone except at the articulating surfaces. The articulating surfaces are covered with a layer of cartilage. The periosteum is essential for bone growth, repair and nutrition. Bones are richly supplied with blood vessels that pass into them from the periosteum. Near the center of the shaft of long bones, a **nutrient artery** passes obliquely through the compact bone via a **nutrient foramen** into the medullary cavity.

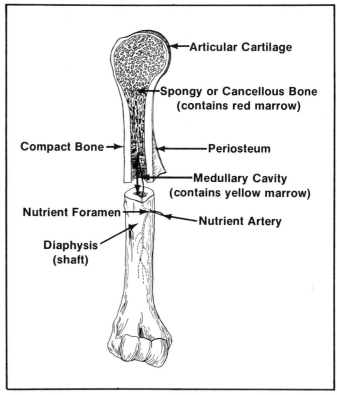

Long Bone   Fig. 1-15

2. Short Bones: Short bones are roughly cuboidal in shape and are only found in the wrists and ankles. Short bones consist mainly of cancellous tissue with a thin outer covering of compact bone. The eight carpal bones of each wrist and the seven tarsal bones of each ankle are all short bones.

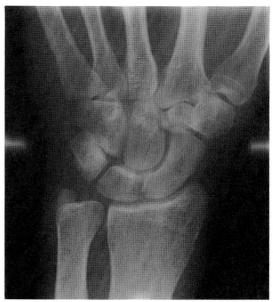

Short Bones (Carpals)   Fig. 1-16

3. Flat Bones: Flat bones consist of two plates of compact bone with cancellous bone and marrow between them. Examples of flat bones are the bones making up the calvarium (skull cap), sternum, ribs and scapulae. The marrow space between the inner and outer table of the flat bones of the cranium is known as diploe. Flat bones provide either protection or broad surfaces for muscle attachment.

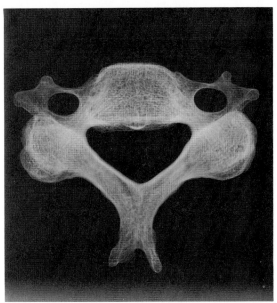

Flat Bones (Calvarium)　Fig. 1-17

4. Irregular Bones: Bones that have peculiar shapes are lumped into the final category of irregular bones. Vertebrae, facial bones, bones of the base of the cranium and bones of the pelvis are examples of irregular bones.

Irregular Bone (Vertebra)　Fig. 1-18

Development of Bones

The process by which bones form in the body is known as **ossification.** The embryonic skeleton is composed of fibrous membranes and hyaline cartilage. Ossification begins about the sixth embryonic week and continues until adulthood.

Two kinds of bone formation are known. When bone replaces membranes, the ossification is termed **intramembranous.** When bone replaces cartilage, the result is **endochondral** or **intracartilaginous** ossification.

Intramembranous Ossification: Intramembranous ossification occurs rapidly and takes place in bones that are needed for protection, such as the flat bones of the skullcap.

Endochondral Ossification: Endochondral ossification occurs much slower than intramembranous ossification and occurs in most parts of the skeleton, especially in the long bones. The first center of ossification is termed the primary center and occurs in the midshaft area. This **primary center of ossification** becomes the **diaphysis.**

Secondary centers of ossification appear near the ends of long bones. Most secondary centers appear after birth, while most primary centers appear before birth. Each **secondary center of ossification** is termed an **epiphysis.** Epiphyses of the distal femur and the proximal tibia are the first to appear and may be present at birth in the term newborn. Cartilaginous plates termed **epiphyseal plates** are found between the diaphysis and each epiphysis until skeletal growth is complete.

The area near each epiphyseal plate on the diaphysis side is termed the **metaphysis.** Longitudinal growth of the long bone occurs in the region of the metaphysis. Once all of the cartilage has been replaced by bone, growth of the skeleton is complete. The time for each bone to complete growth varies for different regions of the body. In addition, the female skeleton usually matures more quickly than does the male skeleton. Extensive charts that list the normal growth patterns of the skeleton are available.

Figure 1-20 shows a radiograph of the legs of a nine-month-old child. Primary and secondary centers of ossification are well shown. Note that cartilage does not radiograph as white since there is no calcium in this area, as yet.

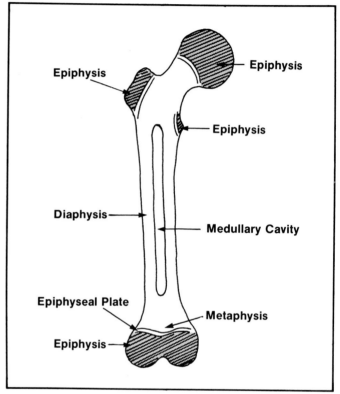

Endochondral Ossification   Fig. 1-19

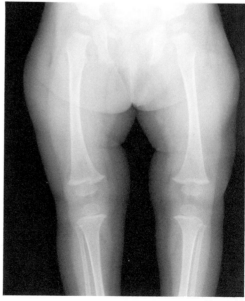

Femur   Fig. 1-20

D. Arthrology (Joints)

The study of joints is termed arthrology. Joints are divided into three main groups, depending on the amount of motion possible at the joint. A joint that is immovable is termed a **synarthrosis.** A joint that is slightly movable is termed an **amphiarthrosis.** Most joints of the body are freely movable and are termed **diarthroses.** Diarthrodial joints are enclosed within a fibrous envelope or capsule. The joint capsule contains synovial fluid, which serves to lubricate the articular cartilage found at the ends of the bones making up the joint.

Synarthrodial Joints

Two examples of synarthrodial or immovable joints are the sutures of the adult skull and the epiphyseal plate between an epiphysis and the diaphysis. Complete fusion of both types of synarthrodial joints occurs in the adult.

Amphiarthrodial Joints

Amphiarthrodial joints are slightly movable. Examples are the joints between any two vertebral bodies, the distal tibiofibular joint and the joints of the pelvis. The pelvic joints are the symphysis pubis in front and the two sacro-iliac joints posteriorly.

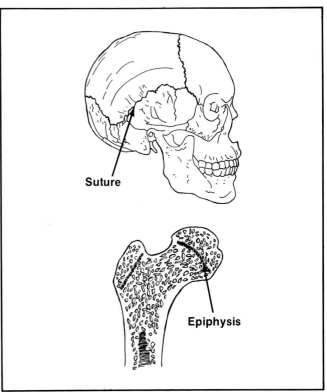

Synarthroses   Fig. 1-21

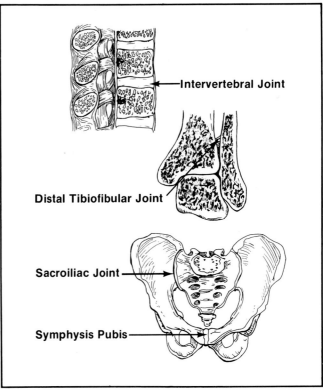

Amphiarthroses   Fig. 1-22

Diarthrodial Joints

All joints of the extremities, with the single exception of the distal tibiofibular joint, are freely movable joints. Since there are a large number of freely movable joints, they are further subdivided into six specific movement types.

Type	Example
1. Ball and Socket	Hip Joint
2. Hinge	Elbow Joint
3. Condyloid	Wrist Joint
4. Pivot	C1-C2 Articulation
5. Saddle	1st Carpometacarpal Joint
6. Gliding	Intercarpal Joints

Ball and Socket Joints: The ball and socket type of joint allows the greatest freedom of motion. Movements such as flexion and extension, abduction and adduction, medial and lateral rotation, and circumduction are possible in these joints. The hip joint and the shoulder joint are examples of the ball and socket joint.

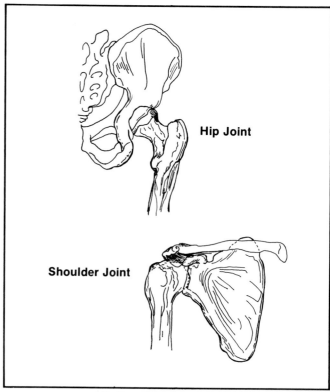

Ball and Socket Joints   Fig. 1-23

Hinge Joints: The hinge joint is a strong joint, firmly secured by strong collateral ligaments, that permits only the motions of flexion and extension. Examples of hinge joints include the interphalangeal joints, elbow joints, knee joints and ankle joints.

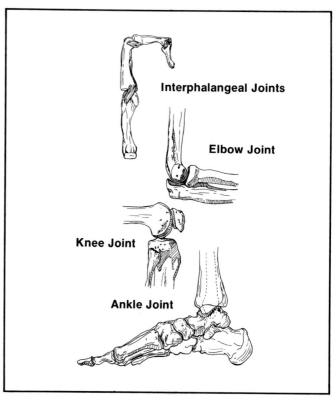

Hinge Joints   Fig. 1-24

Condyloid Joints: The condyloid joint allows motion in four directions. In addition to the flexion and extension of the hinge joint, these joints can abduct and adduct. Examples of condyloid joints are the wrist and the second through the fifth metacarpophalangeal joints.

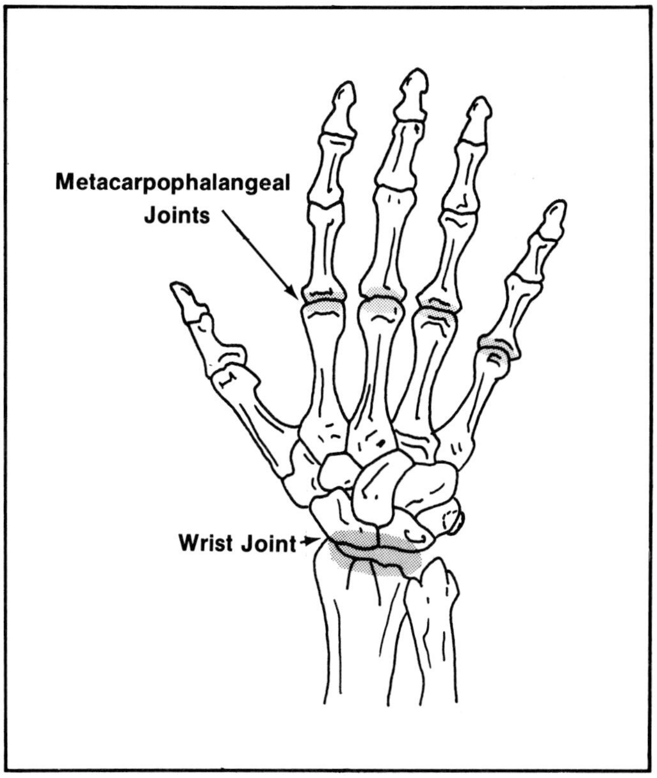

Condyloid Joints

Fig. 1-25

Pivot Joints: Pivot joints allow a rotational movement around a long axis. Both the proximal and distal radioulnar joints are pivot joints, allowing the rotational movements of the forearm and wrist. The joint between the first and second cervical vertebrae allows the head to rotate on the rest of the vertebral column.

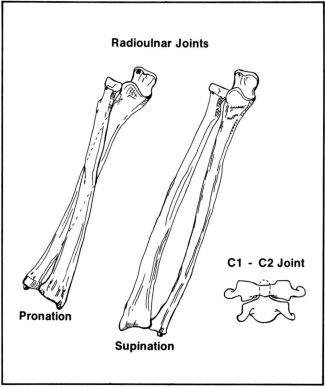

Pivot Joints

Fig. 1-26

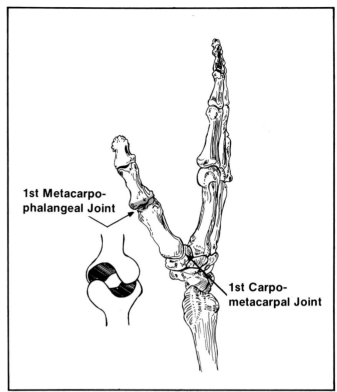

Saddle Joints: Saddle joints are unique to the thumb. These joints allow movement in several directions. The first carpometacarpal joint is the best example of a saddle joint, although the first metacarpophalangeal joint is also classified as a saddle joint.

1st Metacarpophalangeal Joint

1st Carpometacarpal Joint

Saddle Joints
Fig. 1-27

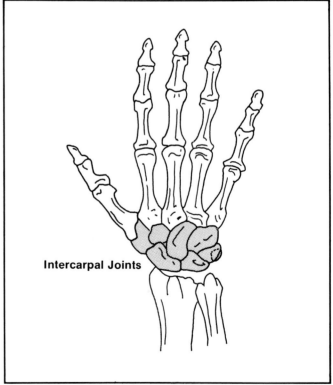

Gliding Joints: The final type of diarthrodial joint is the gliding type. There are numerous gliding joints that permit only a sliding or gliding motion between the articulating surfaces. Examples include the intercarpal joints and the intertarsal joints.

Intercarpal Joints

Gliding Joints
Fig. 1-28

Summary of Joint Classification

Classification	Movement	Examples
Synarthrodial	immovable	skull sutures, epiphyses
Amphiarthrodial	slightly movable	intervertebral joints, distal tibiofibular joints, sacroiliac joints, symphysis pubis
Diarthrodial	freely movable	-----------
Ball and Socket	freely movable	hip and shoulder joints
Hinge	freely movable	elbow, knee, ankle, interphalangeal joints
Condyloid	freely movable	wrist and metacarpophalangeal (2nd to 5th) joints
Pivot	freely movable	radioulnar, C1-C2 joints
Saddle	freely movable	1st carpometacarpal and 1st metacarpophalangeal joints
Gliding	freely movable	intercarpal and intertarsal joints

Part II. Terminology and Basic Principles of Radiographic Positioning

It is basic and essential that each person planning to work as a medical radiographer clearly understands the terminology commonly used in medical radiographic positioning. This part of Chapter 1 lists, describes and illustrates those primary terms used in radiographic positioning.

Also described and illustrated later in this chapter are two general rules or principles used in all medical radiographic positioning. Understanding and applying these principles enable one to quickly and easily determine what routine projections or positions are necessary to demonstrate radiographically on x-ray film body parts, such as the chest, hand, wrist or elbow.

A. Terminology

The following terms, commonly used in radiographic positioning, are defined in clear and precise language to allow easy understanding. Wherever possible, illustrations are included to further clarify meanings and definitions.

General Terms

1. Radiograph
- An x-ray film containing an image of an anatomical part of a patient

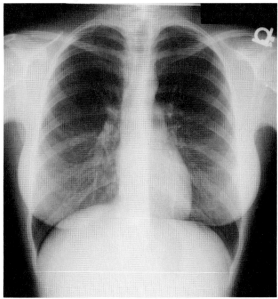

Chest Radiograph   Fig. 1-29

2. Radiographic Examination (of chest)
- A radiographer is shown positioning the patient for a routine chest exam.
- A radiographic examination of the chest includes:
  (a) correct positioning of the body part,
  (b) proper exposure of the film by x-rays passing through the chest structures, and
  (c) processing (developing) of the film.

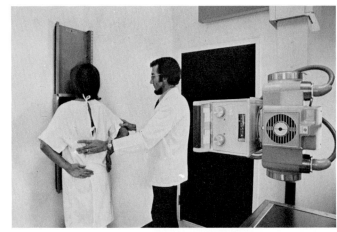

Radiographic Examination   Fig. 1-30

3. Anatomical Position
- A specific body position used as a reference for other positioning terms
- Upright position, arms down, palms forward, head directed straight ahead, feet extended and toes down

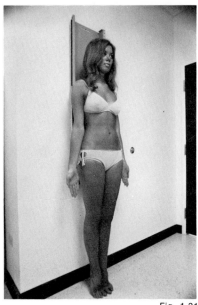

Fig. 1-31
Anatomical
Position

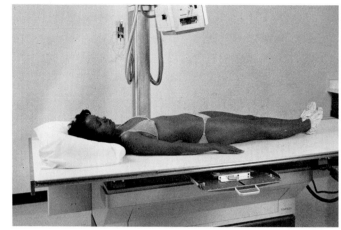

Supine   Fig. 1-32

4. Supine
  - A body position
  - Lying on back, facing upward

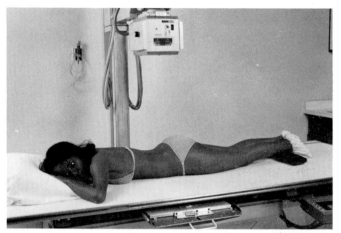

Prone   Fig. 1-33

5. Prone
  - A body position
  - Lying on abdomen, facing downward (head may be turned to one side)

6. Recumbent (Reclining)
  - A body position
  - Lying down in any position (prone, supine, on side, etc.)

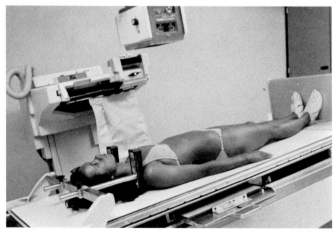

Trendelenburg   Fig. 1-34

7. Trendelenburg
  - A body position
  - A recumbent position with body plane tilted so head is lower than feet

8. Posterior (Dorsal)
- Refers to the back half of patient, includes bottom of feet (refer to anatomical position)

9. Anterior (Ventral)
- Refers to front half of patient

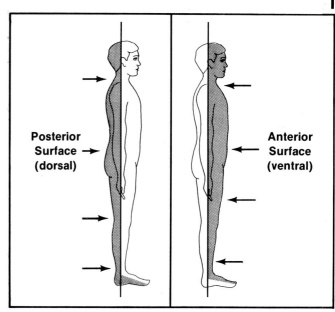

Posterior vs. Anterior   Fig. 1-35

10. Posteroanterior (P.A.)
- A projection of the x-ray beam
- Combines two terms, posterior and anterior
- Refers to direction which x-ray beam travels, called a projection, enters at posterior surface and exits at anterior (P.A. projection)

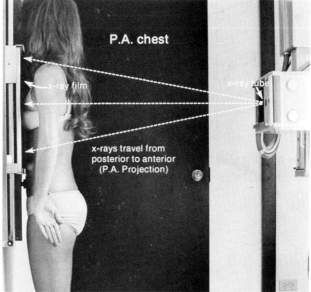

P.A. Projection   Fig. 1-36

11. Anteroposterior (A.P.)
- A projection of the x-ray beam
- Combines two terms, anterior and posterior
- Direction of travel of x-ray beam, enters at anterior surface and exits at posterior (A.P. projection)

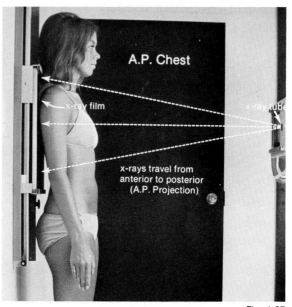

A.P. Projection   Fig. 1-37

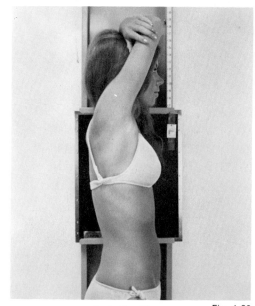

Lat. Position   Fig. 1-38

12. Lateral (Lat.)
- A body position
- Refers to "the side of," a side view
- A true lateral will always be rotated 90° (¼ turn) from a true A.P. or P.A.
- A true lateral is said to be perpendicular or at right angles to a true A.P. or P.A.

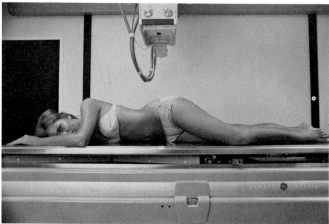

Obli. Position   Fig. 1-39

13. Oblique (Obli.)
- A body position
- A position in which the body plane does not form a right angle (Lat.) or is not parallel (P.A. or A.P.) to film, somewhere between a P.A. (A.P.) and Lat.

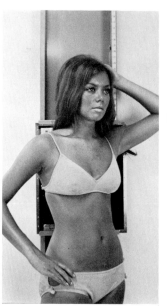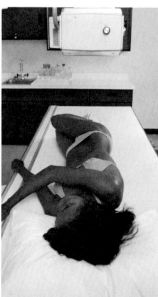

14. Left Posterior Oblique (L.P.O.)
- That position in which the left posterior aspect of body is closest to film

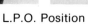

L.P.O. Position   Fig. 1-40

15. Right Anterior Oblique (R.A.O.)

- That position in which the right anterior aspect of body is closest to film

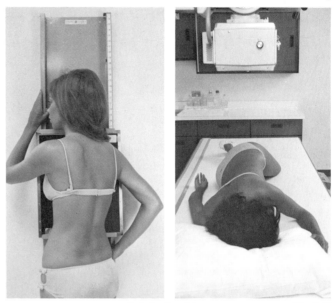

R.A.O. Position   Fig. 1-41

16. Decubitus (Decub.)

- A body position
- Refers to the patient lying down on one of the following body surfaces: back (dorsal), front (ventral), side (right or left lateral)
- Always used with a horizontal x-ray beam

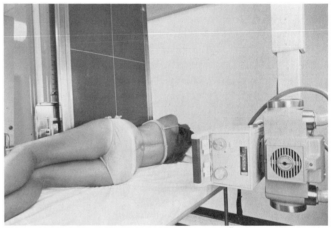

Decub. Position   Fig. 1-42

17. Left Lateral Decubitus

- The body position described as lying on left side with x-ray beam directed horizontally (similar to a left lateral position **except** the x-ray beam is directed horizontally and the image is an A.P. or P.A.).

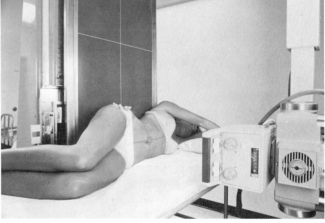

Left Lat. Decub.   Fig. 1-43

18. Dorsal Decubitus

- The body position described as lying on the dorsal (posterior) surface with x-ray beam directed horizontally (similar to a supine position **except** the x-ray beam is directed horizontally and the image is a lateral).

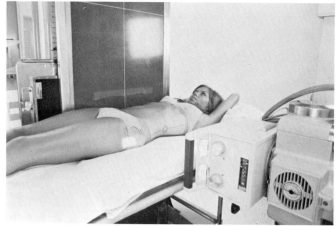

Dorsal Decub.   Fig. 1-44

Common Positioning Terms

The following three positioning terms, **projection, position** and **view,** are often used incorrectly in practice, resulting in confusion and error. It is important that these terms be understood and used correctly.

19. Projection

- The path of the x-ray beam, from entrance to exit (A.P. or P.A.)

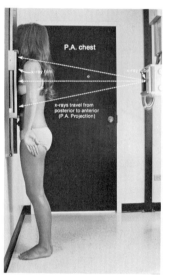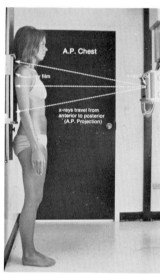

P.A. Projection   A.P. Projection ^{Fig. 1-45}

20. Position

- A specific body position (supine, prone, recumbent, erect)
- Describes lateral and oblique positions used in reference to the body part closest to film (right or left lateral, right or left anterior or posterior obliques)

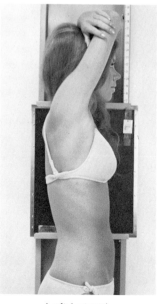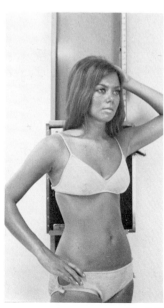

Left Lateral   Left Posterior ^{Fig. 1-46}
Position   Oblique Position

21. View
  - Should only be used in discussing the radiograph or image. View is **not** a positioning term.

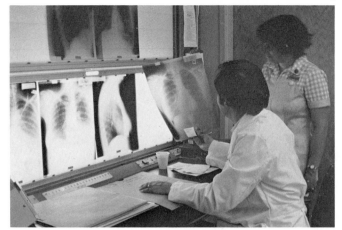

Viewing Radiographs Fig. 1-47

Relationship Terms

22. Cephalic (Superior)
  - Toward head end of body
    vs.

23. Caudal (Inferior)
  - Away from head end of body (toward feet)

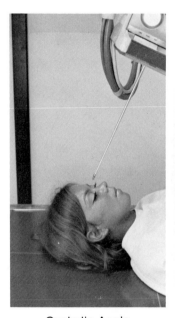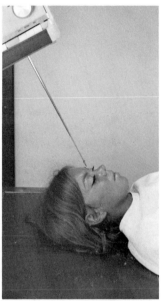

Cephalic Angle   Caudal Angle Fig. 1-48

24. Proximal
  - Near source or beginning (elbow is proximal to wrist)
    vs.

25. Distal
  - Away from source or beginning (ankle is distal to knee)

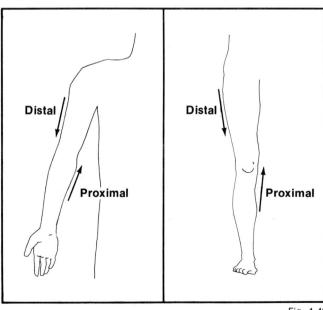

Proximal - Distal Fig. 1-49

23

26. Lateral
- Away from center or "inside" (in the anatomical position, the thumb is on the lateral aspect of hand)
vs.

27. Medial
- Toward center or "inside" (in the anatomical position, the medial aspect of the ankle joint is the "inside" part)

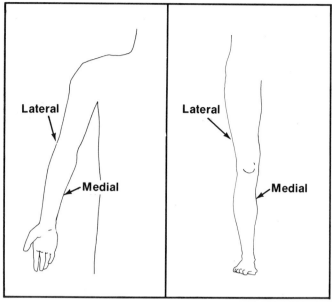

Lateral - Medial

Fig. 1-50

Terms Related to Movement of Joints

28. Flexion
- In flexing or bending a joint, the angle between parts is decreased.
vs.

29. Extension
- In extending or straightening a joint, the angle between parts is increased.

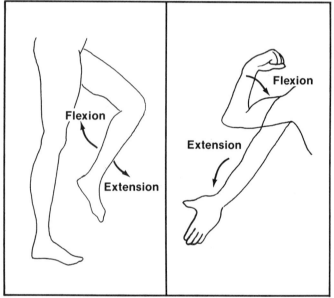

Flexion - Extension

Fig. 1-51

30. Hyperextension
- Extending a joint beyond the straight or neutral position
  Example: A hyperextended elbow or knee results when the joint is extended beyond the straightened or neutral position

NOTE: A special use of flexion and extension involves the spine. Flexion is bending forward and extension is returning to the neutral position. A backward bending beyond the neutral position is hyperextension.

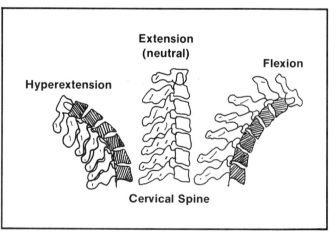

Hyperextension

Fig. 1-52

31. Abduction
- A movement of arm or leg **away** from body, a lateral movement
  vs.

32. Adduction
- A movement of arm or leg **toward** body

NOTE: A memory aid is to associate the <u>d</u> in towar<u>d</u> with the <u>d</u> in a<u>d</u>duction.

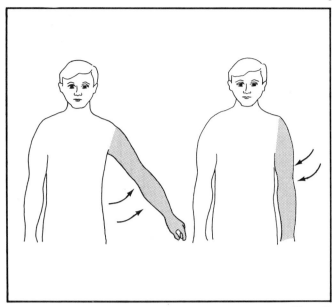

| Abduction (away from) | Adduction (toward) | Fig. 1-53 |

Movements of Foot and Ankle

33. Eversion
- An outward movement of the foot at the ankle joint. The leg does **not** rotate, and stress is applied to the medial aspect of the ankle joint.

  vs.

34. Inversion
- An inward movement of the foot at the ankle joint. The leg does **not** rotate, and stress is applied to the lateral aspect of the ankle joint.

NOTE: Correctly used, these terms refer to stress movements as described, and not to the usual rotational movement.

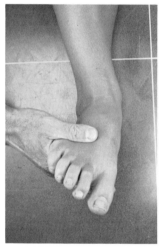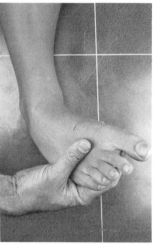

Eversion　　　　Inversion　　Fig. 1-54

Movements of Hand

35. Supination
- A rotation of hand into the anatomical position (palm up in supine position or forward in erect position)
  vs.

36. Pronation
- A rotation of hand into the opposite of the anatomical position (palm down or back)

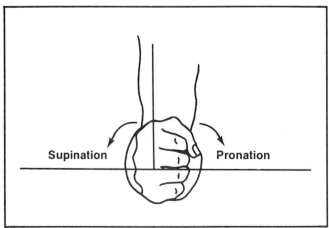

Movements of Hand　　　　Fig. 1-55

Surfaces of Extremities

37. Plantar
- Refers to the sole of foot (posterior)
vs.

38. Dorsum (Dorsum Pedis)
- Refers to the top of foot (anterior)

NOTE: The dorsoplantar projection is the same as an A.P. The plantodorsal projection would be the same as a P.A.

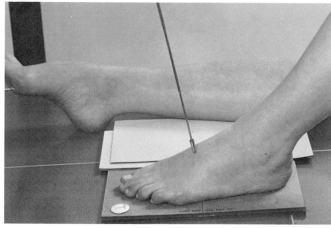

Dorsoplantar (A.P.) Projection   Fig. 1-56

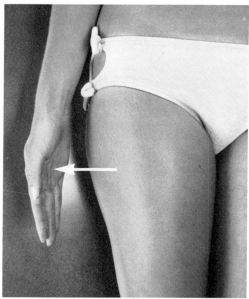

39. Palmar (Volar)
- Refers to the palm of hand (anterior)

Palmar (Volar) Surface   Fig. 1-57

Body Planes

40. Midsagittal
- The plane dividing body into right and left halves
vs.

41. Midcoronal (Midaxillary)
- The plane dividing body into anterior and posterior halves

42. Transverse
- The plane passing through body at right angles to midsagittal and midcoronal planes, dividing body into superior and inferior portions

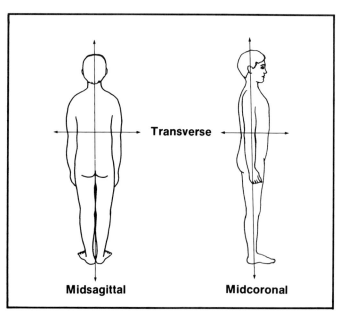

Body Planes   Fig. 1-58

B. General Principles or Rules of Positioning

If one understands and remembers the following two principles, the routine or basic projections or positions required for most body parts can be quickly and easily determined. It should be noted, however, that these are general principles and that exceptions in certain examinations will be encountered.

1. Reasons for a minimum of *two* projections as near 90° from each other as possible

Problem of anatomical structures being superimposed: In general, a single projection should never be taken for any routine radiographic examination because of the superimposition of body parts. For this reason, certain pathological conditions such as small chip fractures, small tumors, etc., may not be visualized on one projection only.

EXAMPLE: A small chest lesion is shown posteriorly on the lateral chest radiograph on the right. This lesion is not visible on the P.A. projection on the left, because it is superimposed by the dense heart shadow.

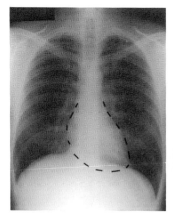

P.A. Radiograph   Lateral   Fig. 1-59
                       Radiograph
Superimposition

Localization of lesions or foreign bodies: A minimum of two projections, taken at 90° or as near right angles from each other as possible, are essential in determining the location of any lesion or foreign body.

EXAMPLE: Foreign steel fragments (white spots) are embedded in tissues of the hand. Note that both the P.A. and lateral projections are necessary to determine the exact location of steel fragments in the hand.

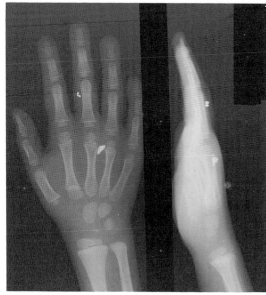

Foreign Bodies   Fig. 1-60

Determination of alignment of fractures: Any fracture requires a minimum of two projections, taken at 90° or as near right angles as possible, both to visualize fully the fracture site and to determine alignment of the fractured parts.

EXAMPLE: Two positions or projections of this fractured lower leg, 90° from each other, are required to allow the physician to determine alignment (also to straighten any misalignment) of the fractured tibia and fibula.

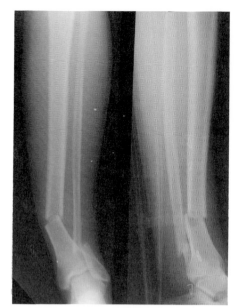

Fracture Alignment   Fig. 1-61

2. Radiographing body parts where joints or articulations are in the prime interest area usually requires three positions or projections, A.P. or P.A., lateral and oblique.

Examples of exams requiring three positions or projections (joint is included)

- fingers
- toes
- hand
- wrist
- elbow
- ankle
- foot
- knee

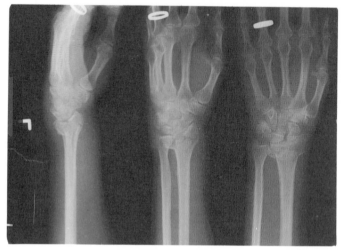

Wrist Examination   Fig. 1-62

Examples of exams requiring two positions or projections (long bones and chest)

- forearm
- humerus
- femur
- tibia-fibula
- chest

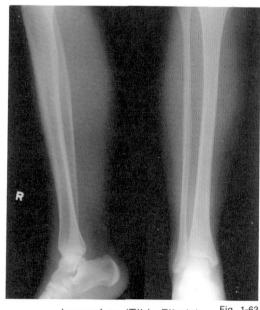

Lower Leg (Tibia-Fibula)   Fig. 1-63
Examination

CHAPTER 2
Radiographic Anatomy and Positioning of the Chest

Part I. Radiographic Anatomy of the Chest

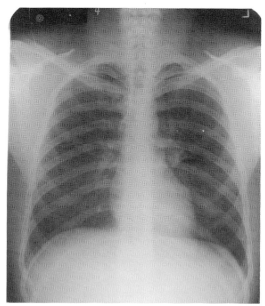

P.A. Chest Radiograph

Fig. 2-1

Chest

That anatomy of the chest most important in chest radiography includes the **respiratory system, heart and major blood vessels,** and the **bony thorax.** The respiratory system includes those parts through which air moves as it passes from the nose or mouth into the lungs.

Bony Thorax

The **bony thorax** is a cagelike structure framing and protecting the thoracic cavity. It consists of the **sternum** (breastbone) anteriorly, the **two clavicles** (collarbones) connecting the sternum to the two **scapulae** (shoulder blades), the **twelve pairs of ribs** circling the bony thorax and the **twelve thoracic vertebrae** posteriorly. A detailed study of all parts of the bony thorax will be presented in Chapter 15.

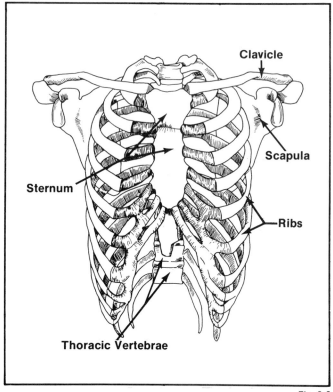

Bony Thorax

Fig. 2-2

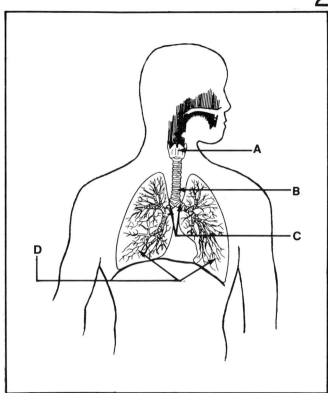

Respiratory System Fig. 2-3

Respiratory System

The four parts of the respiratory system important in chest radiography are **(A)** the **larynx** (voice box), **(B)** the **trachea, (C)** the **right and left bronchi,** and **(D)** the **lungs.** The larynx, trachea and bronchi form a continuous, tubular structure through which air can pass from the nose and mouth into the lungs.

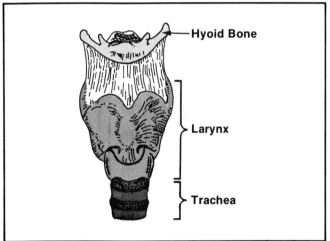

Larynx Fig. 2-4

A. Larynx (voice box)

The larynx is a cagelike, cartilaginous structure approximately 1½ in. or 4 cm. in length. It is suspended from a small bone called the **hyoid,** located in the region of the upper neck just below the tongue or floor of the mouth. The larynx serves as the organ of voice. Sounds are made as air passes through the vocal cords located within the larynx. The upper margin of the larynx is at the approximate level of **C-4** (fourth cervical vertebra). Its lower margin, where the larynx junctions with the trachea, is at the level of **C-6** (sixth cervical vertebra).

The framework of the larynx consists of nine cartilages, the largest of which is called the **thyroid cartilage** (Adam's apple). This cartilage is a prominent structure that is easy to locate; therefore, it becomes an important positioning landmark. The thyroid cartilage is located at approximately the level of **C-5** (fifth cervical vertebra) and is an excellent topographical reference for locating specific skeletal structures in this region.

A small structure known as the **epiglottis** acts as a lid for the slanted opening of the larynx. During the act of swallowing, the epiglottis covers the laryngeal opening and prevents food and fluid from entering the respiratory system.

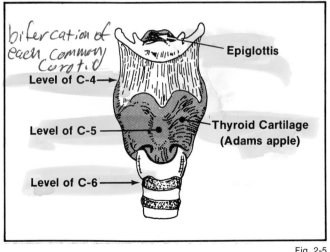

Larynx Fig. 2-5

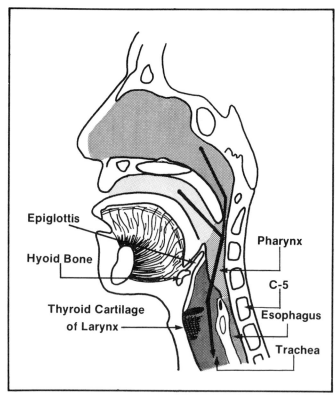

Figure 2-6 is a lateral drawing showing the epiglottis (located over the opening into the larynx) and the anterior protrusion of the thyroid cartilage at the approximate level of **C-5.** The hyoid bone is shown in cross section at the upper margin of the larynx.

This drawing shows an area termed the pharynx, which is located between the nose and mouth, and the trachea. This area serves as a passageway for food and fluid, as well as air, making it common to both the digestive and respiratory systems; therefore, it is not considered part of the respiratory system proper.

Note also the relationship of the esophagus to the larynx. The esophagus is directly posterior to the larynx, beginning at the approximate level of **C-5,** which is also the approximate level of the thyroid cartilage anteriorly.

Upper Airway   Fig. 2-6

B. Trachea

The **trachea** makes up the second division of the respiratory system proper. It is a fibrous muscular tube about ¾ in. or 2 cm. in diameter and 4½ in. or 11 cm. long. Approximately twenty C-shaped rings of cartilage are embedded in its walls providing greater rigidity. The trachea joins the larynx at the level of **C-6** and extends to T-4 or T-5 (fourth or fifth thoracic vertebra).

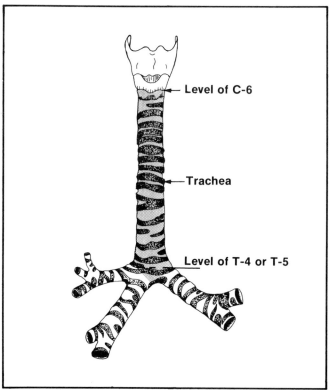

Trachea   Fig. 2-7

C. Right and Left Bronchi

The third part of the respiratory system consists of the right and left **bronchi.** As seen in *Fig. 2-8*, the two **primary** or **main stem bronchi** extend inferiorly and laterally from the lower margin of the trachea. Each of the primary bronchi further divide into **secondary bronchi** within the right and left lungs.

The differences in size and shape between the two primary bronchi are important in radiology because food or other foreign matter that happens to enter the respiratory system is more likely to enter and lodge in the right bronchus. The right bronchus is larger and more vertical in position than is the left bronchus.

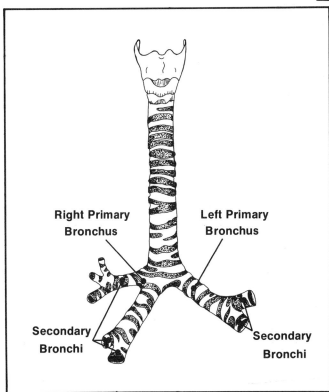

Bronchi   Fig. 2-8

Another important difference between the right and left bronchi is that the right bronchus divides into **three** secondary bronchi, but the left divides into only **two.** Each of these secondary bronchi enter individual lobes of the lungs. Thus the right lung contains **three lobes** and the left contains **two lobes,** as demonstrated in *Figs. 2-9* and *2-10*. These secondary bronchi continue to subdivide into smaller branches that spread to all parts of each lobe.

Each of these small branches of the bronchi terminates or ends in small air sacs or air spaces called **alveoli.** Oxygen and carbon dioxide are exchanged with the blood through the thin walls of the alveoli.

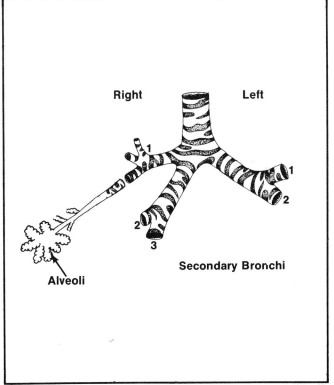

Bronchi and Alveoli   Fig. 2-9

D. Lungs

The fourth and last division of the respiratory system is made up of the two large, spongy **lungs,** located on each side of the thoracic cavity. The lungs fill all of the space not occupied by other structures. It is important to remember that the right lung is made up of three lobes, the **upper, middle** and **lower lobes;** while the left lung has only two lobes, the **upper** and **lower.**

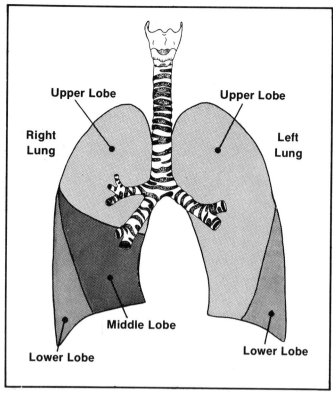

Lungs

Fig. 2-10

Chest Radiograph

Enormous amounts of medical information can be obtained from a properly exposed and carefully positioned P.A. chest radiograph. Although the technical factors are designed to optimally visualize the lungs and other soft tissues, the bony thorax can be seen. The clavicles, scapulae and ribs can be identified by carefully studying the chest radiograph in *Fig. 2-11.* The sternum and thoracic vertebrae are superimposed along with mediastinal structures such as the heart and great vessels; therefore, the sternum and vertebrae are not well visualized on a P.A. chest radiograph. The lungs and trachea of the respiratory system are well shown, although usually the bronchi are not easily seen. The fourth portion of the respiratory system, the larynx, is usually above the top border of the radiograph and cannot be seen. The heart and large blood vessels, and the diaphragm, are also well visualized.

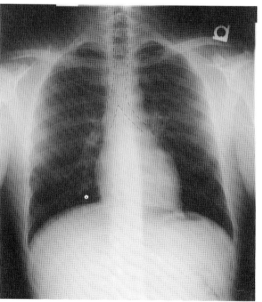

P.A. Chest Radiograph

Fig. 2-11

Parts of Lungs

Other parts of the lungs important radiographically include the **hilus** or **hilum**, which is the central, wedge-shaped area of each lung where the bronchi, blood vessels, lymph vessels and nerves enter and leave the lungs. The **apex** of each lung is that rounded upper area above the level of the clavicles. The **base** of each lung is the lower concave area of each lung that rests on the **diaphragm**. The diaphragm is a muscular partition separating the thoracic and abdominal cavities. The **costophrenic angle** refers to the extreme outermost corner of each lung where the diaphragm meets the ribs. The **pleura** is a double-walled membranous sac enclosing each lung.

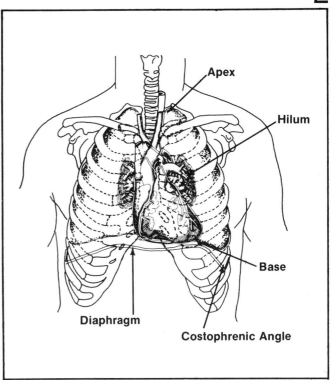

Lungs   Fig. 2-12

The drawing in *Fig. 2-13* shows the left lung as seen from the medial aspect. Since this is the left lung, only two lobes are seen. Note that some of the lower lobe extends above the level of the hilum, while some of the upper lobe extends below the hilum. The posterior part of the diaphragm is the most inferior part of the diaphragm.

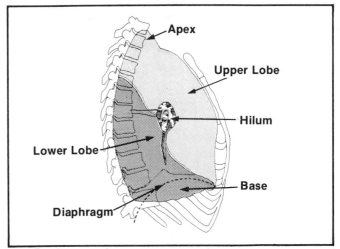

Medial Left Lung   Fig. 2-13

Chest Radiograph

It is of significance, radiographically, to know that the right lung is usually about one inch shorter than the left lung. The reason for this difference is the large space-occupying liver located in the right upper abdomen which pushes up on the right **hemidiaphragm.** (The right half of the diaphragm is termed the right hemidiaphragm.) The right and left hemidiaphragms are seen on the lateral chest radiograph in *Fig. 2-14*. The more superior of the two is the right hemidiaphragm.

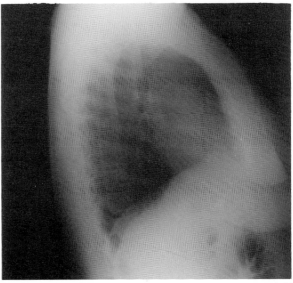

Lateral Chest Radiograph   Fig. 2-14

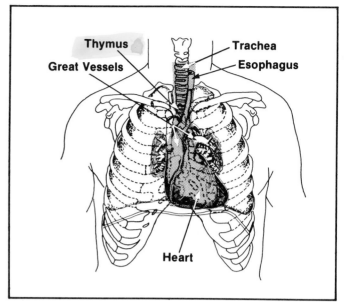

Mediastinum   Fig. 2-15

Mediastinum

The medial portion of the thoracic cavity between the lungs is called the **mediastinum.** Four structures that are radiographically important are located in the mediastinum: the **heart and great vessels,** the **trachea,** the **esophagus,** and the **thymus gland.** The thymus gland, located behind the upper sternum, is said to be a temporary organ because it reaches its maximum size at puberty, then gradually decreases until it almost disappears in the adult.

Chest Radiograph

The heart is located in the lower mediastinum, primarily to the left side as shown on the P.A. chest radiograph in *Fig. 2-16*. If one associates the heart primarily with the left lung, it is easy to remember that, because of the presence of the heart, the left lung only has two lobes as compared to three lobes in the right lung.

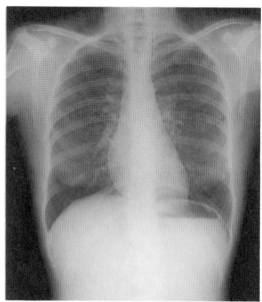

P.A. Chest Radiograph   Fig. 2-16

Degree of Inspiration

In chest radiography it is important to be able to identify and count all twelve pairs of ribs. The first and second pairs are the most difficult to locate. When a chest radiograph is taken, it is important that the patient take as deep a breath as possible and then hold it so as to fully aerate the lungs. The best way to determine the degree of inspiration is to observe how far down the diaphragm has moved and count the pairs of ribs in the lung area above the diaphragm. A general rule for adult patients is to "show" a minimum of ten ribs on a good P.A. chest radiograph. To determine this, start at the top with rib number one and count down to the tenth rib posteriorly. The posterior part of each rib, where it joins a thoracic vertebra, is the most superior part of the rib. You should always check the diaphragm to see that it is below the level of the tenth rib, as shown on the radiograph in *Fig. 2-17*. (On this example, 11 posterior ribs are shown.)

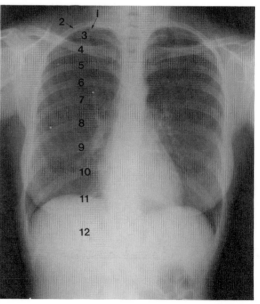

Posterior Ribs   Fig. 2-17

Part II. Radiographic Positioning of the Chest

Patient Preparation

Patient preparation for chest radiography includes the removal of all opaque objects from the chest and neck regions, including clothes with buttons, snaps, hooks or any objects that would be visualized on the radiograph as a shadow. To insure that all such objects are removed from the chest region, the usual procedure is to ask the patient to remove all clothing, including bras, along with necklaces or other objects around the neck. The patient then puts on a hospital gown with the opening in the back.

Long hair braided or tied together in bunches with rubber bands or other fasteners may cause suspicious shadows on the radiograph if it is left superimposing the chest area.

Breathing Instructions

Breathing instructions are very important in chest radiography because any chest or lung movement occurring during the exposure will result in "blurring" of the radiographic image. It is also imperative that chest radiographs be taken on **full** inspiration. This fact needs to be explained to the patient prior to the exposure, as the patient is being positioned. It is often easiest to achieve a full inspiration if the patient is asked to hold the second breath rather than the first. It may be necessary to practice this breathing procedure with the patient before actually making the exposure.

Exposure Factors

The principle exposure factors for chest radiography are:

1. High kVp (above 100) when using grids
   Medium kVp (70 to 90) when using screen cassette only

2. Short exposure time

3. Adequate mAs for sufficient density

Correctly exposed P.A. chest radiographs should faintly visualize the thoracic vertebrae and posterior ribs through the heart shadow. Oblique and lateral positions should be of a similar density.

Erect Chest Radiographs

All chest radiographs should be taken in an erect position if the patient's condition allows it. Cart or stretcher patients may require assistance in sitting up with their legs hanging over the cart or stretcher edge. Various methods for taking chest radiographs of all types of patients are described in this chapter.

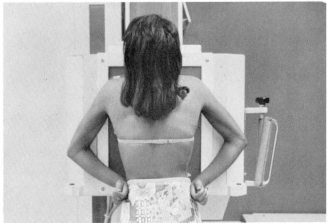

Chest, patient standing   Fig. 2-18

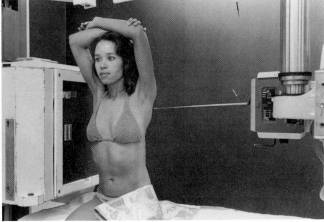

Chest, patient seated   Fig. 2-19

Reasons for Erect Chest Radiographs

Three reasons for taking chest radiographs in an erect position with a 72 in. (183 cm.) focus-film distance (F.F.D.) whenever possible, are the following:

1. To minimize enlargement and distortion of the heart and great vessels

A chest radiograph taken at less than 72 in. (183 cm.) will cause increased magnification of the heart shadow, making it difficult for the radiologist to diagnose any possible cardiac enlargement due to a heart condition or other disease process. This is demonstrated by comparing the heart size on the two chest radiographs of the same patient in *Fig. 2-20.*

2. To allow the diaphragm to move farther down

An erect position causes the liver and other abdominal organs to drop, allowing the diaphragm to move farther down on full inspiration, thus allowing the lungs to fully aerate.

3. To show possible air-fluid levels in the chest

If both air and fluid are present within a lung or within the pleural space, the heavier fluid, such as blood or serum, will always gravitate to the lowest position, while the air will rise. In the recumbent position, a pleural effusion will spread out over the entire posterior surface of the lung, resulting in a hazy appearance of the entire lung. In the upright position, fluid will locate near the base of the lung. The two radiographs of the same patient in *Fig. 2-21* illustrate this principle. The erect chest radiograph shows excess fluid in the right lower thoracic cavity and causes the right costophrenic angle to be obliterated. The supine radiograph shows a generalized hazy appearance of the entire right lung.

Positioning Considerations

P.A. Chest Projection

1. True P.A., NO rotation. Insure that the patient is standing **evenly** on both feet with **both** shoulders rolled forward and downward.

Rotation on chest radiographs can best be determined by carefully examining both sternoclavicular joints for symmetrical appearance in relationship to the spine. On a true P.A. chest without any rotation, both the right and left sternoclavicular joints will be the same distance from the spine. (Note the rotation as demonstrated on the chest radiograph in *Fig. 2-22*. This becomes more obvious on the enlargement of the sternoclavicular area in *Fig. 2-23.)*

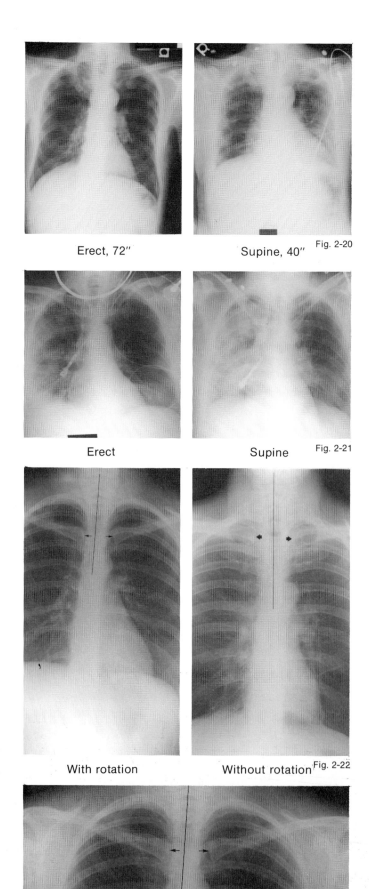

Erect, 72"   Supine, 40"   Fig. 2-20

Erect   Supine   Fig. 2-21

With rotation   Without rotation   Fig. 2-22

Closeup, with rotation   Fig. 2-23

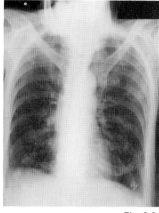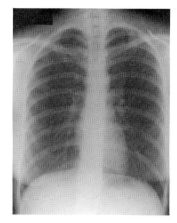

Chin up   Chin down   Fig. 2-24

2. Extending the chin. Sufficiently extending the patient's chin will insure that the chin and neck are not covering up or superimposing the uppermost lung regions, the apices of the lungs. This is demonstrated by the two radiographs in *Fig. 2-24*.

Lateral Chest Position

1. Side closest to the film. The patient's side closest to the film is best demonstrated on the finished radiograph. If the patient's main complaint is in the right lung then a right lateral should be done. If the left side is the primary interest or if no chest problems are indicated, do a left lateral. A left lateral will better demonstrate the heart region because the heart is located primarily in the left thoracic cavity.

2. True lateral, NO rotation. Insure that the patient is standing straight with weight evenly distributed on both feet with arms raised. As a final check against rotation, confirm that the posterior surfaces of both the pelvis and the thorax are perpendicular to the film holder.

Possible rotation on a lateral chest radiograph can be determined by viewing the posterior portion of the ribs. The right and left ribs will be directly superimposed on a true lateral with no rotation. A second way to detect rotation is to determine how nearly the hemidiaphragms and costophrenic angles are superimposed. Both of these effects are illustrated by comparing the true lateral chest radiographs in *Fig. 2-25*.

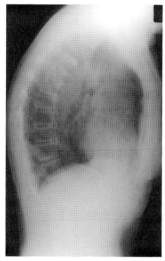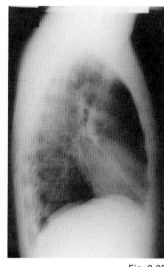

No rotation   With rotation   Fig. 2-25

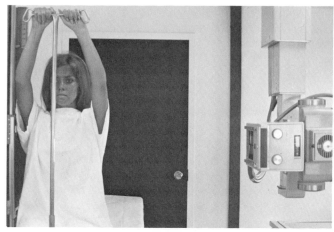

Arms raised high   Fig. 2-26

3. Raise arms high. Insure that the patient raises both arms sufficiently high to prevent superimposition on the chest field. Cart or stretcher patients who are weak or unstable may need to grasp a support, such as an IV stand, placed in front of them. When the patient's arms are not raised sufficiently, the soft tissues of the upper arm will superimpose portions of the lung field as demonstrated in *Fig. 2-27*.

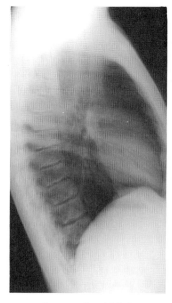
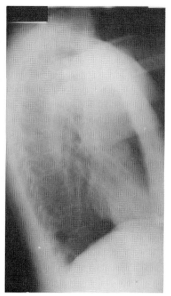

Arms raised high   Arms not raised ^{Fig. 2-27}

Basic and Optional Projections

Certain basic and optional projections or positions for the chest are demonstrated and described on the following pages. Basic projections, also sometimes referred to as routine projections, are those projections commonly taken on average helpful patients. It should be noted that departmental routines (basic projections) vary in different hospitals or departments. Optional projections include those more common projections taken as extra or additional projections to better demonstrate specific body parts or certain pathologic conditions.

Generally, basic projections for a routine radiographic examination of the chest include a P.A. and lateral. Common optional projections may include one or more of the following: A.P. supine or semierect, right and left anterior oblique, right and left posterior oblique, lateral decubitus and A.P. lordotic.

Correct Centering. Accurate centering of the body part to the film and correct central ray location are important to prevent distortion and/or "cutting off" of essential anatomical parts. This is even more critical when phototiming is used because inaccurate centering results in improper film density. To prevent these positioning errors a precise description of the central ray location in relationship to the body part is given, and an x indicating the correct centering point on the film is provided for each projection on the following pages.

Chest
Basic
• P.A.
• Lateral

Chest
Optional
• A.P. Supine or Semierect
• R.A.O. & L.A.O.
• R.P.O. & L.P.O.
• Lateral Decubitus
• A.P. Lordotic

Chest

- **Posteroanterior Projection**
Ambulatory Patient

Film Size:
  14 x 17 in. (35 x 43 cm.)

Bucky:
- Moving or stationary grid.
- Occasionally non-Bucky (screen).

Patient Position:
- Patient erect; feet spread slightly; weight equally distributed on both feet.
- Raise chin and rest on film holder; **no** rotation.
- Hands on lower hips; palms out; elbows partially flexed.
- Shoulders rotated forward and downward as much as possible to allow scapulae to move clear of lung fields.
- Exposure made at end of **full** inspiration.

Part Position:
- Adjust film holder so top of film is 2 to 3 in. (5 to 7.5 cm.) or approximately 3 finger widths above shoulders.
- Center midline of body to midline of film holder.
- **No rotation;** try for a perfect P.A. projection.

Central Ray:
- C.R. perpendicular to and directed to approximately 2 in. above center of film holder (level of T-6).
- 72 in. (183 cm.) F.F.D.

NOTE: • Chin must be elevated so as not to superimpose the apices of the lungs. • The film holder must be sufficiently high to insure that the apices are included on film. • Insure **full** inspiration at exposure by having patient hold breath at end of 2nd inspiration.

Structures Best Shown:
Lungs, including both apices, air-filled trachea, heart and great vessels, diaphragm to include costophrenic angles, and bony thorax. Ribs and vertebral column behind the heart should be just faintly visible.

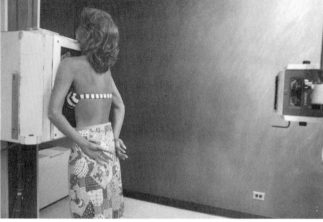

P.A.   Fig. 2-28

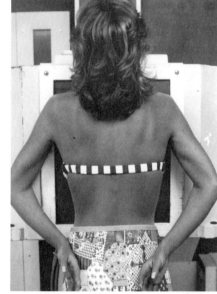

P.A.   Fig. 2-29

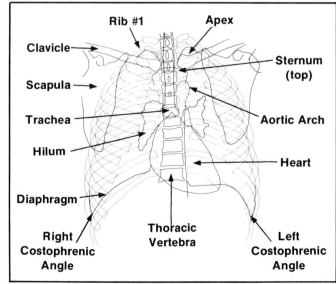

Fig. 2-31   P.A.

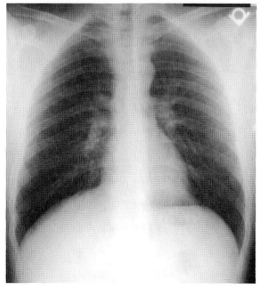

P.A.   Fig. 2-30

Chest
Basic
- **P.A.**
- Lateral

Chest

• **Posteroanterior Projection**
Cart (stretcher) Patient

Film Size:
> 14 x 17 in. (35 x 43 cm.)

Bucky:
- Moving or stationary grid.
- Occasionally non-Bucky (screen).

Patient Position:
- Patient erect, seated on cart.
- Arms around cassette unless a chest film holder is used, then position as for an ambulatory patient.
- Shoulders rotated forward and downward.
- **No** rotation of thorax.
- Exposure made at end of **full** inspiration.

Part Position:
- Adjust film holder so top of film is 2 to 3 in. (5 to 7.5 cm.) above shoulder (approximately 3 finger widths).
- If portable cassette is used, place pillow or padding on lap to raise and support cassette.

Central Ray:
- C.R. perpendicular to and directed to approximately 2 in. above center of film holder (level of T-6).
- 72 in. (183 cm.) F.F.D.

NOTE: • Make exposure upon full inspiration. • Insure that patient is stable and will not waver or move during exposure. • It is best to use a chest film holder, when possible, to provide support for patient.

Structures Best Shown:
Lungs, including both apices, air-filled trachea, heart and great vessels, diaphragm to include costophrenic angles, and bony thorax.

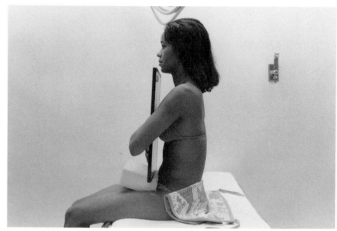

P.A.   Fig. 2-32

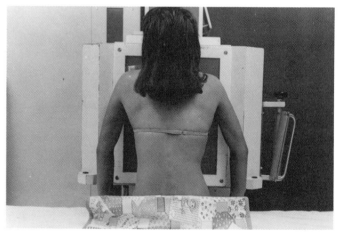

P.A.   Fig. 2-33

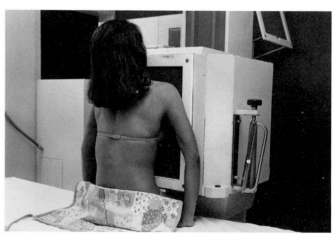

P.A.   Fig. 2-34

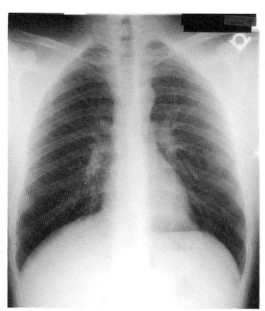

Fig. 2-35   P.A.

<table>
<tr><td>

Chest
Basic
- P.A.
- Lateral

</td></tr>
</table>

Chest

• Lateral Position
Ambulatory Patient

Film Size:
    14 x 17 in. (35 x 43 cm.)

Bucky:
- Moving or stationary grid.
- Occasionally non-Bucky (screen).

Patient Position:
- Patient erect; left side against film (unless patient complaint on right side, then do a right lateral).
- Weight evenly distributed on both feet; look straight ahead; insure that midsagittal plane is vertical and parallel to film.
- Raise arms; cross above head; grasp elbows; keep chin up.
- Exposure made at end of **full** inspiration.

Part Position:
- Top of film holder approximately 2 in. (5 cm.) above shoulders.
- Center patient to film by checking anterior and posterior aspects of thorax.
- Position in a **true lateral** position (check posterior thorax and pelvis for possible rotation).

Central Ray:
- C.R. perpendicular to and directed to approximately 2 in. above center of film holder (level of T-6).
- 72 in. (183 cm.) F.F.D.

NOTE: • Keep chin elevated. • Insure **full** inspiration at exposure. • Hold breath at end of **2nd** inspiration.

Structures Best Shown:
Lungs, trachea, heart and great vessels, diaphragm to include posterior costophrenic angles, and bony thorax.

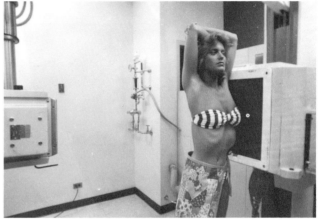
Lateral   Fig. 2-36

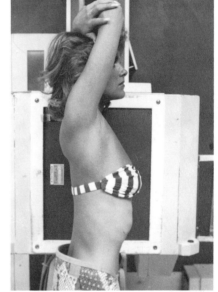
Lateral   Fig. 2-37

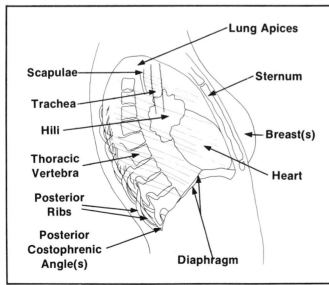

Fig. 2-39   Lateral

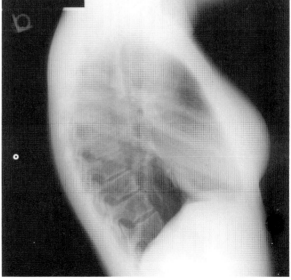
Lateral   Fig. 2-38

Chest
• Lateral Position
Cart (stretcher) Patient

Film Size:
   14 x 17 in. (35 x 43 cm.)

Bucky:
- Moving or stationary grid.
- Occasionally non-Bucky (screen).

Patient Position:
- Patient seated on cart; legs over the edge.
- Arms crossed above head; chin up.
- Exposure made at end of **full** inspiration.

Part Position:
- Top of film approximately 2 in. (5 cm.) above shoulders.
- Center patient to film.
- Insure **no** rotation by viewing patient from tube position.

Central Ray:
- C.R. perpendicular to and directed to approximately 2 in. (5 cm.) above center of film holder.
- 72 in. (183 cm.) F.F.D.

NOTE: • Always attempt to have patient sit completely erect, if possible. However, if patient is in a condition that does not allow this, the head-end of the cart can be raised to the semierect position as demonstrated in *Fig. 2-42*. • Most patients can best sit erect if their legs can be placed down over the edge of the cart, rather than having them extended directly out in front.

Structures Best Shown:
Lungs, trachea, heart and great vessels, diaphragm including posterior costophrenic angles, and bony thorax.

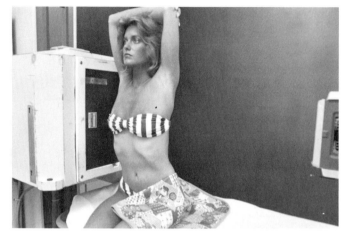
Right Lateral   Fig. 2-40

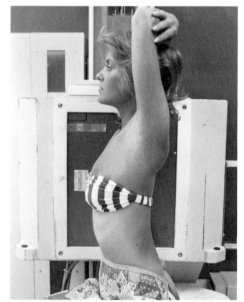
Right Lateral   Fig. 2-41

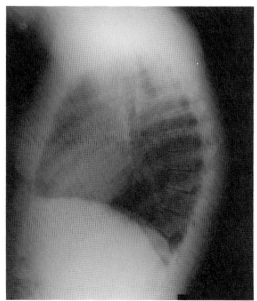
Fig. 2-43
Right Lateral

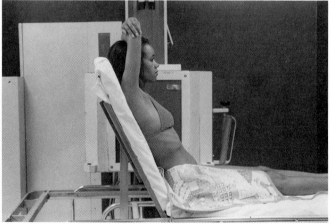
Semierect Left Lateral   Fig. 2-42

Chest

● Anteroposterior Projection
Supine or Semierect

Film Size:
14 x 17 in. (35 x 43 cm.)

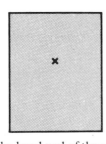

Bucky:
- Stationary grid.
- Often non-Bucky (screen).

Patient Position:
- Patient supine on cart; if possible, the head end of the cart should be raised into a semierect position.
- Roll shoulders forward as much as possible by rotating arms medially.
- Exposure made at end of **full** inspiration.

Part Position:
- Place film holder under or behind patient so top of film holder is about 2 in. (5 cm.) above shoulders.
- Center patient to film holder; check by viewing patient from the top or tube position.

Central Ray:
- C.R. must be perpendicular to the film holder.
- For supine position, raise tube to at least a 40 in. (102 cm.) F.F.D., although more distance is even better.

NOTE: ● For semierect position, some departmental routines ask for a 60 in. (152 cm.) or even 72 in. (183 cm.) F.F.D. if this is possible to obtain. ● Always indicate the F.F.D. used, if the full 72 in. distance is not used; also note projection obtained.

Structures Best Shown:
Lungs, air-filled trachea, bony thorax, diaphragm including costophrenic angles, and heart and great vessels. Heart shadow will be magnified due to shorter F.F.D. and A.P. projection.

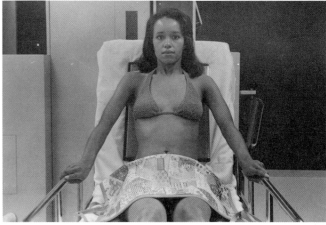
A.P. Supine   Fig. 2-44

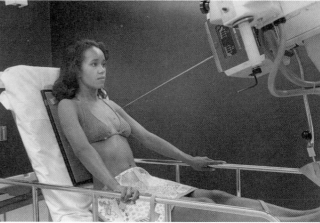
A.P. Semierect   Fig. 2-45

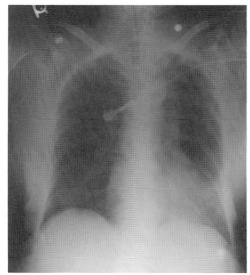
Fig. 2-47
A.P. Supine

A.P. Semierect   Fig. 2-46

Chest

- **Right Anterior Oblique Position**
- **Left Anterior Oblique Position**

Chest
Optional
- A.P. Supine or Semierect
- **R.A.O. & L.A.O.**
- R.P.O. & L.P.O.
- Lateral Decubitus
- A.P. Lordotic

Film Size:
   14 x 17 in. (35 x 43 cm.)

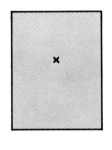

Bucky:
- Moving or stationary grid.

Patient Position:
- Patient erect, rotated 45° with left anterior shoulder against film holder for the L.A.O. and 45° with right anterior shoulder against film holder for the R.A.O.
- Flex the arm nearest film holder and place hand on hip, palm out.
- Raise opposite arm to clear lung field and rest hand on top of head or on chest film holder for support.
- Have patient look straight ahead; keep chin raised.
- Exposure made at end of **full** inspiration.

Part Position:
- Top of film holder 2 to 3 in. (5 to 7.5 cm.) or approximately 3 finger widths above shoulders.
- From the position of the x-ray tube, center the patient to the film.

Central Ray:
- C.R. perpendicular to and directed to level of T-6, approximately 2 in. (5 cm.) above center of film holder.
- 72 in. (183 cm.) F.F.D.

NOTE: • Certain positions for studies of the heart and great vessels require an L.A.O. with more rotation (60°).

Structures Best Shown:
L.A.O. - Left lung, trachea, bony thorax with heart and aorta in front of vertebral column.
R.A.O. - Right lung, trachea, bony thorax, with heart and aorta in front of vertebral column.

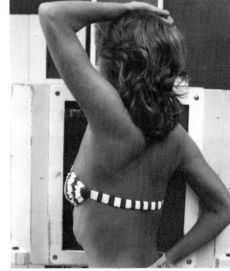

R.A.O.   Fig. 2-48

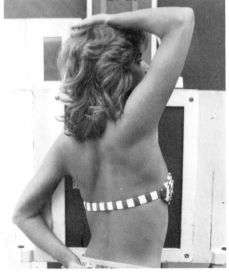

L.A.O.   Fig. 2-49

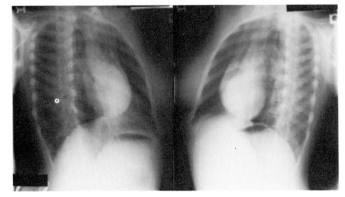

R.A.O.   L.A.O.   Fig. 2-50

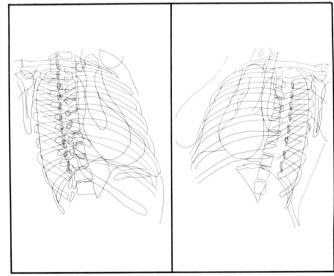

Fig. 2-51
R.A.O.   L.A.O.

Chest

- **Right Posterior Oblique Position**
- **Left Posterior Oblique Position**

Chest
Optional
- A.P. Supine or Semierect
- R.A.O. & L.A.O.
- **R.P.O. & L.P.O.**
- Lateral Decubitus
- A.P. Lordotic

Film Size:
14 x 17 in. (35 x 43 cm.)

Bucky:
- Moving or stationary grid.

Patient Position:
- Patient erect, rotated 45° with right posterior shoulder against film holder for R.P.O. and 45° with left posterior shoulder against film holder for L.P.O.
- Place the backs of both hands on the hips with the elbows flexed.
- Have patient look straight ahead.
- Exposure made at end of **full** inspiration.

Part Position:
- Top of film holder 2 or 3 in. (5 to 7.5 cm.) above shoulders.
- Center thorax to film.

Central Ray:
- C.R. perpendicular to and directed to approximately 2 in. (5 cm.) above center of film.
- 72 in. (183 cm.) F.F.D.

NOTE: • Posterior positions show the same anatomy as the opposite anterior oblique. The L.P.O. position corresponds to the R.A.O. and the R.P.O. to the L.A.O.

Structures Best Shown:
L.P.O. - Right lung, trachea, bony thorax, with heart and aorta in front of vertebral column.
R.P.O. - Left lung, trachea, bony thorax, with heart and aorta in front of vertebral column.

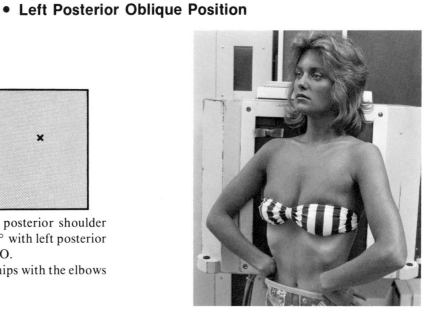

R.P.O.   Fig. 2-52

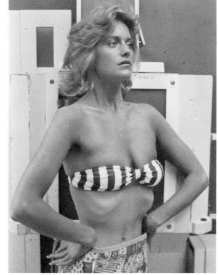

L.P.O.   Fig. 2-53

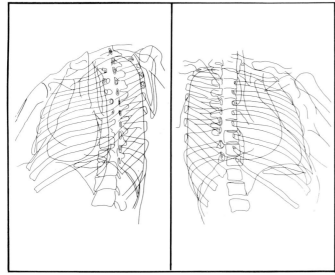

Fig. 2-55   R.P.O.   L.P.O.

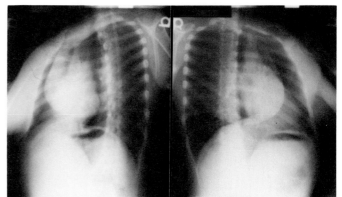

R.P.O.   L.P.O.   Fig. 2-54

Chest
Optional
- A.P. Supine or Semierect
- R.A.O. & L.A.O.
- R.P.O. & L.P.O.
- **Lateral Decubitus**
- A.P. Lordotic

Chest
• **Lateral Decubitus Position**
A.P. Projection

Film Size:
    14 x 17 in. (35 x 43 cm.)
    Lengthwise.

Bucky:
- Moving or stationary grid.

Patient Position:
- Patient lying on right side for right lateral decubitus and on left side for left lateral decubitus.
- Raise both arms above head to clear lung field; place back of patient firmly against film holder.
- Flex knees slightly and insure that pelvis and shoulders are parallel to film with **no** body rotation.
- Exposure made at end of **full** inspiration.

Part Position:
- Adjust height of film holder to center thorax to film.
- Adjust patient and cart so top of film is 2 or 3 in. (5 to 7.5 cm.) above shoulders.

Central Ray:
- C.R. horizontal to and directed to center of film.
- 72 in. (183 cm.) F.F.D.

NOTE: • Suspected side should be the down side. • Insure that the chest nearest the bottom of the film is not cut off.

Structures Best Shown:
Small pleural effusions by demonstrating air-fluid levels in pleural space.

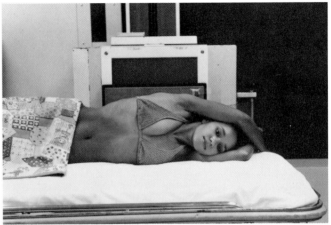

Left Lateral Decubitus Position
(A.P. projection)

Fig. 2-56

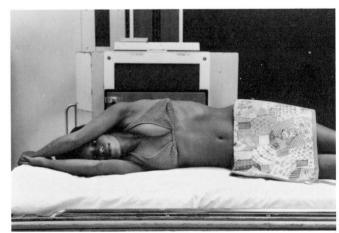

Right Lateral Decubitus Position
(A.P. projection)

Fig. 2-57

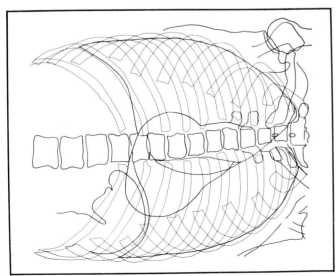

Fig. 2-59

Left Lateral Decubitus

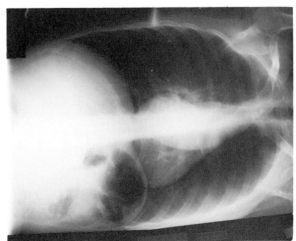

Left Lateral Decubitus

Fig. 2-58

• **Anteroposterior Lordotic Projection**

Chest
Optional
- A.P. Supine or Semierect
- R.A.O. & L.A.O.
- R.P.O. & L.P.O.
- Lateral Decubitus
- **A.P. Lordotic**

Film Size:

    14 x 17 in. (35 x 43 cm.)

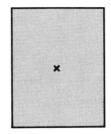

Bucky:

- Moving or stationary grid.

Patient Position:

- Have patient stand about one foot away from film holder and lean back with shoulders, neck and back of head against film holder.
- Rest both hands on hips, palm out; roll shoulders forward.
- Exposure made at end of **full** inspiration.

Part Position:

- Center midsagittal plane to center of film.
- Adjust height of film holder to approximately 3 in. (7.5 cm.) above shoulders.

Central Ray:

- C.R. perpendicular to film, centered to midsternum.
- 72 in. (183 cm.) F.F.D.

Structures Best Shown:

Apices without clavicular superimposition and interlobar effusions.

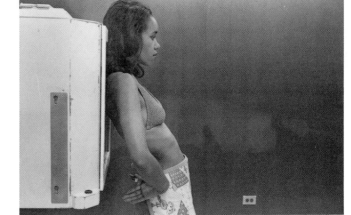

A.P. Lordotic
Fig. 2-60

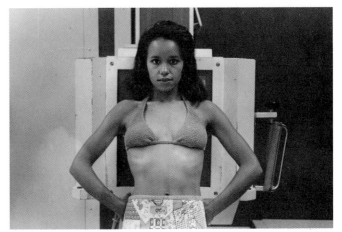

A.P. Lordotic
Fig. 2-61

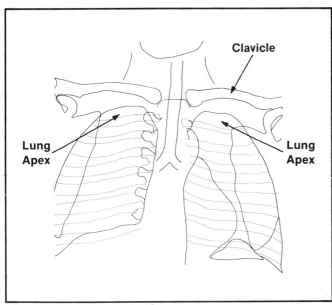

Fig. 2-63
A.P. Lordotic

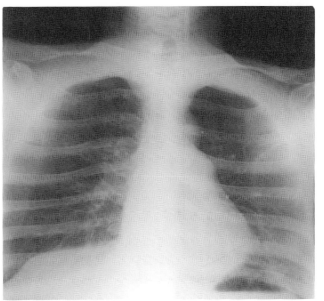

A.P. Lordotic
Fig. 2-62

CHAPTER 3

Radiographic Anatomy and
Positioning of the Abdomen

Part I. Radiographic Anatomy of the Abdomen

Abdominal Radiography

Radiographic study of the abdomen is more difficult and more subtle than that of the chest since there is little air normally found within the abdominopelvic cavity. This fact may be best illustrated by comparing the chest radiograph *(Fig. 3-1)* with the plain abdominal radiograph *(Fig. 3-2)*. The wide density differences in the chest radiograph allow one to observe various margins and borders that are easy to follow and name. In the abdomen, however, organ masses and great vessels merge into a gray shadow, so that many of the individual margins and borders disappear. Contrast media are often ingested, injected or instilled in order to visualize various organs and vessels within the abdominopelvic cavity.

Knowledge of the anatomy of the abdominopelvic cavity, the bony pelvis and the lower spinal column is essential to accurate positioning of the abdomen.

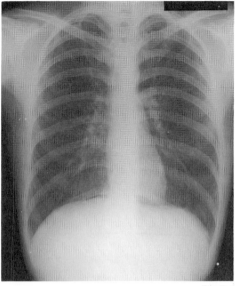

Chest Radiograph   Fig. 3-1

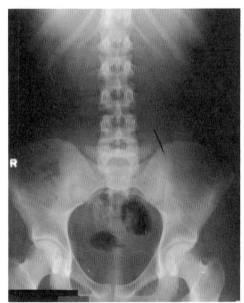

Fig. 3-2

Abdominal Radiograph

A. Topographic Landmarks

One must be able to locate certain bony landmarks on the patient and to use these landmarks to position the patient in relationship to the film for abdominal radiographs. The landmarks are called topographic landmarks and can be located on the patient by careful palpation (light pressure applied by the hand).

The following five palpable landmarks are important in positioning the abdomen:

1. Iliac Crest

The **crest of ilium** (iliac crest) is the upper, curved border of the ilium. The ilium is the large winglike portion of each half of the pelvis. The crest can be felt along its entire length through the lateral wall of the abdomen.

2. Anterior Superior Iliac Spine (A.S.I.S.)

The second important landmark is the prominent anterior end of the iliac crest, known as the **anterior superior iliac spine** or **A.S.I.S.** The A.S.I.S. can be found by locating the iliac crest, then palpating anteriorly until a prominent projection or bump is felt.

3. Symphysis Pubis

The third important topographic landmark is the **symphysis pubis,** the anterior junction of the two pubic bones. The symphysis pubis is a midline structure.

4. Greater Trochanter of Femur

The next important palpable area is the **greater trochanter** of the **femur.** The most superior portion of this large prominence lies about 1½ inches or nearly 4 centimeters above the level of the symphysis pubis. (See radiograph, *Fig. 3-4.*)

5. Ischial Tuberosity

The fifth important topographic landmark is the **ischial tuberosity.** These two bony prominences bear most of the weight of the trunk when a person is seated. Each ischial tuberosity is about 1½ inches or nearly 4 centimeters below the level of the symphysis pubis. One should practice finding these bony landmarks on oneself before attempting to locate them on a patient.

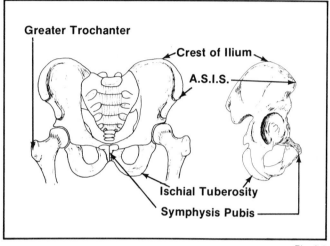

Pelvis   Fig. 3-3

Specific anatomical parts are more difficult to recognize on radiographs than on anatomical drawings. The A.P. pelvis radiograph *(Fig. 3-4)* identifies the five important bony landmarks: **(A)** crest of the ilium, or iliac crest; **(B)** anterior superior iliac spine, or A.S.I.S.; **(C)** greater trochanter of one femur; **(D)** ischial tuberosity; and **(E)** symphysis pubis.

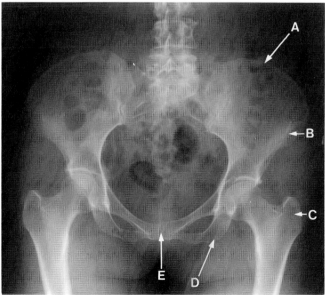

A.P. Pelvis   Fig. 3-4

B. Vertebral Column

The lower vertebral column, which forms the posterior portion of the abdominopelvic cavity, is composed of the lumbar, sacral and coccygeal spine.

The lumbar spine consists of five large vertebrae. The **sa-crum** is made up of five bony segments fused into one bone articulating on either side with the two ilia of the pelvis. Three to five incompletely developed vertebrae fuse in the adult to form the small **coccyx** or tailbone.

Note that the crest of the ilium is at the same level as the disc space between the fourth and fifth lumbar vertebrae.

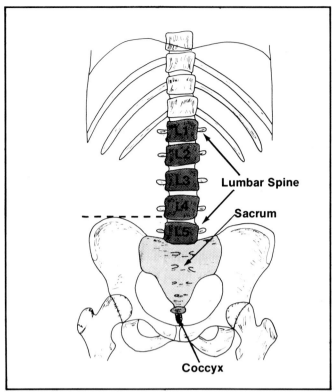

Lower Vertebral Column

Fig. 3-5

C. Abdominal Muscles

There are many muscles associated with the abdominopelvic cavity; however, the following three are the most important in abdominal radiography:

1. **Diaphragm**
2. **Left psoas major**
3. **Right psoas major**

The **diaphragm** is an umbrella-shaped muscle separating the abdominal cavity from the thoracic cavity. The diaphragm must be perfectly motionless during radiography of either the abdomen or the chest. Motion of the patient's diaphragm can be stopped by providing appropriate breathing instructions.

The two **psoas major** muscles are located on either side of the lumbar vertebral column. The lateral borders of these two muscles should be visible on a diagnostic abdominal radiograph.

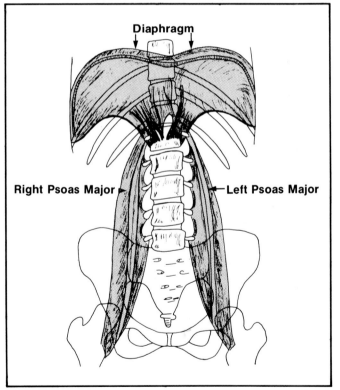

Abdominal Muscles

Fig. 3-6

54

D. Abdominal Organ Systems

The various organ systems found within the abdomino-pelvic cavity are presented only briefly in this chapter. Each of these systems is described in greater detail in later chapters devoted to those specific systems.

The digestive system (as listed) along with its accessory organs (the liver, gallbladder and pancreas) fill much of the abdominal cavity.

Digestive System Organs

1. Mouth
2. Pharynx
3. Esophagus
4. **Stomach**
5. **Small intestine**
6. **Large intestine**

Trachea
C6 to T4 or T5

Mouth, Pharynx and Esophagus. The digestive system begins at the **mouth** and continues as the **pharynx** and **esophagus**. The esophagus is located in the mediastinum of the thoracic cavity.

Stomach. The stomach is the first organ of the digestive system found in the abdominal cavity. The stomach is an expandable reservoir for swallowed food and fluids. The three main subdivisions of the stomach are the **fundus, body** and **pyloric antrum.** The fundus is the proximal portion superior to the esophageal opening. The distal portion, which continues as the small intestine, is the pyloric antrum. The major part of the stomach between the fundus and the pyloric antrum is termed the body. The radiographic and anatomical position of the stomach is highly variable depending on body build, posture and stomach contents.

The two openings of the stomach are guarded by circular sphincter muscles. Between the esophagus and stomach is the **cardiac orifice** or opening, while the **pyloric orifice,** or **pylorus,** is located between the stomach and small intestine. When the stomach is empty it tends to collapse, except for the upper portion or fundus. A gas bubble is usually seen in the fundus, just below the left hemidiaphragm, on a radiograph of an upright person. The empty stomach lining forms longitudinal folds termed **rugae,** which mostly disappear when the stomach is full.

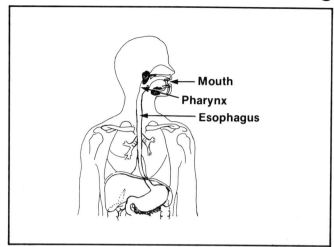

Upper Digestive System   Fig. 3-7

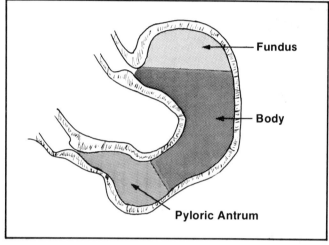

Stomach   Fig. 3-8

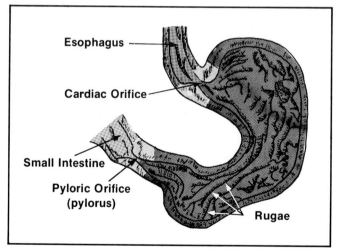

Stomach   Fig. 3-9

Gas Bubble in Fundus of Stomach

Due to the gas bubble that rises to the top of the stomach, the fundus is all that is visible on a plain abdominal radiograph in the upright position *(Fig. 3-10)*. Note that the fundus of the stomach lies just below the left hemidiaphragm. The rest of the stomach blends in with other abdominal structures and is not readily visible.

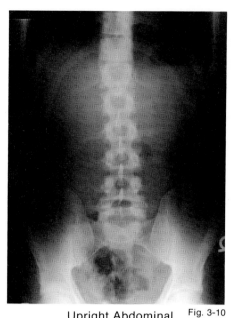

Upright Abdominal Radiograph   Fig. 3-10

Barium Sulfate in Stomach

A dense suspension of barium sulfate and water has been ingested by the patient in *Fig. 3-11,* resulting in the entire stomach being visualized. The parts of the stomach as labeled on the radiograph are: **(A)** fundus, **(B)** body, **(C)** pyloric antrum, **(D)** pyloric orifice or pylorus, and **(E)** cardiac orifice.

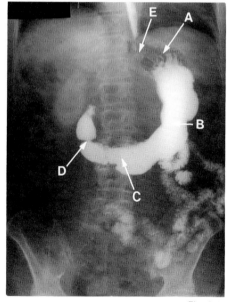

Stomach Radiograph   Fig. 3-11

Small Intestine. The next portion of the digestive tract, the small intestine, consists of three parts:

1. **Duodenum**
2. **Jejunum**
3. **Ileum**

The small intestine begins at the pyloric orifice and extends 15 to 18 feet (4.5 to 5.5 meters), then joins the large intestine at the ileocecal valve.

The first portion of the small intestine, the **duodenum,** is the shortest of the three segments. It is about 10 inches, or 25 centimeters, in length. When filled with contrast medium, the duodenum looks like a letter **C.** The proximal portion of the duodenum is called the duodenal bulb or cap. It has a certain characteristic shape, usually well seen on barium studies of the upper gastrointestinal tract. Ducts from the liver, gallbladder and pancreas drain into the duodenum.

The remainder of the small bowel lies in the central and lower abdomen. The first two-fifths following the duodenum is termed the **jejunum,** while the distal three-fifths is called the **ileum.** Note the spelling of ileum as compared to the superior portion of the hip bone, which is spelled i-l-i-u-m.

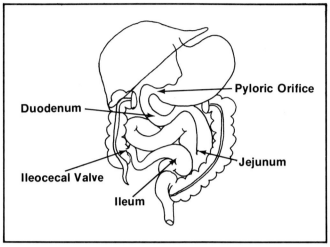

Small Intestine

Fig. 3-12

Radiograph of Small Intestine

Air is seldom seen within the entire small intestine on a plain abdominal radiograph of a healthy, ambulatory adult. The radiograph in *Fig. 3-13* visualizes the stomach, small intestine and proximal large intestine because they are filled with radiopaque barium sulfate. The identified general areas are: **(A)** the duodenum, **(B)** the jejunum, **(C)** the ileum, and **(D)** the ileocecal valve.

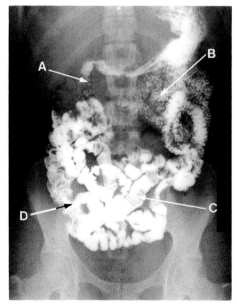

Small Intestine
Radiograph

Fig. 3-13

Large Intestine

The large intestine begins in the lower right quadrant at the junction with the small intestine. That portion of the large intestine below the **ileocecal valve** is a saclike area termed the **cecum.** The **appendix** is attached to the postero-medial aspect of the cecum. The vertical portion of the large bowel above the cecum is the **ascending colon,** which joins the **transverse colon** at the **hepatic flexure.** The transverse colon joins the **descending colon** at the **splenic flexure.** The descending colon continues as the S-shaped **sigmoid colon** in the lower left abdomen. The **rectum** is the final 6 inches, or 15 centimeters, of the large intestine. The rectum ends at the **anus,** the sphincter muscle at the terminal opening of the large intestine.

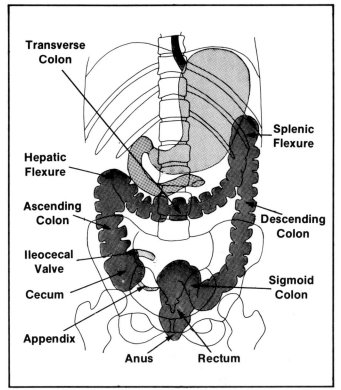

Large Intestine

Fig. 3-14

Radiograph of Large Intestine

Portions of the large intestine can usually be seen on a plain abdominal radiograph due to contained fecal matter and varying amounts of gas. In addition, the muscles of the large bowel cause the formation of large saclike divisions termed **haustra,** which give the large bowel a different internal appearance than the small bowel. Radiopaque contrast medium must be added to the clean large bowel during the radiographic examination, termed a barium enema, in order to visualize all of the large intestine. A barium enema radiograph *(Fig. 3-15)* shows the following labeled anatomy: **(A)** anus, **(B)** rectum, **(C)** sigmoid colon, **(D)** descending colon, **(E)** splenic flexure, **(F)** transverse colon, **(G)** hepatic flexure, **(H)** ascending colon, and **(I)** cecum.

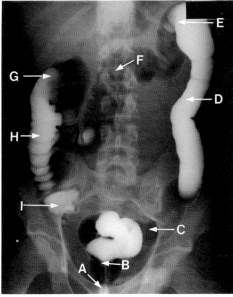

Large Intestine
Radiograph

Fig. 3-15

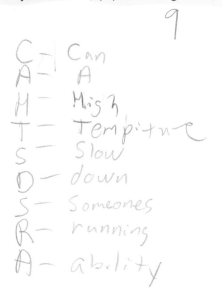

9

C - Can
A - A
H - Migh
T - Tempiture
S - Slow
D - down
S - Someones
R - running
A - ability

Accessory Digestive Organs

Certain accessory organs of digestion also located in the abdominal cavity are:
1. Pancreas
2. Liver
3. Gallbladder

Pancreas. The pancreas is an elongated gland located posterior to the stomach and near the posterior abdominal wall, between the duodenum and the spleen. The head of the pancreas is nestled in the **C**-loop of the duodenum. The body and tail of the pancreas extend toward the upper left abdomen. The pancreas, not seen on a plain abdominal radiograph, manufactures several digestive juices that move to the duodenum via a main pancreatic duct, as needed, for digestion. In addition, the pancreas produces certain hormones, such as insulin, that are necessary to normal well-being.

Liver. The liver is the largest solid organ in the body, occupying most of the upper right quadrant. One of its numerous functions is the production of bile, which assists in the digestion of fats. If bile is not needed for digestion, it is stored and concentrated for future use in the gallbladder.

Gallbladder. The gallbladder is a pear-shaped sac located beneath the liver. The primary functions of the gallbladder are to store and concentrate bile, and to contract and release bile when stimulated by an appropriate hormone.

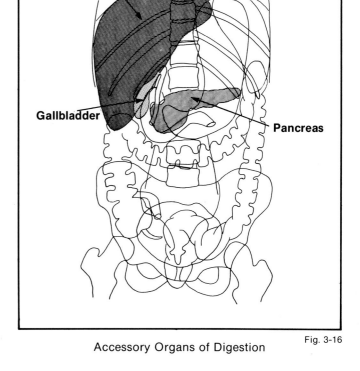

Accessory Organs of Digestion   Fig. 3-16

Bile Ducts

Bile formed in the liver travels to one of the main hepatic ducts and, finally, into the **common hepatic duct.** Bile then travels to the gallbladder to be stored via the **cystic duct.** When needed for digestion, concentrated bile from the gallbladder travels back through the cystic duct to the **common bile duct** and finally into the duodenum. The common bile duct may join the main pancreatic duct before emptying into the duodenum.

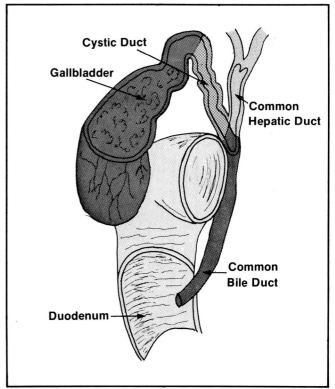

Biliary System   Fig. 3-17

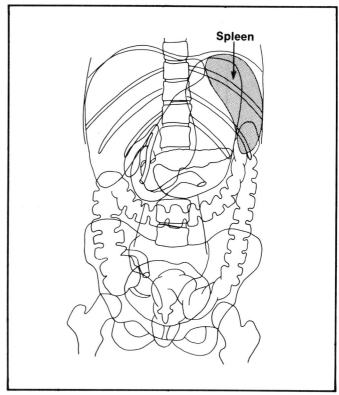

Spleen   Fig. 3-18

(Spleen). The spleen is not associated with the digestive system, but does occupy a space to the left of the stomach in the upper left quadrant. The spleen is often visualized on plain abdominal radiographs, particularly if the organ is enlarged. It is a very fragile organ and is sometimes lacerated during trauma to the lower left rib cage.

E. Urinary System

The urinary system is composed of

1. two **kidneys,**
2. two **ureters,**
3. one **urinary bladder,**
4. one **urethra.**

Each of the **kidneys** drains by way of its own **ureter** to the single **urinary bladder.** The bladder, situated above and behind the symphysis pubis, serves to store urine. Under voluntary control, the stored urine passes to the exterior via the **urethra.** The two **adrenal glands** of the endocrine system are located at the superomedial portion of each kidney. The bean-shaped kidneys are located on either side of the lumbar vertebral column. The right kidney is usually situated a little lower than the left one, due to the presence of the large liver on the right. Waste materials and excess water are eliminated from the blood by the kidneys and are transported through the ureters to the urinary bladder.

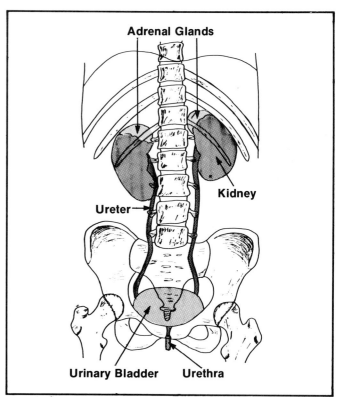

Urinary System   Fig. 3-19

Excretory Urogram

The kidneys are usually seen on a plain abdominal radiograph due to a fatty capsule that surrounds each kidney. The contrast medium examination shown in *Fig. 3-20* is termed an excretory urogram, which is one radiographic examination of the urinary system. During this examination the hollow organs of this system are visualized. The organs labeled are: **(A)** left kidney, **(B)** left ureter, **(C)** urinary bladder, and **(D)** the area of the right adrenal gland.

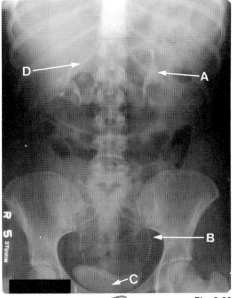

Excretory Urogram

prostate

Fig. 3-20

F. Quadrants and Regions

Four Abdominal Quadrants

If two imaginary perpendicular planes were passed through the abdomen at the umbilicus or navel, they would divide the abdomen into four quadrants. One plane would be transverse through the abdomen at the level of the umbilicus, while the second plane would coincide with the midsagittal plane and would pass through both the umbilicus and the symphysis pubis. These two planes would divide the abdominopelvic cavity into four quadrants: the right upper quadrant (R.U.Q.), the left upper quadrant (L.U.Q.), the right lower quadrant (R.L.Q.), and the left lower quadrant (L.L.Q.).

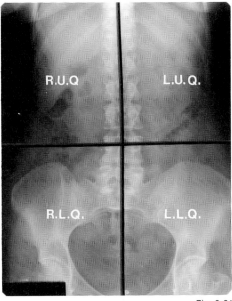

Fig. 3-21

Four Abdominal Quadrants

Nine Abdominal Regions

The abdominopelvic cavity can be further divided into nine regions by using two horizontal (or transverse) and two vertical imaginary planes. The two vertical planes would be parallel to the midsagittal plane, and midway between it and each anterior superior iliac spine. One tranverse plane would be located at the lower border of the first lumbar vertebra and the second at the level of the body of the fifth lumbar vertebra. These four imaginary planes divide the abdominopelvic cavity into the nine regions.

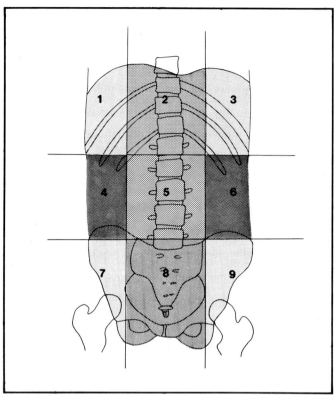

Nine Abdominal Regions   Fig. 3-22

The names of these nine regions are listed in *Fig. 3-23*. The upper three regions are the right and left hypochondriac regions and the epigastric region. The middle three are the right and left lateral regions, formerly known as lumbar regions, and the umbilical region. The bottom three are the right and left inguinal regions, formerly known as iliac regions, and the pubic, formerly known as the hypogastric region.

The four-quadrant system is generally adequate for use in radiographically localizing any particular organ, but the nine regions also need to be known and understood.

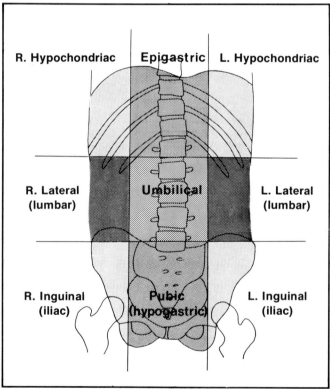

Nine Abdominal Regions   Fig. 3-23

Part II. Radiographic Positioning
of the Abdomen

A. Patient Preparation

Patient preparation for abdominal radiography includes removal of all clothing and any opaque objects in the area to be radiographed. A hospital gown should be put on with the opening and ties in the back. Shoes and socks may remain on the feet.

Some abdominal radiographs, particularly those requiring contrast media, necessitate special instructions to the patient prior to the examination. Instructions may include such things as fasting or a laxative the night before, but the abdominal radiograph is usually taken "as is."

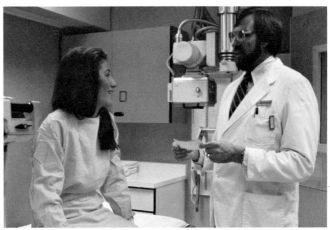

Patient Preparation   Fig. 3-24

B. Breathing Instructions

Most abdominal radiographs are taken on expiration. The patient is instructed to "take in a deep breath — let it all out and hold it — don't breathe." Before making the exposure, it is important to observe patients to be sure they are following instructions.

C. Exposure Factors

The principle exposure factors for abdominal radiographs are:

1. Medium kVp (70-90)
2. Short exposure time (½ second or less)
3. Adequate mAs for sufficient density

Correctly exposed abdominal radiographs should visualize the lateral borders of the psoas muscles, lower liver margin, kidney outlines and lumbar vertebrae transverse processes.

D. General Positioning Procedures

Make the patient as comfortable as possible on the radiographic table. A pillow under the head and support under the knees will enhance the patient's comfort. Cover the table with clean linen. Adjust the midsagittal plane to coincide with the midline of the table or the midline of the film holder. Be sure that the pelvis is not rotated, and adjust the arms at the patient's sides, away from the abdomen. Most abdominal radiographs are centered to the iliac crest with the symphysis pubis showing at the bottom edge of the radiograph. Collimation should be visible along the lateral margins of the finished radiograph.

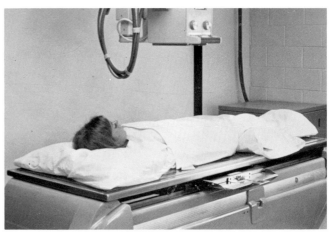

General Positioning Procedures   Fig. 3-25

Basic and Optional Projections/Positions

Certain basic and optional projections or positions for the abdomen are demonstrated and described on the following pages. **Basic projections,** also referred to as routine projections, are those projections commonly taken on average helpful patients. It should be noted that departmental routines or basic projections vary in different hospitals or departments. **Optional** projections include the more common projections taken as extra or additional projections to better demonstrate specific anatomical parts or certain pathologic conditions. Optional positioning may be necessary if the patient is uncooperative or cannot cooperate.

Generally, basic projections or positions for a routine radiographic examination of the abdomen include an A.P. supine radiograph, and occasionally both an A.P. supine and an A.P. upright abdominal radiograph. A horizontal beam radiograph, such as an upright or a decubitus, is necessary to visualize any air-fluid levels. Presence or absence of air-fluid levels is an important diagnostic determination. The basic fetogram is a P.A. projection in the prone position. Common optional projections may include one or more of the following: P.A., lateral decubitus and dorsal decubitus.

Correct Centering

Accurate centering of the body part to the film and correct central ray location are important to prevent distortion and/or "cutting off" of essential anatomical parts. This is even more critical when phototiming is used because inaccurate centering results in improper film density. To prevent these positioning errors a precise description of the central ray location in relationship to the body part is given, and an x indicating the correct centering point on the film is provided for each projection on the following pages.

Abdomen		**Abdomen**	**Abdomen**	**Acute Abdomen**	**Fetogram**
Basic	**or**	Basic	Optional	Basic	Basic
• A.P. (K.U.B.)		• A.P. (K.U.B.)	• P.A.	• A.P. Recumbent	• P.A.
		• Erect A.P.	• Lat. Decub.	• A.P. Erect	
			• Dorsal Decub.	• P.A. Chest Erect	
				Optional	
				• Left Lat. Decub.	

Abdomen

• **Anteroposterior Projection**
K.U.B.

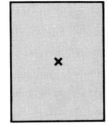

Film Size:
14 x 17 in. (35 x 43 cm.)

Bucky:
- Moving or stationary grid.

Patient Position:
- Supine with midsagittal plane of body centered to midline of table and/or film.
- Legs extended, not crossed, with support under the knees.
- Arms at patient's sides, away from body.

Part Position:
- Trunk of body, including pelvis, comfortable — not rotated.

Central Ray:
- C.R. perpendicular to film holder.
- Center to level of **iliac crests** and to midsagittal plane.
- 40 in. (102 cm.) F.F.D.

NOTE: • **Psoas muscle** outline, lower **liver, kidneys,** and **lumbar transverse processes** should be visible. • **Symphysis pubis** should be visible near bottom of radiograph. • Closely **collimate** lateral margins. • Use **gonadal shield** on males. • Expose on suspended **expiration.**

Structures Best Shown:
Liver, spleen, kidneys and any abnormal masses, calcifications or accumulations of gas. Pelvis, lumbar spine and lower ribs are well shown.

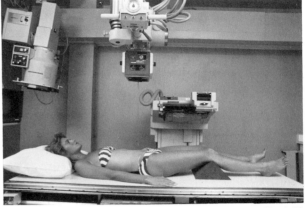

A.P.   Fig. 3-26

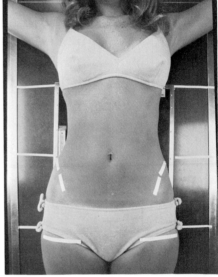

A.P.   Fig. 3-27

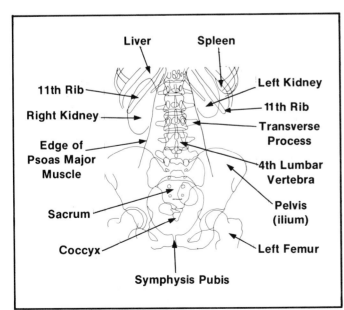

Fig. 3-29   A.P.

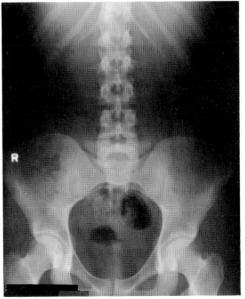

A.P.   Fig. 3-28

Abdomen

• Erect Anteroposterior Projection

Abdomen
Basic
• A.P. (K.U.B.)
• Erect A.P.

Film Size:
14 x 17 in. (35 x 43 cm.)

Bucky:
- Moving or stationary grid.

Patient Position:
- Upright with midsagittal plane of body centered to midline of table and/or center of film.
- Table is vertical or, rarely, tilted slightly toward horizontal, if patient has difficulty standing.
- Legs extended; knees stabilized by compression band, if necessary.
- Hands grasping table or hand-holds; body weight equally distributed.

Part Position:
- Trunk of body, including pelvis, NOT rotated.

Central Ray:
- C.R. perpendicular to film holder (**horizontal,** if table is tilted).
- Center to level of **iliac crests** and to midsagittal plane.
- 40 in. (102 cm.) F.F.D.

NOTE: • **Symphysis pubis** should be visible near bottom of radiograph. • Patient should be upright a minimum of **5 minutes** before exposure. • X-ray beam must be **horizontal.** • Use **gonadal shield** on males. • Closely **collimate** lateral margins. • Expose on suspended **expiration.**

Structures Best Shown:
Liver, spleen, kidneys and any abnormal masses, calcifications or accumulations of gas. Air-fluid levels, if present.

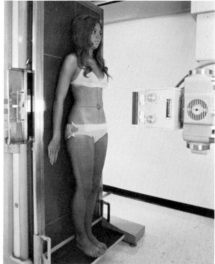

Erect A.P.   Fig. 3-30

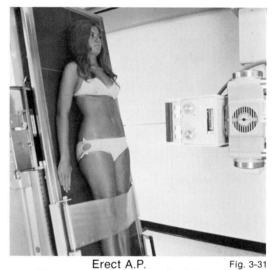

Erect A.P.   Fig. 3-31
(Slight table tilt, horizontal C.R.)

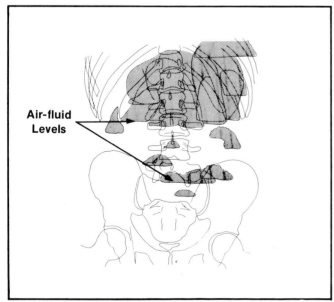

Air-fluid Levels

Fig. 3-33
Erect A.P.

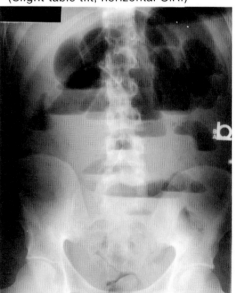

Erect A.P.   Fig. 3-32

Abdomen

• Posteroanterior Projection

Film Size:
14 x 17 in. (35 x 43 cm.)

Bucky:
- Moving or stationary grid.

Patient Position:
- Prone with midsagittal plane of body centered to midline of table and/or film.
- Legs extended with support under ankles.
- Arms up, beside head.

Part Position:
- Trunk of body, including pelvis, comfortable and not rotated.

Central Ray:
- C.R. perpendicular to film holder.
- Center to level of **iliac crests** and to midsagittal plane
- 40 in. (102 cm.) F.F.D.

NOTE: • **Psoas muscle** outline, lower **liver, kidneys** and **lumbar transverse processes** should be visible. • **Symphysis pubis** should be visible near bottom of radiograph. • Closely **collimate** lateral margins. • Expose on suspended **expiration.**

Structures Best Shown:
Liver, spleen, kidneys and any abnormal masses, calcifications or accumulations of gas. Pelvis, lower spine and lower ribs are well shown.

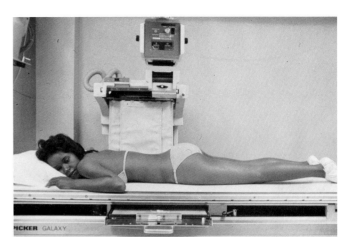

P.A.   Fig. 3-34

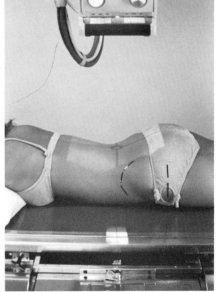

P.A.   Fig. 3-35

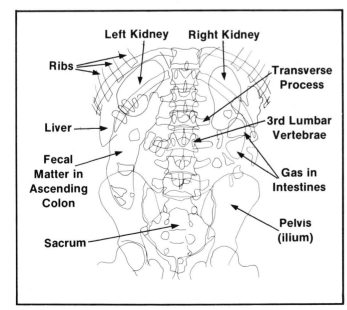

Fig. 3-37   P.A.

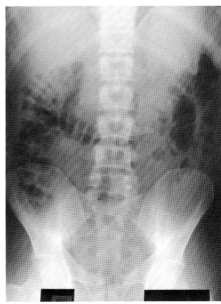

P.A.   Fig. 3-36

Abdomen
• **Lateral Decubitus Position**
A.P. Projection

Film Size:
   14 x 17 in. (35 x 43 cm.)

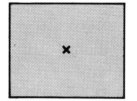

Bucky:
- Moving or stationary grid.

Patient Position:
- Lateral recumbent.
- Knees partially flexed, one on top of the other.
- Arms up, near head.

Part Position:
- Trunk of body, including pelvis, not rotated.

Central Ray:
- C.R. perpendicular to film holder.
- Center to level of **iliac crests** and to midsagittal plane.
- 40 in. (102 cm.) F.F.D.

NOTE: • Table or grid cassette vertical. • **A.P.** projection more comfortable for patient. • Patient should be on side a minimum of **5 minutes** before exposure. • **Left lateral decubitus** will best demonstrate free air within abdominal cavity. • **Collimate** to film size. • Expose on suspended **expiration.** • X-ray beam must be **horizontal.**

Structures Best Shown:
Liver, spleen, kidneys and any abnormal masses, accumulations of gas or free intra-abdominal air.

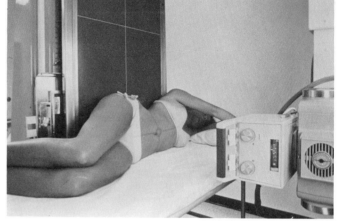

Left Lat. Decub.   Fig. 3-38

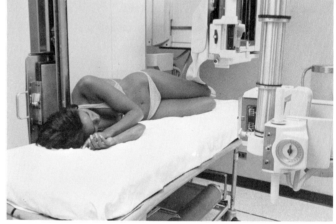

Right Lat. Decub.   Fig. 3-39

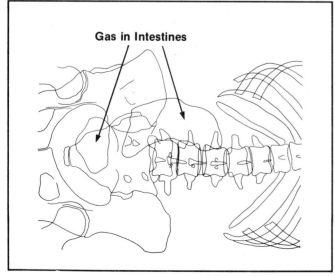

Gas in Intestines

Fig. 3-41   Left Lat. Decub.

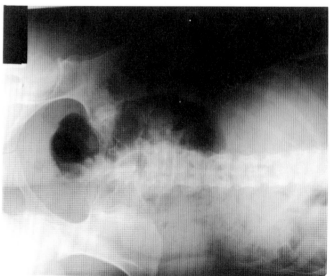

Left Lat. Decub.   Fig. 3-40

Abdomen
Optional
- P.A.
- **Lat. Decub. (P.A.)**
- Dorsal Decub.

Abdomen

• **Lateral Decubitus Position**
P.A. Projection

Film Size:
14 x 17 (35 x 43 cm.)

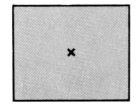

Bucky:
- Moving or stationary grid.

Patient Position:
- Lateral recumbent.
- Knees partially flexed, one on top of the other.
- Arms up, near head.

Part Position:
- Trunk of body, including pelvis, not rotated.

Central Ray:
- C.R. perpendicular to film holder.
- Center to level of **iliac crests** and to midsagittal plane.
- 40 in. (102 cm.) F.F.D.

NOTE: • Table or grid cassette **vertical.** • Less comfortable than A.P. projection. • Patient should be on side a minimum of **5 minutes** before exposure. • **Collimate** to film size. • Expose on suspended **expiration.** • X-ray beam must be **horizontal.**

Structures Best Shown:
Liver, spleen, kidneys and any abnormal masses, accumulations of gas or free intra-abdominal air.

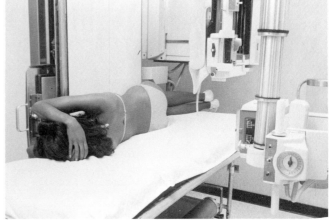
Left Lat. Decub. (P.A.)   Fig. 3-42

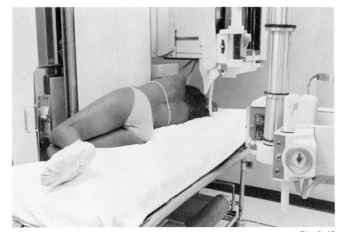
Right Lat. Decub. (P.A.)   Fig. 3-43

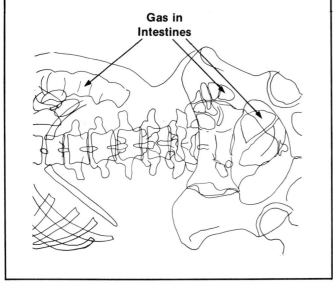

Gas in Intestines

Fig. 3-45
Right Lat. Decub.

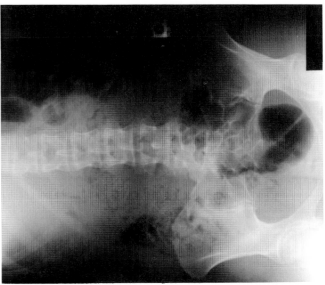
Right Lat. Decub.   Fig. 3-44

Abdomen

• Dorsal Decubitus Position

Abdomen
Optional
• P.A.
• Lat. Decub.
• **Dorsal Decub.**

Film Size:
14 x 17 in. (35 x 43 cm.)

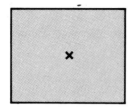

Bucky:
- Moving or stationary grid.

Patient Position:
- Supine.

Part Position:
- Trunk of body, including pelvis, not rotated.

Central Ray:
- C.R. perpendicular to film holder.
- Center to **iliac crests** and to midaxillary plane.
- 40 in. (102 cm.) F.F.D.

NOTE: • Table or grid cassette **vertical.** • **Collimate** to film size. • Expose on suspended **expiration.** • X-ray beam must be **horizontal.**

Structures Best Shown:
Abnormal masses, accumulations of gas, free intra-abdominal air and umbilical hernias.

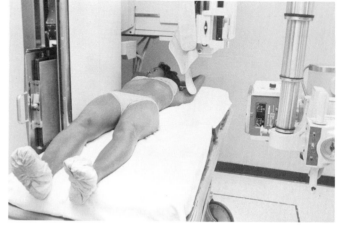

Dorsal Decub.   Fig. 3-46

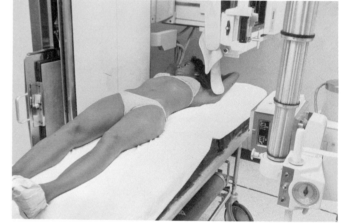

Dorsal Decub.   Fig. 3-47

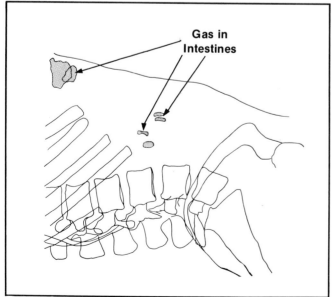

Gas in Intestines

Fig. 3-49
Dorsal Decub.

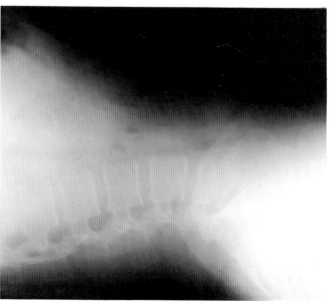

Dorsal Decub.   Fig. 3-48

Abdomen

● Acute Abdominal Series
Three-way Abdomen

Acute Abdomen
Basic
● A.P. Recumbent
● A.P. Erect
● P.A. Chest
Optional
● Left Lat. Decub.

Film Size:

14 x 17 in. (35 x 43 cm.)

Same as described on preceding pages.

Bucky:

- Moving or stationary grid.

- Same as described on preceding pages.

Patient and Part Position:

- Same as described on preceding pages.

Central Ray:

- Same as described on preceding pages.

Common Reasons for Series:

(1) Perforated hollow viscus

(2) Obstruction

(3) Infection

NOTE: Left lateral decubitus replaces erect position, if the patient is too ill to stand. ● **Horizontal beam** is necessary to visualize air-fluid levels. ● **Upright chest** best visualizes free air under diaphragm. ● Patient should be upright or on side for a minimum of **five minutes** before exposure.

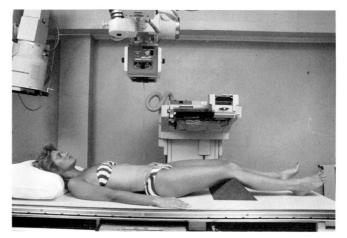

A.P. Recumbent   Fig. 3-50

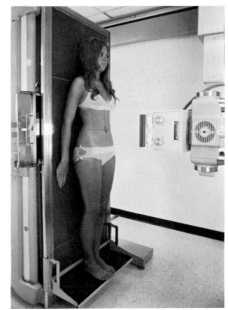

A.P. Erect   Fig. 3-51

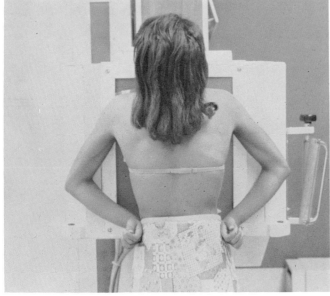

Fig. 3-53

P.A. Chest

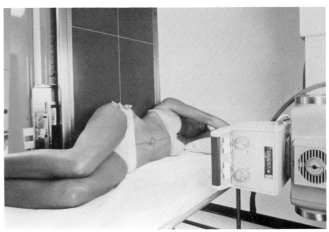

Left Lat. Decub. (Optional)   Fig. 3-52

71

Fetogram
Basic
• **P.A.**

Fetogram

• **Posteroanterior Projection**

NOTE: See Chapter 9 (Pelvis) for pelvimetry exam.

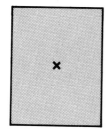

Film Size:
14 x 17 in. (35 x 43 cm.)

Bucky:
- Moving or stationary grid.

Patient Position:
- Prone with midsagittal plane of body centered to midline of table and/or film.
- Legs extended with support under ankles, pelvis and chest.
- Arms up, beside thorax.

Part Position:
- Trunk of body, including pelvis, as comfortable as possible without rotation.
- Supports under chest and pelvis aid patient in maintaining this position without rotation.

Central Ray:
- C.R. perpendicular to film holder.
- Center to level of **iliac crests** and to midsagittal plane.
- 40 in. (102 cm.) F.F.D.

NOTE: • **Prone** position places fetus closer to film and helps to control fetal motion. • Suspend respiration on expiration after **several** deep breaths. • Use **fast film — fast screens,** if possible.

Structures Best Shown:
Age, presentation and position of fetus or fetuses.

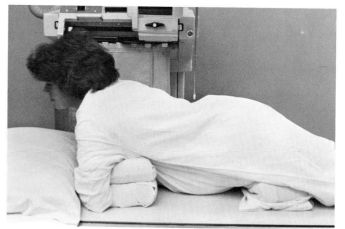

P.A.   Fig. 3-54

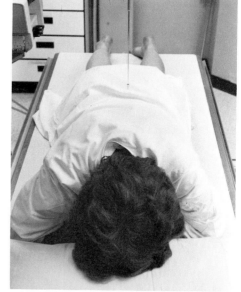

P.A.   Fig. 3-55

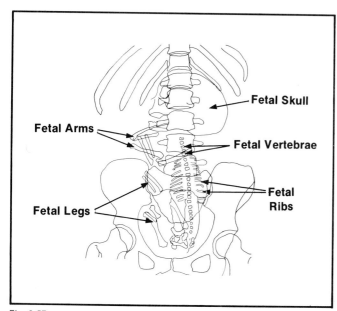

Fig. 3-57   P.A.

Fetal Skull

Fetal Arms

Fetal Vertebrae

Fetal Legs

Fetal Ribs

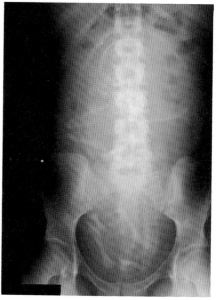

P.A.   Fig. 3-56

CHAPTER 4

Radiographic Anatomy and Positioning of the Hand and Wrist

Part I. Radiographic Anatomy of the Hand and Wrist

Hand and Wrist

The 27 bones of one hand and wrist are divided into three groups:

Phalanges (fingers and thumb)	14
Metacarpals (palm)	5
Carpals (wrist)	8
Total	27

The most distal bones of the hand are the **phalanges,** which make up the digits (fingers and thumb). The second group of bones are the **metacarpals,** which make up the palm of each hand. The third group of bones, the **carpals,** compose the bones of the wrist.

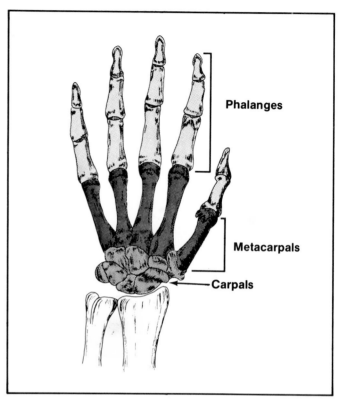

Hand and Wrist

Fig. 4-1

Phalanges - Fingers and Thumb (digits)

Each finger and thumb is called a digit, and each digit consists of two or three separate small bones called phalanges (singular is **phalanx**). The digits are numbered starting with the thumb as number one and ending with the little finger as digit number five.

Each of the four fingers (digits two, three, four and five) are made up of three phalanges; the **proximal, middle** and **distal.** The thumb, or first digit, has just two phalanges, the proximal and distal.

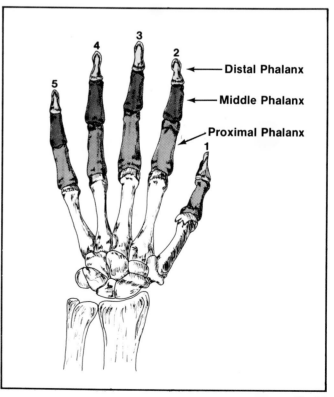

Phalanges

Fig. 4-2

74

Joints of the Hand and Wrist

The joints or articulations between the individual bones of the extremities are important in radiology because small chip fractures may occur near the joint spaces. Therefore, accurate identification of all joints of the phalanges, metacarpals and carpals of the hand and wrist is required.

Thumb (first digit). The thumb has only two phalanges, so the joint between them is called the **interphalangeal** or **I.P. joint.** The joint between the first metacarpal and the proximal phalanx of the thumb is called the **first metacarpophalangeal** or **M.P. joint.** Note that the name of this joint consists of the names of the two bones making up this joint. The more proximal bone is named first, followed by the name of the more distal bone.

Fingers (second through fifth digits). The second through fifth digits have three phalanges, therefore they would also have three joints each. Starting from the most distal portion of each digit, the joints are the **distal interphalangeal** or **D.I.P. joint,** then the **proximal interphalangeal** or **P.I.P. joint** and, most proximally, the **metacarpophalangeal** or **M.P. joint.**

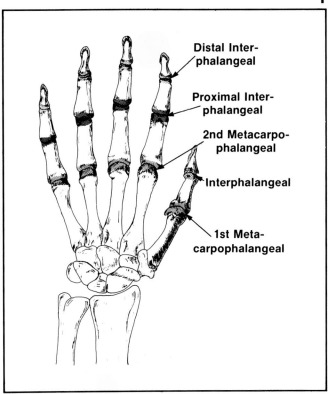

Joints of the Hand and Wrist

Fig. 4-3

In identifying joints of the hand, it is important to remember that the specific digit and hand must be included in descriptions of these joints. A radiograph of a hand *(Fig. 4-4)* demonstrates the phalanges and joints that have been described. Part **A** is the proximal phalanx of the second digit of the right hand; **B** is the distal interphalangeal joint of the second digit of the right hand; **C** is the distal phalanx of the third digit of the right hand; **D** is the middle phalanx of the fourth digit of the right hand; and **E** is the proximal interphalangeal joint of the fourth digit of the right hand.

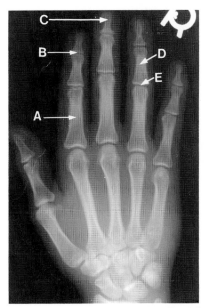

Radiograph of the Hand

Fig. 4-4

Metacarpals (palm)

The second group of bones of the hand, making up the palm, are the five metacarpals. These bones are numbered in the same way the digits are numbered, with the first metacarpal being on the thumb or lateral side when the hand is in the anatomical position.

Joints of the Metacarpals. The metacarpals articulate with the phalanges at their distal ends and are called **meta-carpophalangeal** or **M.P. joints.** At the proximal end, the metacarpals articulate with the respective carpals and are called **carpometacarpal** or **C.M. joints.**

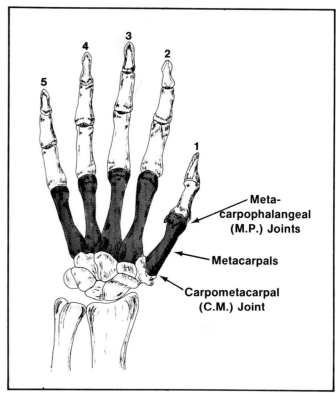

Metacarpals

Fig. 4-5

The metacarpal joints usually are not identified with a digit, only with the number of that metacarpal. Therefore, parts labeled in *Fig. 4-6* are: **(A)** the first carpometacarpal joint of the right hand; **(B)** the first metacarpal of the right hand; **(C)** the second metacarpal of the right hand; **(D)** the fifth metacarpophalangeal joint of the right hand; and **(E)** the fifth metacarpal of the right hand.

It should be noted that radiographs of hands or feet should always be placed on an illuminator with the fingers or toes up, as in *Fig. 4-6*.

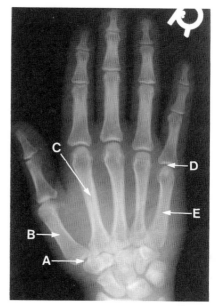

Radiograph of the Hand

Fig. 4-6

Carpals (wrist)

Proximal Row

The third group of bones of the hand and wrist are the carpals. The eight carpals form two rows of four bones each. It is easiest to learn the names of these eight carpals by beginning on the thumb side of the proximal row with the **navicular** or **scaphoid.** This bone is the most important, radiographically, because it is the most frequently fractured carpal bone.

It should be noted that one of the tarsal bones of the foot is also called the navicular or scaphoid. Correct terminology dictates that the tarsal bone of the **foot** should be called the **navicular,** while the carpal bone of the **wrist** should be called the **scaphoid.** However, it is common practice to call both the carpal of the wrist and the tarsal of the foot the navicular.

The second carpal in the proximal row is the **lunate** or **semilunar.** The third carpal is the **triangular** or **cuneiform,** occasionally called the **triquetrum.** The fourth and last carpal in the proximal row is the **pisiform,** the only carpal with just one name. The first name given for these carpals is the most common, but the other names should also be learned.

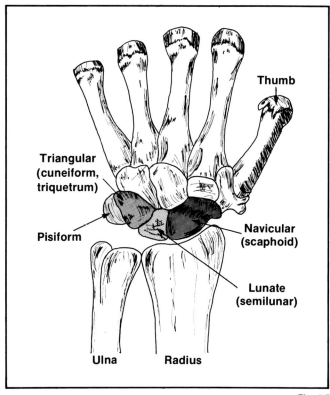

Carpals, proximal row

Fig. 4-7

Distal Row

The second, more distal row of carpal bones is also made up of four carpals. Starting on the lateral or thumb side is the **greater multangular** or **trapezium.** Next is the **lesser multangular** or **trapezoid,** followed by the **capitate** or **os magnum.** The fourth and last carpal in the distal row is the **hamate** or **unciform.**

The names of these eight carpals can be more easily remembered by utilizing the following mnemonic: **N**ever **L**ower **T**illie's **P**ants; **G**randma **M**ight **C**ome **H**ome.

(1) **N**ever	-	Navicular or scaphoid
(2) **L**ower	-	Lunate or semilunar
(3) **T**illie's	-	Triangular or cuneiform (triquetrum)
(4) **P**ants	-	Pisiform
(5) **G**randma	-	Greater Multangular or trapezium
(6) **M**ight	-	lesser **M**ultangular or trapezoid
(7) **C**ome	-	Capitate or os magnum
(8) **H**ome	-	Hamate or unciform

lesser is trapped

Hammate Hook & Unciform
Unicorn's horn

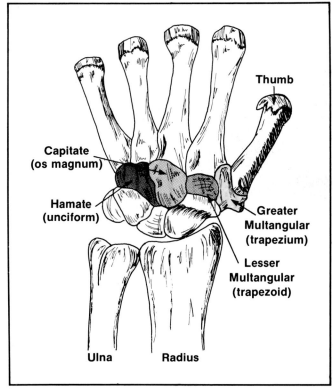

Carpals, distal row

Fig. 4-8

Carpal Canal

Figure 4-9 is a drawing of the carpals as they would appear looking tangentially down the wrist and arm from the palm or volar side of a hyperextended wrist. This drawing demonstrates the carpal canal formed by the concave anterior surface of the carpals. The pisiform and hamate are best visualized on this view. The term hamate means hooked, describing the shape of the hamate as seen in the drawing.

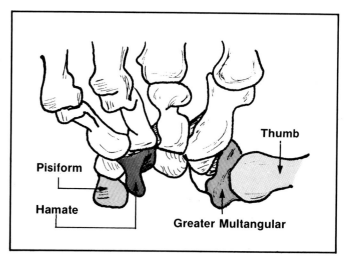

Carpal Canal

Fig. 4-9

Lateral Radiograph of the Wrist

The greater multangular and the pisiform are located in almost the same vertical plane in a true lateral position of the wrist, as shown on the radiograph in *Fig. 4-10.* **A** is the pisiform and **B** is the greater multangular. The other carpals are difficult to identify in a lateral position because they are primarily superimposed.

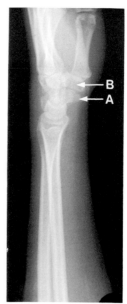

Fig. 4-10
Lateral Radiograph
of the Wrist

Wrist Joint and Distal Radioulnar Joint

The two bones of the forearm are the radius (laterally) and the ulna (medially). The lower or distal end of the radius is broad and has a conical projection on its lateral end called the **radial styloid process.** A similar conical projection extends from the ulna on the medial side and is called the **ulnar styloid process.** The rounded distal portion of the ulna, proximal to the styloid process, is called the **head** of the ulna.

The distal radius and ulna articulate with each other at a joint called the **distal radioulnar joint.**

Of the two bones of the forearm, only the radius articulates directly with carpal bones. This articulation is called the **radiocarpal** joint or the wrist joint proper. The three carpals involved in the wrist joint are the scaphoid or navicular, the lunate and the triangular. The carpals also articulate with adjacent carpals and, distally, with the metacarpals.

Classification of Joints

All joints of the hand and wrist are freely movable and are classified as diarthrodial joints. The wrist joint proper, the radiocarpal joint, is a condyloid-type joint with movements in four directions. These movements are flexion, extension, abduction and adduction. The intercarpal joints between the various carpals have only a gliding-type movement. Both the first carpometacarpal joint and the first metacarpophalangeal joint involving the thumb are saddle type joints, although the proximal joint allows more motion and is the classic saddle joint. These saddle type joints involving the thumb are unique in that they have the four movements of the condyloid type joint in addition to an axial rotational movement. No other joints of the body have this type of movement.

The second through fifth carpometacarpal joints only allow gliding movements. The second through fifth metacarpophalangeal joints (the base of the fingers) are condyloid joints that allow movement in four directions. All interphalangeal joints of the fingers are hinge type joints with movements in two directions only, flexion and extension.

Summary of Hand and Wrist Joints

1. Radiocarpal Joint — Wrist
   - *Diarthrodial (condyloid)*
2. Intercarpal Joints
   - *Diarthrodial (gliding)*
3. Carpometacarpal Joints
   - *Diarthrodial*
     First digit (thumb) — saddle
     Second - fifth digits — gliding
4. Metacarpophalangeal Joints
   - *Diarthrodial*
     First digit (thumb) — saddle
     Second - fifth digits — condyloid
5. Interphalangeal Joints
   - *Diarthrodial (hinge)*

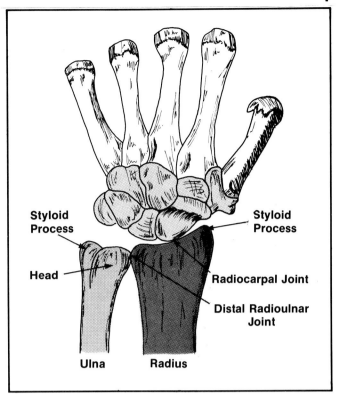

Wrist Joint

Fig. 4-11

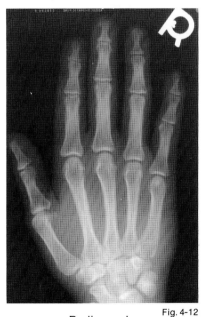

Fig. 4-12

Radiograph
of the Hand and Wrist

Motions of the Wrist Joint

Confusing terminology involving the wrist joint includes radial deviation or ulnar flexion, and ulnar deviation or radial flexion. Flexion of the wrist joint involves the anterior surface of the wrist. Ulnar or radial flexion involves a lateral bending at the wrist joint. If the hand is forced toward the ulnar side of the forearm with the hand pronated, the wrist joint near the distal ulna will be flexed. This motion is termed **ulnar flexion** or **radial deviation,** and serves to open up the carpal joints on the opposite side of the wrist. The carpals primarily involved are the scaphoid, lunate, greater multangular and lesser multangular. This motion is often used to obtain a better view of the scaphoid or navicular.

If the hand is forced toward the radial side of the forearm with the hand pronated, the wrist joint near the distal radius will be flexed. This motion is termed **radial flexion** or **ulnar deviation,** and serves to open up the carpal joints on the little finger side of the wrist. The carpals involved are the triangular, pisiform, capitate and hamate.

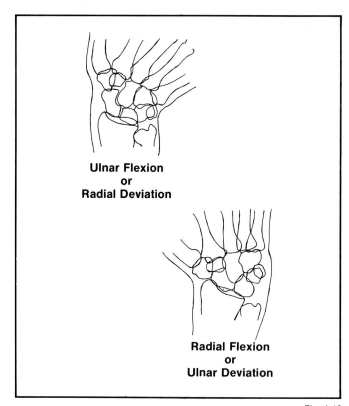

**Ulnar Flexion
or
Radial Deviation**

**Radial Flexion
or
Ulnar Deviation**

Motions of the Wrist Joint

Fig. 4-13

Part II. Radiographic Positioning of the Hand and Wrist

Basic and Optional Projections/Positions

Certain basic and optional projections or positions for the hand and wrist are demonstrated and described on the following pages. **Basic projections,** also sometimes referred to as routine projections, are those projections commonly taken on average helpful patients. It should be noted that departmental routines (basic projections) vary in different hospitals or departments. **Optional projections** include those more common projections taken as extra or additional projections to better demonstrate specific anatomical parts or certain pathological conditions.

Radiographic examination of the thumb, fingers, hand or wrist involves joints; therefore, three projections or positions are generally required. The hand is an exception that may require only two projections, a P.A. and an oblique. The lateral position of the hand superimposes the metacarpals and is of limited value.

The basic projections described for the thumb include an A.P. and a lateral of the thumb only, with the oblique thumb as part of a P.A. hand projection. This is a common routine for the thumb, but an alternative routine sometimes used is taking the oblique of the thumb only, rather than including the entire P.A. hand.

In addition to the three basic projections described for the wrist, an optional projection is illustrated and described for use when an additional view of the navicular is required.

Two post reduction projections of the wrist or forearm with cast are also illustrated and described. These projections are taken after the anatomical parts of the fractured wrist and forearm have been "reduced" or aligned, and a cast has been applied.

Correct Centering

Accurate centering of the body part to the film and correct central ray location are important to prevent distortion and/or "cutting off" of essential anatomical parts. This is even more critical when phototiming is used because inaccurate centering results in improper film density. To prevent these positioning errors a precise description of the central ray location in relationship to the body part is given, and an x indicating the correct centering point on the film is provided for each projection on the following pages.

| **Thumb**
Basic
• A.P.
• Lateral
• Oblique (P.A. hand)
Optional
• Oblique (thumb only) | **Fingers**
Basic
• P.A. (hand)
• Lateral
• Oblique | **Hand**
Basic
• P.A.
• Oblique | **Wrist**
Basic
• P.A.
• Oblique
• Lateral
Optional
• Ulnar Flexion
  (radial deviation) | **Wrist or Forearm**
(Post Reduction)
• P.A.
• Lateral |

Thumb (1st digit)
• Anteroposterior Projection
• Lateral Position

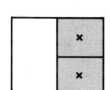

Thumb
Basic
- A.P.
- Lateral
- Oblique (P.A. hand)

Optional:
- Oblique (thumb only)

Film Size:
> 10 x 12 in. (24 x 30 cm.)
> 8 x 10 in. (18 x 24 cm.)
> for small hand
> Use half of film.

Non-Bucky:
- Detail screen or CBH.

Patient Position:
- Patient seated at end of x-ray table with hand and forearm resting on tabletop (place lead shield over patient's lap).

Part Position:
A.P.
- Internally rotate hand until posterior surface of thumb is on film holder.
- Hold fingers with opposite hand.
- Demonstrate correct position for patient.

Lateral
- Start with hand pronated, then rotate thumb into true lateral position.
- Entire lateral aspect of thumb should be in contact with film holder.

Centray Ray:
- C.R. perpendicular to film holder.
- To first metacarpophalangeal (M.P.) joint.
- 40 in. (102 cm.) F.F.D.

NOTE: • Avoid motion by using short exposure time (high mA, short time). • Use small focal spot, close collimation and CBH or detail screens for optimum definition. • Be sure to include all of first metacarpal on film.

Structures Best Shown:
Distal and proximal phalanges and metacarpal of first digit, along with associated joints.

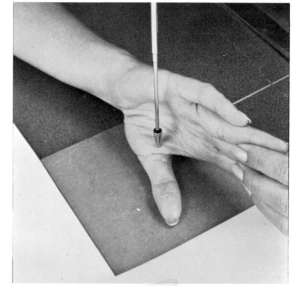
A.P.   Fig. 4-14

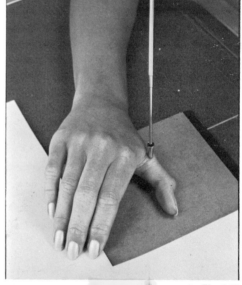
Lateral   Fig. 4-15

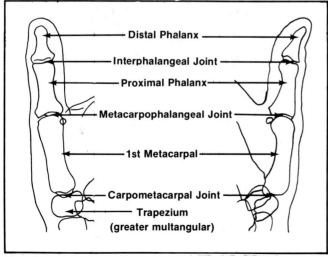

Distal Phalanx
Interphalangeal Joint
Proximal Phalanx
Metacarpophalangeal Joint
1st Metacarpal
Carpometacarpal Joint
Trapezium
(greater multangular)

Fig. 4-17   A.P.   Lateral

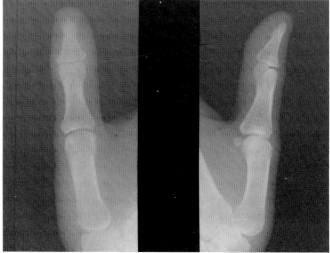
A.P.   Lateral   Fig. 4-16

Thumb

• Oblique Position (P.A. hand)
Optional: Oblique (thumb only)

Thumb
Basic
• A.P.
• Lateral
• **Oblique (P.A. hand)**
Optional
• Oblique (thumb only)

Film Size:
    10 x 12 in. (24 x 30 cm.)
    8 x 10 in. (18 x 24 cm.)
      for small hand
    Use half of film.

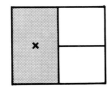

Non-Bucky:
- Detail screen or CBH.

Patient Position:
- Patient seated at end of table with hand and forearm resting on tabletop (place lead shield over patient's lap).

Part Position:
- Pronate hand with palmar surface in contact with film holder. (This will naturally place the thumb into a 45° oblique position.)

Central Ray:
- C.R. perpendicular to film holder.
- 40 in. (102 cm.) F.F.D.
  Oblique (P.A. hand)
  - To 3rd metacarpophalangeal (M.P.) joint.
  Oblique (thumb only)
  - To 1st metacarpophalangeal (M.P.) joint.

NOTE: • The reason for including the total hand on the oblique thumb position is that a patient with a primary injury to the thumb often has secondary injury to other parts of the hand.

Structures Best Shown:
Phalanges and metacarpals of hand, and all associated joints.

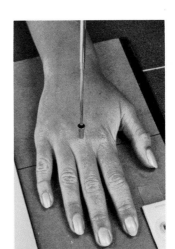

Oblique Thumb   Fig. 4-18
(including P.A. hand)

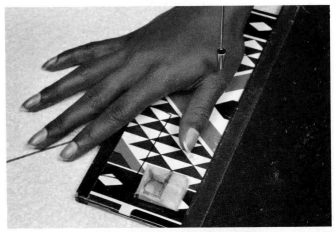

Optional Projection: Oblique (thumb only)   Fig. 4-19

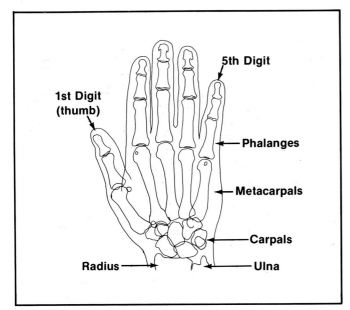

Fig. 4-21   P.A. Hand -
Oblique Thumb

Labels in diagram: 1st Digit (thumb), 5th Digit, Phalanges, Metacarpals, Carpals, Radius, Ulna

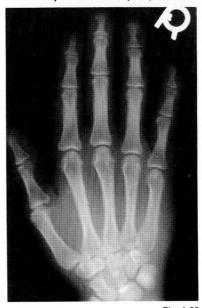

P.A. Hand -   Fig. 4-20
Oblique Thumb

Fingers
Basic
• P.A. (hand)
• **Lateral**
• Oblique

Fingers (2nd - 5th digits)

• **Lateral Position**

Film Size:

    10 x 12 in. (24 x 30 cm.)
    8 x 10 in. (18 x 24 cm.)
    for small hand
    Use one quarter of film.

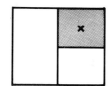

Non-Bucky:

- Detail screen or CBH.

Patient Position:

- Patient seated at end of table with hand and forearm resting on tabletop (place lead shield over patient's lap).

Part Position:

- Hand and fingers in lateral position.
- Flex unaffected fingers.
- Use sponge block or similar device to support finger and prevent motion.
- **Be sure** that the long axis of the finger is parallel to the film.

Central Ray:

- C.R. perpendicular to film holder.
- To proximal interphalangeal (P.I.P.) joint.
- 40 in. (102 cm.) F.F.D.

NOTE: • It is always very important for the finger being radiographed to be parallel to the film to "open up" and clearly visualize the interphalangeal spaces for possible fracture fragments (avulsion or "chip" fracture).

Structures Best Shown:

Phalanges and interphalangeal joints.

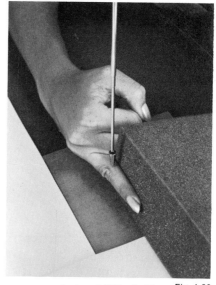

Lateral (4th digit)   Fig. 4-22

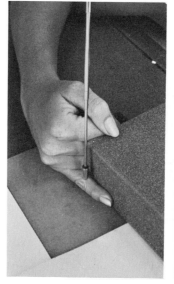

Lateral (5th digit)

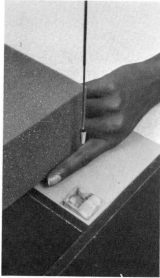

Lateral (2nd digit)   Fig. 4-23

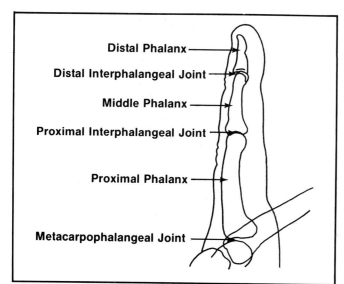

Fig. 4-25

Lateral
(2nd digit)

Distal Phalanx

Distal Interphalangeal Joint

Middle Phalanx

Proximal Interphalangeal Joint

Proximal Phalanx

Metacarpophalangeal Joint

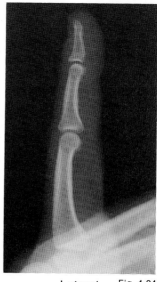

Lateral   Fig. 4-24
(2nd digit)

Fingers
Basic
- P.A. (hand)
- Lateral
- Oblique

Fingers (2nd - 5th digits)

• Oblique Position

Film Size:

10 x 12 in. (24 x 30 cm.)
8 x 10 in. (18 x 24 cm.)
for small hand
Use one quarter of film.

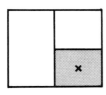

Non-Bucky:

- Detail screen or CBH.

Patient Position:

- Patient seated at end of table with forearm and hand resting on tabletop (place lead shield over patient's lap).

Part Position:

2nd digit

- Hand and finger rotated **medially** into 45° oblique with finger in direct contact with film.
- Unaffected fingers and thumb flexed to prevent superimposition of injured digit.

3rd - 5th digits

- Hand and fingers rotated **laterally** using 45° sponges or other radiolucent support.
- Fingers separated.

Central Ray:

- C.R. perpendicular to film holder.
- To proximal interphalangeal (P.I.P.) joint.
- 40 in. (102 cm.) F.F.D.

NOTE: • The finger being radiographed must be parallel to film holder.

Structures Best Shown:

Phalanges and interphalangeal joints.

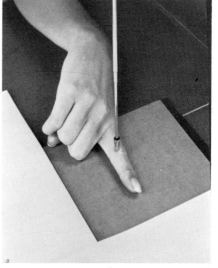

Medial Oblique   Fig. 4-26
(2nd digit)

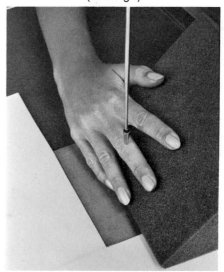

Lateral Oblique   Fig. 4-27
(3rd digit)

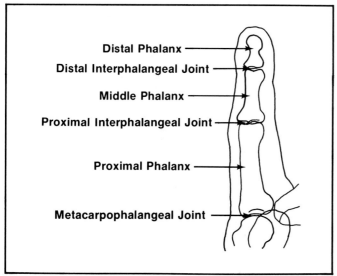

Fig. 4-29

Oblique (2nd digit)

Distal Phalanx
Distal Interphalangeal Joint
Middle Phalanx
Proximal Interphalangeal Joint
Proximal Phalanx
Metacarpophalangeal Joint

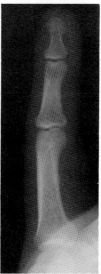

Fig. 4-28
Oblique (2nd digit)

Hand
Basic
• P.A.
• Oblique

Hand

- ## Posteroanterior Projection
- ## Oblique Position (semipronation)

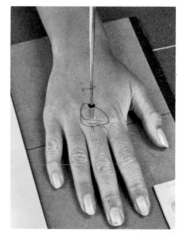

P.A. Fig. 4-30

Film Size:
   10 x 12 in. (24 x 30 cm.)
   8 x 10 in. (18 x 24 cm.)
    for small hand
   Divide film in half.

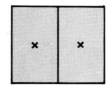

Non-Bucky:
- Detail screen or CBH.

Patient Position:
- Patient seated at end of table with hand and forearm resting on tabletop (place lead shield over patient's lap).

Part Position:

P.A.
- Pronate hand with palmar surface in contact with film holder.
- Insure that all digits are included on the radiograph.

Oblique
- Pronate hand and rotate laterally 45°.
- Separate and flex fingers partially to lightly rest finger tips and thumb on film holder.

Central Ray:
- C.R. perpendicular to film holder.
- To third metacarpophalangeal joint.
- 40 in. (102 cm.) F.F.D.

NOTE: • If digits are an area of primary interest, **extend the fingers and thumb,** and rest hand against 45° sponge block as shown on *Fig. 4-31,* right side.

Structures Best Shown:
Phalanges, metacarpals and all joints of hand.

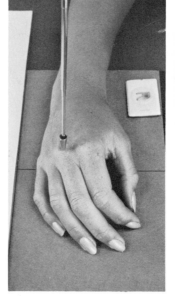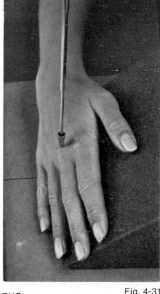

Oblique Fig. 4-31

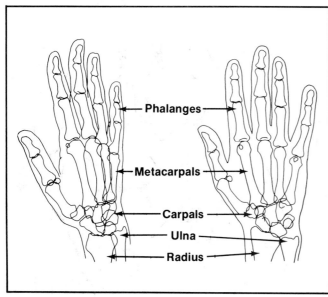

Fig. 4-33   Oblique   P.A.

Labels: Phalanges, Metacarpals, Carpals, Ulna, Radius

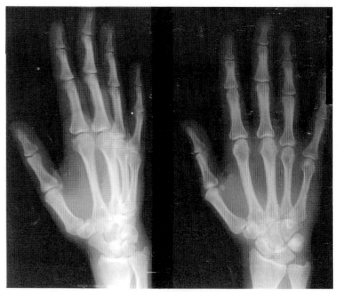

Oblique   P.A.   Fig. 4-32

Wrist
Basic
- P.A.
- Oblique
- Lateral

Optional
- Ulnar Flexion
  (radial deviation)

Wrist

- **Posteroanterior Projection**
- **Oblique Position** (semipronation)

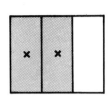
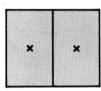

Film Size:

    10 x 12 in. (24 x 30 cm.)
    Divide film into thirds.
      or
    One 10 x 12 in. and one
    8 x 10 in. for large patient.

Non-Bucky:

- Detail screen or CBH.

Patient Position:

- Patient seated at end of table with hand and forearm resting on tabletop (place lead shield over patient's lap).

Part Position:

- Position forearm and wrist parallel to long axis of film.

P.A.

- Pronate hand.
- Flex digits and arch hand to allow wrist to be in contact with film holder.

Oblique

- From prone position, rotate laterally 45°.
- For stability, partially flex digits and arch hand to lightly rest finger tips on film holder.

Central Ray:

- C.R. perpendicular to film holder.
- To midcarpal area.
- 40 in. (102 cm.) F.F.D.

NOTE: • Be sure that wrist is rotated laterally far enough so that wrist and distal forearm are truly 45° from film holder.

Structures Best Shown:

Proximal metacarpals, eight carpals, distal radius and ulna, plus intercarpal and wrist joints.

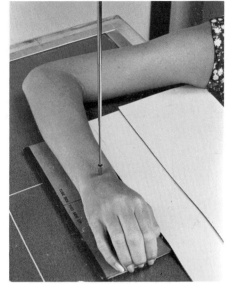

P.A.   Fig. 4-34

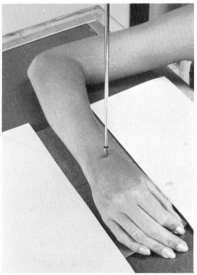

Oblique   Fig. 4-35

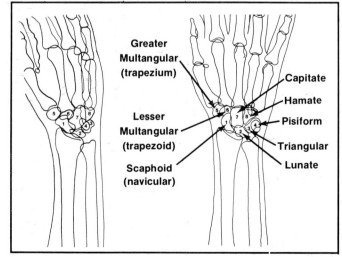

Greater Multangular (trapezium)

Capitate

Hamate

Lesser Multangular (trapezoid)

Pisiform

Triangular

Scaphoid (navicular)

Lunate

Fig. 4-37   Oblique   P.A.

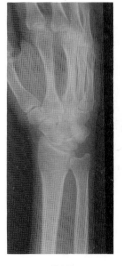
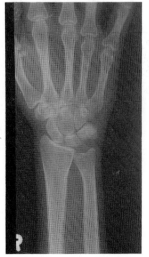

Oblique   P.A.   Fig. 4-36

Wrist

• Lateral Position

Wrist
Basic
- P.A.
- Oblique
- **Lateral**

Optional
- Ulnar Flexion (radial deviation)

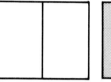

Film Size:

    10 x 12 in. (24 x 30 cm.)
    Divide film into thirds.
    or
    One 10 x 12 in. (24 x 30 cm.)
      and
    One 8 x 10 in. (18 x 24 cm.)
      for large patient.

Non-Bucky:

- Detail screen or CBH.

Patient Position:

- Patient seated at end of table with elbow flexed about 90°, and hand and forearm resting on tabletop (place lead shield over patient's lap).

Part Position:

- Rotate hand and forearm 90° to film holder, into a true lateral position.
- Extend digits and support against a radiolucent support block.

Central Ray:

- C.R. perpendicular to film holder.
- To wrist joint.
- 40 in. (102 cm.) F.F.D.

NOTE: • Carefully examine the wrist and distal forearm to insure that they are in a **true lateral** position.

Structures Best Shown:

Superimposed proximal metacarpals, carpals, distal radius and ulna, and wrist joint.

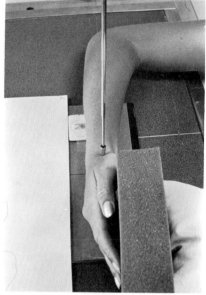

Lateral   Fig. 4-38

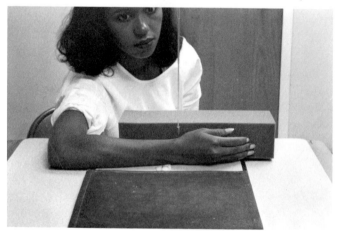

Lateral   Fig. 4-39

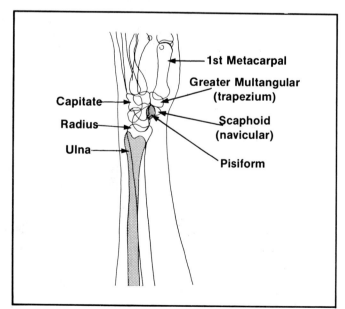

Fig. 4-41   Lateral

- 1st Metacarpal
- Greater Multangular (trapezium)
- Capitate
- Radius
- Ulna
- Scaphoid (navicular)
- Pisiform

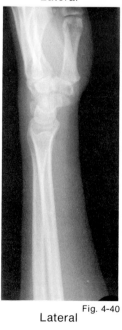

Lateral   Fig. 4-40

<table>
<tr><td>

Wrist

Basic
- P.A.
- Oblique
- Lateral

Optional
- **Ulnar Flexion**
  (radial deviation)

</td></tr>
</table>

Wrist

• **Ulnar Flexion**
(radial deviation)

Film Size:
    8 x 10 in. (18 x 24 cm.)

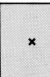

Non-Bucky:
- Detail screen or CBH.

Patient Position:
- Patient seated at end of table with hand and forearm resting on tabletop (place lead shield over patient's lap).

Part Position:
- Pronate hand completely.
- Without moving forearm, gently move hand laterally (ulnar flexion) as far as possible without lifting or obliquing forearm.

Central Ray:
- Direct C. R. **20°** **toward elbow** and center to scaphoid (carpal navicular) bone.
- 40 in. (102 cm.) F.F.D.

NOTE: • The purpose of the 20° angle toward the elbow is to **direct the C.R. perpendicular to the scaphoid** (carpal navicular). • For another special view of the scaphoid, this angle may be increased to more than 20° to elongate the scaphoid.

Structures Best Shown:
Scaphoid without foreshortening.

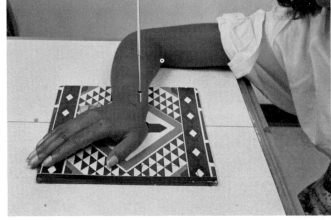

Ulnar Flexion
with Tube Angulation   Fig. 4-42

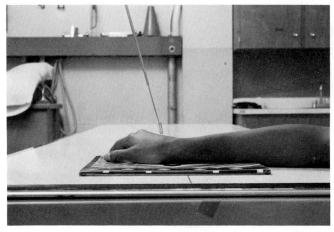

Ulnar Flexion
with Tube Angulation   Fig. 4-43

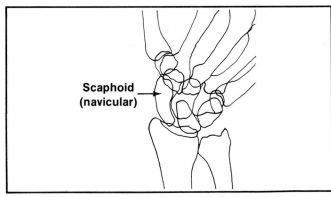

Fig. 4-45

Ulnar Flexion

Scaphoid
(navicular)

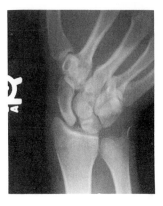

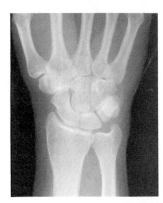

Ulnar Flexion
with Tube Angulation   Routine P.A.   Fig. 4-44

Wrist
(Post Reduction)
- P.A.
- Lateral

Wrist
(Post Reduction, in cast)
- **Posteroanterior Projection**
- **Lateral Position**

Film Size:

    10 x 12 in. (24 x 30 cm.)
    Divide film in half, lengthwise.
    or
    Two 8 x 10's (18 x 24 cm.)

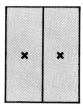
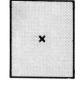

Non-Bucky:
- Detail screen or CBH.

Patient Position:
- Patient seated at end of table with hand and forearm resting on tabletop (place lead shield over patient's lap).
- Patient may also be supine on cart.

Part Position:

P.A.
- Pronate hand and wrist into true prone position.

Lateral
- Rotate hand and wrist into true lateral position.

Central Ray:
- C.R. perpendicular to film holder.
- To wrist joint.
- 40 in. (102 cm.) F.F.D.

NOTE: ● These two projections must be at 90° to each other to check for correct alignment.

Structures Best Shown:
Distal forearm and wrist to check for alignment of fracture fragments.

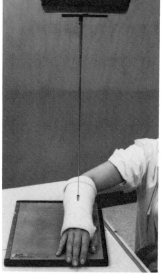
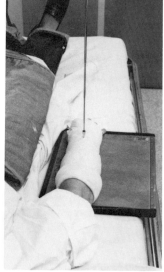

P.A.   Fig. 4-46

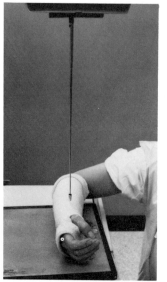
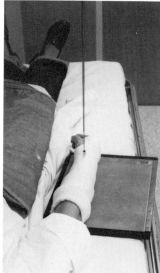

Lateral   Fig. 4-47

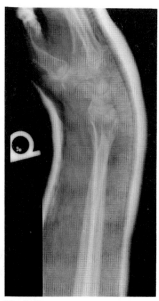
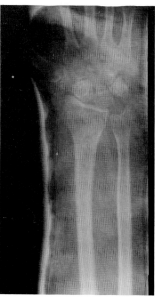

Fig. 4-49

Lateral   P.A.

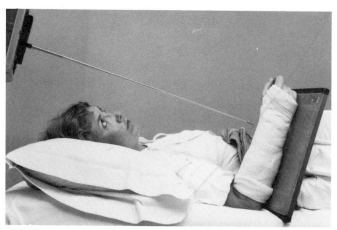

Lateral   Fig. 4-48

get one joint in closest to fracture

| **Wrist or Forearm** |
| (Post Reduction) |
| • P.A. |
| • Lateral |

Wrist or Forearm
(Post Reduction, in cast)
• Posteroanterior Projection
• Lateral Position

Film Size:
10 x 12 in. (24 x 30 cm.)
Divide film in half, lengthwise.

Non-Bucky:
- Detail screen or CBH.

Patient Position:
- Patient seated or standing with wrist and forearm resting on tabletop.
- Patient may also be supine on cart.

Part Position:

P.A.
- Pronate hand and forearm into prone position.
- Include joint nearest injury on film.

Lateral
- Position wrist and forearm into lateral position.
- Include joint nearest injury on film.

Central Ray:
- C.R. perpendicular to film holder.
- To center of film holder.
- 40 in. (102 cm.) F.F.D.

NOTE: • The position of wrist and forearm in the cast makes the P.A. projection relatively easy to position. The lateral position, however, may require angling of the tube to get a true lateral position.

Structures Best Shown:
Radius and ulna to check for alignment of fracture fragments.

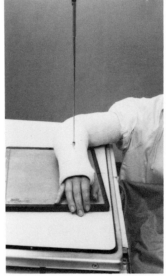
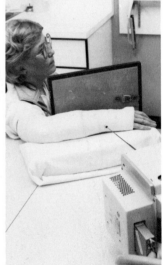

P.A.   Fig. 4-50

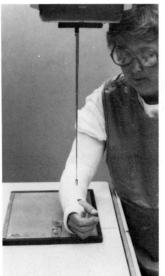
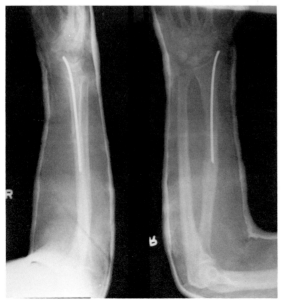

Lateral   Fig. 4-51

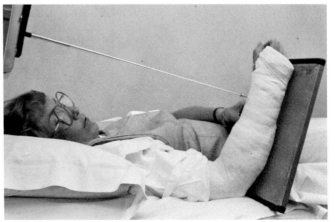

Fig. 4-53
Lateral   P.A.   Lateral   Fig. 4-52

CHAPTER 5

Radiographic Anatomy and Positioning of the
Forearm, Elbow and Humerus

Part I. Radiographic Anatomy
Forearm, Elbow and Humerus

Each upper extremity (upper limb) includes the shoulder girdle, upper arm, elbow, forearm, wrist and hand.

The single bone of the upper arm is the **humerus.** The humerus articulates with the **scapula** (shoulder blade) at the shoulder joint. Each shoulder girdle is composed of a scapula and a clavicle (collarbone). The bones of the shoulder girdle are described in detail in Chapter 6.

The two bones of the forearm are the **radius** on the lateral side (thumb side) and the **ulna** on the medial side. The radius, ulna and humerus comprise the elbow joint.

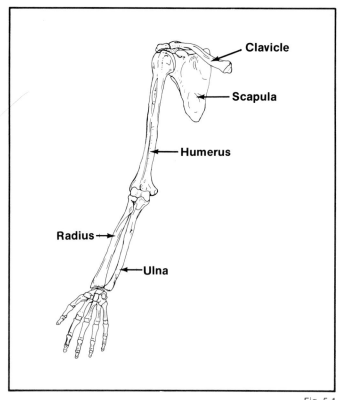

Upper Extremity

Fig. 5-1

Forearm — Radius and Ulna

Small conical projections termed **styloid processes** are located at the extreme distal end of both the radius and the ulna. The radial styloid process can be palpated on the thumb side of the wrist joint. The radial styloid process extends 2 cm. more distally than does the ulnar styloid process. The **ulnar notch** is a small depression on the medial aspect of the distal radius. The head of the ulna fits into the ulnar notch.

The **head of the ulna** is located near the wrist at the **distal** end of the ulna. When the hand is pronated, the ulnar head is easily felt and seen on the little finger side of the distal forearm. The **head of the radius** is located at the **proximal** end of the radius near the elbow joint. The long midportion of both the radius and the ulna is termed the **shaft.**

The radius is the shorter of the two bones of the forearm and is the only one of the two involved in the wrist joint. During the act of pronation, the radius is the bone that rotates around the more stationary ulna. The proximal radius demonstrates the round disclike head, and the **neck** of the radius, a tapered constricted area directly below the head. The rough oval process on the medial side of the radius, just distal to the neck, is the **radial tuberosity.**

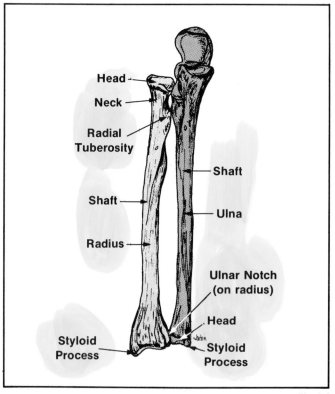

Radius and Ulna

Fig. 5-2

Ulna

The ulna is the longer of the two bones of the forearm and is primarily involved in the formation of the elbow joint. The two beaklike processes of the proximal ulna are termed the **olecranon** and **coronoid** processes. The olecranon process can be easily palpated on the posterior aspect of the elbow joint.

The large, concave depression or notch articulating with the distal humerus is the **semilunar notch.** The small, shallow depression located on the lateral aspect of the proximal ulna is the **radial notch.** The head of the radius articulates with the ulna at the radial notch. This joint or articulation is the proximal radioulnar joint that combines with the distal radioulnar joint to allow rotation of the forearm during pronation. During the act of pronation the radius crosses over the ulna near the upper third of the forearm.

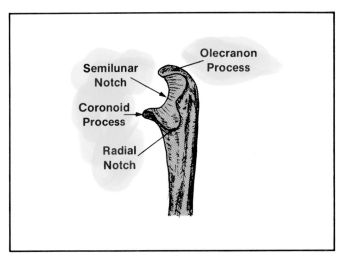

Proximal Ulna   Fig. 5-3

Radiographs of the Forearm

Anatomical parts of the radius and ulna are more difficult to identify on radiographs than on drawings. The radiograph of the forearm in *Fig. 5-4* demonstrates the following: **(A)** olecranon process of the ulna (as seen through the distal humerus), **(B)** coronoid process of the ulna, **(C)** shaft of the ulna, **(D)** head of the ulna, **(E)** styloid process of the ulna, **(F)** head of the radius, **(G)** neck of the radius, **(H)** radial tuberosity, **(I)** shaft of the radius, and **(J)** radial styloid process.

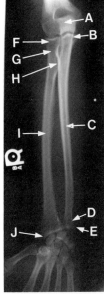

Radiograph Fig. 5-4
of Forearm

The lateral radiograph of the elbow and proximal forearm demonstrates: **(A)** olecranon process of the ulna, **(B)** semilunar notch of the ulna, **(C)** coronoid process of the ulna, **(D)** shaft of the radius, and **(E)** shaft of the ulna.

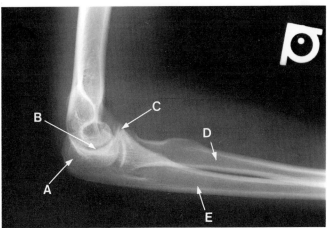

Lateral Radiograph of Elbow   Fig. 5-5

Arm — Humerus

The single bone of the upper arm is the humerus, articulating with the ulna at the elbow joint and with the scapula at the shoulder joint.

Distal Humerus

The distal humerus is shown in *Fig. 5-6.* The entire distal end of the humerus is the **humeral condyle.** The articular portion of the humeral condyle is divided into two parts. They are the **trochlea,** located on the medial side and articulating with the ulna, and the **capitellum,** located on the lateral side and articulating with the head of the radius. (A memory aid is to associate the capitellum, "cap," with the "head" of the radius.)

The small projection on the lateral edge of the distal humerus above the capitellum is the **lateral epicondyle** (prefix "epi" means upon). The **medial epicondyle** is larger and more prominent than the lateral and is located on the medial edge of the distal humerus proximal to the trochlea. The **shaft** of the humerus is the long center section.

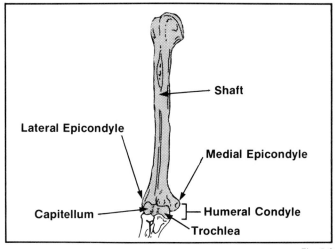

Humerus   Fig. 5-6

The drawing in *Fig. 5-7* shows two depressed areas of the distal humerus. The shallow anterior depression is the **coronoid fossa.** The coronoid process of the ulna fits into the coronoid fossa of the humerus when the arm is flexed.

The deep posterior depression is the **olecranon fossa.** The olecranon process of the ulna fits into this depression when the arm is fully extended.

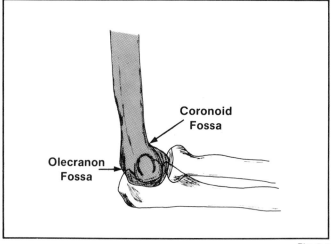

Lateral Humerus   Fig. 5-7

Radiograph of the Elbow

Anatomical parts of the distal humerus labeled on the A.P. radiograph of the elbow in *Fig. 5-8* are: **(A)** shaft of the humerus, **(B)** medial epicondyle, **(C)** trochlea, **(D)** capitellum ("cap" over head of radius), and **(E)** lateral epicondyle.

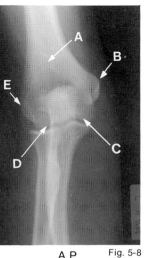

A.P.   Fig. 5-8
Radiograph
of Elbow

96

Proximal Humerus

The proximal humerus is that part of the upper arm that articulates with the scapula, making up the shoulder joint. The most proximal part is the rounded **head** of the humerus. The slightly constricted area directly below the head is the **anatomical neck.** The process directly below the anatomical neck on the anterior surface is the **lesser tuberosity,** and the larger lateral process is the **greater tuberosity.** The groove between these two tuberosities is the **bicipital groove.** The tapered area below the head and tuberosities is the **surgical neck,** and distal to the surgical neck is the long **shaft** of the humerus.

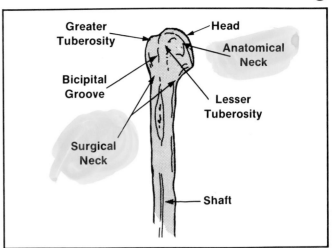

Humerus   Fig. 5-9

Radiograph of the Shoulder

Figure 5-10 is an A.P. radiograph of the shoulder with the anatomical parts of the proximal humerus labeled. Some of these parts are difficult to clearly visualize on radiographs, but a good understanding of locations and relationships between various anatomical parts aids in this identification.

Part **(A)** is the head of the humerus; **(B)** is the greater tuberosity; **(C)** is the bicipital groove; **(D)** is the lesser tuberosity; **(E)** is the anatomical neck (which has been enhanced); **(F)** is the surgical neck; and **(G)** is the shaft of the humerus.

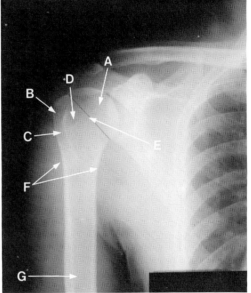

A.P. Radiograph   Fig. 5-10
of Shoulder

Classification of Joints

Radioulnar Joints

All joints of the forearm, elbow and humerus are classified as **diarthrodial** joints because they are freely movable. Both the proximal and distal radioulnar joints involve a rotational movement, indicating a **pivot** joint. During pronation, this rotational movement causes the radius to cross over the ulna at the upper third of the forearm. This is why a frontal position (A.P. projection) of the forearm must be obtained in the supinated or palm-up position.

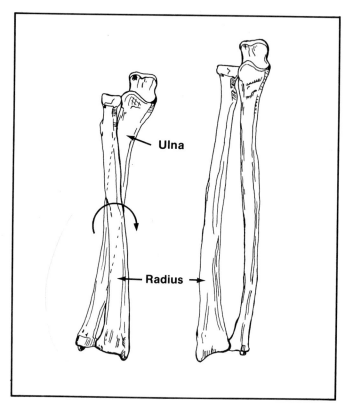

Forearm Rotational Movements   Fig. 5-11

Elbow Joint

The elbow joint is generally considered a **hinge type** joint with flexion and extension movements between the humerus, and the ulna and radius. The complete elbow joint, however, includes three joints enclosed in one capsule. In addition to the hinge joints between the humerus and ulna and the humerus and radius, the proximal radioulnar joint (pivot type) is also considered part of the elbow joint.

Shoulder Joint

The shoulder joint, described in more detail in Chapter 6, is a diarthrodial joint of the **ball and socket** type, allowing movement in all directions.

Summary of Forearm, Elbow and Humerus Joints

1. Proximal and Distal Radioulnar Joints
   - *Diarthrodial (pivot type)*

2. Elbow Joint
   - *Diarthrodial (hinge type)*
   (proximal radioulnar joint - pivot type)

3. Shoulder Joint
   - *Diarthrodial (ball and socket type)*

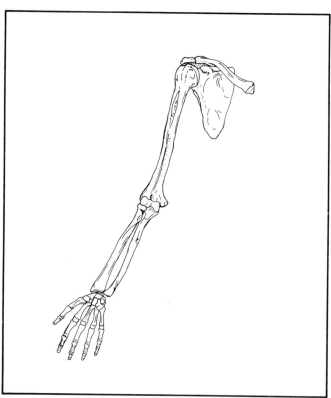

Forearm, Elbow and Humerus   Fig. 5-12

Part II. Radiographic Positioning
Forearm, Elbow and Humerus

Positioning Considerations

Radiography of the long bones of the humerus and forearm requires two projections or positions. At least one joint must be included and well-visualized on the finished radiograph. This joint should be the one nearest the patient's injury. If the injury is in the area of the distal forearm, then locate the film holder so at least 1½ to 2 inches (4 to 5 centimeters) of the film is below the wrist joint. If the injury is closer to the elbow joint, then include the elbow joint on the film.

Some department routines, however, require that both ends of the long bones in question be visible on the finished radiograph. For the forearm or humerus, this requires a sufficiently long film, such as a 7 x 17 in. (18 x 43 cm.) or 14 x 17 in. (35 x 43 cm.) divided in half.

Radiographs of extremities measuring less than 9 centimeters in thickness generally are taken using cardboard film holders or cassettes with detail screens for better definition. On average patients, this procedure includes the distal humerus, elbow and forearm, while the proximal humerus and the shoulder are taken on cassettes with average screens or cassettes with a grid. An exception to the use of cardboard film holders for extremities is when patients are uncooperative or can't hold still. Cassettes with screens can then be used to shorten exposure times and reduce the chance of motion.

Basic Projections/Positions

Certain basic and optional projections or positions for the forearm, elbow and humerus are demonstrated and described on the following pages. **Basic projections,** sometimes referred to as routine projections, are those commonly taken on average cooperative patients. It should be remembered, however, that basic or routine projections vary in different hospitals or departments.

Optional projections include those more common or more useful projections taken as extra or additional projections to better demonstrate specific anatomical parts. Examples of optional projections are the Coyle positions of the elbow — special angled projections for trauma patients to better demonstrate specific parts of the elbow — as demonstrated and described in this chapter. (Courtesy of George F. Coyle, R.T., as described and submitted to the publisher, 1980).

Correct Centering

Accurate centering of the body part to the film and correct central ray location are important to prevent distortion and/or "cutting off" of essential anatomical parts. This is even more critical when phototiming is used because inaccurate centering results in improper film density. To prevent these positioning errors a precise description of the central ray location in relationship to the body part is given, and an x indicating the correct centering point on the film is provided for each projection on the following pages.

Forearm	**Elbow**	**Humerus** (to include shoulder)	**Humerus**
Basic	Basic	Basic	Basic
• A.P.	• A.P.	(Trauma Routine)	(Nontrauma Routine)
• Lateral	• Oblique	• A.P.	• A.P.
	• Lateral	• Transthoracic Lateral	• Lateral
	Optional	(Nontrauma Routine)	
	• Coyle Trauma Positions	• A.P. with internal	
	1. For radial head	and external rotation	
	2. For coronoid process	Optional	
		• Transaxillary Lateral	

Forearm
Basic
• **A.P.**
• Lateral

Film Size:
- Include one joint routine.
    10 x 12 in. (24 x 30 cm.)
    Divide in half, lengthwise.

or

- Alternate routine; both joints.
    7 x 17 in. (18 x 43 cm.)

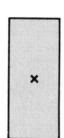

Non-Bucky:
- Detail screen or CBH.

Patient Position:
- Patient seated at end of table with hand and forearm extended, resting on tabletop.
- Support hand to prevent motion (place lead shield over patient's lap).

Part Position:
- Fully extend elbow and **supinate** hand.
- Have patient lean laterally, if necessary, to get proximal forearm and elbow in true frontal position.
- Include joint nearest injury site on film (for alternate routine, include both joints).

Central Ray:
- C.R. perpendicular to center of film holder.
- 40 in. (102 cm.) F.F.D.

NOTE: • Remember, for an A.P. projection of the forearm, **supinate** the hand (pronation will result in an oblique view of the forearm with the radius rotated over the ulna).

Structures Best Shown:
Radius and ulna, plus wrist and/or elbow joint.

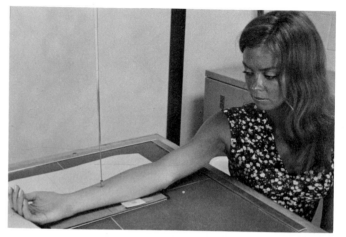

A.P. (one joint included)   Fig. 5-13

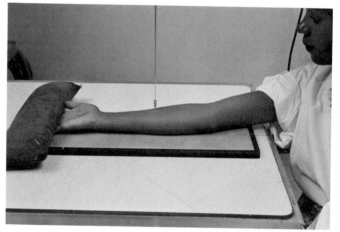

Alternate Routine (A.P., include both joints) Fig. 5-14

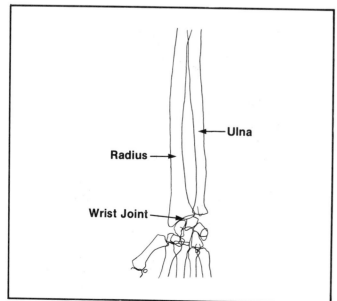

Fig. 5-16   A.P. (wrist joint)

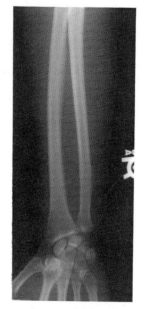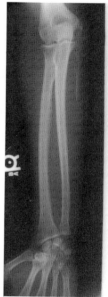

A.P. (wrist joint)   A.P. (both joints)
Fig. 5-15

| Forearm |
| Basic |
| • A.P. |
| • Lateral |

Forearm

• **Lateral Position**

Film Size:
- Include one joint only routine.
    10 x 12 in. (24 x 30 cm.)
    Divide in half, lengthwise.

    or

- Alternate routine; both joints.
    7 x 17 in. (18 x 43 cm.)

Non-Bucky:
- Detail screen or CBH.

Patient Position:
- Patient seated at end of table with elbow flexed 90°.
- Drop shoulder to rest humerus on tabletop (place lead shield over patient's lap).

Part Position:
- Flex elbow 90°.
- Forearm and humerus in same plane.
- Thumb must be up.
- Wrist and elbow in true lateral position.
- Support hand to prevent motion.
- Include joint nearest in**jury** site on film (for alternate routine, include **both** joints).

Central Ray:
- C.R. perpendicular to center of film holder.
- 40 in. (102 cm.) F.F.D.

NOTE: • Thumb must be up and elbow flexed 90°.

Structures Best Shown:
Superimposed radius and ulna, plus wrist and/or elbow joint.

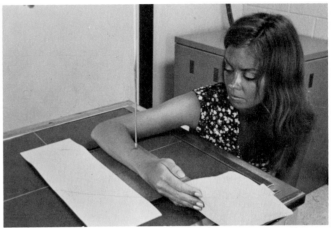

Lateral (one joint included)   Fig. 5-17

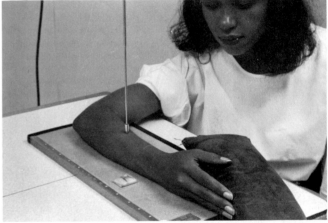

Alternate Routine   Fig. 5-18
(Lateral, both joints included)

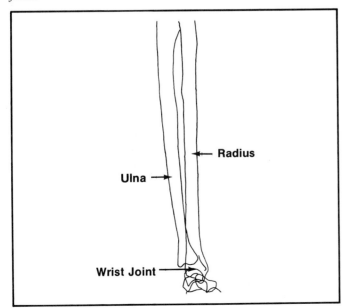

Fig. 5-20   Lateral (wrist joint)

Radius

Ulna

Wrist Joint

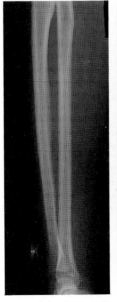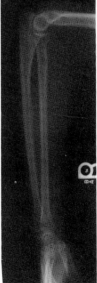

Lateral (wrist joint)   Lateral (both joints)
Fig. 5-19

Elbow

• Anteroposterior Projection

Elbow
Basic
• **A.P.**
• Oblique
• Lateral
Optional
• Coyle Trauma Positions
  1. For radial head
  2. For coronoid process

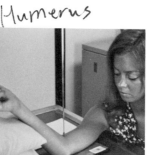

Film Size:
    10 x 12 in. (24 x 30 cm.)
    Divide in half, crosswise.

Non-Bucky:
- Detail screen or CBH.

Patient Position:
- Patient seated at end of table with elbow fully extended, if possible.
- Lower shoulder to same plane as tabletop (place lead shield over patient's lap).

Part Position:
Fully extended
- Extend elbow and **supinate** hand.
- Have patient lean laterally, as necessary, for true A.P. projection.
- Place support over hand to prevent motion.

Partially Flexed
- **Supinate** hand.
- **Two** A.P. projections required; one with **forearm parallel** to film holder, one with **humerus parallel** to film holder.
- Place support under forearm for projection with humerus parallel to film holder.
- Increase exposure 4 to 6 kVp.

Central Ray:
- C.R. to elbow joint, perpendicular to film.
- 40 in. (102 cm.) F.F.D.

NOTE: • If, due to injury, patient cannot extend elbow at least partially and the elbow is flexed to near 90°, angle the C.R. 10 to 15° into elbow joint to allow for visualization of the joint. • Do **not** angle C.R. if elbow is extended to more than 90° as shown in *Fig. 5-22* (angling of C.R. will cause distortion of bony structures).

Structures Best Shown:
Distal humerus, and proximal portions of radius and ulna.

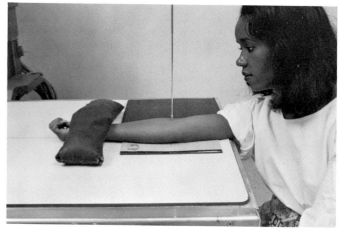

A.P. (fully extended)   Fig. 5-21

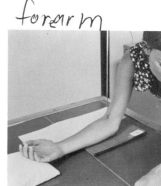

A.P. (partially flexed)   Fig. 5-22

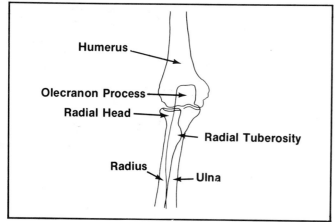

Fig. 5-24   A.P. (extended)

Humerus — Radius — Olecranon Process — Radial Head — Radial Tuberosity — Radius — Ulna

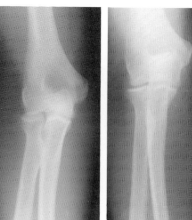

A.P. (extended)   A.P. (partially flexed)   Fig. 5-23

Elbow

• **Oblique Position**

Elbow
Basic
• A.P.
• **Oblique**
• Lateral
Optional
• Coyle Trauma Positions
 1. For radial head
 2. For coronoid process

Film Size:
 10 x 12 in. (24 x 30 cm.)
 Divide in half, crosswise.

Non-Bucky:
- Detail screen or CBH.

Patient Position:
- Patient seated at end of table with elbow extended.
- Pronate hand for internal oblique, and have patient lean laterally.
- Supinate hand for external oblique (place lead shield over patient's lap).

Part Position:
Internal oblique
- Pronate hand into natural palm-down position.
- Take care that distal humerus and anterior surface of elbow joint are **not** rotated more than 45°.
- Lower shoulder to same plane as tabletop.

External oblique
- Supinate hand.
- Laterally rotate entire arm so that anterior surface of elbow joint is 45° to film holder.
- Patient will need to lean over and drop shoulder onto tabletop.

Central Ray:
- C.R. to mid elbow joint, perpendicular to film holder.
- 40 in. (102 cm.) F.F.D.

NOTE: • Most department routines include the **internal** oblique **unless** the radial head and neck are a prime area of interest; then the **external** oblique should be taken.

Structures Best Shown:

Internal oblique	**External oblique**
- **Coronoid process** of ulna.	- **Radial head** and **neck** region.

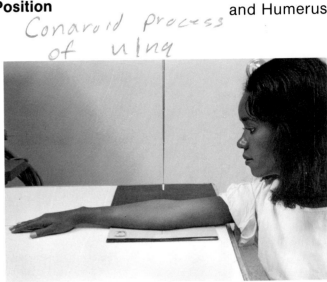

Oblique - Internal rotation   Fig. 5-25

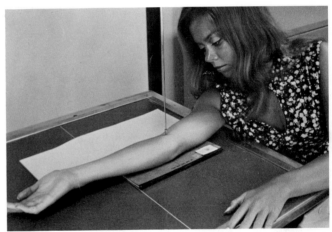

Oblique - External rotation   Fig. 5-26

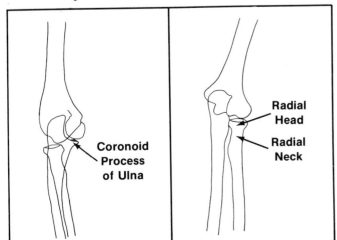

Fig. 5-28 Internal Oblique   External Oblique

**Coronoid
Process
of Ulna**

**Radial
Head**

**Radial
Neck**

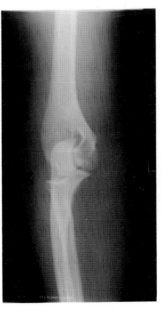
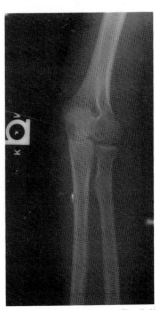

Internal Rotation   External Rotation Fig. 5-27

Elbow

• Lateral Position

Elbow
Basic
• A.P.
• Oblique
• **Lateral**
Optional
• Coyle Trauma Positions
  1. For radial head
  2. For coronoid process

Film Size:

8 x 10 in. (18 x 24 cm.)
Use full film, crosswise.

Non-Bucky:

- Detail screen or CBH.

Patient Position:

- Patient seated at end of table with elbow flexed 90°.
- Drop shoulder to rest humerus on tabletop (place lead shield over patient's lap).

Part Position:

- Flex elbow 90°, if possible.
- Forearm and humerus in same plane.
- Thumb must be up.
- Wrist and elbow in true lateral position.
- Support hand and wrist to prevent motion.

Central Ray:

- C.R. to mid elbow joint, perpendicular to film holder
- 40 in. (102 cm.) F.F.D.

NOTE: • Thumb must be up. • Elbow should be flexed 90°, if possible.

Structures Best Shown:

Lateral view of distal humerus and proximal forearm. Clearly visualizes olecranon process.

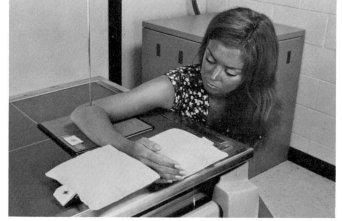

Lateral   Fig. 5-29

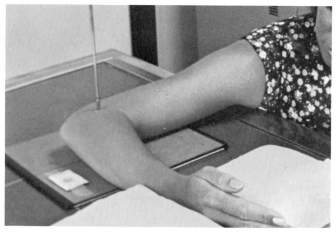

Lateral (close-up)   Fig. 5-30

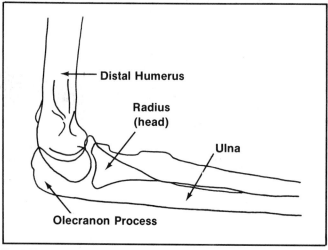

Distal Humerus

Radius (head)

Ulna

Olecranon Process

Fig. 5-32   Lateral

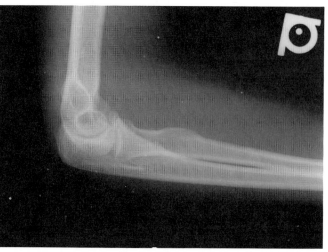

Lateral   Fig. 5-31

Elbow

- **Coyle Trauma Positions**
  1. For radial head
  2. For coronoid process

Film Size:
   8 x 10 in. (18 x 24 cm.)

Non-Bucky:
- Detail screen or CBH.

Patient Position:
- Supine.

Part Position:
1. Radial Head
   - Elbow flexed 90°.
   - Hand pronated.

2. Coronoid Process
   - Elbow flexed 80° from extended position (more than 80° will obscure coronoid process).
   - Hand pronated.

Central Ray:
1. Radial Head
   - Angle 45° toward shoulder, centered to radial head.

2. Coronoid Process
   - Angle 45° toward the brachial crease from the shoulder.

- 40 in. (102 cm.) F.F.D.

NOTE: • Increase basic technical factors because of angled C.R. • Effective with or without splint. • Support and immobilize elbow.

Structures Best Shown:
1. Radial head and capitellum.
2. Coronoid process and trochlea.

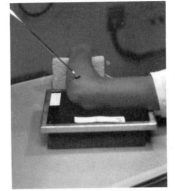
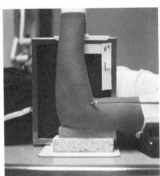

Angled for Radial Head   Fig. 5-33

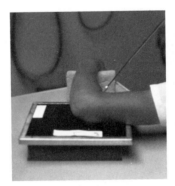
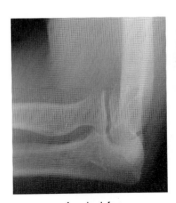

Angled for Coronoid Process   Fig. 5-34

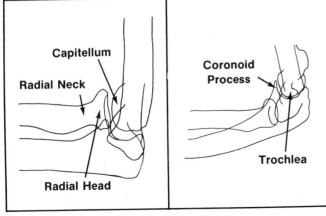

Fig. 5-36   Angled for Radial Head   Angled for Coronoid Process

Capitellum
Radial Neck
Radial Head
Coronoid Process
Trochlea

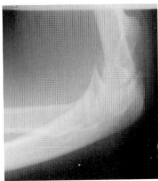

Angled for Radial Head   Angled for Coronoid Process   Fig. 5-35

Humerus

(Nontrauma Routine)
• Anteroposterior Projection
• Lateral Position

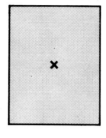 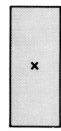

Humerus
Basic
(Nontrauma Routine)
• A.P.
• Lateral

Film Size:
Film lengthwise.
Two 14 x 17 in. (35 x 43 cm.)
   or
Two 7 x 17 in. (18 x 43 cm.)

Non-Bucky:
- Screen, detail screen or CBH.

Patient Position:
- May be taken erect or supine, depending on condition of patient. (If fracture is suspected, see **NOTE** below for alternate routine.)

Part Position:

A.P. (erect or supine)
- Rotate body toward affected side as needed to place humerus in contact with film holder.
- Supinate hand, unless patient is in severe pain.

Lateral (erect)
- Taken same as A.P. erect, except internally rotate arm so epicondyles of elbow are at right angles to film.

Lateral (supine)
- Abduct arm and partially flex elbow.
- Rotate humerus 90° medially from A.P. projection; superimpose epicondyles.
- It may be necessary to elevate film holder with support blocks to keep humerus in contact with film holder (Fig. 5-38).

Central Ray:
- C.R. perpendicular to film holder.
- C.R. to center of film holder or mid humerus.
- 40 in. (102 cm.) F.F.D.

NOTE: • Do **NOT** attempt these A.P. and lateral projections if patient is in severe pain or if a fracture is suspected. Instead, take A.P. and transthoracic lateral projections to include shoulder as shown on the following page.
• If injury is to distal third of humerus, take elbow routine.

Structures Best Shown:
Frontal and lateral views of entire humerus.

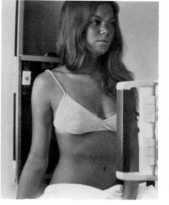 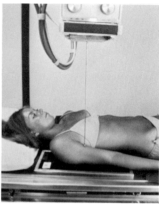
A.P. erect   A.P. supine   Fig. 5-37

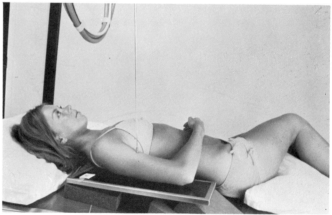
Lateral   Fig. 5-38

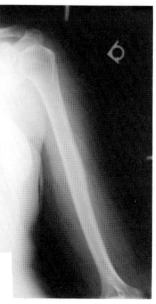 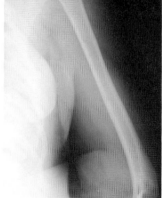
A.P.   Lateral   Fig. 5-39

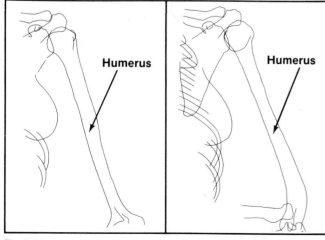
Fig. 5-40   A.P.   Lateral

<table>
</table>

Humerus

(Trauma Routine)
- **Anteroposterior Projection**
  - **Transthoracic Lateral**

Film Size:
Two 10 x 12 in. (24 x 30 cm.)
Film lengthwise.

Bucky:
- Moving or stationary grid.

Patient Position: (Trauma Routine)
- The erect position is generally more comfortable for patients with trauma and pain to the shoulder region.
- Patient seated or standing, as illustrated.
- Suspend respiration during exposure.
- For transthoracic lateral, a breathing technique with a long exposure may be used to blur out lung structures.

Part Position:
A.P.
- Position patient with back against film holder.
- Rotate patient slightly toward affected side to place proximal humerus in contact with film holder.
- Place hand at patient's side in neutral position (palm of hand against thigh).
C.R.
- C.R. to surgical neck (midfilm), perpendicular to film holder.
- 40 in. (102 cm.) F.F.D.
Lateral
- Seat or stand patient in lateral position with affected arm in neutral position against film holder.
- Raise opposite arm; rest hand on top of head.
C.R.
- Direct C.R. through thorax to surgical neck with **10 to 15° cephalic** angle to better visualize proximal humerus.
- 40 in. (102 cm.) F.F.D.

NOTE: • If patient is not in too much pain and can elevate uninjured arm and shoulder higher and drop injured shoulder, cephalic angle of C.R. is not required.

Structures Best Shown:
Frontal and lateral views of proximal two-thirds of humerus.

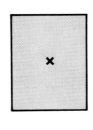

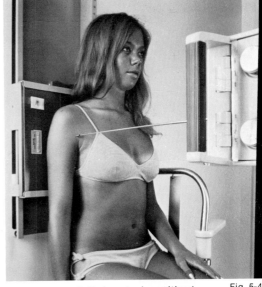

A.P. (neutral position)   Fig. 5-41

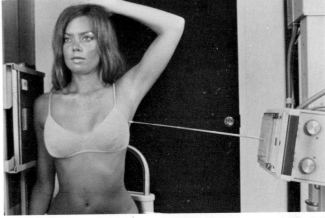

Lateral (Transthoracic)   Fig. 5-42

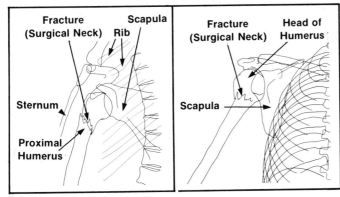

Fig. 5-44
Lateral (Transthoracic)   A.P. (neutral position)

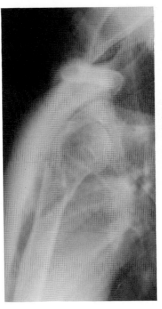
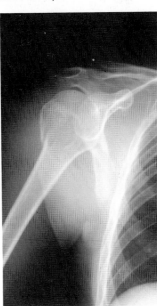

Lateral (Transthoracic)   A.P. (neutral position)   Fig. 5-43

Humerus

Humerus (to include shoulder)
Basic
(Trauma Routine)
• A.P.
• Transthoracic Lateral
(Nontrauma Routine)
• **A.P. with internal and
external rotation**
Optional
• Transaxillary Lateral

• **Anteroposterior Projection**
With Internal and External Rotation

**Warning: Never attempt rotation views
if fracture or dislocation is suspected.**

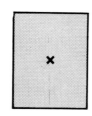

Film Size:
Two 10 x 12 in. (24 x 30 cm.)
Film lengthwise.

Bucky:
- Moving or stationary grid.

Patient Position: (Non-trauma Routine)
- Seat or stand patient with back of affected shoulder against film holder. (May be done supine if patient's condition necessitates.)
- Suspend respiration during exposure.

Part Position:
- Position patient with back firmly against film holder.
- Slightly rotate patient toward affected side to place proximal humerus and shoulder against film holder.
- Adjust height of film holder to about 2 in. (5 cm.) above shoulder.

Internal Rotation
- Rotate arm internally as far as possible, keeping proximal humerus against film holder.

External Rotation
- Rotate arm externally as far as possible. (Maximum internal and external rotation on most patients results in two views approximately 90° from each other.)

Central Ray:
- Directed perpendicular to center of film holder.
- 40 in. (102 cm.) F.F.D.

NOTE: • This positioning routine is primarily for the proximal humerus. If the area of interest is primarily in the shoulder, including the scapula and clavicle, see Chapter 6 for shoulder routines.

Structures Best Shown:
Two views of proximal humerus 90° from each other.
External rotation — Greater tuberosity is in profile.

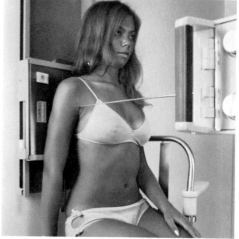

A.P. - Internal rotation   Fig. 5-45

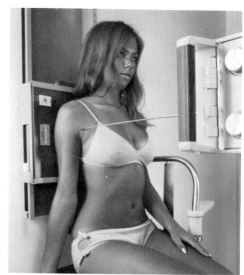

A.P. - External rotation   Fig. 5-46

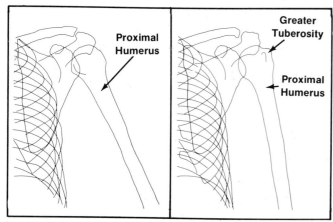

Fig. 5-48 Internal rotation   External rotation

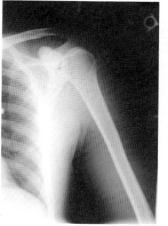

Internal rotation

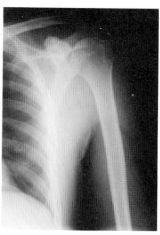

External rotation Fig. 5-47

Skip

Humerus

Humerus (to include shoulder)
Basic
(Trauma Routine)
- A.P.
- Transthoracic Lateral
(Nontrauma Routine)
- A.P. with internal and
  external rotation
Optional
- **Transaxillary Lateral**

- **Transaxillary Lateral**
(Inferosuperior Projection)
**Warning: Never attempt this projection if fracture
or dislocation of proximal humerus is suspected.**

Film Size:
  8 x 10 in. (18 x 24 cm.)
  Film crosswise.

Bucky:
- Stationary grid.

Patient Position:
- Supine with affected arm abducted.
- Suspend respiration during exposure.

Part Position:
- Abduct arm 90° from body; keep arm in external rotation (palm up).
- Place support under wrist and hand.
- Place nonopaque support under shoulder.
- Rotate head away from affected side.
- Rest film holder on table surface as close to neck as possible. Use sandbags or other support to hold film holder in place.

Central Ray:
- Direct C.R. horizontally to axilla.
- Position x-ray tube next to patient's body.
- 40 in. (102 cm.) F.F.D.

NOTE: • This is an excellent lateral projection of the neck and head region of the humerus, visualizing the shoulder joint well. • This may also be used as a post reduction lateral projection when the arm is placed in a cast or otherwise immobilized in this position.

Structures Best Shown:
Lateral view of head and neck of proximal humerus, and relationship to glenoid fossa of scapula. Also visualizes the coracoid process and, to some degree, the acromioclavicular articulation (superimposed by the humeral head).

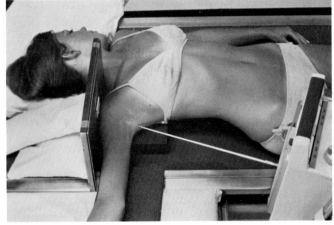

Transaxillary Lateral   Fig. 5-49

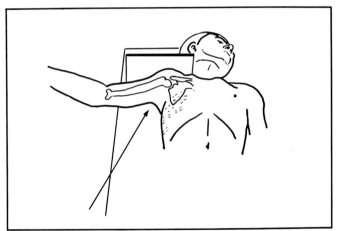

Transaxillary Lateral   Fig. 5-50

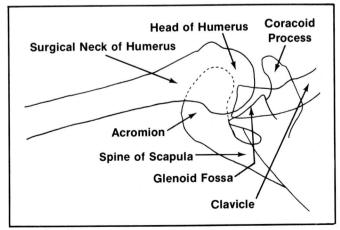

Head of Humerus
Coracoid Process
Surgical Neck of Humerus
Acromion
Spine of Scapula
Glenoid Fossa
Clavicle

Fig. 5-52   Transaxillary Lateral

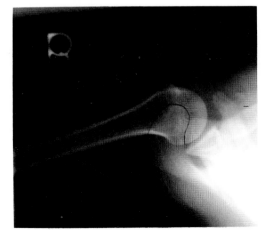

Transaxillary Lateral   Fig. 5-51

CHAPTER 6
Radiographic Anatomy and Positioning
of the
Shoulder Girdle

Part I. Radiographic Anatomy
Shoulder Girdle

The shoulder girdle consists of two bones, the **clavicle** and the **scapula.** The function of the clavicle and scapula is to connect each upper limb (extremity) to the trunk. Each shoulder girdle and upper limb connect at the shoulder joint between the scapula and the humerus. Each clavicle is located over the upper, anterior rib cage, and each scapula is situated over the upper, posterior rib cage. The upper margin of the scapula is at the level of the second posterior rib and the lower margin is at the level of the posterior seventh rib.

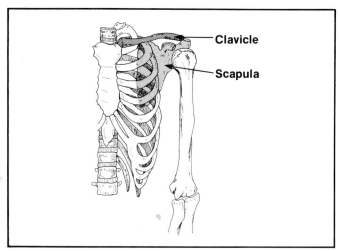

Shoulder Girdle

Fig. 6-1

Clavicle (collarbone)

The clavicle is a long bone with a double curvature having three main parts, the two ends and the long central portion. The **acromial end** (extremity) of the clavicle articulates with the acromion of the scapula. The **sternal end** (extremity) articulates with the upper part of the sternum. The **shaft** or **body** of the clavicle is the elongated portion between the two ends.

The acromial end of the clavicle is flattened and has a downward curvature at its attachment with the acromion. The sternal end is more triangular in shape and is also directed downward to articulate with the sternum.

In general, there is a difference in size and shape of the clavicle between male and female. The female clavicle is usually shorter and less curved than is the male clavicle. The clavicle in the male tends to be thicker and more curved in shape, usually being most curved in heavily muscled males.

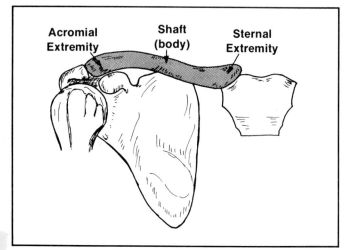

Clavicle

Fig. 6-2

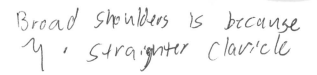

Broad shoulders is because
4 . straighter clavicle

Radiograph of the Clavicle

The A.P. radiograph of the clavicle in *Fig. 6-3* identifies the three parts of the clavicle. Part **A** is the **sternal end;** **B** is the **shaft or body;** and **C** is the **acromial end.** The acromial end is the most lateral portion of the clavicle. It is difficult to identify on radiographs because it has less tissue surrounding it and appears dark.

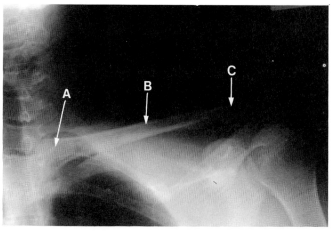

A.P. Radiograph of Clavicle

Fig. 6-3

112

Scapula (Shoulder Blade)

The scapula, which forms the posterior part of the shoulder girdle, is a flat triangular bone with three borders, three angles and two surfaces. The three borders include the **vertebral border**, which is the long edge or border near the vertebrae; the **superior border**, the uppermost margin of the scapula; and the **axillary border**, the border nearest the axilla. Axilla is the medical term for the armpit.

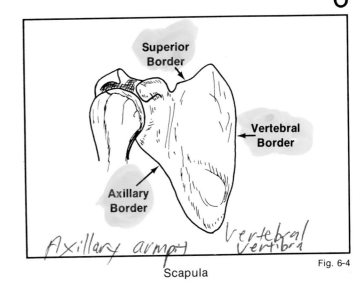

Scapula

Fig. 6-4

Scapula (anterior view)

The three corners of the triangularly shaped scapula are called angles. The **lateral angle,** sometimes called the head of the scapula, is the thickest part of the scapula and ends in a shallow depression called the **glenoid fossa.** The humerus articulates with the glenoid fossa of the scapula to form the shoulder joint.

The **superior** and **inferior angles** refer to the upper and lower ends of the vertebral border. The **body** of the scapula is arched for greater strength. The thin, flat, lower part of the body is sometimes referred to as the "wing" of the scapula, although this is not a correct anatomical term.

The **acromion** is a long, curved process extending laterally over the head of the humerus. The **coracoid process** is a thick, beaklike process projecting anteriorly beneath the clavicle. The **scapular notch** is a notch on the superior border partially formed by the base of the coracoid process.

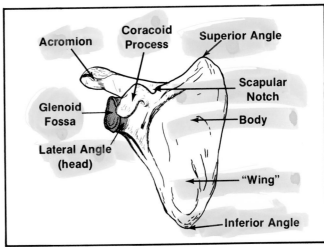

Scapula (anterior surface)

Fig. 6-5

Scapula (posterior view)

Figure 6-6 shows a prominent structure on the dorsal or posterior surface of the scapula, called the **spine.** The elevated spine of the scapula starts at the vertebral border as a smooth triangular area and continues laterally to end at the **acromion.** The acromion overhangs the shoulder joint posteriorly. The spine separates the posterior surface into an **infraspinatus fossa** and a **supraspinatus fossa.** Large muscles attach in these fossae.

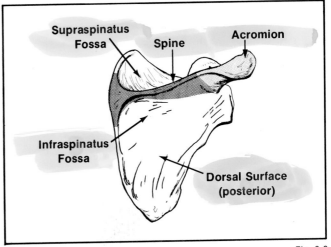

Scapula (posterior surface)

Fig. 6-6

The lateral view of the scapula, shown in *Fig. 6-7,* demonstrates relative positions of the various parts of the scapula. The thin scapula looks like the letter Y in this position. The **acromion** is the expanded distal end of the spine extending superiorly and posteriorly to the **glenoid fossa.** The **coracoid process** is located more anteriorly in relationship to the glenoid fossa or shoulder joint.

The posterior surface or back portion of the scapula is called the **dorsal surface.** The spine extends from the dorsal surface at its upper margin. The anterior surface is called the **ventral** or **costal surface.** Costal refers to ribs. The lower part of the thin body ends at the **inferior angle.**

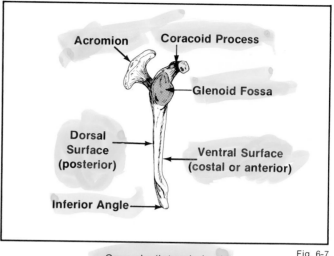

Scapula (lateral view)

Fig. 6-7

Radiographs of the Scapula

Figure 6-8 is an A.P. radiograph of the scapula with various anatomical parts labeled.

Part **A** is the **acromion; B** is the **coracoid process; C** is the **scapular notch; D** is the **superior angle; E** is the **vertebral border; F** is the **inferior angle; G** is the **axillary border;** and **H** is the **glenoid fossa.**

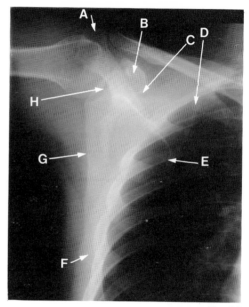

A.P. Radiograph of Scapula

Fig. 6-8

In a lateral radiograph of the scapula, as shown in *Fig. 6-9,* it is more difficult to recognize all the structures identified on previous drawings. Knowing the anatomical relationships of these parts makes identification easier.

A is the **acromion; B** is the **coracoid process; C** is the **inferior angle;** and **D** is the **spine** of the scapula.

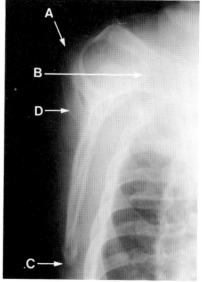

Fig. 6-9

Lateral Radiograph
of Scapula

Transaxillary Position

A transaxillary position of the shoulder is shown in *Fig. 6-10.* The transaxillary position results in a lateral view of the head and neck of the humerus. It also demonstrates the relationship of the humerus to the glenoid fossa. This position, as described in Chapter 5, is **NEVER** taken if a fracture or dislocation of the head of the humerus is suspected.

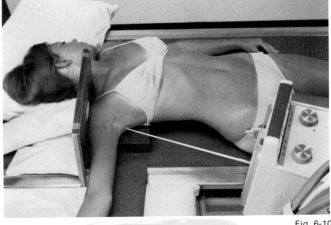

Transaxillary Position   Fig. 6-10

The anatomy shown on a radiograph of the scapula in the transaxillary position *(Fig. 6-11)* is rather confusing. Identification of the anatomy can only be accomplished by associating various prominent structures with other stuctures.

Part **A** is the **coracoid process,** which is located anterior to the shoulder joint and would, therefore, be uppermost on the radiograph since the anterior shoulder would be at the top in this position. Part **B** is the **glenoid fossa,** which articulates with the head of the humerus; **C** is the **spine** of the scapula; and **D** is the **acromion.**

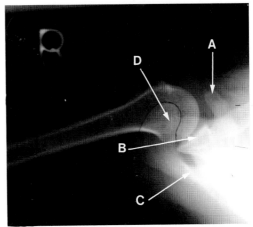

Fig. 6-11

Transaxillary Position

Classification of Shoulder Girdle Joints

The **shoulder joint** involves articulation between the head of the humerus and the glenoid fossa of the scapula. This joint was described in Chapter 5 as a diarthrodial joint of the ball and socket type, which allows movement in all directions.

The shoulder girdle also includes two joints involving both ends of the clavicle. These are the sternoclavicular and acromioclavicular joints. These joints are also classified as diarthrodial joints. The **sternoclavicular joint** is a gliding type joint involving the clavicle and sternum, as well as the first rib. This joint allows a limited amount of gliding motion in nearly every direction. The **acromioclavicular joint** allows both gliding and rotary movements, but is generally termed a gliding type joint.

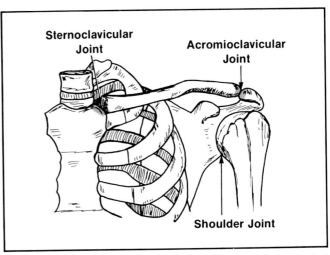

Joints of Shoulder Girdle   Fig. 6-12

Summary of Shoulder Girdle Joints

1. Shoulder Joint
   - *Diarthrodial (ball and socket type)*
2. Sternoclavicular Joint
   - *Diarthrodial (gliding type)*
3. Acromioclavicular Joint
   - *Diarthrodial (gliding type)*

Part II. Radiographic Positioning
Shoulder Girdle

Positioning Considerations

Chapter 5 presented a description and demonstration of the projections for the proximal humerus, including the shoulder joint. Chapter 6 includes projections of the shoulder joint, but these require different central ray locations and different film positions than those described for the proximal humerus. The shoulder girdle usually measures more than 9 centimeters and, therefore, requires the use of cassettes with screens, or preferably a moving or stationary grid, rather than cardboard film holders. If grids are used, they must be positioned with the length of the grid in the same direction as the tube angle to prevent grid cutoff.

Basic and Optional Projections/Positions

Certain basic and optional projections or positions for the shoulder girdle including the clavicle, the acromioclavicular joints (A.C. joints) and the scapula are demonstrated and described on the following pages. **Basic projections,** sometimes referred to as routine projections, are those commonly taken on average patients. Positioning of the shoulder girdle requires a routine for nontrauma patients — those patients not suspected of having suffered a fracture and/or a dislocation. A different routine must be used on trauma patients, in which case the humerus must not be moved or rotated unnecessarily. Forced movement or rotation would not only cause pain for the patient, but also might displace fractured parts in such a way that reduction or realignment would be very difficult or even impossible without surgery.

Certain **optional projections** are also described and demonstrated as extra or additional projections to better demonstrate specific body parts or certain pathological conditions. Examples of optional projections include a transaxillary lateral and an A.P. with body rotation to better demonstrate the glenoid fossa, head of the humerus and shoulder joint.

Correct Centering

Accurate centering of the body part to the film and correct central ray location are important to prevent distortion and/or "cutting off" of essential anatomical parts. This is even more critical when phototiming is used because inaccurate centering results in improper film density. To prevent these positioning errors a precise description of the central ray location in relationship to the body part is given, and an x indicating the correct centering point on the film is provided for each projection on the following pages.

Shoulder (Nontrauma Routine) Basic • A.P. Int. Rotation • A.P. Ext. Rotation Optional • Transaxillary Lateral • A.P. for glenoid fossa	**Shoulder** (Trauma Routine) Basic • A.P. Neutral • Transthoracic Lateral Optional • A.P. for glenoid fossa	**Clavicle** Basic • A.P. (cephalic angulation) or • P.A. (caudal angulation)

A.C. Joints Basic • A.P. without weights • A.P. with weights	**Scapula** Basic • A.P. • Lateral

Shoulder

(Nontrauma Routine)
Basic
- **A.P. Int. Rotation**
- A.P. Ext. Rotation

Optional
- Transaxillary Lateral
- A.P. for glenoid fossa

Shoulder (Nontrauma)

• **Anteroposterior Projection**

Internal Rotation

Warning: Do not rotate the humerus if fracture or dislocation is suspected.

Film Size:
> 10 x 12 in. (24 x 30 cm.) Crosswise.

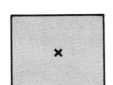

Bucky:
- Moving or stationary grid.

Patient Position:
- Supine or erect.
- Suspend respiration during exposure.

Part Position:
- Position shoulder against tabletop or film holder.
- Rotate patient toward side of interest, as necessary, to place shoulder in contact with tabletop or film holder.
- Top of film is 2 in. (5 cm.) above top of shoulder.
- Rotate arm internally (pronate hand) until epicondyles of distal humerus are **perpendicular** to film.

Central Ray:
- C.R. perpendicular to film holder, centered to coracoid process.
- 40 in. (102 cm.) F.F.D.

NOTE: • If symptoms indicate a possible fracture or dislocation of proximal humerus, do **NOT** take rotation positions, but use A.P. neutral rotation and transthoracic lateral.

Structures Best Shown:
Proximal humerus, scapula and relationship of humeral head to glenoid fossa. Also demonstrates possible calcium deposits in muscles, tendons or bursal structures of shoulder.

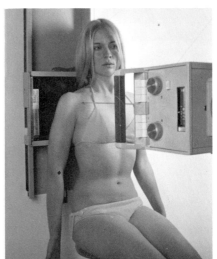

A.P. Shoulder, Internal Rotation   Fig. 6-13

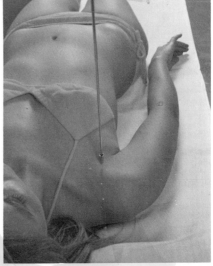

A.P. Shoulder, Internal Rotation   Fig. 6-14

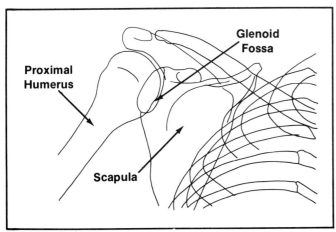

Fig. 6-16
A.P. Shoulder, Internal Rotation

Glenoid Fossa

Proximal Humerus

Scapula

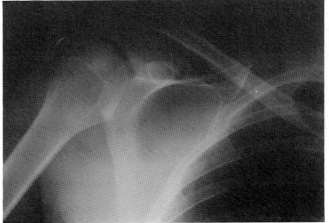

A.P. Shoulder, Internal Rotation   Fig. 6-15

117

Shoulder
(Nontrauma Routine)
Basic
- A.P. Int. Rotation
- **A.P. Ext. Rotation**
Optional
- Transaxillary Lateral
- A.P. for glenoid fossa

Shoulder (Nontrauma)

• Anteroposterior Projection
External Rotation
Warning: Do not rotate the humerus if
fracture or dislocation is suspected.

Film Size:
   10 x 12 in. (24 x 30 cm.)
   Crosswise.

Bucky:
- Moving or stationary grid.

Patient Position:
- Supine or erect.
- Suspend respiration during exposure.

Part Position:
- Position shoulder against tabletop or film holder.
- Rotate patient toward side of interest, as necessary, to place shoulder in contact with tabletop or film holder.
- Top of film is 2 in. (5 cm.) above top of shoulder.
- Rotate arm externally (supinate hand) until epicondyles of distal humerus are **parallel** to tabletop.

Central Ray:
- C.R. perpendicular to film holder, centered to coracoid process.
- 40 in. (102 cm.) F.F.D.

NOTE: • If symptoms indicate a possible fracture or dislocation of proximal humerus, do **NOT** take rotation positions, but use A.P. neutral rotation and transthoracic lateral.

Structures Best Shown:
Proximal humerus including greater tuberosity in profile, scapula and relationship of humeral head to glenoid fossa. Also demonstrates possible calcium deposits in muscles, tendons or bursal structures of shoulder.

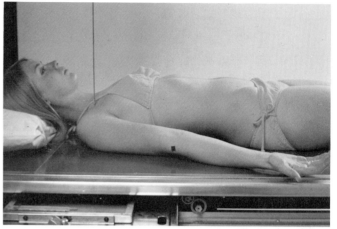

A.P. Shoulder, External Rotation   Fig. 6-17

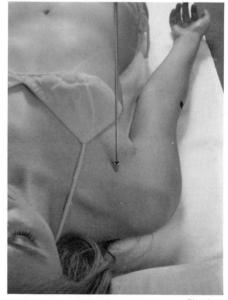

A.P. Shoulder,   Fig. 6-18
External Rotation

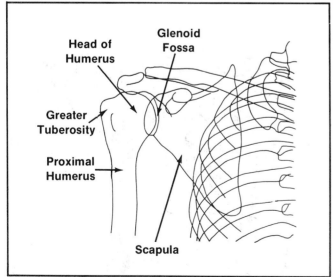

Fig. 6-20

A.P. Shoulder, External Rotation

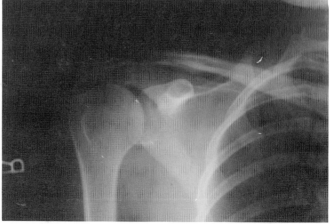

A.P. Shoulder, External Rotation   Fig. 6-19

Shoulder
(Nontrauma Routine)
Basic
- A.P. Int. Rotation
- A.P. Ext. Rotation
Optional
- **Transaxillary Lateral**
- A.P. for glenoid fossa

Shoulder (Nontrauma)

- **Transaxillary Lateral Position**
(Inferosuperior Projection)

Warning: Do not attempt this position if fracture
or dislocation of proximal humerus is suspected.

Film Size:

8 x 10 in. (18 x 24 cm.)
Crosswise.

Bucky:
- Stationary grid.

Patient Position:
- Supine.
- Abduct arm on side of interest.
- Suspend respiration during exposure.

Part Position:
- Abduct arm 90° from body; keep arm in external rotation (palm up).
- Place support under wrist and hand.
- Place nonopaque support under shoulder.
- Rotate head toward opposite side.
- Rest film holder on table as close to neck as possible. Use sandbags or other supports to hold film holder in place.

Central Ray:
- Direct C.R. horizontally to axilla.
- Position x-ray tube as close to patient's body as possible.
- 40 in. (102 cm.) F.F.D.

NOTE: • This is an excellent lateral of neck and head region of humerus for **nontrauma** patients. A.P. and transthoracic lateral should be used on trauma patients.

Structures Best Shown:
Lateral view of head and neck of proximal humerus, and relationship of proximal humerus to glenoid fossa. Also visualizes the coracoid process and the acromioclavicular articulation.

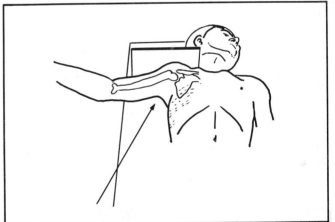

Transaxillary Lateral

Fig. 6-21

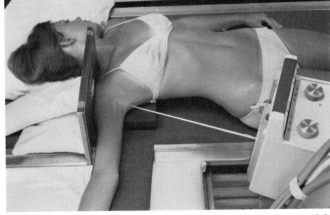

Transaxillary Lateral

Fig. 6-22

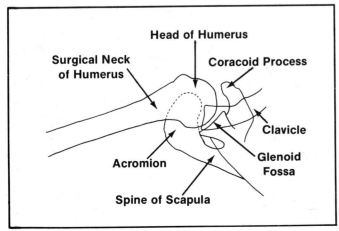

Fig. 6-24

Transaxillary Lateral

Head of Humerus
Surgical Neck of Humerus
Coracoid Process
Clavicle
Glenoid Fossa
Acromion
Spine of Scapula

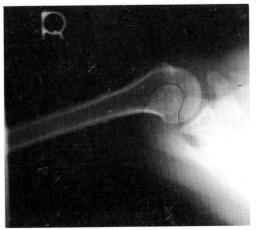

Transaxillary Lateral

Fig. 6-23

Shoulder

● Glenoid Fossa Position
(Glenohumeral Joint Space)

Shoulder
(Nontrauma Routine)
Basic
● A.P. Int. Rotation
● A.P. Ext. Rotation
Optional
● Transaxillary Lateral
● **A.P. for glenoid fossa**

Film Size:

8 x 10 in. (18 x 24 cm.)
Crosswise.

Bucky:

- Moving or stationary grid.

Patient Position:

- Erect or supine.
- Rotate body approximately 35°.

Part Position:

- Rotate approximately 35° toward side of interest, which places the scapula parallel to the film.
- Posterior aspect of arm and shoulder should be in contact with film holder or tabletop.
- If patient cannot stand or sit in erect position, this can be done tabletop with patient rolled up 35° toward side of interest.
- Place supports under elevated shoulder and hip.
- Abduct arm slightly.

Central Ray:

- C.R. perpendicular to film holder.
- Center to shoulder joint (glenohumeral joint space).
- 40 in. (102 cm.) F.F.D.

NOTE: ● The degrees of patient rotation may vary depending on how flat- or square-shouldered the patient is. Rounded shoulders require more rotation to place scapula parallel to film.

Structures Best Shown:

Glenoid fossa in profile and joint space between humeral head and glenoid fossa (shoulder joint).

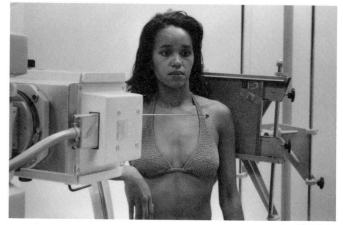

Glenoid Fossa Position

Fig. 6-25

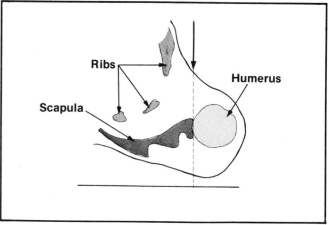

Glenoid Fossa Position

Fig. 6-26

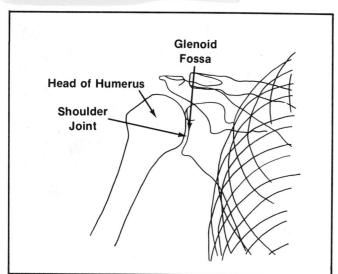

Fig. 6-28

Glenoid Fossa Position

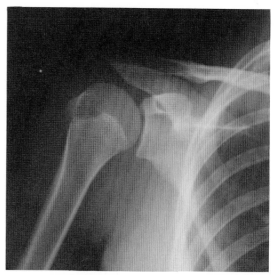

Glenoid Fossa Position

Fig. 6-27

Shoulder (Trauma Routine)

• Anteroposterior Projection

(Neutral Position, no rotation of arm)

Shoulder
(Trauma Routine)
Basic
• **A.P. Neutral**
• Transthoracic Lateral
Optional
• A.P. for glenoid fossa

Film Size:

   10 x 12 in. (24 x 30 cm.)
   Crosswise.

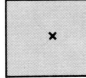

Bucky:

- Moving or stationary grid.

Patient Position:

- Supine or erect.
- Suspend respiration during exposure.

Part Position:

- Position shoulder against tabletop or film holder.
- Rotate patient toward side of interest, as necessary, to place shoulder in contact with tabletop or film holder.
- Top of film is 2 in. (5 cm.) above top of shoulder.
- Patient's arm is placed at side in neutral position, no rotation of arm.

Central Ray:

- C.R. perpendicular to film holder, centered to coracoid process.
- 40 in. (102 cm.) F.F.D.

NOTE: • Do not attempt to rotate arm; this routine is primarily for patients suspected of either dislocation or fracture of proximal humerus, or fracture to scapula in the area of the glenoid fossa.

Structures Best Shown:

Proximal humerus, scapula and relationship of humeral head to glenoid fossa.

A.P. Shoulder, Neutral Position, Erect

Fig. 6-29

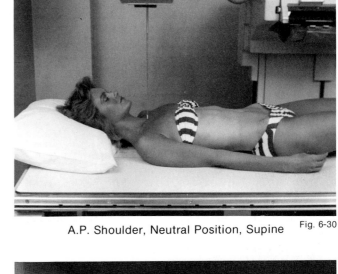

A.P. Shoulder, Neutral Position, Supine

Fig. 6-30

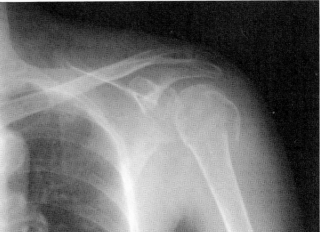

Coracoid Process

Scapula

Fracture
(Surgical Neck)

Proximal
Humerus

Fig. 6-32

A.P. Shoulder, Neutral Position
(Note fracture)

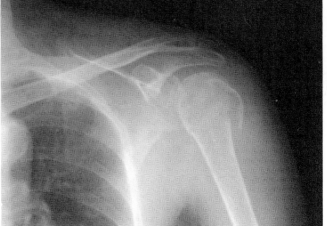

Fig. 6-31

A.P. Shoulder, Neutral Position
(Note fracture)

Shoulder (Trauma Routine)

• Transthoracic Lateral Position

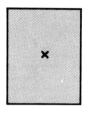

Film Size:

> 10 x 12 in. (24 x 30 cm.)
> Verticle or crosswise.

Bucky:

- Moving or stationary grid.

Patient Position:

- Erect or supine. The erect position may be more comfortable.

- Suspend respiration during exposure or use breathing technique with a long exposure to blur out lung structures and better visualize humerus.

Part Position:

Erect

- Seat or stand patient in lateral position with side of interest against film holder in neutral position.
- Raise opposite arm and place hand on top of head.
- Position top of film about 3 in. (7.5 cm.) above top of shoulder.

Supine

- Center humerus in question to midline of film holder.
- Raise opposite arm.

Central Ray:

- Center to surgical neck of humerus with a 10 to 15° cephalic angle of the tube.
- 40 in. (102 cm.) F.F.D.

NOTE: • Be sure that patient is in true lateral position so humerus is not superimposed by thoracic vertebrae or sternum.

Structures Best Shown:

Proximal humerus and relationship of glenohumeral joint.

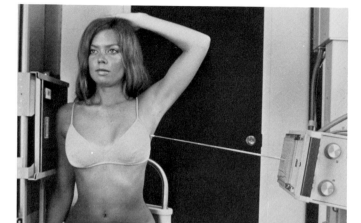

Erect Transthoracic Lateral   Fig. 6-33

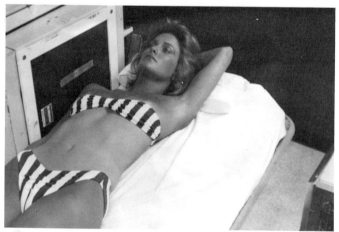

Supine Transthoracic Lateral   Fig. 6-34

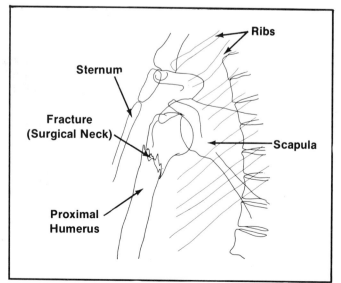

Fig. 6-36

Transthoracic Lateral

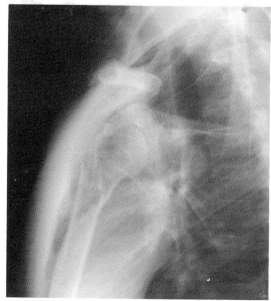

Transthoracic Lateral   Fig. 6-35

Clavicle
Basic
- **A.P.** (cephalic angulation)
  or
  P.A. (caudal angulation)

Clavicle

• Anteroposterior Projection
or
Posteroanterior Projection

Film Size:
10 x 12 in. (24 x 30 cm.) Crosswise.

Bucky:
- Moving or stationary grid.

Patient Position:
- Erect with arms at sides; supine (A.P.) or prone (P.A.).
- **Warning:** Do **NOT** attempt prone position in cases of obvious fracture or trauma to clavicle area.
- Suspend respiration during exposure.

Part Position:

A.P.
- Position patient with posterior shoulder in contact with film holder, without rotation of body.
- Angle 10 to 15° **cephalad.**
- Supine tabletop positioning similar to erect.

P.A.
- Position patient facing film without rotation of body.
- Turn head away from side of interest to allow anterior shoulder to be in contact with film holder.
- Center clavicle to film.
- Angle 10 to 15° **caudad**.
- Prone tabletop position similar to erect position.

Central Ray:
- C.R. to mid clavicle, 10 to 15° caudal (P.A.), 10 to 15° cephalic (A.P.).
- 40 in. (102 cm.) F.F.D.

NOTE: • Patient with thin shoulders, angle 15°. With thick shoulders, decrease angle to 5 or 10°. • The P.A. projection may be preferred for patients with kyphosis.

Structures Best Shown:
Clavicle and acromioclavicular joint.

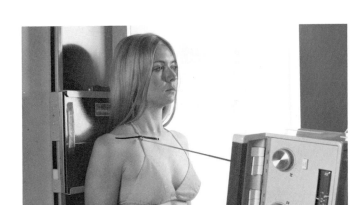

A.P. 10 to 15° cephalic   Fig. 6-37

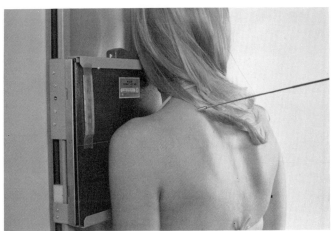

P.A. 10 to 15° caudal   Fig. 6-38

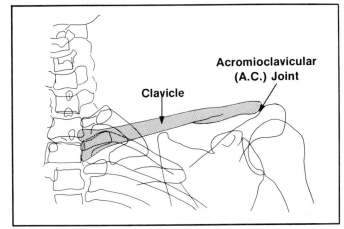

Fig. 6-40

Acromioclavicular (A.C.) Joint

Clavicle

A.P. Clavicle

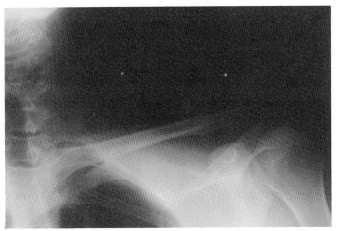

A.P. Clavicle   Fig. 6-39

A.C. Joints
Basic
• A.P. with weights
• A.P. without weights

A.C. Joints

• **Anteroposterior Projection**

(Bilateral — with and without weights)

Film Size:

> One 7 x 17 in. (18 x 43 cm.)
> Crosswise.
> **or**
> Two 8 x 10 in. (18 x 24 cm.)
> Crosswise.

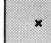

Non-Bucky:

- Screen.

Patient Position:

- Erect with equal weight on both feet, arms at sides, no rotation of trunk. Look straight ahead.
- Suspend respiration during exposure.

Part Position:

- Position posterior aspect of both shoulders against film holder.
- Position film holder vertically so center of film is approximately 2 in. (5 cm.) above top of shoulders (center A.C. joints to vertical midline of film).
- For average patient, use one 7 x 17 in. cassette, crosswise, to include both A.C. joints on same exposure.
- For broad-shouldered patient, use two 8 x 10 in. cassettes, crosswise.
- Two exposures are usually required, one with about 10 lbs. of weight in each hand and one with no weights.

Central Ray:

- Use a 72 in. (183 cm.) F.F.D. with C.R. perpendicular to center of film(s).

NOTE: • Weights will tend to pull shoulders down and demonstrate separation of a dislocated A.C. joint. • It is important that both A.C. joints be included on radiograph(s) in exactly the same position. • A.P. projections without weights are taken in same position as with weights.

Structures Best Shown:

Both A.C. joint spaces for comparison with and without stress.

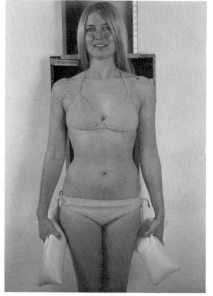

A.P. with Weights   Fig. 6-41
(one 7 x 17 in. - 18 x 43 cm.)

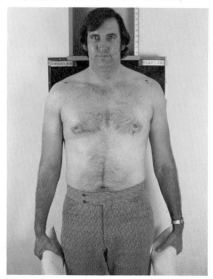

A.P. with Weights   Fig. 6-42
(two 8 x 10 in. - 18 x 24 cm.)

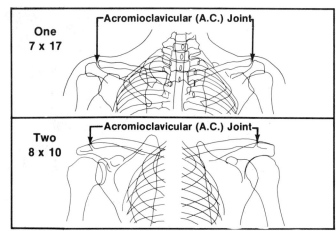

Fig. 6-44
A.P. Acromioclavicular Joints

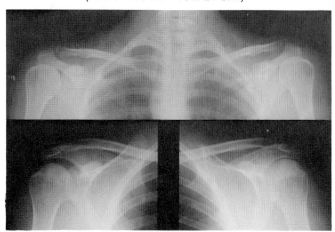

A.P. Acromioclavicular Joints   Fig. 6-43

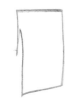

Scapula
Basic
- A.P.
- Lateral

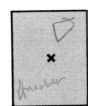

Scapula
- **Anteroposterior Projection**

Film Size:
10 x 12 in. (24 x 30 cm.)
Vertical.

Bucky:
- Moving or stationary grid.

Patient Position:
- Supine or erect position with posterior shoulder in direct contact with tabletop or film holder.

Part Position:
- Abduct arm on side of interest 90° and supinate hand.
- In erect position, support arm to lessen chance of motion during exposure.

Central Ray:
- Direct C.R. to mid scapula, 2 in. (5 cm.) below coracoid process and perpendicular to film holder.
- 40 in. (102 cm.) F.F.D.

NOTE: • Erect position may be more comfortable for patient. • Abduction of the arm tends to pull the scapula laterally to clear thoracic structures. • Generally, shoulder routines are taken before specific projections of the scapula.

Structures Best Shown:
Scapula with the lateral border free from rib superimposition.

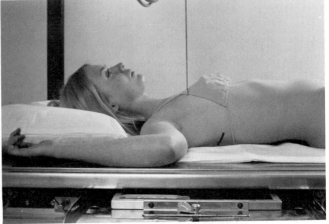

A.P. (supine) Fig. 6-45

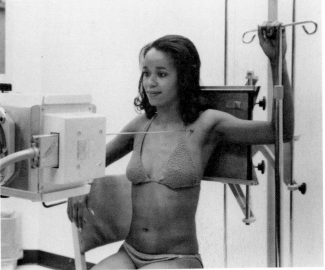

A.P. (erect) Fig. 6-46

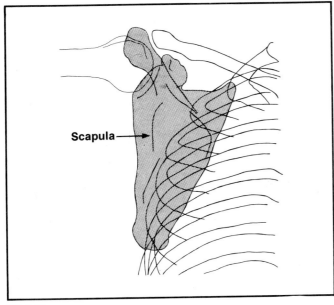

Fig. 6-48

A.P. Scapula

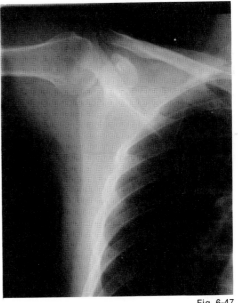

Fig. 6-47

A.P. Scapula

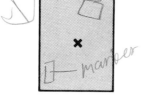

Scapula
Basic
• A.P.
• Lateral

Scapula
• Lateral Position

Film Size:
10 x 12 in. (24 x 30 cm.)

Bucky:
- Moving or stationary grid.

Patient Position:
- Erect, facing the film holder in an anterior oblique with arm on side of interest crossed in front of patient and hand resting on opposite shoulder.

Part Position:
- Palpate the borders of the scapula and rotate the patient until the scapula is in a true lateral position. (The flat posterior surface of the scapula should be perpendicular to the film.)
- The average patient will be rotated approximately 30° from the lateral position.
- Place top of film holder about 2 in. (5 cm.) above top of shoulder.

Central Ray:
- Direct C.R. to midvertebral border of scapula and perpendicular to film holder.
- 40 in. (102 cm.) F.F.D.

NOTE: • A posterior oblique (60°) can be done with the patient recumbent if the condition of the patient requires, but the erect position is usually less painful to the patient.

Structures Best Shown:
Lateral scapula projected free of rib cage. A fracture of the body of the scapula is best demonstrated on this lateral position.

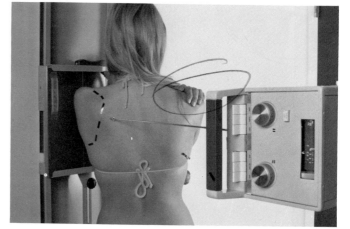

Lateral   Fig. 6-49

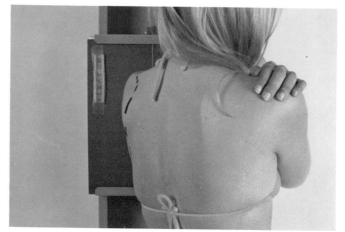

Lateral (view from tube)   Fig. 6-50

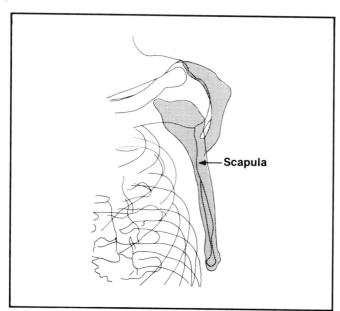

Fig. 6-52
Lateral Scapula

Scapula

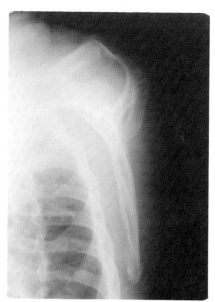

Lateral Scapula   Fig. 6-51

CHAPTER 7

Radiographic Anatomy and Positioning of the Foot and Ankle

Part I. Radiographic Anatomy
Foot and Ankle

Foot and Ankle

The 26 bones of one foot and ankle are divided into three groups:

Phalanges (Toes)	14
Metatarsals (Instep)	5
Tarsals	7
Total	26

The most distal bones of the foot are the **phalanges,** which make up the digits or toes. Each of the digits is made up of three bones with the exception of the first digit, which has only two. Each of the individual bones of the digits is termed a **phalanx.** Since the first toe has two phalanges, and digits two through five have three apiece, there are **14** phalanges in each foot.

The second group of bones are the **metatarsals,** consisting of **five** separate bones which make up the instep of the foot. The third group of bones, the **tarsals,** make up the proximal portion of the foot. The **seven** bones are sometimes referred to as the ankle bones although only one of the tarsals, the **talus,** is directly involved in the ankle joint. Thus fourteen phalanges, five metatarsals and seven tarsals make up the 26 bones of each foot.

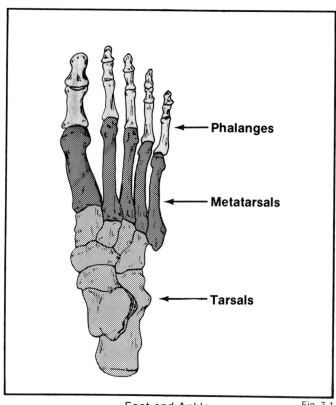

Foot and Ankle   Fig. 7-1

Phalanges - Toes (digits)

The five digits of each foot are numbered one through five starting on the medial or big toe side of the foot. Note that the large toe or first digit has only two phalanges. These are the **proximal phalanx** and the **distal phalanx.** Each of the second, third, fourth and fifth digits has a **middle phalanx** in addition to a proximal and a distal phalanx. When describing any of the bones of the foot, it is important to state which digit and which foot is involved. For instance the distal phalanx of the first digit of the right foot would leave no doubt as to which bone is in question. It should be noted that the distal phalanges of the second through fifth toes are very small and may be difficult to identify as separate bones on a good radiograph.

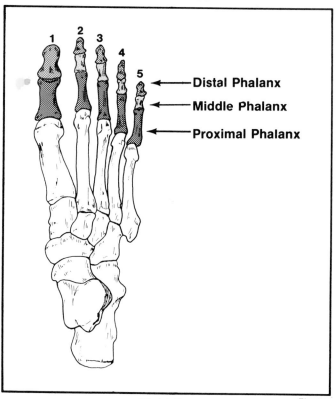

Right Foot   Fig. 7-2

Joints of Digits. The joints or articulations of the digits of the foot are important to identify since fractures may involve the joint surfaces. Each joint of the foot has a name derived from the two bones on either side of that joint. Between the proximal and distal phalanges is the **interphalangeal** or **I.P. joint.** Between the first metatarsal and the proximal phalanx is the **metatarsophalangeal** or **M.P. joint** of the first digit.

Since digits two through five each have one more bone, these digits have three joints each. Between the middle and distal phalanges is the **distal interphalangeal joint** or **D.I.P. joint.** Between the proximal and middle phalanges is the **proximal interphalangeal joint** or **P.I.P. joint.** The joint between each metatarsal and its respective proximal phalanx is the same for all five digits. This joint is the **metatarsophalangeal** or **M.P. joint.**

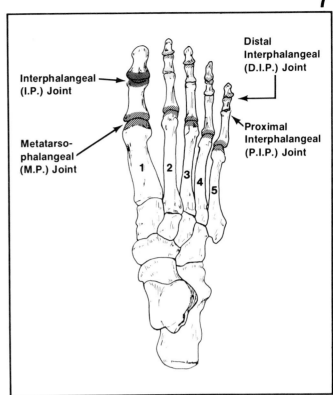

Right Foot

Fig. 7-3

Metatarsals

The five bones of the instep are the **metatarsal** bones. These are numbered as the digits are with number one on the medial side and number five on the lateral side. Each of the metatarsals is composed of three parts. The small, rounded, distal part of each metatarsal is the **head.** The centrally located, long, slender portion is termed the **shaft** or **diaphysis.** The expanded, proximal end of each metatarsal is the **base.**

Radiographs of the hands or feet should always be placed on an illuminator with the toes or fingers pointing up. Remembering this, the head of each metatarsal or metacarpal will always be up and the base will be toward the bottom of the radiograph.

Joints of metatarsals. Each of the joints at the head of each metatarsal is a **metatarsophalangeal** or **M.P. joint,** while each of the joints at the base of each metatarsal is a **tarsometatarsal joint** or **T.M. joint.** The base of the third metatarsal or the third tarsometatarsal joint is important, because this is the centering point for an A.P. foot.

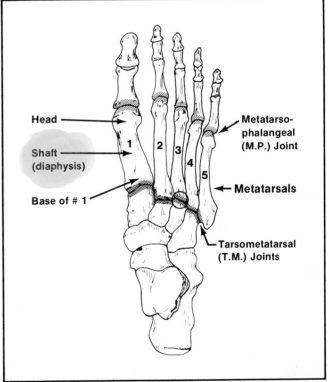

Metatarsals

Fig. 7-4

Sesamoid Bones

Several small detached bones, called **sesamoid** bones, are often found in the feet and hands. These extra bones are often present near various joints. The two sesamoid bones illustrated in *Fig. 7-5* are almost always present on the posterior or plantar surface of the first metatarsophalangeal joint. Sesamoid bones may also be found near other joints of the foot. Sesamoid bones are important radiographically, because it is possible to fracture these small bones. Due to their plantar location, they can be quite painful and cause discomfort. Special positioning is necessary to demonstrate a fracture of a sesamoid bone.

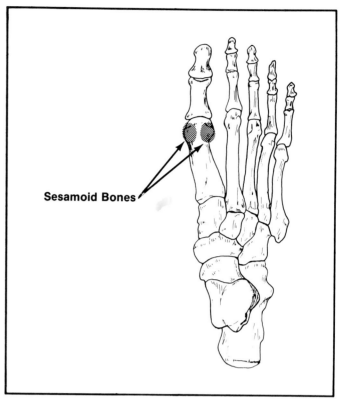

Sesamoid Bones

Fig. 7-5

Tarsals

The seven large bones of the proximal foot are termed tarsal bones. The names of the tarsals can be remembered with the aid of a mnemonic; **C**ome **T**o **C**olorado (the) **N**ext **3** Christmases.

(1) **C**ome	-	**C**alcaneus or Os Calcis
(2) **T**o	-	**T**alus or Astragalus
(3) Colorado	-	**C**uboid
(4) **N**ext	-	**N**avicular or Scaphoid
(5-6-7) **3** Christmases	-	**1st, 2nd** and **3rd C**uneiforms

Note that the calcaneus, talus, and navicular bones are also known by the alternative names; os calcis, astragalus, and scaphoid. Correct usage dictates that the tarsal bone of the foot should be called the navicular, while the carpal bone of the wrist, which has a similar shape, should be called the scaphoid. The carpal bone, unfortunately, is more often called the navicular than it is the scaphoid.

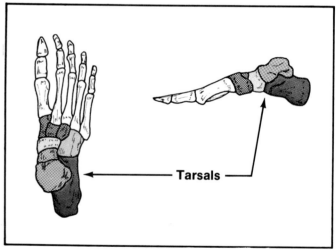

Tarsals

Fig. 7-6

The largest of the tarsal bones is the heelbone, properly termed the **calcaneus or os calcis.** The second largest tarsal bone is the **talus** or **astragalus.** The talus is located superior to the calcaneus and is the only tarsal bone involved in formation of the ankle joint.

Distal to the talus on the medial side of the foot is the **navicular** or **scaphoid.**

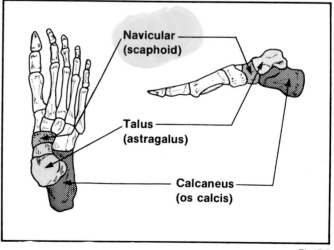

Navicular (scaphoid)

Talus (astragalus)

Calcaneus (os calcis)

Tarsals

Fig. 7-7

The remaining four tarsal bones are those which articulate with the five metatarsals. The **cuboid** is on the lateral side of the foot and articulates distally with the fourth and fifth metatarsals, and proximally with the calcaneus.

The three cuneiforms are identified starting on the medial side of the foot. The cuneiform articulating with the first metatarsal is termed the **first cuneiform** or **internal cuneiform.** The middle cuneiform is the **second** or **middle cuneiform** and articulates with the second metatarsal. The **third** or **external cuneiform** articulates with the third metatarsal. The proximal articulation of all three cuneiforms is with the navicular.

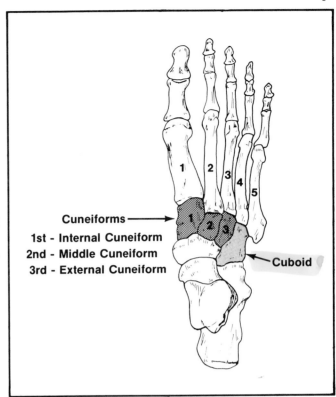

Tarsals

Fig. 7-8

Arches

The bones of the foot are arranged in **longitudinal** and **transverse arches,** providing a strong support for the weight of the body. The springy, longitudinal arch is composed of a medial and a lateral component, while the transverse arch is located mainly along the plantar surface of the tarsometatarsal joints.

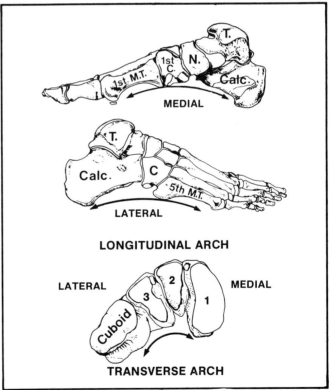

Arches

Fig. 7-9

Ankle Joint

Ankle Joint (frontal view)

The **ankle joint** is formed by three bones; the two long bones of the lower leg, the **tibia** and **fibula,** and one tarsal bone, the **talus.** The expanded distal end of the slender fibula is termed the **lateral malleolus.** The lower end of the larger, stronger tibia has a broad articular surface for the superior talus and also presents an elongation along the medial end termed the **medial malleolus.** The inferior portions of the tibia and fibula form a deep socket or mortise into which the upper talus fits.

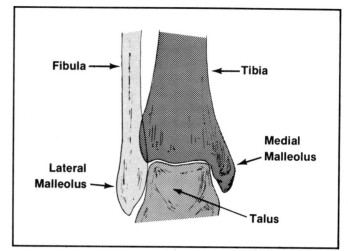

Ankle Joint   Fig. 7-10

Ankle Joint (lateral view)

An ankle joint in the lateral position is shown in *Fig. 7-11.* Note that the medial and lateral malleoli superimpose. The more slender lateral malleolus usually extends lower than its medial counterpart, however.

Posterior malleolus is a radiographic term describing the posterior articular margin of the tibia. Serious fractures of the ankle may involve all three malleoli and would be termed a trimalleolar fracture.

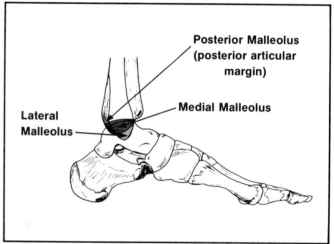

Ankle Joint   Fig. 7-11

Subtalar Joint

The important joint between the talus and the calcaneus is termed the **subtalar joint.** This is an irregular joint with three areas for articulation. Since any articular surface is termed a facet, we can say that the subtalar joint has three facets.

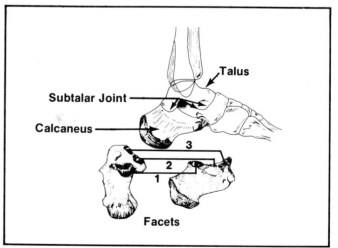

Subtalar Joint   Fig. 7-12

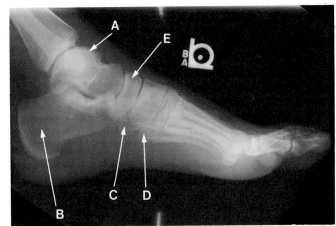

Radiographs of Foot and Ankle

Lateral Foot

Figure 7-13, a radiograph of a left foot in the lateral position, demonstrates five important anatomical features. Part **A** is the talus or astragalus; **B** is the calcaneus or os calcis; **C** is the cuboid; **D** is the base of the fifth metatarsal; and **E** is the navicular or scaphoid.

Oblique Foot

The oblique position of the foot shows more anatomy without superimposition than does the A.P. or lateral. Part **A** is the talus or astragalus; **B** is the navicular or scaphoid; **C** is the first metatarsal; **D** is the cuboid; and **E** is the calcaneus.

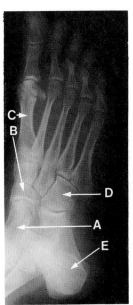

Oblique Fig. 7-14
Right Foot

Oblique Foot

The toes are well shown on a radiograph of the foot in the oblique position. Note the small size of the middle and distal phalanges of the second through fifth digits. They can be difficult to differentiate at times. Part **A** is the metatarsophalangeal (M.P.) joint of the first digit; **B** is the interphalangeal (I.P.) joint of the first digit; **C** is the middle phalanx of the second digit; **D** is the proximal phalanx of the fifth digit; and **E** is the base of the fifth metatarsal. Fractures of the base of the fifth metatarsal are fairly common. Note how the base of the fifth metatarsal sticks out, forming a palpable bony prominence.

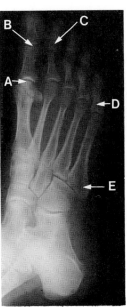

Oblique Fig. 7-15
Right Foot

A.P. Ankle

The ankle joint is well shown on this A.P. projection of the ankle *(Fig. 7-16)*. The labeled parts are: (**A**) distal fibula, (**B**) lateral malleolus, (**C**) talus, (**D**) medial malleolus, and (**E**) distal tibia.

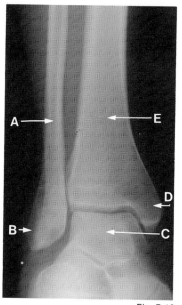

A.P. Right Ankle   Fig. 7-16

Classification of Joints

The joints of the foot and ankle are all freely movable joints classified as diarthrodial joints. The **ankle** and the **interphalangeal** joints have the most motion; but their motion is primarily limited to flexion and extension, movements associated with **hinge** joints, so that these are classified as **hinge** type joints.

The **intertarsal** joints, including the subtalar joint, have limited motion and are classified as **gliding** type joints along with the **tarsometatarsal** joints. The **metatarsophalangeal** joints are **condyloid** joints, as are the similar joints of the hands; however, the amount of toe motion is far less than comparable movement in the joints of the hand.

Summary of Foot and Ankle Joints

1. Ankle Joint
   - *Diarthrodial (hinge)*
2. Intertarsal Joints (including subtalar)
   - *Diarthrodial (gliding)*
3. Tarsometatarsal Joints
   - *Diarthrodial (gliding)*
4. Metatarsophalangeal Joints
   - *Diarthrodial (condyloid)*
5. Interphalangeal Joints
   - *Diarthrodial (hinge)*

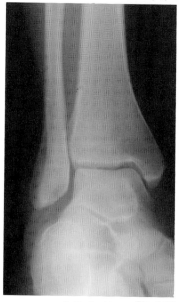

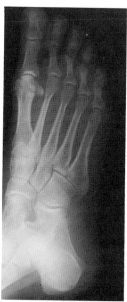

Oblique Foot   Fig. 7-17

A.P. Ankle   Fig. 7-18

Surfaces of the Foot

The surfaces of the foot are sometimes confusing in that the top or **anterior surface** of the foot is called **dorsum.** Dorsal is usually the posterior part of the body. Dorsum, in this case, comes from the term **dorsum pedis** which refers to the upper surface or the surface opposite the sole of the foot.

The sole of the foot is the **posterior** surface or **plantar surface.** Using these terms one can describe the common projections of the foot. The **anteroposterior** or **A.P. projection** is the same as a **dorsoplantar projection.** The less common **posteroanterior** or **P.A. projection** could be called a **plantodorsal projection.**

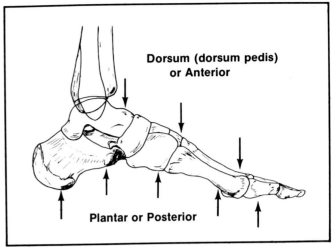

Surfaces of Foot   Fig. 7-19

Motions of Foot and Ankle

Other confusing terminology involving the ankle and intertarsal joints are: **dorsiflexion, plantarflexion, inversion,** and **eversion.** To decrease the angle (flex) between the dorsum pedis and the anterior part of the lower leg is to dorsiflex at the ankle joint. Extending the ankle joint or pointing the foot and toes downward with respect to the normal position is termed plantarflexion.

Inversion is an inward turning of the ankle and subtalar joints, while eversion is an outward turning. The lower leg does not rotate during inversion or eversion. Most sprained ankles result from an accidental and forced inversion or eversion.

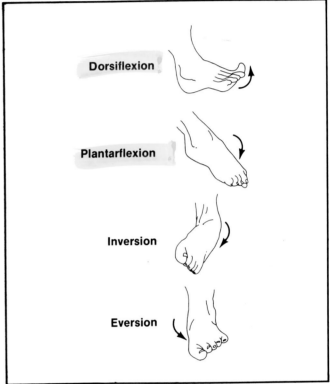

Motions of Foot and Ankle   Fig. 7-20

Part II. Radiographic Positioning
Foot and Ankle

Basic and Optional Projections/Positions

Certain basic projections or positions for the toes, foot and ankle are demonstrated and described on the following pages. **Basic projections,** sometimes referred to as routine projections, are those projections commonly taken on average, helpful patients. It should be noted that departmental routines on basic projections vary in different hospitals or departments.

Radiographic examination of the toes, foot or ankle involves joints, so that three positions or projections are required. Radiography specifically of the calcaneus requires only a lateral position and a plantodorsal projection, however. Two common routines exist for radiography of the toes. One routine calls for three positions or projections of the toe only, while the more common routine calls for an A.P. projection of the foot followed by an oblique and a lateral of the toe in question.

| Toe
Basic
• A.P.
  - Include foot
• Oblique
  - Toe only
• Lateral
  - Toe only | **or** | Toe
Basic
• A.P.
• Oblique
• Lateral | | Foot
Basic
• A.P.
• Oblique
• Lateral | | Calcaneus
Basic
• Plantodorsal
• Lateral | | Ankle
Basic
• A.P.
• Oblique
• Lateral |

<table>
<tr><td>

Toe
Basic
- **A.P.**
  - Toe only
  - Include foot
- Oblique
- Lateral

</td></tr>
</table>

Toe

- **Anteroposterior Projection**
Injured toe only

Film Size:
8 x 10 in. (18 x 24 cm.)
Divide into thirds.

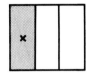

Non-Bucky:
- Detail screen or CBH.

Patient Position:
- Patient supine with knee flexed.

Part Position:
- Plantar surface of foot resting on film holder.
- Flex knee so that foot rests firmly and easily on film holder.

Central Ray:
- C.R. perpendicular to film holder.
- 1st toe — interphalangeal joint.
- 2nd - 5th toes — proximal interphalangeal joint.
- 40 in. (102 cm.) F.F.D.

NOTE: • One routine calls for an A.P. of only the toe of interest, while a second routine calls for an A.P. of the entire foot (next page).

Structures Best Shown:
Phalanges of digit in question to include distal metatarsal.

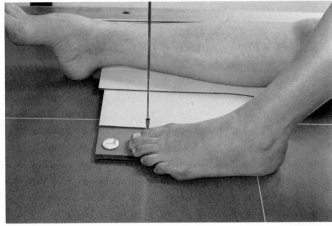

A. P. - 1st Toe   Fig. 7-21

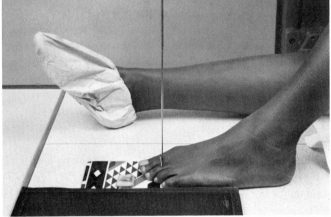

A. P. - 3rd Toe   Fig. 7-22

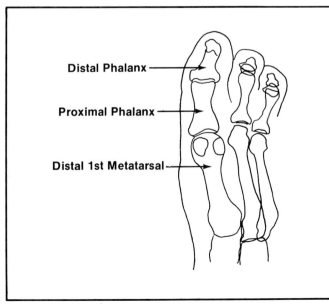

Fig. 7-24   A.P. - 1st Toe

Distal Phalanx
Proximal Phalanx
Distal 1st Metatarsal

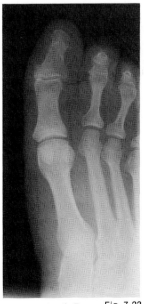

A.P. -   Fig. 7-23
1st Toe

Toe
Basic
• **A.P.**
- Toe only
- **Include foot**
• Oblique
• Lateral

• **Anteroposterior Projection**
Include foot

Film Size:

    10 x 12 in. (24 x 30 cm.)
    Divide in half, lengthwise.

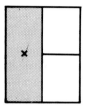

Non-Bucky:

- Detail screen or CBH.

Patient Position:

- Patient supine with knee flexed.

Part Position:

- Plantar surface (sole) of foot resting on film holder.
- Flex knee so that foot rests firmly and easily on film holder.

Central Ray:

- Center to base of 3rd metatarsal.
- Angle 10° toward the heel.
- 40 in. (102 cm.) F.F.D.

NOTE: • Use CBH or detail screen.

Structures Best Shown:

Phalanges, metatarsals, cuneiforms, cuboid and navicular.

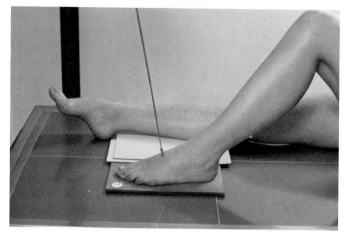

A.P. Foot   Fig. 7-25

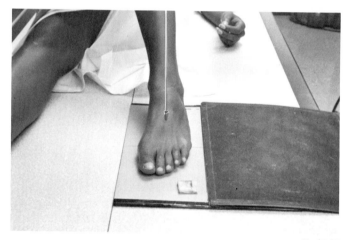

A.P. Foot   Fig. 7-26

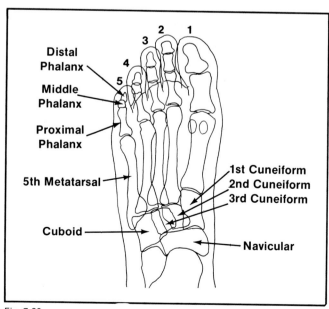

Fig. 7-28   A.P. Foot

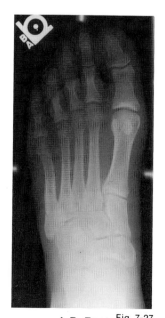

A.P. Foot   Fig. 7-27

Toe

- **Oblique Position**

Toe
Basic
- A.P.
  - Toe only
  - Include foot
- **Oblique**
- Lateral

Film Size:
Toes only routine.
   8 x 10 in. (18 x 24 cm.)
   Use middle third.

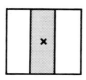

Include foot routine.
   10 x 12 in. (24 x 30 cm.)
   Use half of second half.

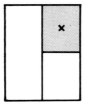

Non-Bucky:
- Detail screen or CBH.

Patient Position:
- Patient supine with knee flexed.

Part Position:
- 45° medial oblique for 1st, 2nd and 3rd digits.
- 45° lateral oblique for 4th and 5th digits.

Central Ray:
- C.R. perpendicular to film holder.
- 1st toe — interphalangeal joint.
- 2nd - 5th toes — P.I.P. joint.
- 40 in. (102 cm.) F.F.D.

NOTE: • Use 45° block to support foot and minimize motion. • Use CBH or detail screen.

Structures Best Shown:
Phalanges of digit in question, to include distal metatarsal.

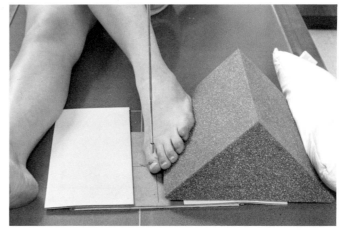
Oblique - 1st Toe   Fig. 7-29

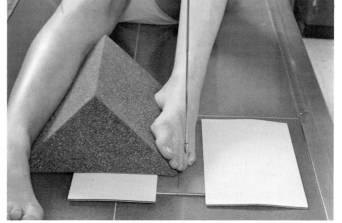
Oblique - 4th Toe   Fig. 7-30

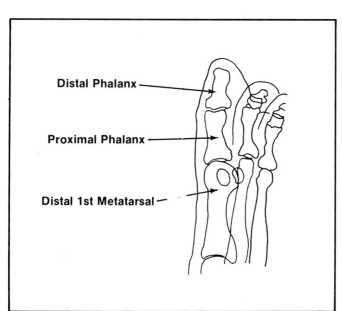

Distal Phalanx

Proximal Phalanx

Distal 1st Metatarsal

Fig. 7-32
Oblique - 1st Toe

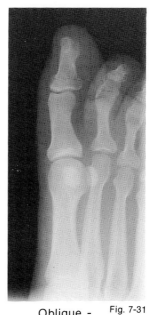
Oblique -   Fig. 7-31
1st Toe

Toe
Basic
- A.P.
  - Toe only
  - Include foot
- Oblique
- **Lateral**

- **Lateral Position**

Film Size:
Toes only routine
8 x 10 in. (18 x 24 cm.)
Use final third.

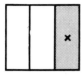

Include foot routine
10 x 12 in. (24 x 30 cm.)
Use remaining fourth.

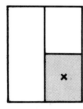

Non-Bucky:
- Detail screen or CBH.

Patient Position:
- Lateral recumbent.

Part Position:
- Rotate leg medially for 1st, 2nd and 3rd toes.
- Rotate leg laterally for 4th and 5th toes.

Central Ray:
- C.R. perpendicular to film holder.
- 1st toe — interphalangeal joint.
- 2nd - 5th toes — P.I.P. joint
- 40 in. (102 cm.) F.F.D.

NOTE: • Use tape, gauze, tongue blade or sandbags to control unaffected toes. • Sandbag cannot be in field of interest. • Occlusal film decreases part-film distance, but does not show all of proximal phalanx.

Structures Best Shown:
Phalanges of digit in question free of superimposition.

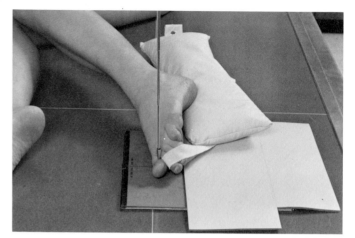

Lateral - 1st Toe   Fig. 7-33

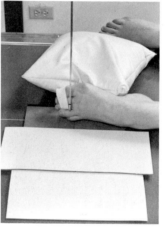
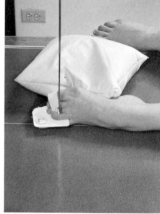

Lateral - 4th Toe

Fig. 7-34

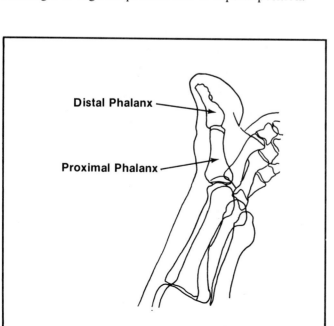

Distal Phalanx

Proximal Phalanx

Fig. 7-36

Lateral - 1st Toe

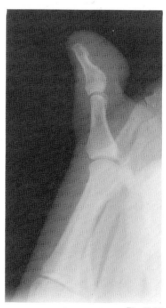

Lateral -   Fig. 7-35
1st Toe

<table>
<tr><td>

Foot
Basic
- **A.P.**
- Oblique
- Lateral

</td></tr>
</table>

Foot

• Anteroposterior Projection
Dorsoplantar Projection

Base of 3rd metatarsal (handwritten)

Film Size:
  10 x 12 in. (24 x 30 cm.)
  Divide in half lengthwise.

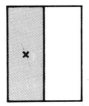

Non-Bucky:
- Detail screen or CBH.

Patient Position:
- Patient supine with knee flexed.

Part Position:
- Plantar surface (sole) of foot resting on film holder.
- Flex knee so that foot rests firmly and easily on holder.

Central Ray:
- Center to base of 3rd metatarsal.
- Angle 10° toward the heel. Angle may vary from 5 to 15° so that C.R. is perpendicular to metatarsals.
- 40 in. (102 cm.) F.F.D.

NOTE: • May need angle block under film holder so foot can rest on holder.

Structures Best Shown:
Phalanges, metatarsals, cuneiforms, cuboid and navicular.

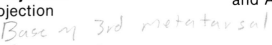

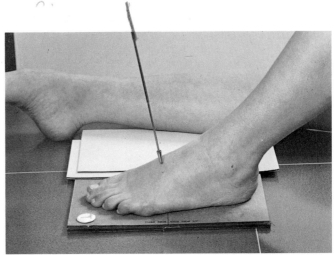

A.P. Foot   Fig. 7-37

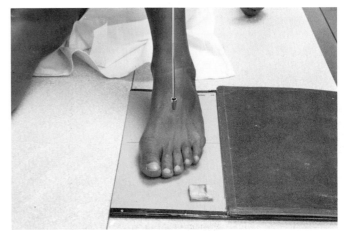

A.P. Foot   Fig. 7-38

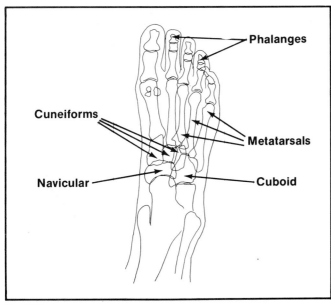

Fig. 7-40   A.P. Foot

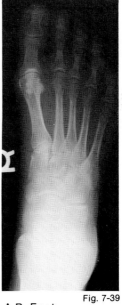

A.P. Foot   Fig. 7-39

Foot
Basic
• A.P.
• **Oblique**
• Lateral

Foot

• **Medial Oblique Position**

Straight down

45°

Film Size:

10 x 12 in. (24 x 30 cm.)
Divide in half, lengthwise.

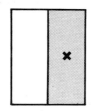

Non-Bucky:

- Detail screen or CBH.

Patient Position:

- Patient supine with knees flexed and body slightly turned away from side in question.

Part Position:

- Foot rotated medially 45°.

Central Ray:

- C.R. perpendicular to film holder, centered to base of 3rd metatarsal.
- 40 in. (102 cm.) F.F.D.

NOTE: • Use 45° block to support foot and minimize motion. • May need a pillow or other support between legs.

Structures Best Shown:

Phalanges, metatarsals, cuboid, 3rd cuneiform, navicular and distal calcaneus.

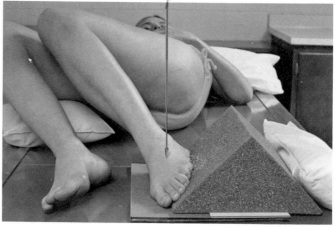

Medial Oblique Foot   Fig. 7-41

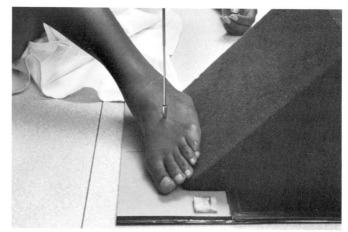

Medial Oblique Foot   Fig. 7-42

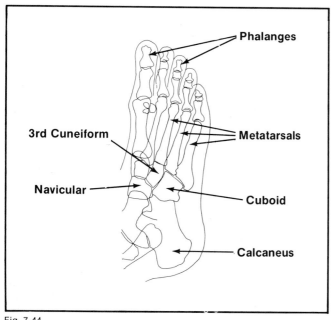

Phalanges

3rd Cuneiform

Metatarsals

Navicular

Cuboid

Calcaneus

Fig. 7-44

Medial Oblique Foot

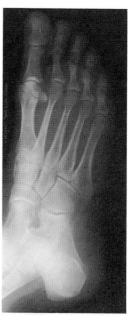

Medial   Fig. 7-43
Oblique Foot

Foot

Base of 3rd metatarsal *Straight down*

• **Lateral Position**
Mediolateral Projection

Foot
Basic
● A.P.
● Oblique
● **Lateral**

Film Size:
8 x 10 in. (18 x 24 cm.)

or

10 x 12 in. (24 x 30 cm.)
(for large foot)

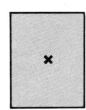

Non-Bucky:
- Detail screen or CBH.

Patient Position:
- Lateral recumbent.

Part Position:
- Turn toward affected side until leg and foot are in a true
  lateral position.
- Support must be placed under knee in order to maintain
  lateral position.

Central Ray:
- C.R. perpendicular to film holder, centered to base of 3rd
  metatarsal.
- 40 in. (102 cm.) F.F.D.

NOTE: ● Plantar surface of the foot must be perpendicular to film holder. ● Distal metatarsals as well as tibia and
fibula should superimpose on the radiograph.

Structures Best Shown:
Tarsals, ankle joint and subtalar joint. Metatarsals and
phalanges are superimposed.

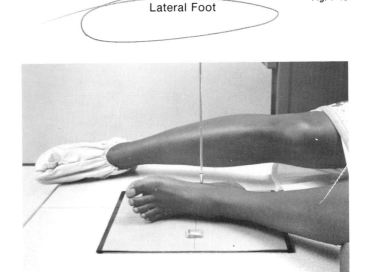

Fig. 7-45

Lateral Foot

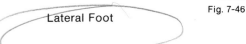

Fig. 7-46

Lateral Foot

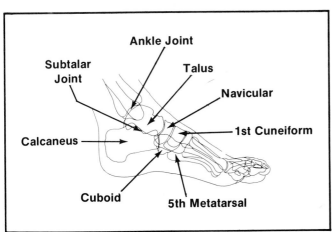

Ankle Joint

**Subtalar
Joint**

Talus

Navicular

1st Cuneiform

Calcaneus

Cuboid

5th Metatarsal

Fig. 7-48

Lateral Foot

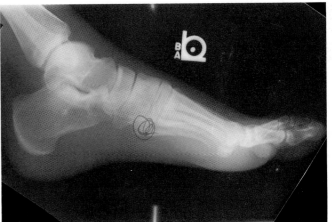

Lateral Foot

Fig. 7-47

Film Size:
 8 x 10 in. (18 x 24 cm.)
 Divide in half.

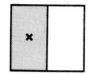

Non-Bucky:
- Detail screen or CBH.

Patient Position:
- Patient supine or seated with leg fully extended.

Part Position:
- Plantar surface must be perpendicular to film holder.
- Place heel near bottom of film so that calcaneus is projected to middle of film.
- Closely collimate.

Central Ray:
- C.R. forms a 40° angle with long axis of foot and enters at the base of the 3rd metatarsal.
- 40 in. (102 cm.) F.F.D.

NOTE: • May be necessary to loop tape or gauze around ball of foot and have the patient pull toward him. • Requires more exposure than other foot projections.

Structures Best Shown:
Calcaneus.

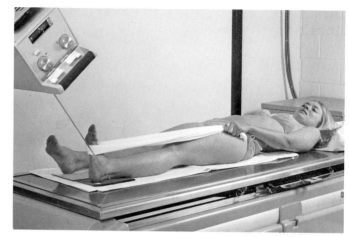

Plantodorsal Calcaneus   Fig. 7-49

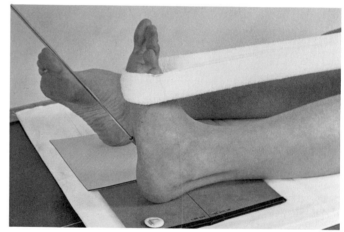

Plantodorsal Calcaneus   Fig. 7-50

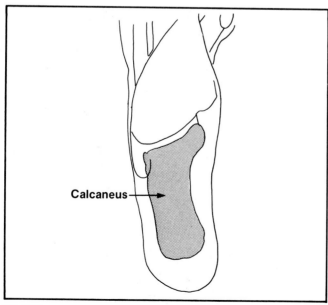

Fig. 7-52

Plantodorsal Calcaneus

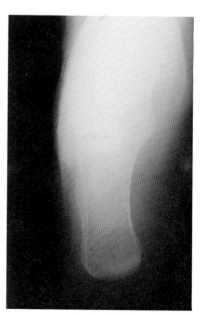

Plantodorsal   Fig. 7-51
Calcaneus

Film Size:
8 x 10 in. (18 x 24 cm.)
Divide in half.

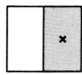

Non-Bucky:
- Detail screen or CBH.

Patient Position:
- Lateral recumbent.

Part Position:
- Turn toward affected side until leg and foot are in a true lateral position.
- Place support under knee.
- Closely collimate.

Central Ray:
- C.R. perpendicular to film holder, centered to mid calcaneus.
- 40 in. (102 cm.) F.F.D.

NOTE: • This position is similar to a lateral foot or ankle except for the centering point.

Structures Best Shown:
- Calcaneus, talus and subtalar joint.

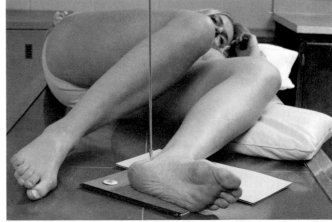

Lateral Calcaneus

Fig. 7-53

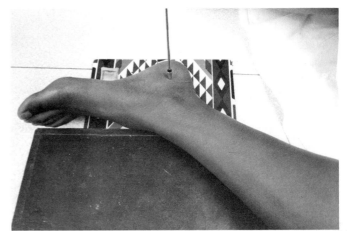

Lateral Calcaneus

Fig. 7-54

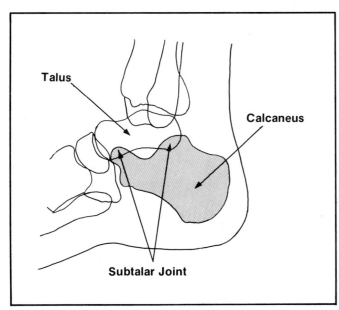

Fig. 7-56

Lateral Calcaneus

Labels: Talus, Calcaneus, Subtalar Joint

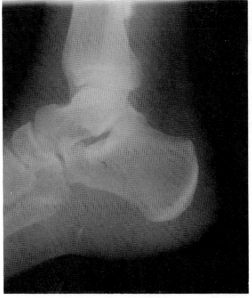

Lateral Calcaneus

Fig. 7-55

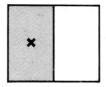

Ankle
Basic
- **A.P.**
- Oblique
- Lateral

Ankle

• **Anteroposterior Projection**

Film Size:
   10 x 12 in. (24 x 30 cm.)
   Divide in half.

Non-Bucky:
- Detail screen or CBH.

Patient Position:
- Supine.

Part Position:
- Plantar surface should be perpendicular to film holder.
- Place support under knee and against ball of foot.
- Internally rotate the leg 5 to 15° to place intermalleolar
  line parallel to film holder.

Central Ray:
- C.R. perpendicular to film holder, centered to mid ankle
  joint.
- 40 in. (102 cm.) F.F.D.

NOTE: • **Entire leg** must be **internally** rotated 5 to 15°
for a true A.P. of ankle.

Structures Best Shown:
Distal tibia and fibula, talus and ankle joint.

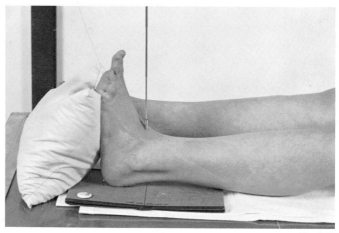

A.P. Ankle   Fig. 7-57

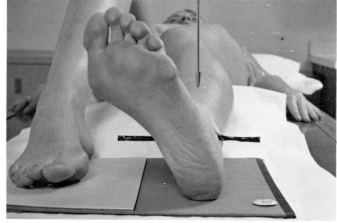

A.P. Ankle   Fig. 7-58

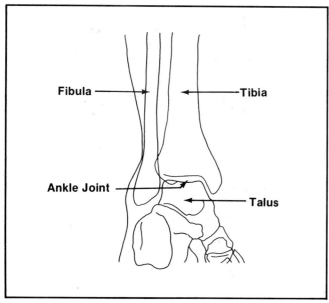

Fig. 7-60
            A.P. Ankle

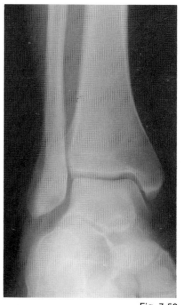

A.P. Ankle   Fig. 7-59

Ankle

• **Medial Oblique Position**

Film Size:
- 10 x 12 in. (24 x 30 cm.)
  Divide in half.

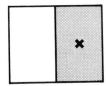

Non-Bucky:
- Detail screen or CBH.

Patient Position:
- Patient supine with body and leg rotated away from side of interest.

Part Position:
- Intermalleolar line forms an angle of 45° with film holder.
- Entire leg must be internally rotated.
- Closely collimate.

Central Ray:
- C.R. perpendicular to film holder, centered to mid ankle joint.
- 40 in. (102 cm.) F.F.D.

NOTE: • Support knee and foot.

Structures Best Shown:
Lateral malleolus, distal tibia, ankle joint and distal tibio-fibular joint.

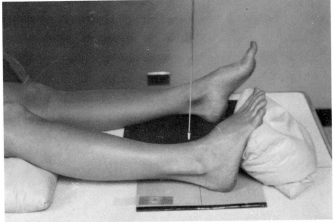

Medial Oblique Ankle   Fig. 7-61

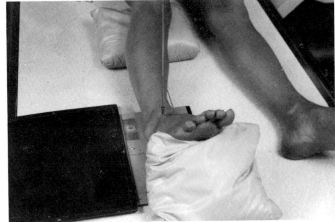

Medial Oblique Ankle   Fig. 7-62

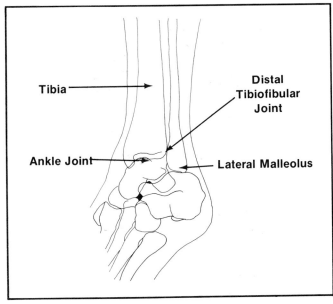

Fig. 7-64
Medial Oblique Ankle

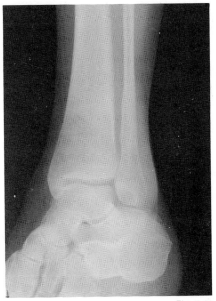

Medial
Oblique Ankle   Fig. 7-63

Ankle

- **Lateral Position**

Film Size:
8 x 10 in. (18 x 24 cm.)

Non-Bucky:
- Detail screen or CBH.

Patient Position:
- Lateral recumbent.

Part Position:
- Turn toward affected side until leg and foot are in a true lateral position.
- Place support under knee.
- Closely collimate.

Central Ray:
- C.R. perpendicular to film holder, centered to medial malleolus.
- 40 in. (102 cm.) F.F.D.

NOTE: • If both foot and ankle are to be radiographed, combine the two lateral views on one exposure. • Center midway between ankle joint and base of 3rd metatarsal.

Structures Best Shown:
Distal tibia and fibula, ankle joint, talus and calcaneus.

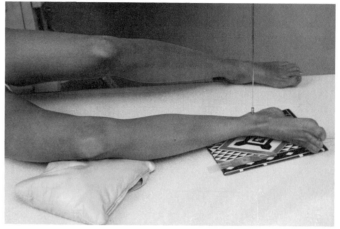

Lateral Ankle

Fig. 7-65

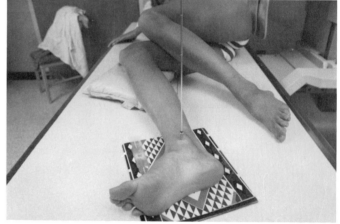

Lateral Ankle

Fig. 7-66

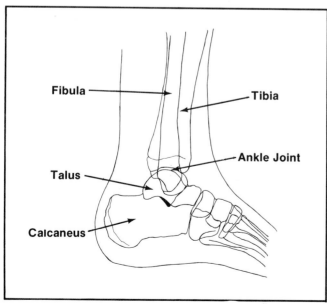

Fig. 7-68

Lateral Ankle

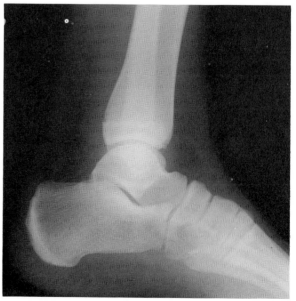

Lateral Ankle

Fig. 7-67

CHAPTER 8

Radiographic Anatomy and Positioning of the
Leg, Knee, Patella and Femur

Part I. Radiographic Anatomy
Leg, Knee, Patella and Femur

Leg

There are four bones found in each leg between the hip joint and the ankle joint. These bones are: (1) the **femur**, (2) the **tibia**, (3) the **fibula**, and (4) the **patella.** The strong femur is the single bone of the thigh, while the tibia and fibula are the two bones of the lower leg. The tibia, which is located medially, is the larger of the two bones of the lower leg. The smaller fibula is located laterally. The patella is a large sesamoid bone that protects the anterior part of the knee.

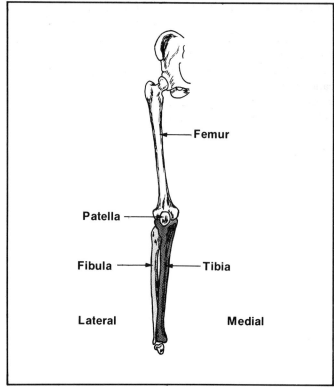

Right Leg   Fig. 8-1

Tibia

The entire proximal end of the tibia of the lower leg is termed the **head** of the tibia. The head of the tibia consists primarily of four parts: (1) **medial condyle,** (2) **lateral condyle,** (3) **tibial plateau,** and (4) **tibial spine.** The medial and lateral condyles are the two large processes making up the medial and lateral aspects of the proximal tibia. The tibial spine, also called the intercondyloid eminence, includes two small pointed prominences located on the superior surface of the tibial head between the two condyles. The upper articular surface of the condyles is referred to as the tibial plateau. The two surfaces of the tibial plateau articulate with the femur.

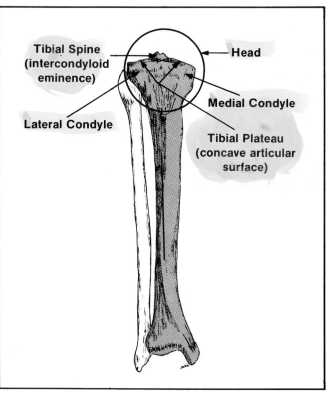

Tibia   Fig. 8-2

Tibia

The **tibial tuberosity** is a rough-textured prominence located on the midanterior surface of the tibia just distal to the condyles. This tuberosity is the distal attachment of the patellar tendon, which connects to the large muscle of the anterior thigh. Sometimes in young persons, the tibial tuberosity separates from the shaft of the tibia, a condition known as Osgood-Schlatter disease. The **shaft** or **diaphysis** is the long portion of the tibia between the head and the distal end. Along the anterior surface of the shaft, extending from the tibial tuberosity to the medial malleolus, is a sharp ridge called the **anterior crest** or **border**. This sharp anterior crest is just under the skin surface and is often referred to as the shin or shin bone. The **medial malleolus** is the prominence on the medial aspect of the distal tibia, which assists in formation of the ankle joint or mortise.

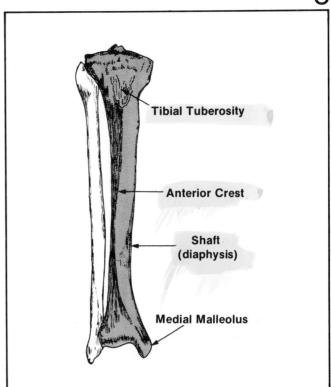

Tibia

Fig. 8-3

Fibula

The **fibula** or calf bone is a long slender bone located on the lateral aspect of the lower leg. The upper end of the fibula is expanded much like the tibia into a **head,** which articulates with the lateral aspect of the posteroinferior surface of the lateral condyle of the tibia. The extreme proximal aspect of the head is pointed and is known as the **styloid process** or **apex** of the head of the fibula. The tapered area just below the head is the **neck** of the fibula. The **shaft** or **diaphysis** is the long, slender portion of the fibula between the two ends. The enlarged distal end of the fibula can be felt as a distinct bump on the lateral aspect of the ankle joint, and is known as the **lateral malleolus.**

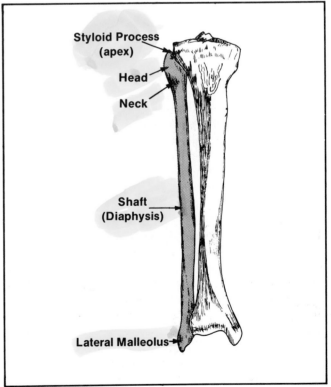

Fibula

Fig. 8-4

Femur

The **femur** or thigh bone is the longest and strongest bone in the entire body. The femur is the only long bone between the **hip joint** and the **knee joint.** Similar to all long bones, the **shaft** or **diaphysis** of the femur is the slender, elongated portion of the bone.

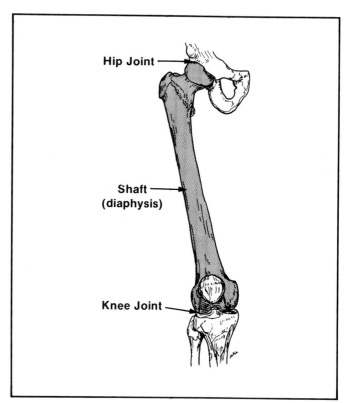

Femur (anterior)   Fig. 8-5

Proximal Femur

The prominent structures of the proximal femur are best seen from the posterior, as illustrated in *Fig. 8-6.* The **head** of the femur is the smooth, rounded portion that fits into the acetabulum of the hip bone to form the hip joint. The constricted segment distal to the head is the **neck** of the femur. Two processes, called trochanters, are located at the junction of the shaft and the neck of the femur. The more obvious process is the **greater trochanter,** located at the upper lateral aspect of the femur. The greater trochanter is so prominent that it can usually be palpated in the soft tissues of the lateral thigh. The **lesser trochanter** is a smaller process located posteriorly and medially on the femur. A ridge of bone known as the **intertrochanteric crest** or **ridge** extends between the two trochanters posteriorly. Common areas for fractures are the neck and intertrochanteric crest of the proximal femur, especially in elderly persons.

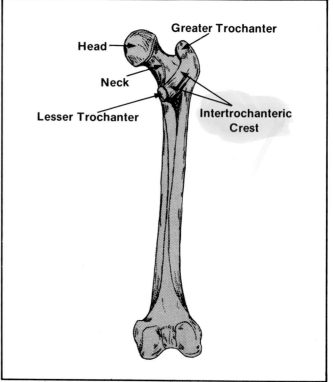

Femur (posterior)   Fig. 8-6

Distal Femur (posterior)

The distal femur consists of two prominent condyles separated by a deep depression or notch. The two articular condyles are the **medial** and **lateral condyles,** and the deep depression between the two is termed the **intercondylar fossa** or **notch.** The **medial** and **lateral epicondyles** are rough prominences located on the upper, outer extremes of the condyles. Muscles attach to these epicondyles. Note that the intercondylar fossa is located primarily on the posterior aspect of the femur.

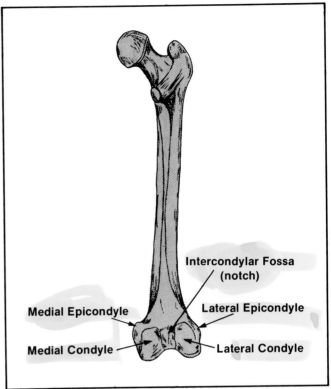

Femur (posterior)   Fig. 8-7

Distal Femur (lateral)

Figure 8-8 is a lateral view of the distal femur and knee joint, showing the usual location of the **patella.** The patella is classified as a **sesamoid bone** and, in fact, is the largest sesamoid bone found in the human body. The patella is located anterior to the distal femur. The smooth surface on the femur beneath the patella is termed the **patellar surface** of the femur. Note that the most inferior part of the patella is above the actual knee joint by approximately 1 centimeter.

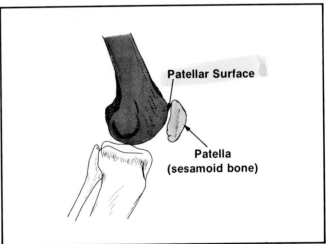

Distal Femur (lateral)   Fig. 8-8

Distal Femur (end view)

An end view of the distal femur is shown in *Fig. 8-9*. The **intercondylar fossa** or **notch** is a very deep notch on the posterior aspect of the femur. The **epicondyles** are rough prominences on the outer tips of the **condyles.** The **patella** fits smoothly along the **patellar surface** of the femur.

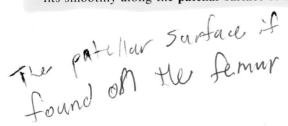
The patellar surface is found on the femur

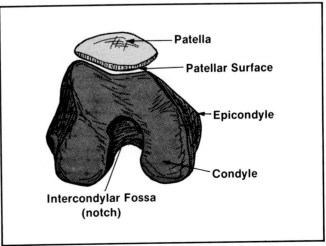

Distal Femur (end view)   Fig. 8-9

Patella

The **patella** is roughly triangular in shape with the pointed **apex** located along the inferior border. The **base** of the patella is the upper border. The patella serves to protect the anterior aspect of the knee joint and acts as a pivot to increase the leverage of the large upper anterior leg muscle. The patella is somewhat movable when the leg is extended, but it becomes locked into position when the leg is flexed.

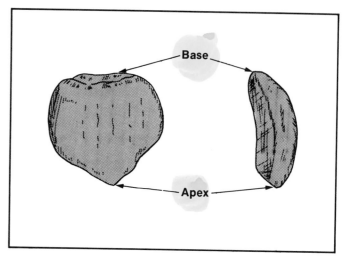

Patella   Fig. 8-10

Knee Joint

The knee joint is a hinge joint that is enclosed in an articular capsule. Numerous ligaments, which stretch from one bone to another bone, bind the tibia and femur together. Four very strong **ligaments** help to stabilize the knee joint. Two cartilaginous pads, the **medial and lateral menisci,** are located on the tibial plateau at the proximal end of the tibia and function as shock absorbers for the knee. Trauma to the knee joint may damage ligaments or cartilage (meniscus) requiring further medical treatment. The area directly posterior to the knee joint is termed the **popliteal** region. Note that the knee joint involves only the tibia and the femur; the patella and the fibula are not involved.

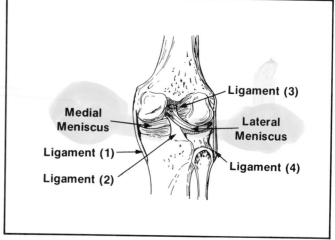

Knee Joint (popliteal surface)   Fig. 8-11

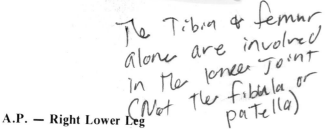

The Tibia & femur alone are involved in the knee Joint (Not the fibula or patella)

A.P. — Right Lower Leg

The radiograph in *Fig. 8-12* is an A.P. projection of a lower right leg. Those parts labeled are: (A) medial condyle of the tibia, **(B)** shaft or diaphysis of the tibia, **(C)** medial malleolus, **(D)** lateral malleolus, **(E)** shaft or diaphysis of the fibula, **(F)** neck, **(G)** head, **(H)** styloid process or apex of the head of the fibula, **(I)** lateral condyle of the tibia, and **(J)** tibial spine or intercondylar eminence.

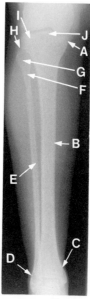

Fig. 8-12
Lower Leg
Radiograph (A.P.)

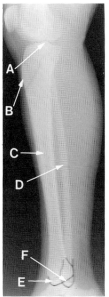

Lower Leg Fig. 8-13
Radiograph (lateral)

Lateral — Right Lower Leg

A lower right leg in the lateral position is illustrated in *Fig. 8-13*. Labeled are the: **(A)** tibial spine, **(B)** tibial tuberosity, **(C)** shaft of the tibia, **(D)** shaft of the fibula, **(E)** medial malleolus, and **(F)** lateral malleolus.

fibula (feminine) on outside (Lateral) and extends the most posteriorly

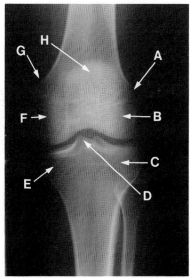

Knee Radiograph Fig. 8-14
(A.P.)

A.P. — Left Knee

Labeled in *Fig. 8-14* are: **(A)** lateral epicondyle of femur, **(B)** lateral condyle of femur, **(C)** lateral condyle of tibia, **(D)** tibial spine or intercondylar eminence, **(E)** medial condyle of tibia, **(F)** medial condyle of femur, **(G)** medial epicondyle of femur, and **(H)** patella.

Lateral — Left Knee

Labeled in *Fig. 8-15* are: **(A)** the base of the patella, **(B)** the apex of the patella, **(C)** tibial tuberosity, **(D)** neck of fibula, **(E)** head of fibula, and **(F)** tibial spine or intercondylar eminence.

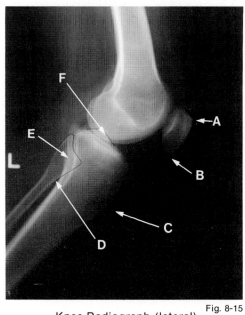

Fig. 8-15
Knee Radiograph (lateral)

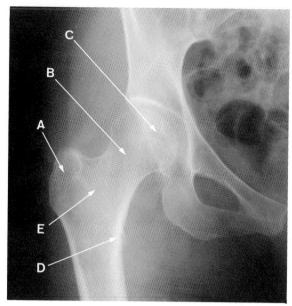

Hip Radiograph (A.P.)

Fig. 8-16

A.P. — Right Hip

Labeled in *Fig. 8-16* are: **(A)** the greater trochanter of the femur, **(B)** neck of femur, **(C)** head of femur, **(D)** lesser trochanter, and **(E)** the intertrochanteric crest.

Classification of Joints

The joints of the leg are all freely movable, with one exception. The freely movable joints are the **hip, knee,** and **proximal tibiofibular joint** — all diarthrodial joints. The **distal tibiofibular joint** is held together by strong fibrous bands that allow only limited motion, so it is an amphiarthrodial joint.

The hip joint is similar to the shoulder joint, allowing movement in all directions, typical of a ball and socket joint. The knee joint allows flexion and extension and is termed a hinge joint. Remember that the knee joint involves only the femur and tibia. The proximal tibiofibular joint allows a gliding type of motion that helps in rotational movements of the lower leg.

Summary of Leg Joints

1. Hip Joint
   Diarthrodial (Ball and Socket)
2. Knee Joint
   - *Diarthrodial (Hinge)*
3. Proximal Tibiofibular Joint
   - *Diarthrodial (Gliding)*
4. Distal Tibiofibular Joint
   - *Amphiarthrodial*

Prox Tib-Fib is die
Distal Tib-Fib is Amp

156

Part II. Radiographic Positioning
Leg, Knee, Patella and Femur

Basic Projections/Positions

Radiography of the long bones of the leg requires two positions or projections. At least one joint must be well visualized on the finished radiograph. If only one joint is required on the radiograph, include that joint closest to the patient's injury. If the injury is near the ankle joint, then locate the film so that at least 2 inches (5 centimeters) of the film is below the ankle joint. If the injury is closer to the knee, then include the knee joint. Some departmental routines require that both ends of long bones in question be visible on the finished radiograph.

Radiographs of extremities measuring more than 9 centimeters in thickness usually require the use of a cassette with screens or a cassette and grid, rather than a cardboard film holder, due to the production of large amounts of scatter radiation in larger body parts. The grid can mean a portable grid, a grided cassette or a fixed or movable grid in a radiographic table.

Basic positioning for the leg, knee, patella and femur follow.

Lower Leg
Basic
- A.P.
- Lateral

Knee
Basic
- A.P.
- Oblique
- Lateral

Patella
Basic
- P.A.
- Oblique
- Lateral
- Axial

Knee — Intercondyloid Fossa
Basic
- Semiaxial P.A.

Distal Femur
Basic
- A.P.
- Lateral

Lower Leg

• Anteroposterior Projection

Film Size:
7 x 17 in. (18 x 43 cm.)

or

14 x 17 in. (35 x 43 cm.)
Divide in half.

Bucky: (to include knee)
- Moving or stationary grid.

Non-Bucky: (to include ankle)
- Detail screen or CBH.

Patient Position:
- Supine.

Part Position:
- Adjust pelvis and leg so that entire extremity is not rotated.
- Position lower leg and foot so intermalleolar line is parallel to film holder.
- Place sandbag against foot.
- Place lead shield over pelvis.

Central Ray:
- C.R. perpendicular to film holder.
- Center to film holder to include joint nearest injury.
- Film should extend beyond joint by approx. 2 in. (5 cm.).
- 40 in. (102 cm.) F.F.D.

NOTE: • To insure a true A.P. projection, check lower leg and ankle to be sure the intermalleolar line is parallel to film holder.

Structures Best Shown:
Tibia and fibula, including either the ankle or knee joint.

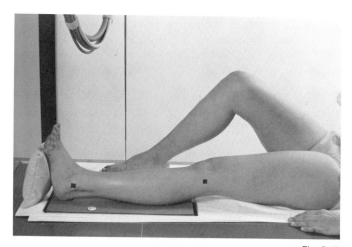

A.P. (to include ankle joint)   Fig. 8-17

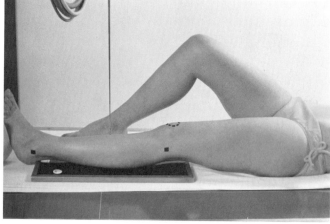

A.P. (to include knee joint)   Fig. 8-18

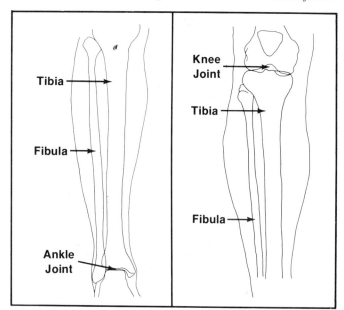

Fig. 8-20

A.P. (include ankle)   A.P. (include knee)

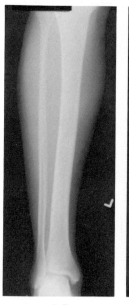 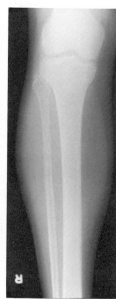

A.P.
(include ankle)

A.P. Fig. 8-19
(include knee)

Lower Leg
Basic
- A.P.
- Lateral

Lower Leg

• Lateral Position

Film Size:
7 x 17 in. (18 x 43 cm.)

or

14 x 17 in. (35 x 43 cm.)
Divide in half.

Bucky: (to include knee)
- Moving or stationary grid.

Non-Bucky: (to include ankle)
- Detail screen or CBH.

Patient Position:
- Lateral recumbent.

Part Position:
- Turn patient toward affected side.
- Be sure leg is in a true lateral position.
- Place unaffected leg posterior to side being radiographed.
- Place lead shield over pelvis.

Central Ray:
- C.R. perpendicular to film holder.
- Center to film holder to include joint nearest injury.
- Film should extend beyond joint by approx. 2 in. (5 cm.).
- 40 in. (102 cm.) F.F.D.

NOTE: • To insure a true lateral position, check to see that an imaginary line between femoral epicondyles and the intermalleolar line are perpendicular to film holder.

Structures Best Shown:
Tibia and fibula, including either the ankle or knee joint.

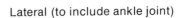

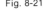

Lateral (to include ankle joint)

Fig. 8-21

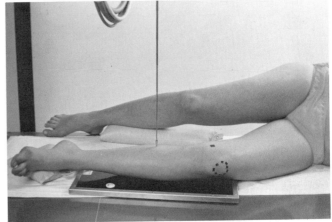

Lateral (to include knee joint)

Fig. 8-22

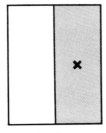

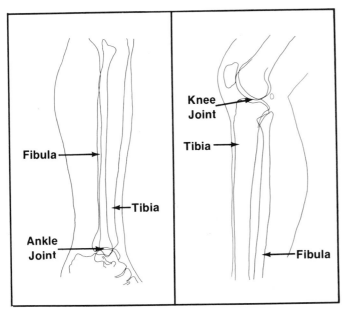

Fibula

Tibia

Ankle
Joint

Knee
Joint

Tibia

Fibula

Fig. 8-24
Lateral (include ankle)

Lateral (include knee)

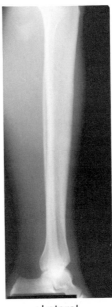

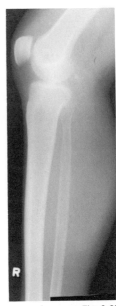

Lateral
(include ankle)

Lateral
(include knee)

Fig. 8-23

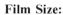

Knee
Basic
• **A.P.**
• Oblique
• Lateral

Knee

• Anteroposterior Projection

Film Size:
    8 x 10 in. (18 x 24 cm.)

Bucky:
- Moving or stationary grid.

Patient Position:
- Supine.

Part Position:
- Internally rotate the leg slightly to place intermalleolar line and line between femoral epicondyles parallel to table.
- Sandbag the ankle and foot.
- Collimate closely and place lead shield over pelvis.

Central Ray:
- Angle C.R. cephalad 5°.
- C.R. enters **1 cm. inferior** to apex of patella.
- 40 in. (102 cm.) F.F.D.

NOTE: • The most common positioning error for a knee is to center too high. • Center to the knee joint, 1 cm. inferior to apex of patella. • May be done non-Bucky if part measures less than 9 cm.

Structures Best Shown:
Distal femur, proximal tibia and fibula, and knee joint.

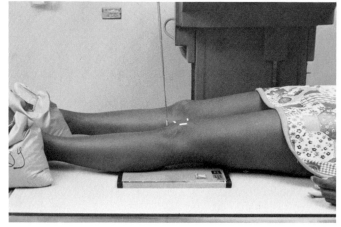

A.P.   Fig. 8-25

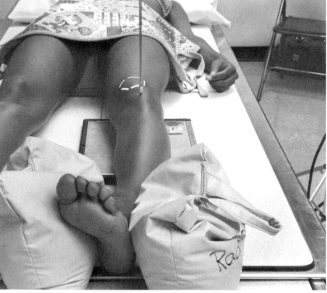

A.P.   Fig. 8-26

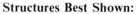

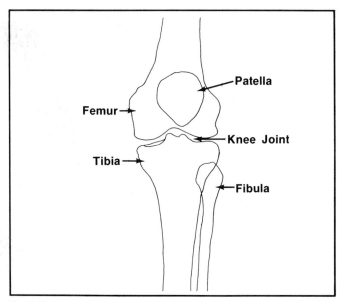

Fig. 8-28
    A.P. Knee

Patella —
Femur →
Knee Joint
Tibia →
Fibula

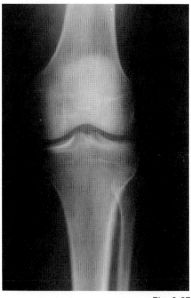

A.P. Knee   Fig. 8-27

Knee

• Medial Oblique Position

Film Size:

8 x 10 in. (18 x 24 cm.)

Bucky:
- Moving or stationary grid.

Patient Position:
- Semisupine with body and entire leg rotated away from side of interest.

Part Position:
- Leg should be rotated internally 45°.
- Place support under elevated hip.
- Immobilize foot and ankle.
- Collimate closely and place lead shield over pelvis.

Central Ray:
- Angle C.R. cephalad 5°.
- C.R. enters **1 cm. inferior** to apex of patella.
- 40 in. (102 cm.) F.F.D.

NOTE: • Difficult position for some patients. • May have to tolerate some part-film distance. • May be done non-Bucky if part measures less than 9 cm.

Structures Best Shown:
Head and neck of fibula and proximal tibiofibular joint.

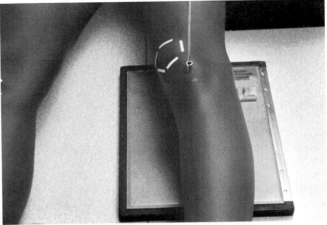

Medial Oblique

Fig. 8-29

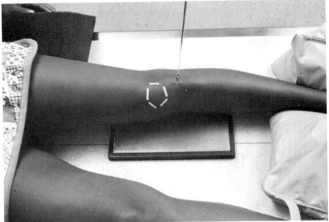

Medial Oblique

Fig. 8-30

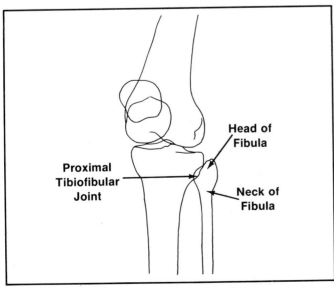

Fig. 8-32

Medial Oblique Knee

Proximal
Tibiofibular
Joint

Head of
Fibula

Neck of
Fibula

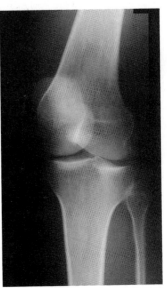

Fig. 8-31

Medial
Oblique Knee

Knee

Knee
Basic
- A.P.
- Oblique
- **Lateral**

• Lateral Position

Film Size:
    8 x 10 in. (18 x 24 cm.)

Bucky:
- Moving or stationary grid.

Patient Position:
- Lateral recumbent.

Part Position:
- Turn toward affected side until knee is in a true lateral position.
- Flex knee about 45°.
- Elevate ankle with sandbag.
- Place unaffected leg posterior to affected side.
- Collimate closely and place lead shield over pelvis.

Central Ray:
- Angle C.R. cephalad 5°.
- C.R. enters **1 cm. distal** to medial epicondyle.
- 40 in. (102 cm.) F.F.D.

NOTE: • Space between patella and femur should be opened up. • 5° cephalic angle superimposes condyles of distal femur. • May be done non-Bucky if part measures less than 9 cm.

Structures Best Shown:
Distal femur, proximal tibia and fibula, and patella.

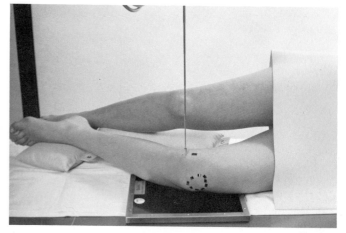

Lateral   Fig. 8-33

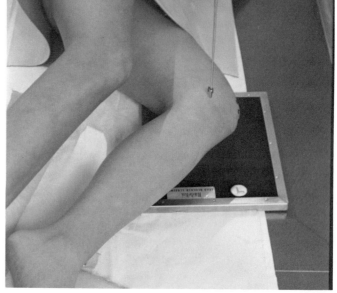

Lateral   Fig. 8-34

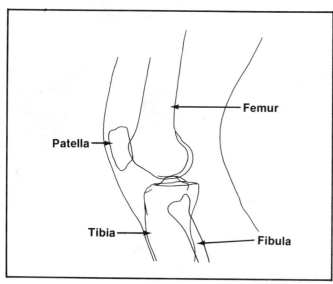

Fig. 8-36

Lateral Knee

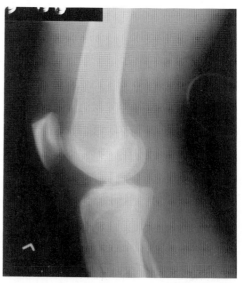

Lateral Knee   Fig. 8-35

Patella
Basic
• **P.A.**
• **Oblique**
• Lateral
• Axial

Patella

- ● **Posteroanterior Projection**
- ● **Medial Oblique Position**

Film Size:
   8 x 10 in. (18 x 24 cm.)

Bucky:
- Moving or stationary grid.

Patient Position:
- P.A. — prone.
- Medial oblique — semiprone.

Part Position:
P.A.
- Line through femoral epicondyles should be parallel to table.
Medial Oblique
- Rotate entire leg **internally** 45°.

- Collimate closely and place lead shield over pelvis.
- Place sandbag under ankle.

Central Ray:
- C.R. perpendicular to film holder, centered to mid patella.
- 40 in. (102 cm.) F.F.D.

NOTE: ● Do not flex knee until transverse fracture of patella is ruled out. ● May be done non-Bucky if part measures less than 9 cm.

Structures Best Shown:
Patella and distal femur.

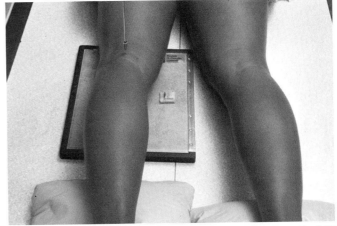

P.A.

Fig. 8-37

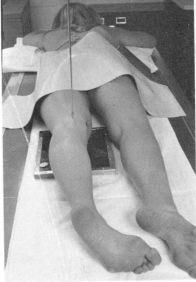

Medial Oblique

Fig. 8-38

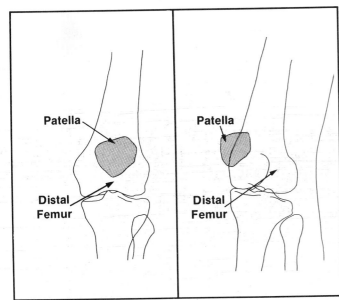

Fig. 8-40

P.A. Patella   Medial Oblique Patella

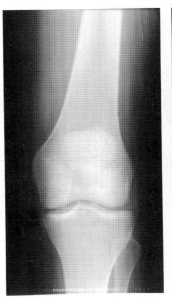
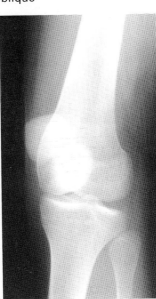

P.A. Patella   Medial Oblique Patella

Fig. 8-39

Patella
Basic
• P.A.
• Oblique
• **Lateral**
• Axial

Patella

• **Lateral Position**

Film Size:
    8 x 10 in. (18 x 24 cm.)

Bucky:
- Moving or stationary grid.

Patient Position:
- Lateral recumbent.

Part Position:
- Turn toward affected side until knee is in a true lateral position.
- Do **NOT** flex knee more than 5°.
- Collimate closely and place lead shield over pelvis.

Central Ray:
- C.R. perpendicular to film holder, centered to medial epicondyle.
- 40 in. (102 cm.) F.F.D.

NOTE: • Do **NOT** flex knee until transverse fracture of patella has been ruled out. • May be done non-Bucky if part measures less than 9 cm.

Structures Best Shown:
Patella, distal femur, and space between femur and patella.

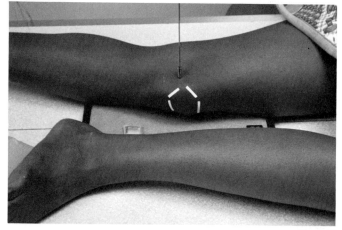

Lateral   Fig. 8-41

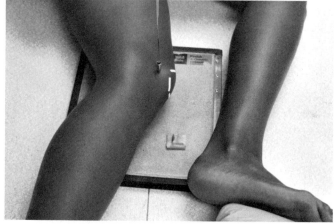

Lateral   Fig. 8-42

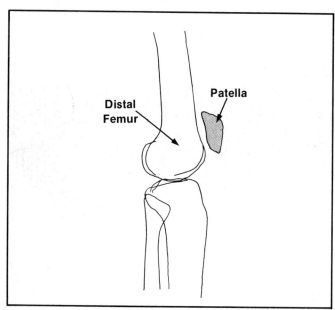

Fig. 8-44

Lateral Patella

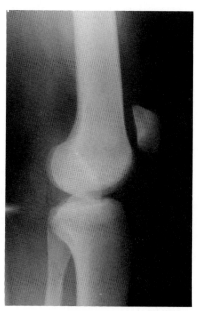

Lateral Patella   Fig. 8-43

Patella

• Axial Projection
Settegast, Sunrise or Skyline Position

Patella
Basic
• P.A.
• Oblique
• Lateral
• **Axial**

Film Size
  8 x 10 in. (18 x 24 cm.)

Non-Bucky:
- Detail screen or CBH.

Patient Position:
- Prone.

Part Position:
- Slowly flex knee as far as possible.
- Tape, gauze or sheet is used to hold leg in position.
- Be sure entire leg is in a vertical plane.

Central Ray:
- Angle cephalad so that a 45° angle exists between lower leg and C.R.
- Center to space between femur and patella.
- 40 in. (102 cm.) F.F.D.

NOTE: • Do **NOT** use this position if a transverse fracture of patella exists. • Never force leg into this position.

Structures Best Shown:
Patella and space between patella and femur.

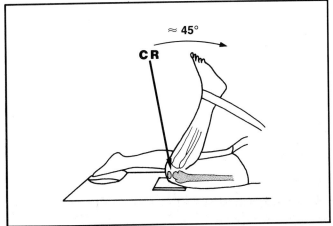

Axial Projection   Fig. 8-45

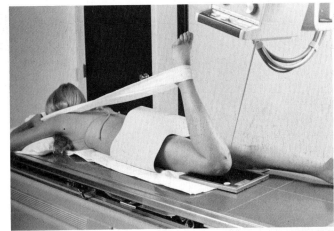

Axial Projection   Fig. 8-46

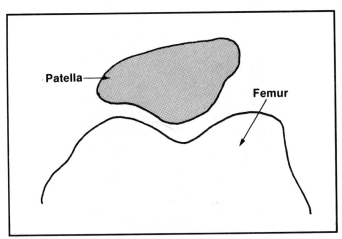

Fig. 8-48   Axial Projection

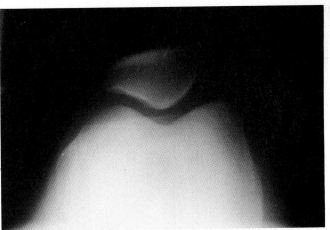

Axial Projection   Fig. 8-47

<table>
<tr><td>

Knee - Intercondyloid Fossa
Basic
• Semiaxial P.A.
</td></tr>
</table>

• Semiaxial P.A. Projection
Tunnel Position

Film Size:
    8 x 10 in. (18 x 24 cm.)

Bucky:
- Moving or stationary grid.

Patient Position:
- (1) Prone or (2) kneeling.

Part Position:
(1) Prone
- Flex knee about 40°.
- Rest foot on support, such as a footboard.
(2) Kneeling
- From "all-fours" position, patient leans forward to shift femur and buttocks out of the central ray.
- Most of the patient's weight is supported on the opposite leg.

Central Ray:
- C.R. through knee joint and **perpendicular** to lower leg.
- 40 in. (102 cm.) F.F.D.

NOTE: • Kneeling position is best, but may be difficult for some patients.

Structures Best Shown:
Intercondyloid fossa, distal femur, tibial spine, tibial plateau and knee joint.

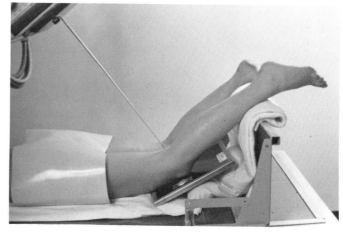

Semiaxial P.A. Projection   Fig. 8-49

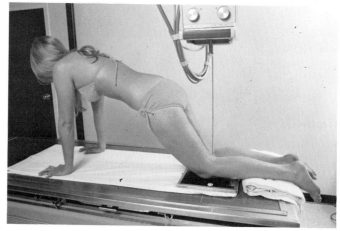

Semiaxial P.A. Projection   Fig. 8-50

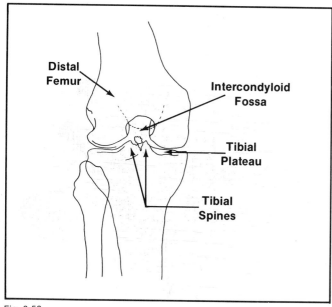

Fig. 8-52
Semiaxial P.A. Projection

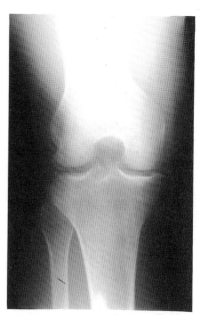

Semiaxial Fig. 8-51
P.A. Projection

Distal Femur

• Anteroposterior Projection

Film Size:
  7 x 17 in. (18 x 43 cm.)

  or

  14 x 17 in. (35 x 43 cm.)
  Divided in vertical halves.

Bucky:
- Moving or stationary grid.

Patient Position:
- Supine.

Part Position:
- Line between femoral epicondyles must be parallel to table.
- Include knee joint on film.
- Center femur to midline of table (femur is in lateral part of thigh).
- Collimate closely and use lead gonadal shield.

Centray Ray:
- C.R. perpendicular to and centered to film holder.
- Be sure to include 5 cm. distal to knee joint on film.
- 40 in. (102 cm.) F.F.D.

NOTE: • Shielding very important since gonads could be in primary beam.

Structures Best Shown:
Mid and distal femur.

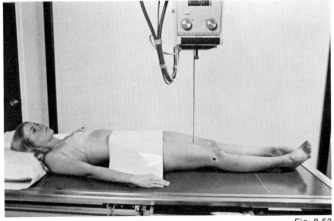

A.P.   Fig. 8-53

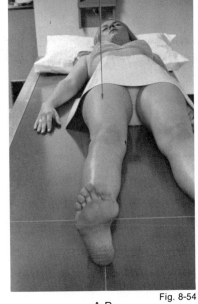

A.P.   Fig. 8-54

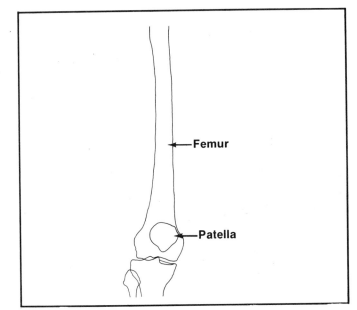

Fig. 8-56

A.P. Distal Femur

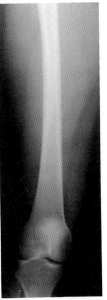

A.P. Fig. 8-55
Distal Femur

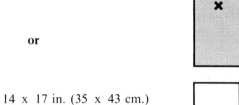

Distal Femur
Basic
- A.P.
- Lateral

Distal Femur

- **Lateral Position**

Film Size:
7 x 17 in. (18 x 43 cm.)

or

14 x 17 in. (35 x 43 cm.)
Divided in vertical halves.

Bucky:
- Moving or stationary grid.

Patient Position:
- Lateral recumbent or supine.

Part Position:
- Line between femoral epicondyles must be perpendicular to film.
- When laterally recumbent, place unaffected leg posterior to affected one.
- Include knee joint on film.
- Center femur to film holder (femur is in anterior part of thigh).
- Collimate closely and use lead gonadal shield.

Central Ray:
- C.R. perpendicular to and centered to film holder.
- Be sure to include 5 cm. distal to knee joint on film.
- 40 in. (102 cm.) F.F.D.

NOTE: • With possible fractured femur, patient must remain supine.

Structures Best Shown:
Mid and distal femur.

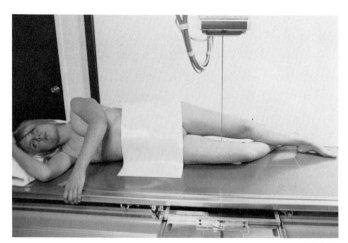

Lateral   Fig. 8-57

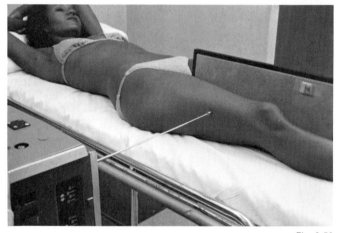

Lateral (horizontal beam)   Fig. 8-58

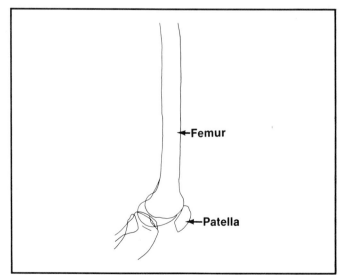

Fig. 8-60
Lateral Distal Femur

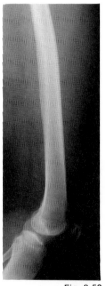

Fig. 8-59
Lateral Distal Femur

CHAPTER 9

Radiographic Anatomy and Positioning of the Hips and Pelvis

Part I. Radiographic Anatomy
Hips and Pelvis

Pelvic Girdle

The **pelvic girdle** consists of four bones: two **hip bones** or **ossa coxae,** one **sacrum** and one **coccyx.** The sacrum and coccyx form the posterior portion of the pelvic girdle, while each hip bone forms the lateral, anterior and inferior portions of the girdle.

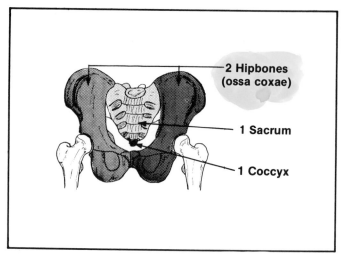

Pelvic Girdle

Fig. 9-1

Hip Bone

Each hip bone is composed of three divisions: **ilium, ischium** and **pubis.** In a child, these three divisions are separate bones, but they fuse in the adult into one bone. The fusion occurs in the area of the **acetabulum.** The acetabulum is a deep, cup-shaped cavity that accepts the head of the femur to form the hip joint. The ilium is the largest of the three divisions and is located superior to the acetabulum. The ischium is inferior and posterior to the acetabulum, while the pubis is inferior and anterior.

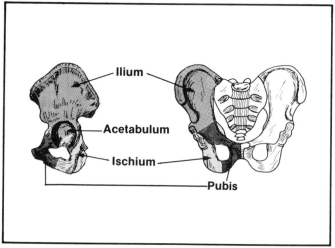

Hip Bone (os coxa)

Fig. 9-2

Ilium. Each large **ilium** is composed of a **body** and an **ala** or wing. The body of the ilium is the more inferior portion near the acetabulum and includes the upper two-fifths of the acetabulum. The ala or wing portion is the thin, flared, upper part of the ilium. The **crest** of the ilium is the upper margin of the ala and extends from the **anterior superior iliac spine** (A.S.I.S.) to the **posterior superior iliac spine** (P.S.I.S.). In radiographic positioning, the uppermost peak of the crest is often referred to as the iliac crest, but it actually extends between the A.S.I.S. and P.S.I.S. Below the anterior superior iliac spine is a less prominent projection referred to as the **anterior inferior iliac spine.** Similarly, inferior to the posterior superior iliac spine is the **posterior inferior iliac spine.** The most important positioning landmarks of these borders and projections are the crest of the ilium and the anterior superior iliac spine (A.S.I.S.).

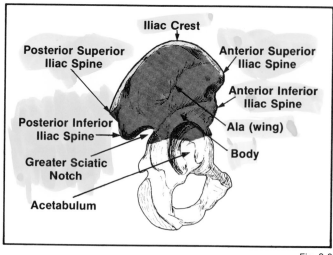

Ilium

Fig. 9-3

170

Ischium. The **ischium** is that part of the hip bone inferior and posterior to the acetabulum. Each ischium is divided into a **body** and two **rami.** The body of the ischium is near the acetabulum and includes the posteroinferior two-fifths of the acetabulum. Extending downward and backward from the body is the **superior ramus.** Projecting anteriorly from the superior ramus is the **inferior ramus.** The rounded, roughened area near the junction of the superior and inferior rami is an important landmark termed the **tuberosity of the ischium** or **ischial tuberosity.** The ischial tuberosities bear most of the weight of the body when one sits and can be palpated through the soft tissues of each buttock when one is prone.

Directly posterior to the acetabulum is a bony projection termed the **spine** of the ischium or **ischial spine.** Directly above the ischial spine is a deep notch termed the **greater sciatic notch.** Below the ischial spine is a smaller notch termed the **lesser sciatic notch.**

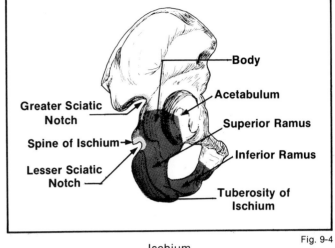

Ischium   Fig. 9-4

Pubis. The last of the three divisions of one hip bone is the **pubis** or **pubic bone.** The **body** of the pubis is anterior and inferior to the acetabulum and includes the anteroinferior one-fifth of the acetabulum. Extending anteriorly and medially from the body of each pubis is a **superior ramus.** The two superior rami meet in the midline to form a slightly movable joint, the **symphysis pubis.** Each **inferior ramus** passes down and posterior from the symphysis pubis to join the inferior ramus of the respective ischium. The **obturator foramen** is a large opening formed by the rami of each ischium and pubis. The obturator foramen is the largest foramen in the human skeletal system.

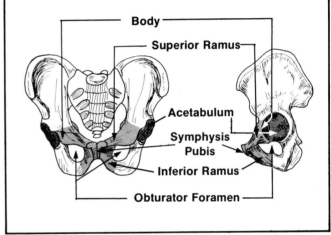

Pubis (Pubic Bone)   Fig. 9-5

Pelvis (summary)

The most important structures and landmarks of the pelvis in *Fig 9-6* are labeled for review purposes. These are: **(A)** iliac crest, **(B)** anterior superior iliac spine (A.S.I.S.), **(C)** symphysis pubis, **(D)** inferior ramus of pubis, **(E)** obturator foramen, **(F)** inferior ramus of ischium, **(G)** ischial tuberosity, **(H)** superior ramus of ischium, **(I)** superior ramus of pubis and **(J)** ischial spine.

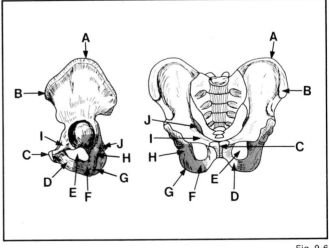

Pelvis   Fig. 9-6

A.P. - Pelvis

Study the radiograph of an A.P. pelvis *(Fig. 9-7)*. The labeled parts are: **(A)** the iliac crest, **(B)** the anterior end of the crest, which is termed the anterior superior iliac spine or A.S.I.S., **(C)** the superior ramus of the left ischium, **(D)** the ischial tuberosity, **(E)** the symphysis pubis, **(F)** the inferior ramus of the right pubis, **(G)** the superior ramus of the right pubis, **(H)** the right ischial spine, and **(I)** the ala or wing of the right ilium.

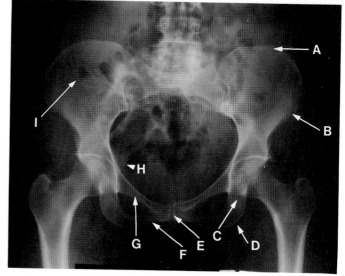

Pelvis — A.P.   Fig. 9-7

True and False Pelvis

A plane through the **brim** of the pelvis divides the pelvic area into two cavities. The pelvic brim is defined by the upper part of the symphysis pubis anteriorly and the upper, prominent part of the sacrum posteriorly. The general area above the oblique plane through the pelvic brim is termed the **greater** or **false pelvis.** The flared portion of the pelvis formed primarily by the alae or wings of the ilia form the lateral and posterior limits of the greater or false pelvis, while the abdominal muscles of the anterior wall define the anterior limits. The lower abdominal organs and a fetus within the pregnant uterus rest on the floor of the greater pelvis.

The area inferior to a plane through the pelvic brim is termed the **lesser** or **true pelvis.** The lesser or true pelvis is a cavity completely surrounded by bony structures. The size and shape of the true pelvis is of greatest importance during the birth process since the true pelvis forms the actual birth canal.

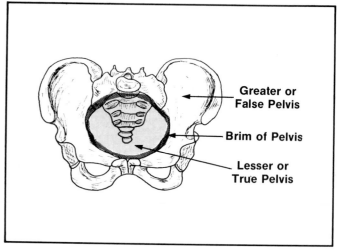

Pelvic Cavities   Fig. 9-8

Greater or False Pelvis

Brim of Pelvis

Lesser or True Pelvis

True Pelvis

The oblique plane defined by the brim of the pelvis is termed the **inlet** of the true pelvis. The **outlet** of the true pelvis is defined by the two ischial tuberosities and the tip of the coccyx. The three sides of the triangularly shaped outlet are formed by a line between the ischial tuberosities and two lines between each ischial tuberosity and the coccyx. The area between the inlet and outlet of the lesser or true pelvis is termed the **cavity** of the true pelvis. During the birth process, the baby must travel through the inlet, cavity and outlet of the true pelvis.

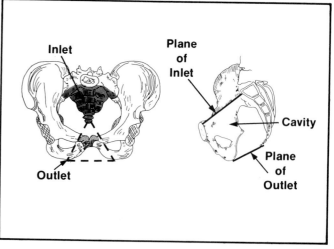

Inlet

Plane of Inlet

Cavity

Outlet

Plane of Outlet

Lesser or True Pelvis   Fig. 9-9

Birth Canal

The **pelvimetry** or, more properly, **cephalopelvimetry,** is a radiographic examination of a pregnant female to determine the actual measurements of both the maternal pelvis and the baby's head. Front to back and side to side measurements of the inlet, midpelvis and outlet (as shown on an A.P. and a lateral radiograph of the mother's pelvis) are made to insure that adequate room for a routine delivery does exist. During a routine delivery, the baby's head first travels through the pelvic inlet, then to the midpelvis, and finally through the outlet to exit in a forward direction.

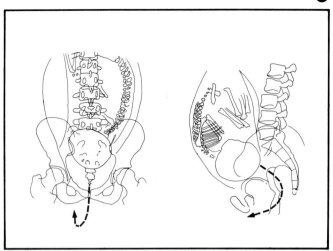

Birth Canal

Fig. 9-10

Male vs. Female Pelvis

The general shape of the female pelvis varies enough from the male pelvis to enable one to discriminate one from the other on pelvic radiographs. In general, the **female pelvis** is broader and more flared, while the **male pelvis** is narrower and less flared. In overall appearance, the female pelvis is deeper. Another major difference is the angle of the pubic arch, formed by the inferior rami of the pubes just below the symphysis pubis. In the female, this angle is usually obtuse or greater than 90 degrees, while in the male the pubic arch usually forms an acute angle, less than 90 degrees. Another difference is the general shape of the inlet. The inlet of the female pelvis is usually round, while in the male it is usually more oval or heart-shaped. The general shape of the pelvis does vary considerably from one individual to another, so that the pelvis of a slender female may resemble a male pelvis. In general, however, the differences are usually obvious enough that one can determine the sex of the patient from a pelvis radiograph.

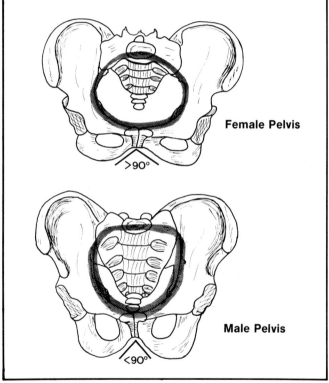

Female Pelvis

Male Pelvis

Pelvis — Male versus Female

Fig. 9-11

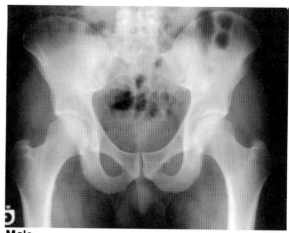

Male

Pelvis Radiographs

Radiographs of a male pelvis and a female pelvis are shown in *Fig. 9-12*. The male pelvis is deeper, narrower, less flared, and presents an acute angle at the pubic arch. Compared to the male pelvis, the female pelvis is shallower, broader, more flared, and shows an obtuse angle at the pubic arch. In addition, the female inlet is rounder than the inlet of the male pelvis.

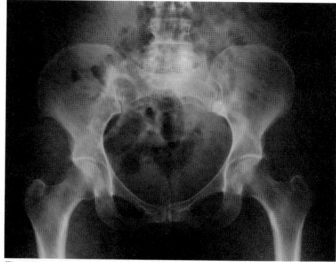

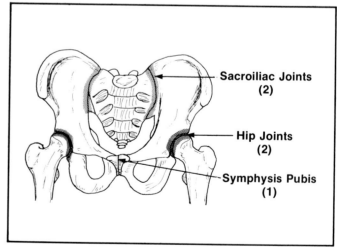

Female　　　　Pelvis Radiographs　　　　Fig. 9-12

Joints of the Pelvic Girdle

Five joints or articulations of the pelvic girdle are:

Sacroiliac Joints	(2)	— *Amphiarthrodial*
Symphysis Pubis	(1)	— *Amphiarthrodial*
Hip Joints	(2)	— *Diarthrodial (ball and socket)*

The **sacroiliac joints** are wide, flat joints located obliquely between the sacrum and each ilium. The sacroiliac articulations are classified as amphiarthrodial joints, indicating that they are only slightly movable. Because these joints are situated at an unusual angle, special positioning is required to visualize the joint space radiographically. The anterior junction of the two pubic bones is the **symphysis pubis.** This joint is also an amphiarthrodial joint, allowing limited expansion during late pregnancy and childbirth. Although the symphysis pubis extends inferiorly for a short distance, radiographic positioning involves palpating the most superior aspect of the joint. Thus the superior margin of the symphysis pubis is used as a positioning landmark.

The **hip joints** are diarthrodial joints, being freely movable, ball and socket type joints. Although both the hip joint and the shoulder joint are ball and socket joints, the hip joint is not as freely movable as the shoulder joint since the head of the femur sits deeply within the acetabulum.

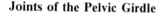

Sacroiliac Joints (2)

Hip Joints (2)

Symphysis Pubis (1)

Joints of the Pelvic Girdle　　　　Fig. 9-13

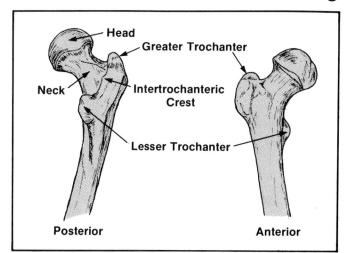

Fig. 9-14

Proximal Femur

Proximal Femur

The proximal femur consists of **head, neck** and **trochanters.** The large **greater trochanter** is located laterally and is palpable. The small **lesser trochanter** is located on the medial aspect of the femur. The ridge of bone connecting the two trochanters on the posterior aspect of the femur is termed the **intertrochanteric crest.**

Male Pelvis

Figure 9-15 is a radiograph of the pelvis of a male subject. Note the oval appearance of the inlet, the acute angle of the pubic arch and the less flared appearance of the ilia. The labeled parts are: **(A)** the sacrum, **(B)** the left sacroiliac joint, **(C)** the greater trochanter, **(D)** the femoral neck, and **(E)** the ischial tuberosity.

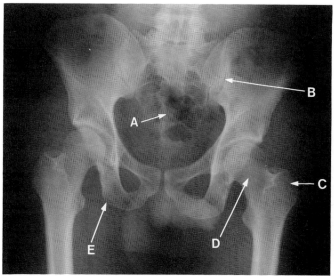

Male Pelvis

Fig. 9-15

Female Pelvis

Figure 9-16 is a radiograph of the pelvis of a female. Note the round appearance of the pelvic inlet, the obtuse angle of the pubic arch and the flared appearance of the ilia. Part **A** is the coccyx; **B** is the acetabulum; **C** is the lesser trochanter; and **D** is the obturator foramen.

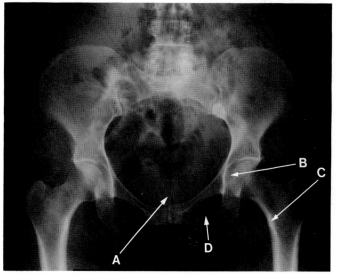

Female Pelvis

Fig. 9-16

Inferosuperior Projection of the Hip Joint

The lateral position or inferosuperior projection of the hip joint is shown in the drawing — *Fig. 9-17*. A good radiograph will appear similar to the left drawing. Part **A** is the acetabulum; **B** is the head of the femur; and **C** is the ischial tuberosity.

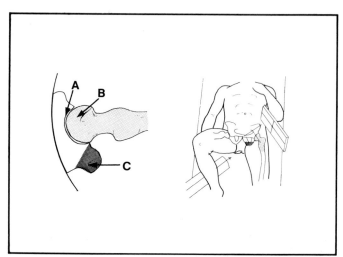

Hip Joint (lateral)   Fig. 9-17

Two lateral hip radiographs are demonstrated in *Fig. 9-18*. Look carefully to determine which is correctly placed and which is upside down. The best way to make this determination is to locate the ischial tuberosity. The ischial tuberosity will be located inferior to the hip joint. When placed on an illuminator correctly, the ischial tuberosity will be near the lower border. The radiograph to the right is displayed correctly. Part **A** is the acetabulum; **B** is the head of the femur; **C** is the neck of the femur; and **D** is the ischial tuberosity.

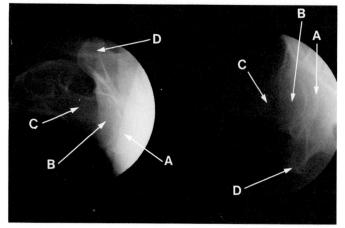

Hip Joint (lateral)   Fig. 9-18

Part II. Radiographic Positioning
Hips and Pelvis

Radiographic positioning of the hip joint is a definite challenge for radiographers. Interrelationships of the pelvic girdle and the hip joint must be thoroughly understood. One must be able to find the exact location of the femoral head and femoral neck by the following positioning landmarks. Two important palpable landmarks are the A.S.I.S. and the upper border of the symphysis pubis. Locate the midpoint of an imaginary line drawn between the A.S.I.S. and the symphysis pubis. The neck of the femur will lie along a line perpendicular to the midpoint of the first line and approximately 2.5 in. (6.25 cm.) below the midpoint. The head of the femur is approximately 1.5 in. (3.75 cm.) below the midpoint of this imaginary line between the A.S.I.S. and the symphysis pubis.

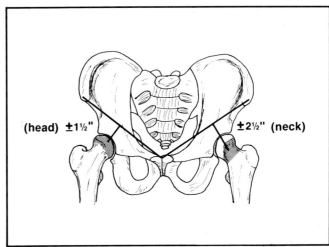

(head) ±1½"   ±2½" (neck)

Head or Neck Localization

Fig. 9-19

When the leg is lying in the true anatomical position, the proximal femur is rotated posteriorly by 15 to 20 degrees. Note that the femoral neck appears shortened and that the lesser trochanter is visible when the leg and ankle are truly A.P. *(Fig. 9-20)*.

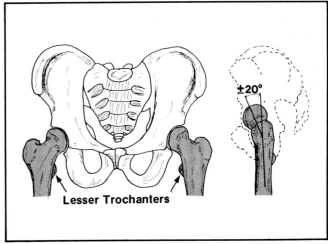

±20°

Lesser Trochanters

Anatomical Position

Fig. 9-20

By **internally rotating** the **entire** leg, the hip joint will be projected in a true A.P. projection. The neck of the femur is now parallel to the imaging surface and will not appear foreshortened *(Fig. 9-21)*. The key to proper placement of the leg is the **lesser trochanter.** If the entire leg is internally rotated 15 to 20 degrees, the outline of the lesser trochanter **cannot** be visualized. If the leg is straight A.P. or externally rotated, then the lesser trochanter is readily visible.

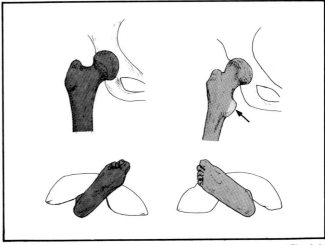

Hip Positioning

Fig. 9-21

Positioning Landmarks

Important positioning landmarks of the pelvis are reviewed in *Fig. 9-22*. The most superior aspect of the iliac crest and the A.S.I.S. are easily palpated. The greater trochanter of the femur can be located in the soft tissues of the upper thigh. Note that the upper margin of the greater trochanter is about 1.5 in. (3.75 cm.) above the upper border of the symphysis pubis, while the ischial tuberosity is about the same distance below the symphysis pubis.

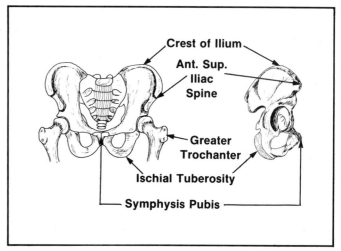

Bony Landmarks

Fig. 9-22

Basic and Optional Projections/Positions

Certain basic and optional projections or positions of the hips and pelvis are demonstrated and described on the following pages. It should be noted that certain positions or projections must not be used on trauma patients with possible hip fractures. For example, the frog leg position or 15° internal rotation of the injured leg on an A.P. hip or pelvis would be very painful for the patient. More importantly, further movement of a fracture could cause additional injury and misalignment of the fracture fragments. This could make proper reduction and treatment more difficult.

An optional translateral position of the hip on a trauma or postop patient who cannot move or rotate the leg or hip of interest is demonstrated and described as a modified translateral (courtesy of Roland W. Clements, R.T., and Harry K. Nakayama, R.T., as described and submitted to the publisher, 1981).

Pelvis
Basic
- A.P.

Bilateral Hip
Basic
- A.P. Pelvis
- Bilateral Frog Leg Position
  or
- Translateral — Both hips

Unilateral Hip
Basic
- A.P. Hip (or Pelvis)
- Unilateral Frog Leg
  or
- Translateral
Optional
- Modified Translateral

Sacroiliac Joints
Basic
- A.P. Pelvis
- Both Posterior Obliques

Pelvimetry
Basic
- A.P.
- Lateral

Pelvis
• Anteroposterior Projection

Film Size:
    14 x 17 in. (35 x 43 cm.)
    Crosswise.

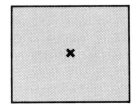

Bucky:
- Moving or stationary grid.

Patient Position:
- Supine.

Part Position:
- Be certain that the pelvis is not rotated; the distance from tabletop to each A.S.I.S. should be equal.
- Except for trauma patients, both legs should be internally rotated 15 to 20 degrees. Do **not** attempt to internally rotate the legs if a hip fracture is suspected.
- Midsagittal plane is centered to film.
- Place supports under knees.
- May need to place sandbag between heels and tape top of feet together.
- Use gonadal shield, if possible.

Central Ray:
- C.R. perpendicular to film holder.
- C.R. midway between symphysis pubis and iliac crest.
- 40 in. (102 cm.) F.F.D.

NOTE: • Lesser trochanter should **NOT** be seen if legs are internally rotated correctly.

Structures Best Shown:
Both hip bones, sacrum and coccyx, plus femoral heads, necks and greater trochanters.

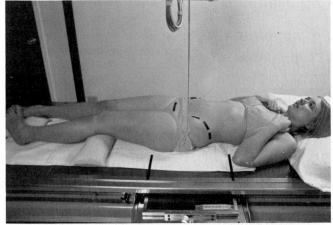

A.P.   Fig. 9-23

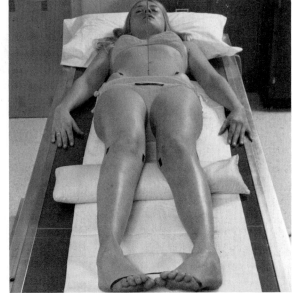

A.P.   Fig. 9-24

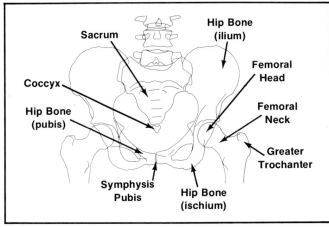

Fig. 9-26   A.P.

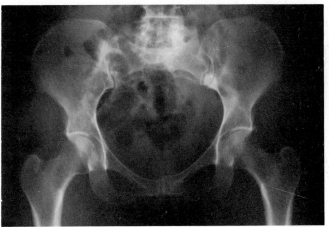

A.P.   Fig. 9-25

Bilateral Hips
Basic
- **A.P. Pelvis**
- Bilateral Frog Leg Position
  or
- Translateral - Both hips

Bilateral Hips

• **Anteroposterior Projection**

Film Size:

14 x 17 in. (35 x 43 cm.)
Crosswise.

Bucky:

- Moving or stationary grid.

Part Position:

- Similar to A.P. pelvis.
- Pelvis should not be rotated.
- Except for trauma patients, both legs should be internally rotated 15 to 20 degrees. Do **NOT** attempt to internally rotate legs if a hip fracture is suspected.
- Midsagittal plane is centered to film.
- Place supports under knees.
- May need to place sandbag between heels and tape top of feet together.
- Use gonadal shield, if possible.

Central Ray:

- C.R. perpendicular to film holder.
- C.R. enters 1 in. (2.5 cm.) cephalad to symphysis pubis.
- 40 in. (102 cm.) F.F.D.

NOTE: • Iliac crests should be visibile near top of radiograph. • Lesser trochanters should **NOT** be visible.

Structures Best Shown:

Femoral heads, necks and greater trochanters, plus both hip bones, sacrum and coccyx.

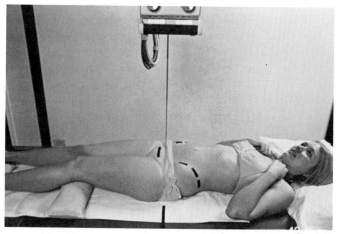

A.P. for Hips   Fig. 9-27

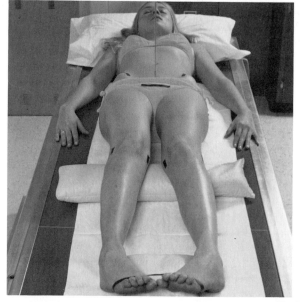

A.P. for Hips   Fig. 9-28

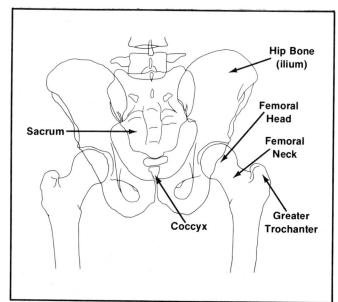

Fig. 9-30

A.P. for Hips

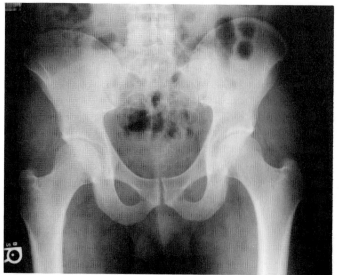

A.P. for Hips   Fig. 9-29

Bilateral Hips
Basic
- A.P. Pelvis
- **Bilateral Frog Leg Position**
  or
- Translateral - Both hips

Bilateral Hips

• **Bilateral Frog Leg Position**
(Nontrauma Routine)

Film Size:
   14 x 17 in. (35 x 43 cm.)
   Crosswise.

Bucky:
- Moving or stationary grid.

Patient Position:
- Supine.

Part Position:
- **This position should NEVER be attempted on the trauma patient.**
- Pelvis must not be rotated.
- Midsagittal plane is centered to film.
- Flex both knees and maximally abduct both hips.
- Plantar surfaces of feet are placed together.

Central Ray:
- C.R. perpendicular to film holder.
- C.R. enters 1 in. (2.5 cm.) cephalad to symphysis pubis.
- 40 in. (102 cm.) F.F.D.

NOTE: • Use gonadal shield, if possible, but do not cover hip joints. • This position is most often used on pediatric patients with possible congenital hip deformities.

Structures Best Shown:
Femoral heads, necks and trochanteric areas on one radiograph for purposes of comparison. Entire pelvis is shown.

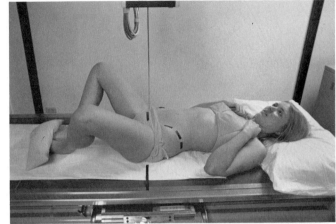

Fig. 9-31

Bilateral Frog Leg Position

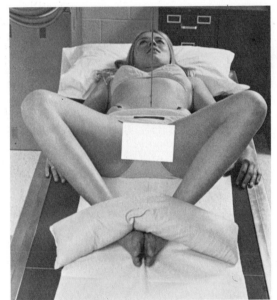

Fig. 9-32

Bilateral Frog Leg Position

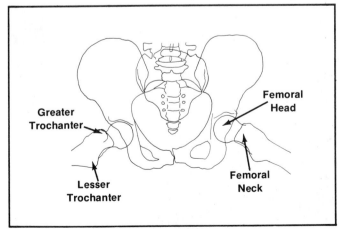

Fig. 9-34

Bilateral Frog Leg Position

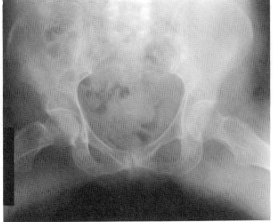

Fig. 9-33

Bilateral Frog Leg Position

Bilateral Hips
Basic
- A.P. Pelvis
- Bilateral Frog Leg Position

 or
- **Translateral — Both hips**

Bilateral Hips
• Translateral Position
Inferosuperior Projection
(Trauma Routine)

Film Size:

  8 x 10 in. (18 x 24 cm.)
  Crosswise.

Bucky:

- Stationary grid cassettes.

Patient Position:

- Supine.

Part Position:

- **This position SHOULD be used on the trauma patient.**
- Each side is done separately.
- To locate femoral neck, draw an imaginary line between A.S.I.S. and symphysis pubis. A second line that perpendicularly bisects the first line will parallel the femoral neck. The neck is about 2.5 in. (6.75 cm.) down from the intersection of the two lines.
- Elevate pelvis 2 in. (5 cm.), if possible, by placing supports under pelvis.
- Flex and elevate unaffected leg.
- Place cassette in crease above iliac crest and parallel to femoral neck. Support with holder or sandbags.
- Internally rotate affected leg 15°, if possible, although on a trauma patient, this is not done.

Central Ray:

- C.R. passes through femoral neck perpendicular to film holder.
- 40 in. (102 cm.) F.F.D.

NOTE: • Same position is used in surgery for a hip nailing.

Structures Best Shown:

Lateral view of femoral head, neck and trochanters to include acetabulum.

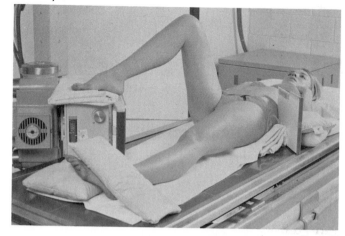

Translateral Hip   Fig. 9-35

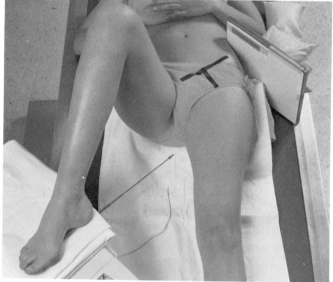

Translateral Hip   Fig. 9-36

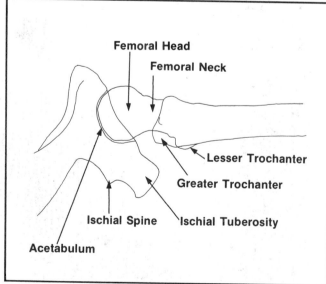

Femoral Head

Femoral Neck

Lesser Trochanter

Greater Trochanter

Ischial Spine   Ischial Tuberosity

Acetabulum

Fig. 9-38

Translateral Hip

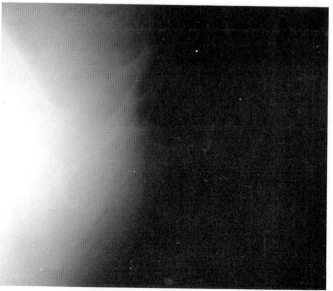

Translateral Hip   Fig. 9-37

Unilateral Hip
• Anteroposterior Projection

Unilateral Hip
Basic
• **A.P. Hip (or Pelvis)**
• Unilateral Frog Leg
or
• Translateral
Optional
• Modified Translateral

Film Size:
   10 x 12 in. (24 x 30 cm.)

Bucky:
- Moving or stationary grid.

Patient Position:
- Supine.

Part Position:
- Pelvis should not be rotated.
- Femoral neck is centered to table. Femoral neck is 2½ in. (6.75 cm.) inferior to perpendicular bisector of line between A.S.I.S. and symphysis pubis.
- Leg on side of interest should be internally rotated 15 to 20° (nontrauma patient).
- Use gonadal shield.

Central Ray:
- Through femoral neck, perpendicular to film holder.
- 40 in. (102 cm.) F.F.D.

NOTE: • The A.P. unilateral hip is done as a follow-up procedure. • The A.P. pelvis must be done during the patient's first examination. Note that slight visualization of the lesser trochanter indicates that the leg was not rotated a full 15 to 20° internally.

Structures Best Shown:
Femoral head, neck and greater trochanter, plus acetabulum.

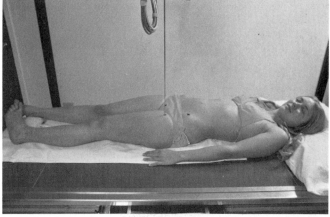

A.P. - Unilateral Hip   Fig. 9-39

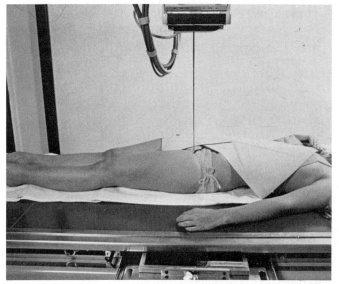

A.P. - Unilateral Hip   Fig. 9-40
(Note lead gonadal shield)

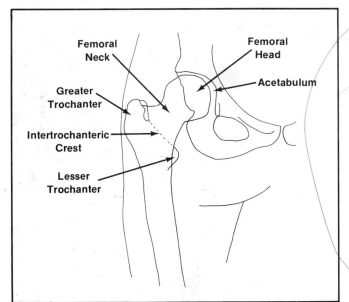

Femoral Neck
Femoral Head
Greater Trochanter
Acetabulum
Intertrochanteric Crest
Lesser Trochanter

Fig. 9-42
A.P. - Unilateral Hip

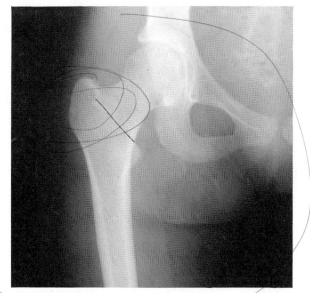

A.P. - Unilateral Hip   Fig. 9-41

Unilateral Hip
Basic
- A.P. Hip (or Pelvis)
- **Unilateral Frog Leg**
  or
- Translateral
Optional
- Modified Translateral

Unilateral Hip
• Frog Leg Position
(Nontrauma Routine)

Film Size:

    10 x 12 in. (24 x 30 cm.)

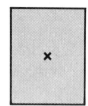

Bucky:

- Moving or stationary grid.

Patient Position:

- Supine.

Part Position:

- **This position should NEVER be attempted on a trauma patient.**
- Rotate slightly toward affected side.
- Flex knee and fully abduct side of interest. Thigh should contact the table.
- Collimate well and use support blocks.
- Use gonadal shield.

Central Ray:

- C.R. through femoral neck, perpendicular to film holder or with 10 to 15° cephalic angle.
- 40 in. (102 cm.) F.F.D.

NOTE: • A 10 to 15° cephalic angle may give a better view of the area of interest.

Structures Best Shown:

Femoral head, neck and trochanteric area, plus acetabulum.

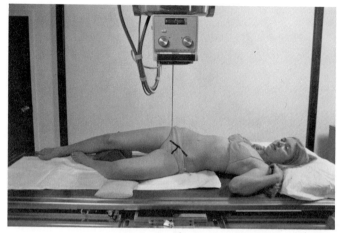

Frog Leg Position - Unilateral, no angle   Fig. 9-43

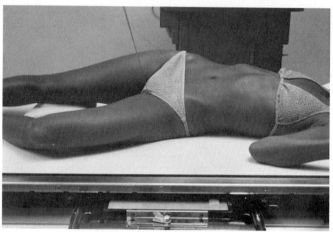

Frog Leg Position with Cephalic Angle   Fig. 9-44

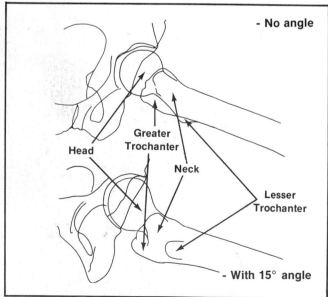

Fig. 9-46

Frog Leg Position - Unilateral

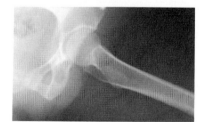

Frog Leg Position
- no angle

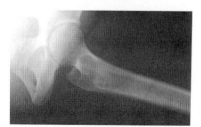

Fig. 9-45

Frog Leg Position
- with 15° angle

Unilateral Hip
Basic
- A.P. Hip (or Pelvis)
- Unilateral Frog Leg
  or
- **Translateral**
Optional
- Modified Translateral

Unilateral Hip

- **Translateral Position**
Inferosuperior Projection
(Trauma Routine)

Film Size:
> 8 x 10 in. (18 x 24 cm.)
> Crosswise.

Bucky:
- Stationary grid cassette.

Patient Position:
- Supine.

Part Position:
- **This position SHOULD be used on the trauma patient.**
- Elevate pelvis 2 in. (5 cm.), if possible, by placing supports under pelvis.
- Flex and elevate unaffected leg.
- Place cassette in crease above iliac crest and parallel to femoral neck. Use cassette holder if available.
- Internally rotate affected leg 15°, if possible, although on a trauma patient this is not done.
- Collimate well.

Central Ray:
- C.R. passes through femoral neck perpendicular to film holder.
- 40 in. (102 cm.) F.F.D.

NOTE: • Use adequate kVp to penetrate the part.

Structures Best Shown:
Femoral head, neck and trochanteric area, plus acetabulum.

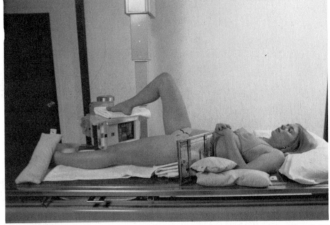

Translateral Hip   Fig. 9-47

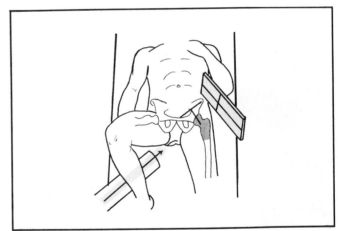

Translateral Hip for Trauma   Fig. 9-48

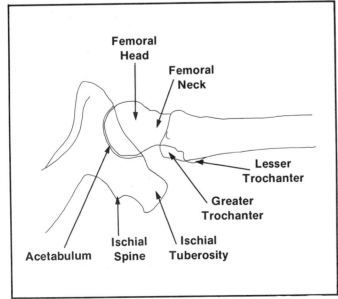

Fig. 9-50
Unilateral Translateral Hip

Unilateral Translateral Hip   Fig. 9-49

Unilateral Hip

Basic
- A.P. Hip (or Pelvis)
- Unilateral Frog Leg
  or
- Translateral

Optional
- **Modified Translateral**

Unilateral Hip

- **Translateral Position**

Inferosuperior Projection

(Clements — Nakayama Position)

Film Size:

8 x 10 in. (18 x 24 cm.)

Bucky:
- Stationary grid cassette.
  (grid vertical, with 15° tilt).

Patient Position:
- Supine with body near edge of table (Bucky tray side).

Part Position:
- This position can be used on any patient who cannot move the hip or leg of interest.
- Both legs remain flat on table.
- Place cassette on Bucky tray with bottom edge below table level and the lead strips vertical.
- Tilt cassette backward 15° from vertical.

Central Ray:
- C.R. is perpendicular to and centered to femoral neck, and angled downward 15°.
- Cassette is centered to central ray.
- 40 in. (102 cm.) F.F.D.

NOTE: • This position is easier to obtain and requires less technique than the standard translateral.

Structures Best Shown:

Femoral head, neck and trochanteric area, and acetabulum.

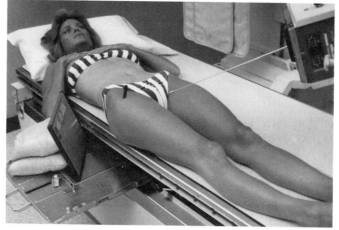

Modified Translateral Position   Fig. 9-51

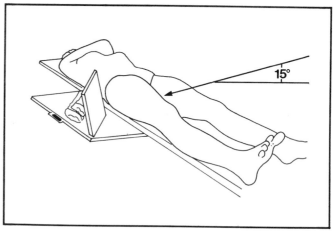

Modified Translateral Position   Fig. 9-52

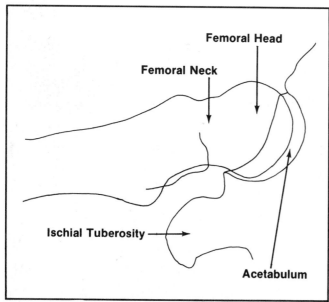

Femoral Head

Femoral Neck

Ischial Tuberosity

Acetabulum

Fig. 9-54

Modified Translateral Hip

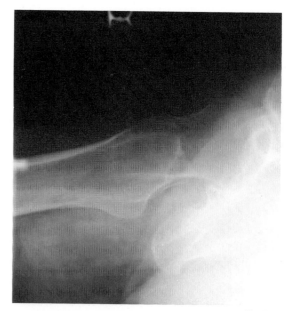

Modified Translateral Position   Fig. 9-53

Sacroiliac Joints
• Anteroposterior Pelvis

Sacroiliac Joints
Basic
● **A.P. Pelvis**
● Both Posterior Obliques

Film Size:
 14 x 17 in. (35 x 43 cm.)
 Crosswise.

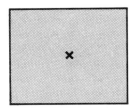

Bucky:
- Moving or stationary grid.

Patient Position:
- Supine.

Part Position:
- Be certain that pelvis is not rotated.
- Midsagittal plane is centered to table.
- Place supports under knees.
- Use gonadal shield, if possible.

Central Ray:
- C.R. perpendicular to film holder.
- C.R. midway between symphysis pubis and iliac crest.
- 40 in. (102 cm.) F.F.D.

NOTE: ● This is the same position as the routine pelvis.

Structures Best Shown:
Both hip bones, sacrum, coccyx and sacroiliac joints.

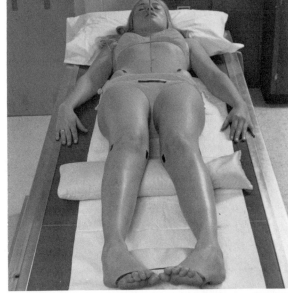

A.P.   Fig. 9-55

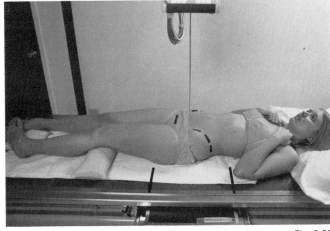

A.P.   Fig. 9-56

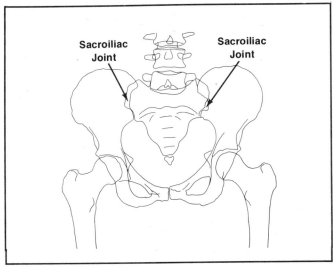

Fig. 9-58   A.P.

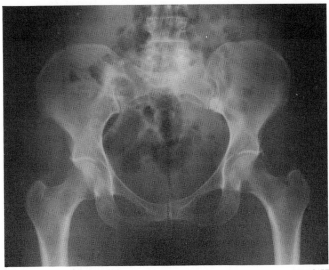

A.P.   Fig. 9-57

Sacroiliac Joints
Basic
• A.P. Pelvis
• Both Posterior Obliques

Sacroiliac Joints

• **Posterior Oblique Position**

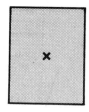

Film Size:
10 x 12 in. (24 x 30 cm.)

Bucky:
- Moving or stationary grid.

Patient Position:
- Semisupine.
- Side of interest is elevated 30°.

Part Position:
- L.P.O. will visualize right joint.
- R.P.O. will visualize left joint.
- Support patient's back.
- Elevated arm should reach across chest to grasp table.
- Adjust sacroiliac joint of interest to center of film.
- Collimate closely.

Central Ray:
- C.R. perpendicular to film holder.
- C.R. enters 1 in. (2.5 cm.) medial to up side A.S.I.S.
- 40 in. (102 cm.) F.F.D.

NOTE: • This position can also be taken semiprone, but the down side joint is then opened. (R.A.O. shows right joint and L.A.O. shows left joint.)

Structures Best Shown:
Profile view of sacroiliac joint. Both sides done for comparison.

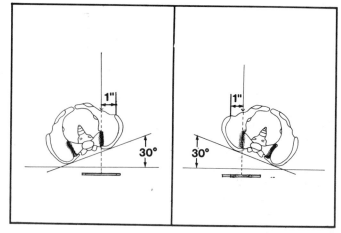

Posterior Oblique Position   Fig. 9-59

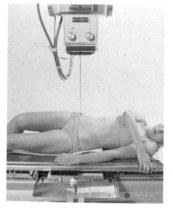

Posterior Oblique Position   Fig. 9-60

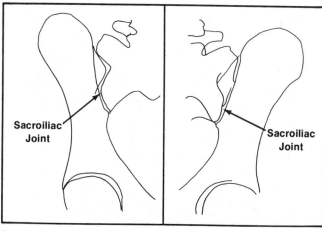

Fig. 9-62

Bilateral Posterior Obliques

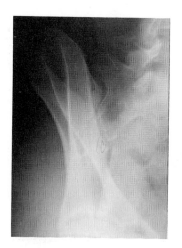

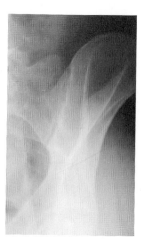

Bilateral Posterior Obliques   Fig. 9-61

Pelvimetry
Basic
- **A.P.**
- Lateral

Cephalopelvimetry

• **Anteroposterior Projection**
Colcher — Sussman Technique

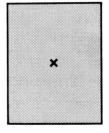

Film Size:
14 x 17 in. (35 x 43 cm.)

Bucky:
- Moving or stationary grid.

Patient Position:
- Supine with midsagittal plane of body centered to midline of table and/or film.
- Legs in bilateral frog leg position with knees abducted as far as possible.
- Plantar surfaces of feet together.

Part Position:
- Pelvis should not be rotated.

Central Ray:
- C.R. perpendicular to film holder.
- C.R. enters 1 in. (2.5 cm.) cephalad to symphysis pubis.
- 40 in. (102 cm.) F.F.D.

NOTE: • Set pelvimeter at level of ischial tuberosities or 10 cm. less than measurement at symphysis pubis. • Pelvimeter must be visible on bottom of radiograph. **DO NOT** cut off ruler. • Use fast screens and fast film. • Cover patient. • Suspend respiration on exhalation after several deep breaths and in between contractions.

Structures Best Shown:
Pelvic landmarks defining inlet, midpelvis, and outlet, plus fetal head unless presentation is breech.

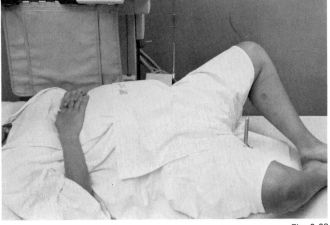

A.P. Cephalopelvimetry   Fig. 9-63

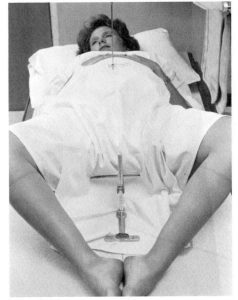

A.P.   Fig. 9-64
Cephalopelvimetry

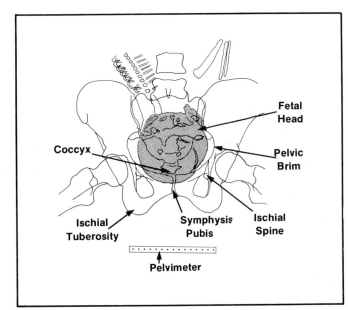

Fig. 9-66

A.P. Cephalopelvimetry

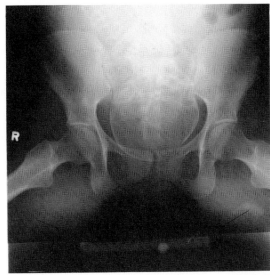

A.P. Cephalopelvimetry   Fig. 9-65

Cephalopelvimetry
• Lateral Position
Colcher — Sussman Technique

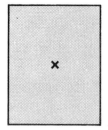

Film Size:
   14 x 17 in. (35 x 43 cm.)

Bucky:
- Moving or stationary grid.

Patient Position:
- Standing lateral preferred.
- Recumbent lateral, if necessary.
- Have patient rotate into a left lateral position.
- Extend legs so femurs will not overlie symphysis pubis.
- Body must be perfectly lateral; check back, pelvis and legs.

Part Position:
- Pelvis must be true lateral.

Central Ray:
- C.R. perpendicular to film holder.
- Center to most palpable part of right greater trochanter.
- 40 in. (102 cm.) F.F.D.

NOTE: • Set pelvimeter at level of gluteal fold and place within upper gluteal fold. • Pelvimeter should be visible on lateral margin of radiograph. **DO NOT** cut off ruler. • Use fast screens and fast film. • Suspend respiration on exhalation after several deep breaths and in between contractions. • Upright position allows fetus to descend maximally into pelvis.

Structures Best Shown:
Pelvic landmarks defining inlet, midpelvis and outlet, plus fetal head unless presentation is breech.

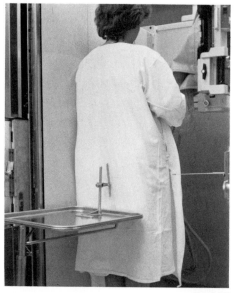

Standing Lateral   Fig. 9-67

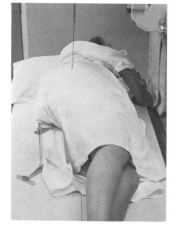
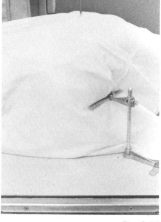

Recumbent Lateral   Fig. 9-68

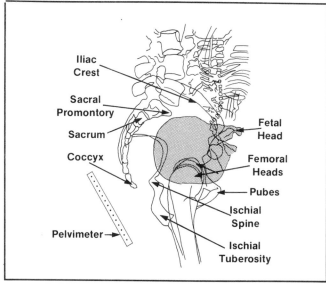

Fig. 9-70

Lateral Cephalopelvimetry

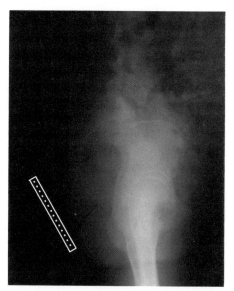

Lateral   Fig. 9-69
Cephalopelvimetry

CHAPTER 10
Radiographic Anatomy and Positioning
of the
Cranium, Sella Turcica
and Petrous Pyramids

Part I. Radiographic Anatomy
Cranium, Sella Turcica and Petrous Pyramids

Skull

The **skull** or bony skeleton of the head is divided into two main portions; the **cranium,** which consists of eight separate bones, and the fourteen **facial bones.** The cranium is that part of the skull that surrounds and protects the brain, while that portion anterior and inferior to the brain case is termed the facial skeleton or the facial bones. The eight cranial bones will be studied in this chapter and will be referred to as the cranium.

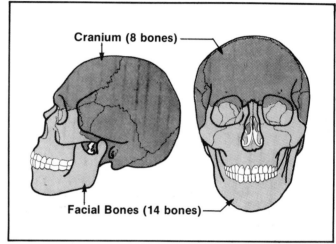

Skull — Bony Skeleton of Head

Fig. 10-1

Cranial Topography (surface landmarks)

Certain surface landmarks and localizing lines must be used for accurate positioning of the cranium. Each of these topographical structures can either be seen or palpated. The smooth prominence between the eyebrows and above the bridge of the nose is the **glabella.** The **acanthion** is the midline point at the junction of the upper lip and the nasal septum. This is the point where the nose and upper lip meet.

A flat triangular area projects forward as the chin in the human. The midpoint of this triangular area of the chin as is appears from the front is termed the **mental point** (see *Fig. 10-2*). Under each eyebrow is a ridge of bone, and slightly above this ridge is a groove or depression termed the **supraorbital groove** or **S.O.G.** The S.O.G. is important because it corresponds to the highest level of the facial bone mass, which is also the level of the floor of the anterior fossa of the cranial vault.

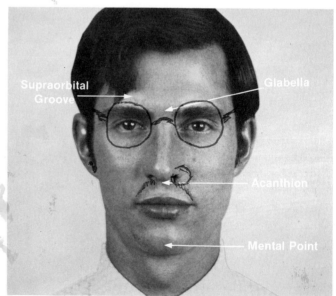

Surface Landmarks

Fig. 10-2

The **glabella, acanthion** and **mental point** are shown in *Fig. 10-3* as seen from the side of the head. The **nasion** is the depression at the bridge of the nose. Anatomically, the nasion is the junction of the two nasal bones and the frontal bone. The **gonion** refers to the lower posterior angle on each side of the jaw or mandible.

The **vertex** is the most superior portion of the skull or the very top of the cranium. The **inion,** also called the **external occipital protuberance,** is the bump along the midline of the lower back of the head. The approximate locations of the vertex and inion are shown in *Fig. 10-3*.

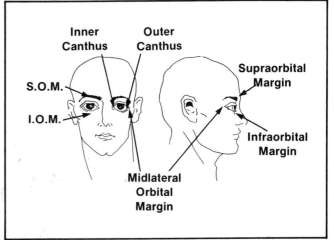

Surface Landmarks   Fig. 10-3

Base of Orbit

Landmarks associated with the eye or base of the bony orbit are shown in *Fig. 10-4*. The base of the orbit is the circle of bone forming the base of the bony socket, termed the orbit. The orbit is conical in shape and extends posteriorly from the base. The junctions of the upper and lower eyelids are termed canthi. Thus the **inner canthus** is where the eyelids meet near the nose, while the more lateral junction of the eyelids is termed the **outer canthus.**

The superior rim of the orbital base is termed the **supraorbital margin** or **S.O.M.,** and the inferior rim is termed the **infraorbital margin** or **I.O.M.** Another important landmark is the **midlateral orbital margin,** that portion of the lateral rim near the outer canthus of the eye.

Surface Landmarks   Fig. 10-4

Ear

Many localizing lines utilize the **external auditory meatus (E.A.M.)** as a reference point. The E.A.M. is the opening of the external ear canal. The **auricle** or **pinna** is that portion of external ear not contained within the head, that is, the flap of the ear. The **top of ear attachment (T.E.A.)** is the most superior attachment of the auricle to the scalp or that point where the side-frames of one's eyeglasses rest. The top of the ear attachment is an important landmark because it corresponds to the level of the petrous ridge on each side.

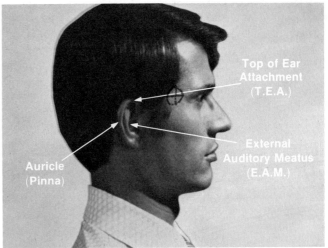

Surface Landmarks   Fig. 10-5

Lines and Planes

The **midsagittal** or median **plane** divides the body into equal left and right halves. This plane is of extreme importance in accurate positioning of the cranium since, for every frontal or lateral position, the midsagittal plane is either perpendicular to or parallel to the plane of the film.

The **interpupillary** or interorbital **line** is a line connecting either the pupils or the outer canthi of the patient's eyes. When the head is placed in a true lateral position, the interpupillary line must be exactly perpendicular to the plane of the film.

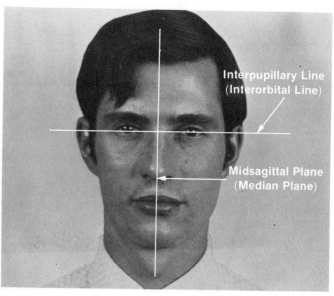

Lines and Planes   Fig. 10-6

Frontal Skull Positioning Lines

Certain positioning lines are important in frontal skull radiography. These lines are formed by connecting certain landmarks to the midpoint of the external auditory meatus (E.A.M.). The most superior of these lines is the **glabellomeatal line,** which is not as precise as the other four since the glabella is an area and not a point. The **orbitomeatal line (O.M.L.)** is a frequently used positioning line located between the outer canthus or midlateral orbital margin and the E.A.M.

The **infraorbitomeatal line (I.O.M.L.)** is formed by connecting the middle of the infraorbital margin to the E.A.M. An older term identifying the same line is Reid's base line. The **acanthiomeatal** and **mentomeatal lines** are important in radiography of the facial bones. These lines are formed by connecting the acanthion and the mental point, respectively, to the E.A.M.

Infraorbital is used on submentovertex

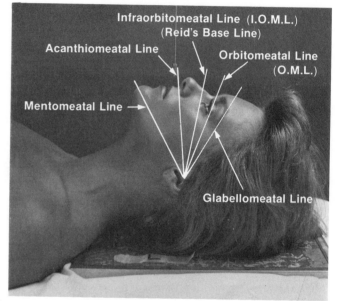

Positioning Lines   Fig. 10-7

Acanthiomeatal in mainly used on facial bones

A straightedge can be used, as shown in *Fig. 10-8,* to accurately position the cranium. In this case, the orbitomeatal line has been placed perpendicular to the film plane by depressing the chin. The chin can be raised or lowered to change the perpendicular reference line to be used.

Mentomeatal (waters) mostly used on sinuses

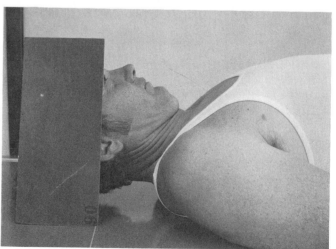

Frontal Positioning   Fig. 10-8

Cranium

The eight bones of the cranium are further divided into calvarium or skull cap, and floor. Each of these areas more or less consists of four bones.

Calvarium (Skull Cap)
(1) Frontal Bone
(2) Left Parietal Bone
(3) Right Parietal Bone
(4) Occipital Bone

Floor
(5) Sphenoid Bone
(6) Ethmoid Bone
(7) Left Temporal Bone
(8) Right Temporal Bone

Frontal Bone

As viewed from the front, the only bone of the calvarium readily visible is the **frontal bone.** This bone, which forms the forehead and the superior part of each orbit, consists of two main parts. The **squamous** or **vertical portion** forms the forehead, while the orbital or horizontal portion forms the superior part of the orbits. The **glabella** is the smooth prominence between the eyebrows and above the bridge of the nose. The **supraorbital groove (S.O.G.)** is the depression above each eyebrow. The superior rim of each orbit is the **supraorbital margin** or **S.O.M.** That ridge of bone beneath each eyebrow is termed the **superciliary arch.** Between the superciliary arches is the glabella. On each side of the squama, above the supraorbital grooves, is a rounded prominence termed the **frontal eminence.**

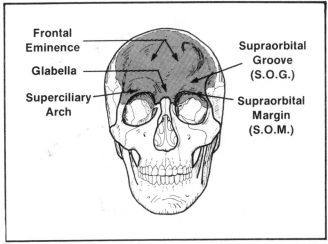

Squamous Portion of Frontal Bone

Fig. 10-9

Inferior View of Frontal Bone

As seen from the inferior aspect, the frontal bone shows primarily the **horizontal** or **orbital portion.** The **supraorbital margins,** the **superciliary arches,** the **glabella** and the **frontal eminences** can all be seen. The **orbital plate** on each side forms the superior part of each orbit. Below the orbital plates lie facial bones, and above the orbital plates is the anterior part of the floor of the brain case. The supraorbital groove is the external landmark at the level of the orbital plates. Each orbital plate is separated from the other by the **ethmoidal notch.** The ethmoid bone, one of the bones of the floor of the cranium, fits into this notch. The **frontal spine** is found at the anterior end of the ethmoidal notch.

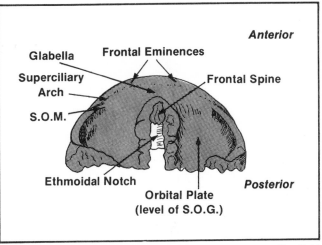

Orbital Portion of Frontal Bone

Fig. 10-10

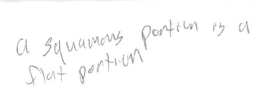
a squamous portion is a flat portion

Parietal Bones

The paired **parietal bones** are well demonstrated on the side and top view drawings in *Fig. 10-11.* The lateral walls of the cranium and part of the roof are formed by the two parietal bones. Each of the parietals is roughly square in shape and has a concave internal surface. The widest portion of the entire skull is located between the **parietal eminences** of the two parietal bones. The frontal bone is primarily anterior to the parietals, the occipital is posterior, and the temporals are inferior.

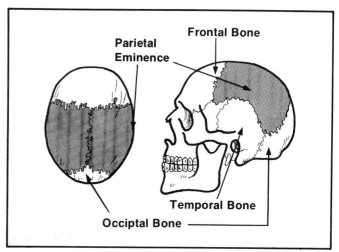

Parietal Bones   Fig. 10-11

Joints of the Cranium (Sutures). Each parietal bone is roughly square in shape. Each of the four sides of one parietal articulates with another bone of the skull. These articulations or joints are called **sutures** and belong in the class of joints termed **synarthrodial** or immovable joints. The **coronal suture** separates the frontal bone from the two parietals. Separating the two parietal bones in the midline is the **sagittal suture.**

Posteriorly, the **lambdoidal suture** separates the two parietals from the occipital bone. The **squamosal suture** is formed by the inferior junction of each parietal bone with the respective temporal bone.

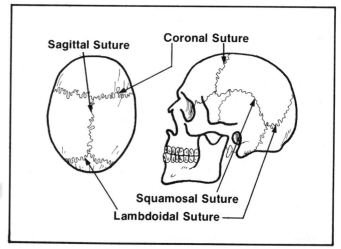

Joints of Cranium   Fig. 10-12

Each end of the sagittal suture is identified as a point or area with a specific name. The anterior end of the sagittal suture is termed the **bregma**, while the posterior end is the **lambda.** The **vertex** is the most superior part of the cranium, usually lying slightly posterior to the bregma. Early in life, the bregma and lambda are not bony, but are soft spots. These soft spots are termed the **anterior** and **posterior fontanels** in the newborn. Later, when bone fills in these areas, they are called the bregma and lambda.

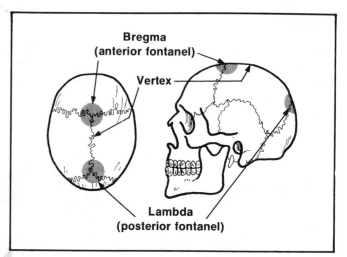

Cranial Landmarks   Fig. 10-13

Occipital Bone

The inferoposterior portion of the calvarium or skull cap is formed by the single occipital bone. The external surface of the occipital bone presents a rounded part termed the **squamous portion.** The squamous portion forms most of the back of the head and is that part of the occipital bone superior to the **foramen magnum.** Foramen magnum literally means "great hole" and is the avenue by which the spinal cord leaves the brain. The prominent bump on the squamous portion of the occipital bone is the **inion** or **external occipital protuberance.**

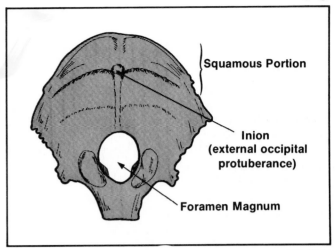

Occipital Bone   Fig. 10-14

Temporal Bones

The paired **temporal bones** are complex structures housing the delicate organs of hearing and balance. As seen from the side in *Fig. 10-15*, the left temporal bone is situated between the sphenoid bone anteriorly and the occipital bone posteriorly. The thin upper portion of each temporal forms part of the wall of the cranium, termed the **squamous** portion. This part of the skull is quite thin and is therefore the most vulnerable portion of the entire skull to fracture, which may result in hemorrhage beneath the bony surface.

Extending anteriorly from the squamous portion of the temporal bone is an arch of bone termed the **zygomatic process.** This process meets the temporal process of the zygomatic or malar bone to form the easily palpated zygomatic arch. Inferior to the zygomatic process and just anterior to the **external auditory meatus** is the **temporomandibular fossa,** into which the mandible fits to form a diarthrodial joint called the **T.M.J.** or **temporomandibular joint.** Between the mandible and the E.A.M. is a slender bony projection called the **styloid process.**

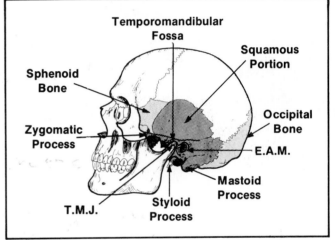

Temporal Bone   Fig. 10-15

The second main portion of the temporal bone is that area posterior to the E.A.M., the **mastoid** portion. Extending downward from this portion is the easily palpated **mastoid process** or **tip.** Many air cells are located within the mastoid process.

The floor of the cranium is well visualized in *Fig. 10-16*. The single occipital bone resides between the paired temporal bones. The third main portion of each temporal bone is the **petrous** portion, often termed the **petrous pyramid** or **pars petrosa.** This pyramid-shaped portion of the temporal bone is the thickest and densest bone in the cranium. The petrous pyramid projects forward and toward the midline from the **external auditory meatus.** The delicate organs of hearing and balance are housed in and protected by the petrous pyramids. The upper edges of the pyramids are often called the **petrous ridges.** The petrous ridge corresponds to the level of the external landmark, the T.E.A. or top of the ear attachment. Medially, each petrous pyramid ends with the **internal auditory meatus,** which serves to transmit the nerves of hearing and equilibrium.

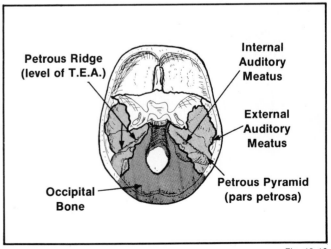

Temporal Bones (superior view)   Fig. 10-16

Sphenoid Bone

The single **sphenoid bone** forms the anchor for all eight cranial bones. The central portion of the sphenoid is the body, which lies in the midline of the floor of the cranium. The central depression on the body is termed the **sella turcica.** This depression looks like a saddle from the side and derives its name from words meaning Turkish saddle. The sella turcica partially surrounds and protects the master gland of the body, the pituitary gland. Posterior to the sella turcica is the back of the saddle, the **dorsum sellae.**

Extending laterally from the body to either side are two pairs of wings. The smaller pair, termed the **lesser wings,** are triangular in shape and are nearly horizontal. They project laterally from the upper, anterior portion of the body and extend to about the middle of each orbit. The **greater wings** extend laterally from the sides of the body and form a portion of the floor of the cranium, as well as a portion of the sides of the cranium.

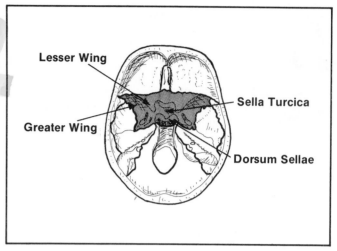

Sphenoid Bone

Fig. 10-17

An oblique drawing of the sphenoid bone in *Fig. 10-18* demonstrates the complexity of this bone. Using one's imagination, the shape of the sphenoid has been compared to a bat with its wings and legs extended as in flight. The centrally located depression, the **sella turcica,** is better seen on this view. The posterior part of the saddle is the **dorsum sellae.** Two small earlike projections of bone are seen extending superiorly from the dorsum sellae. These are termed the **posterior clinoid processes.** Arising from the most posterior aspect of the **lesser wings** are two more bony projections termed **anterior clinoid processes.** The anterior clinoids are somewhat larger and are spread further apart than are the posterior clinoid processes.

Projecting downward from the inferior surface of the body are four processes that correspond to the legs of the imaginary bat. The more lateral, somewhat flat extensions are termed the **pterygoid processes.** Directly medial to these are two more pointed processes called the **pterygoid hamuli.**

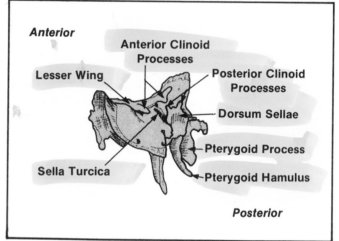

Sphenoid Bone (oblique view)

Fig. 10-18

Sella Turcica (lateral). In a true lateral position, the **sella turcica** would look similar to the drawing in *Fig. 10-19.* Deformity of the sella turcica is often the only clue that a lesion exists intracranially; therefore, radiography of the sella turcica may be very important. The depression of the sella turcica and the **dorsum sellae** are best seen from the side. The **anterior clinoid processes** are seen anterior to the sella turcica, while the **posterior clinoid processes** are demonstrated superior to the dorsum sellae.

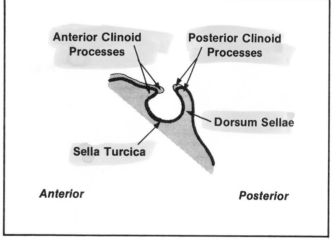

Sella Turcica (lateral)

Fig. 10-19

Ethmoid Bone

The single ethmoid bone lies primarily below the floor of the cranium. The top of the ethmoid is shown on the left in *Fig. 10-20,* situated in the ethmoidal notch of the frontal bone. The horizontal portion of the bone is termed the **cribriform plate** and contains many small openings or foramina through which pass the olfactory nerves, the nerves of smell. Projecting superiorly from the cribriform plate, similar to a rooster's comb, is the **crista galli.**

The major portion of the ethmoid lies beneath the floor of the cranium. Projecting downward in the midline is the **perpendicular plate** which helps to form the bony nasal septum. The two **lateral masses** or **labyrinths** are suspended from the under surface of the cribriform plate on each side of the perpendicular plate. The lateral masses contain many air cells and help to form the medial walls of the orbits and the lateral walls of the nasal cavity. Extending medially and downward from the medial wall of each labyrinth are thin scroll-shaped projections of bone. These projections are termed the **superior** and **middle nasal conchae** or **turbinates.**

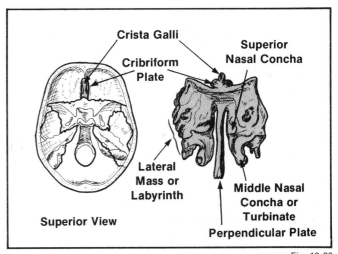

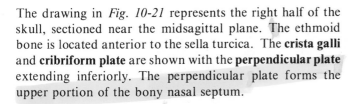

Ethmoid Bone   Fig. 10-20

The drawing in *Fig. 10-21* represents the right half of the skull, sectioned near the midsagittal plane. The ethmoid bone is located anterior to the sella turcica. The **crista galli** and **cribriform plate** are shown with the **perpendicular plate** extending inferiorly. The perpendicular plate forms the upper portion of the bony nasal septum.

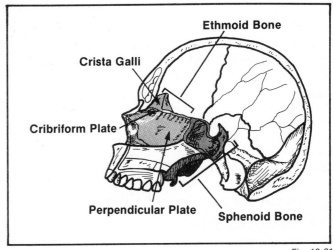

Ethmoid - Sphenoid Bones   Fig. 10-21

Skull Classifications by Shape and Size

Mesocephalic Skull

The shape of the average head is termed **mesocephalic.** The average caliper measurements of the adult skull are 15 centimeters between the parietal eminences, 19 centimeters from frontal eminence to external occipital protuberance, and 23 centimeters from vertex to beneath the chin. While most adults have a skull of the average size and shape, there are exceptions to the rule.

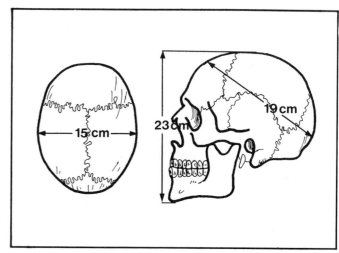

Average Skull (Mesocephalic)   Fig. 10-22

Brachycephalic - Dolichocephalic Skulls

Variations of the average-shaped or mesocephalic skull include the **brachycephalic** and the **dolichocephalic** designations. The short, broad head is termed brachycephalic; while the long, narrow head is called dolichocephalic. The most common radiographic positions and projections are based on the mesocephalic standard, so persons with other skull shapes will require different angulations and rotations than those normally used.

The main variation to remember is the angle difference between the petrous pyramids and the midsagittal plane. In the average-shaped, mesocephalic head, the petrous pyramids form an angle of 45 degrees. An angle greater than 45 degrees (approximately 54 degrees) is found in the brachycephalic skull; while an angle less than 45 degrees (approximately 40 degrees) is found in the dolichocephalic designation.

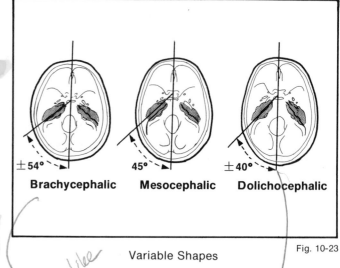

Variable Shapes   Fig. 10-23

Part II. Radiographic Positioning
Cranium, Sella Turcica and Petrous Pyramids

Patient Comfort

Patient motion almost always results in an unsatisfactory radiograph. During skull radiography the head must be placed in precise positions and held there long enough to obtain a motionless exposure. Always remember that there is a patient attached to the other end of the skull being manipulated. If every effort is made to make the body comfortable and to utilize positioning aids such as sponges, sandbags and compression devices, radiographic positioning of the head will be much easier.

Causes of Positioning Errors

When positioning a patient's head, it is necessary to look at various facial features and palpate numerous anatomical landmarks in order to place certain planes precisely in relation to the plane of the film. Although the human body is supposed to be bilaterally symmetrical, that is, the right half is supposed to be exactly like the left half, this supposition is not always true. The ears, nose and jaw are often asymmetrical. The nose frequently deviates to one side of the midsagittal plane, while the ears are not necessarily in the same place nor of the same size on each side. The lower jaw or mandible is also often asymmetrical. Bony parts, such as the mastoid tips and the orbital margins, are safter landmarks to use. While you often look at the patient's eyes during positioning, it is best not to look at the nose in between.

Common Positioning Errors

Rotation and **tilt** are two very common positioning errors. Rotation of the skull almost always results in a retake, therefore it is important that the head is not turned to one side. Tilt is a tipping or slanting to one side, even though rotation is not present. Both rotation and tilt must be avoided in skull positioning.

Basic Projections/Positions

Certain basic projections or positions for the cranium, sella turcica and petrous pyramids are demonstrated and described on the following pages. Departmental routines may vary in different departments or hospitals. **Basic** projections are those projections or positions commonly taken on average, helpful patients. Included in the positioning section is a trauma skull series that can be performed on patients in any condition. A "skull series," which may be relatively easy to perform on a healthy subject, may become very difficult on a sick, injured or uncooperative patient.

Radiographic examination of the cranium requires a minimum of two positions or projections. Four positions or projections of the cranium are considered standard or basic. A trauma skull series requires a minimum of three positions or projections.

Basic positions or projections are also described and demonstrated for visualization of the sella turcica and the petrous pyramids.

Skull Series
Basic
- Lateral
- P.A. (Caldwell)
- Semiaxial A.P.
  (Occipital or Towne)
- Basilar or Submentovertex

Skull Series
Trauma
- Lateral
  Horizontal Beam
- A.P.
- Semiaxial A.P.

Sella Turcica
Basic
- Lateral
- Semiaxial A.P.

Petrous Pyramids
Basic
- Semiaxial A.P.
- Submentovertex

---

infra orbital line is only used on submental vertex

Cranium

• Lateral Position

Skull Series
Basic
- **Lateral**
- P.A. (Caldwell)
- Semiaxial A.P. (Occipital or Towne)
- Basilar or Submentovertex

Film Size:
   10 x 12 in. (24 x 30 cm.) Crosswise.

Bucky:
- Moving or stationary grid.

Patient Position:
- Semiprone or upright with head turned to lateral position.
- Remove all metallic, plastic or other removable objects from head and neck.

Part Position:
- Head in true lateral.
- Interpupillary line perpendicular to table.
- Midsagittal plane parallel to table.
- Radiolucent support under chin.
- Infraorbitomeatal line perpendicular to front edge of cassette.
- Closely collimate and immobilize.
- Side of interest closest to film.

Central Ray:
- For entire cranium, C.R. perpendicular to film, passing through a point 1 in. (2.5 cm.) anterosuperior to the top of the ear attachment (T.E.A.).
- 40 in. (102 cm.) F.F.D.

NOTE: • Routine may include both laterals or one lateral in stereo. • Mandibular rami and orbital roofs should superimpose.

Structures Best Shown:
Lateral cranium closest to film, sella turcica, anterior and posterior clinoid processes, dorsum sellae and sphenoid sinus.

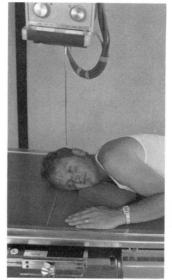
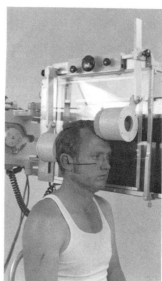

Lateral   Fig. 10-24

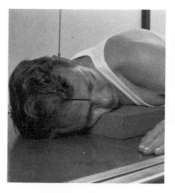
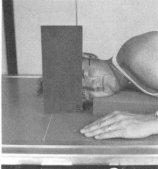

Lateral   Fig. 10-25

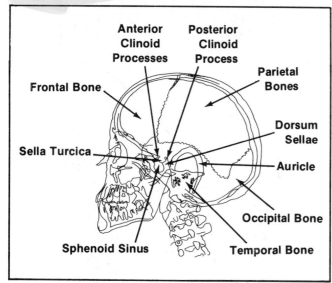

Fig. 10-27

Lateral

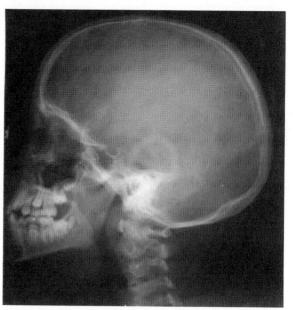

Lateral   Fig. 10-26

Skull Series
Basic
- Lateral
- **P.A.** (Caldwell)
- Semiaxial A.P.
  (Occipital or Towne)
- Basilar or Submentovertex

Cranium
• Posteroanterior (P.A.) Projection
Caldwell Position

Film Size:
    10 x 12 in. (24 x 30 cm.)

Bucky:
- Moving or stationary grid.

Patient Position:
- Prone or upright.

Part Position:
- Orbitomeatal line perpendicular to table.
- Forehead and nose touch table.
- No rotation or tilt.
- Midsagittal plane perpendicular to table.
- Closely collimate and immobilize.

Central Ray:
- Tube angled 15° caudad
- C.R. passes through nasion.
- 40 in. (102 cm.) F.F.D.

NOTE: • Petrous pyramids should fill lower third of orbits. • Distance from midlateral orbital margin to lateral margin of cranium same on both sides.

Structures Best Shown:
Frontal bone, frontal and ethmoid paranasal sinuses, greater and lesser wings of sphenoid, crista galli, petrous ridges and internal auditory canals.

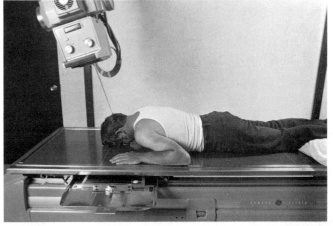

P.A.

Fig. 10-28

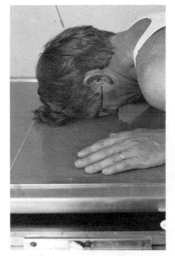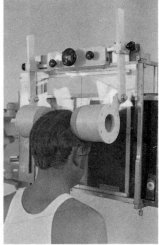

P.A.

Fig. 10-29

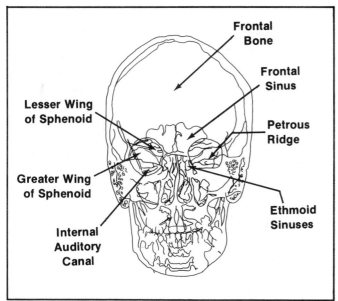

Fig. 10-31   P.A.

Frontal Bone

Frontal Sinus

Lesser Wing of Sphenoid

Petrous Ridge

Greater Wing of Sphenoid

Internal Auditory Canal

Ethmoid Sinuses

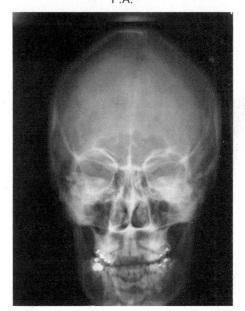

P.A.   Fig. 10-30

Skull Series
Basic
- Lateral
- P.A. (Caldwell)
- **Semiaxial A.P.**
  (Occipital or Towne)
- Basilar or Submentovertex

• Semiaxial Anteroposterior Projection
Occipital or Towne Position

Film Size:
>   10 x 12 in. (24 x 30 cm.)

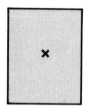

Bucky:
- Moving or stationary grid.

Patient Position:
- Supine or upright.

Part Position:
- Orbitomeatal line perpendicular to table.
- No rotation or tilt.
- Midsagittal plane perpendicular to table.
- Top of film same level as vertex.
- Closely collimate and immobilize.

Central Ray:
- Tube angled 30° caudad.
- C.R. enters at hairline, passing through a line connecting both E.A.M.'s.
- 40 in. (102 cm.) F.F.D.

NOTE: • If infraorbitomeatal line is perpendicular to table, angle tube 37° caudad (See *Fig. 10-33*.). • An angle of **30° between O.M.L. and C.R.** should be achieved.

Structures Best Shown
Occipital bone, petrous pyramids, posterior foramen magnum with dorsum sellae and posterior clinoids in its shadow.

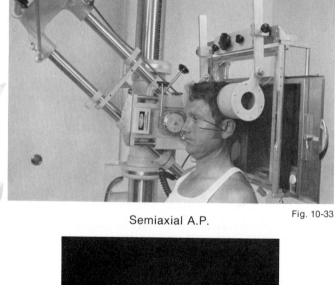

Semiaxial A.P.   Fig. 10-32

Semiaxial A.P.   Fig. 10-33

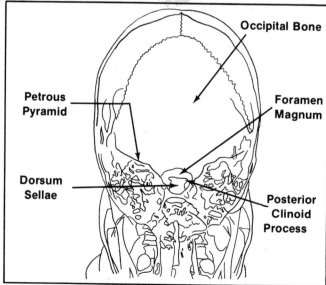

Fig. 10-35

Semiaxial A.P.

Occipital Bone

Petrous Pyramid

Foramen Magnum

Dorsum Sellae

Posterior Clinoid Process

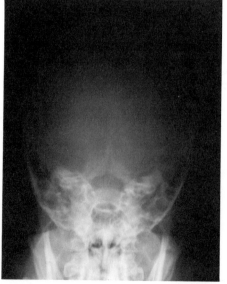

Semiaxial A.P.   Fig. 10-34

Skull Series

Basic
- Lateral
- P.A. (Caldwell)
- Semiaxial A.P. (Occipital or Towne)
- **Basilar or Submentovertex**

Cranium

• Submentovertex Projection
Basilar Position

Film Size:

10 x 12 in. (24 x 30 cm.)

Bucky:
- Moving or stationary grid.

Patient Position:
- Supine (supports under back, knees flexed) or upright.

Part Position:
- Infraorbitomeatal line parallel to table.
- Midsagittal plane perpendicular to table.
- Head rests on vertex.
- Neck hyperextended.
- Closely collimate and immobilize.

Central Ray:
- C.R. must be perpendicular to infraorbitomeatal line.
- C.R. enters midway between gonia, exits at vertex passing through sella turcica.
- 40 in. (102 cm.) F.F.D.

NOTE: • C.R. must be **perpendicular to I.O.M.L.** (tube may have to be angled to accomplish this). • Mandibular condyles must be anterior to petrous pyramids. • Check mandible for asymmetry on radiograph. • Very uncomfortable — patient should be in position a minimum amount of time.

Structures Best Shown:

Cranial base, petrous pyramids, mastoid processes, sphenoid sinus, mandible and foramen magnum.

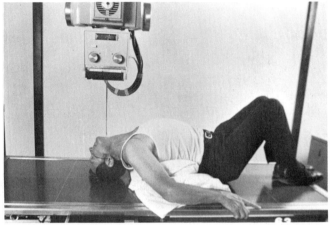

Submentovertex

Fig. 10-36

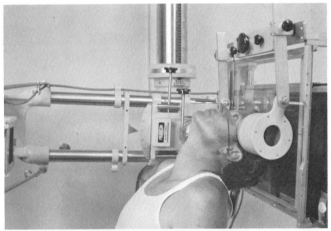

Submentovertex

Fig. 10-37

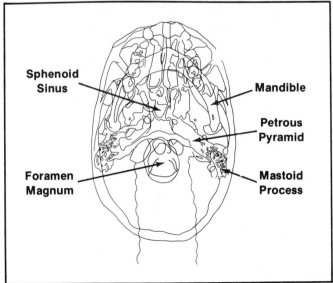

Fig. 10-39

Submentovertex

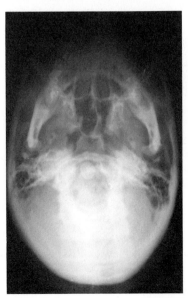

Submentovertex

Fig. 10-38

205

Skull Series
Trauma
• **Lateral -**
   Horizontal Beam
• **A.P.**
• **Semiaxial A.P.**

Film Size:
    10 x 12 in. (24 x 30 cm.)

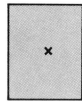

Bucky:
- Moving or stationary grid.

Patient Position:
- Supine.

Part Position:
Lateral
- Head in true lateral.
- Elevate occiput on sponge or towel.
- Side of injury closest to film.
- Use grid cassette placed vertically.
- Horizontal beam essential.
- Center for entire cranium.
A.P.
- No rotation or tilt.
- Center to nasion.
- C.R. forms a 15° cephalic angle with O.M.L.
Semiaxial A.P.
- No rotation or tilt.
- Top of grid cassette level with vertex.
- C.R. forms a 30° caudal angle with O.M.L.
- Caudal angle will be 37° if I.O.M.L. is perpendicular to grid.
- 40 in. (102 cm.) F.F.D.

NOTE: • **Rule out cervical spine fracture or dislocation before** attempting trauma skull series.

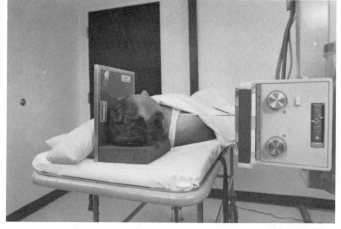

Trauma Lateral   Fig. 10-40

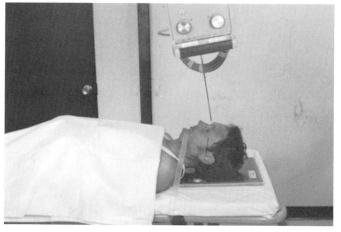

Trauma A.P.   Fig. 10-41

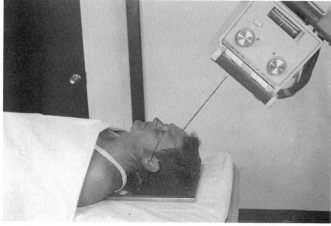

Fig. 10-43   Trauma Semiaxial A.P.

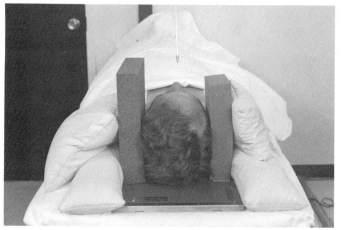

Trauma A.P.   Fig. 10-42

Sella Turcica
Basic
• Lateral
• Semiaxial A.P.

Sella Turcica

• Lateral Position

Film Size:

    8 x 10 in. (18 x 24 cm.)
    Collimated.

Bucky:
- Moving or stationary grid.

Patient Position:
- Semiprone or upright with head turned to lateral position.

Part Position:
- Head in true lateral.
- Interpupillary line perpendicular to table.
- Midsagittal plane parallel to table.

Central Ray
- C.R. perpendicular to film, passing through a point ¾ in. (2 cm.) anterior **and** superior to external auditory meatus (E.A.M.).
- 40 in. (102 cm.) F.F.D.

NOTE: • Enlargement of pituitary gland may cause erosion or enlargement of sella turcica. • A **true lateral** position and **close collimation** are essential.

Structures Best Shown:
Sella turcica, anterior and posterior clinoid processes and dorsum sellae.

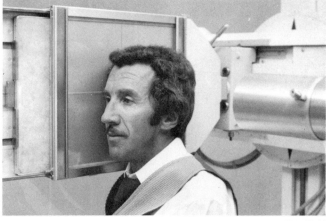

Lateral Sella Turcica

Fig. 10-44

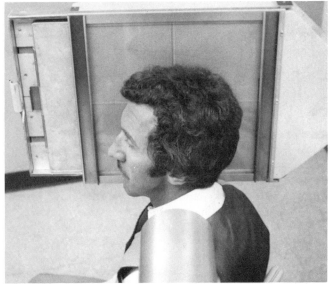

Lateral Sella Turcica

Fig. 10-45

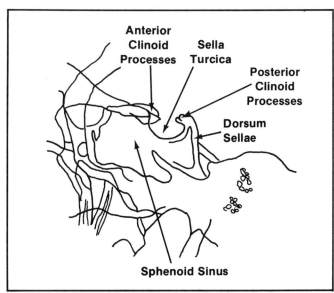

Fig. 10-47

Lateral Sella Turcica

Anterior Clinoid Processes
Sella Turcica
Posterior Clinoid Processes
Dorsum Sellae
Sphenoid Sinus

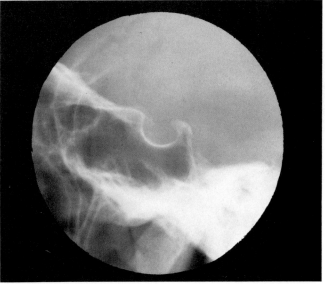

Lateral Sella Turcica

Fig. 10-46

Sella Turcica
Basic
• Lateral
• Semiaxial A.P.

Sella Turcica

• Semiaxial Anteroposterior Projection

Film Size:
    8 x 10 in. (18 x 24 cm.)
    Collimated.

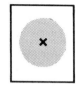

Bucky:
- Moving or stationary grid.

Patient Position:
- Supine or upright.

Part Position:
- O.M.L. perpendicular to table.
- No rotation or tilt.
- Midsagittal plane perpendicular to table.

Central Ray:
- Tube angled 30° caudad.
- C.R. enters at hairline and passes through a line connecting both E.A.M.'s.
- 40 in. (102 cm.) F.F.D.

NOTE: • This projection is the same as for a skull series, but extension cylinder should be used to collimate to area of interest.

Structures Best Shown:
Dorsum sellae and posterior clinoids within shadow of foramen magnum.

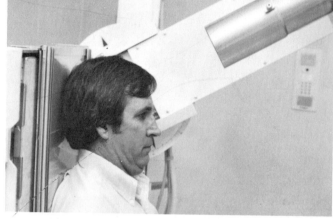

Semiaxial A.P. Sella Turcica   Fig. 10-48

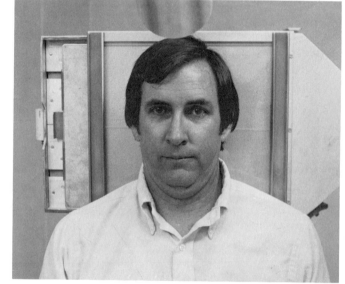

Semiaxial A.P. Sella Turcica   Fig. 10-49

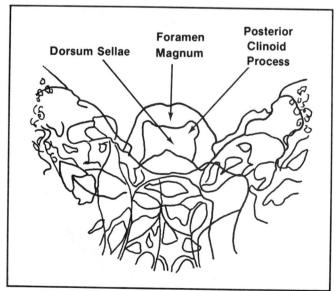

Fig. 10-51

Semiaxial A.P. Sella Turcica

Dorsum Sellae   **Foramen Magnum**   **Posterior Clinoid Process**

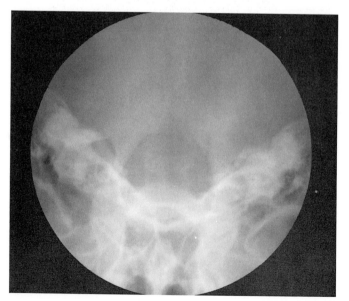

Semiaxial A.P. Sella Turcica   Fig. 10-50

Petrous Pyramids
Basic
- Semiaxial A.P.
- Submentovertex

Petrous Pyramids

- **Semiaxial Anteroposterior Projection**
- **Submentovertex Projection**

Film Size:
   10 x 12 in. (24 x 30 cm.)

Bucky:
- Moving or stationary grid.

Patient Position:
- Supine or upright.

Part Position:
Semiaxial A.P.
- O.M.L. perpendicular to table.
- No rotation or tilt.
- Midsagittal plane perpendicular to table.

Submentovertex
- I.O.M.L. parallel to film.
- No rotation or tilt.
- Midsagittal plane perpendicular to table.

Central Ray:
Semiaxial A.P.
- Tube angled 30° caudad.
- C.R. enters at hairline and passes through a line connecting E.A.M.'s.

Submentovertex
- C.R. perpendicular to I.O.M.L.
- C.R. enters inferior to mentum, exits at vertex and passes through sella turcica.
- 40 in. (102 cm.) F.F.D.

NOTE: • These projections are the same as for a skull series, but collimation is to petrous pyramids. • If infra-orbitomeatal line is perpendicular to table, as in *Fig. 10-52,* angle tube 37° caudad.

Structures Best Shown:
Bilateral petrous pyramids.

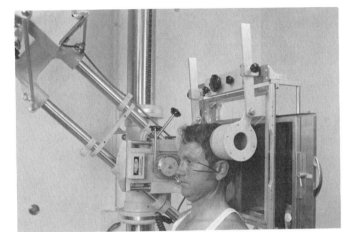
Semiaxial A.P.   Fig. 10-52

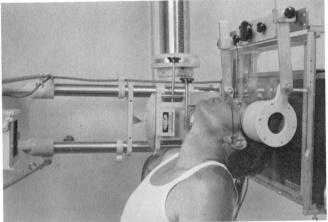
Submentovertex   Fig. 10-53

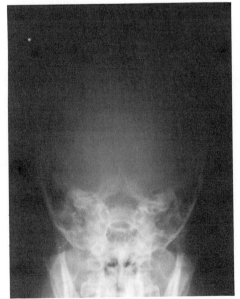
Fig. 10-55
Semiaxial A.P.

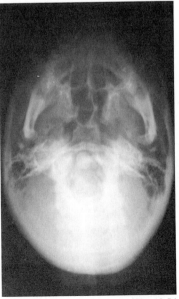
Fig. 10-54
Submentovertex

CHAPTER 11

Radiographic Anatomy and Positioning of the
Facial Bones, Zygomatic Arches and Optic Foramina

Part I. Radiographic Anatomy
Facial Bones, Zygomatic Arches and Optic Foramina

Facial Bones

The skull or bony skeleton of the head consists of **14 facial bones** listed and described in this chapter, and 8 cranial bones described in Chapter 10. The 14 facial bones contribute to the shape and form of a person's face. In addition, the cavities of the orbits, nose and mouth are largely constructed from the bones of the face. Of the 14 bones making up the facial skeleton, only 2 are single bones. The remaining 12 consist of six pairs of bones with similar bones on each side of the face.

Facial Bones

2	-	Maxillae (Upper Jaw) or Maxillary Bones
2	-	Zygomatic or Malar Bones
2	-	Lacrimal Bones
2	-	Nasal Bones
2	-	Inferior Nasal Conchae
2	-	Palatine Bones
1	-	Vomer
1	-	Mandible (Lower Jaw)

____

14   Total

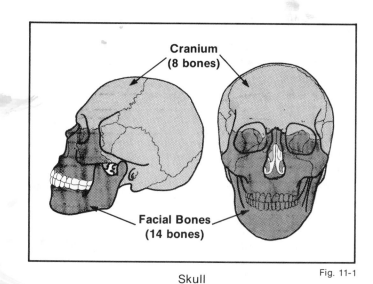

Skull

Fig. 11-1

3M
Never leave positions in vein

Maxillae

The two **maxillae** or **maxillary bones** are the largest immovable bones of the face. The only facial bone that is larger than the maxilla is the movable lower jaw or mandible. All of the other bones of the upper facial area are closely associated with the two maxillae, thus they are structurally the most important bones of the upper face. The right and left maxillary bones are solidly united at the midline below the nasal septum. Each maxilla assists in the formation of three cavities of the face: (1) the mouth, (2) the nasal cavity, and (3) one orbit.

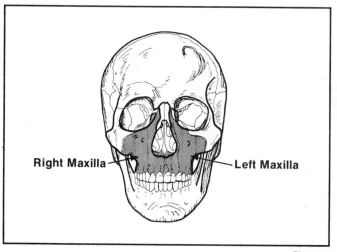

Maxillae

Fig. 11-2

Each maxilla consists of a centrally located **body** and three processes projecting from that body. A fourth process, to be described later in this chapter, can only be seen on the inferior aspect of each maxilla. The body of each maxilla is the centrally located portion that lies lateral to the nose. One of the three processes seen in *Fig. 11-3* is the **frontal process,** which projects upward along the lateral border of the nose toward the frontal bone. The **zygomatic process** projects laterally to unite with the zygomatic or malar bone. The third process, the **alveolar process,** is the inferior or lower aspect of the body of each maxilla. The eight upper teeth on each side are embedded in cavities along the inferior margin of the alveolar process.

The two maxillae are solidly united in the midline anteriorly. At the upper part of this midline union, directly beneath the acanthion, is the **anterior nasal spine.** A blow to the nose sometimes results in this nasal spine being separated from the maxillae.

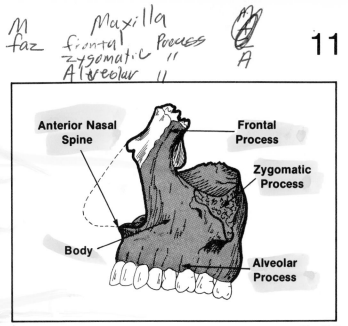

Left Maxilla

Fig. 11-3

The relationship of the two maxillary bones to the remainder of the bones of the skull is well demonstrated in *Fig. 11-4*. Note the three processes seen in a frontal view of the skull. Extending upward toward the frontal bone is the **frontal process.** Extending laterally toward the zygomatic or malar bone is the **zygomatic process,** and supporting the upper teeth is the **alveolar process.** The body of each maxillary bone contains a large air-filled cavity known as a **maxillary sinus.** There are several of these air-filled cavities found in certain bones of the skull. These sinuses communicate with the nasal cavity and are collectively termed paranasal sinuses.

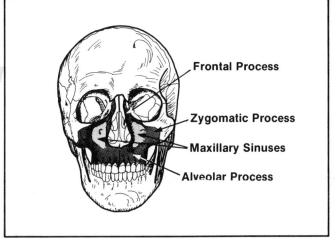

Maxillae

Fig. 11-4

Hard Palate (inferior surface)

The fourth process of each maxillary bone is the **palatine process,** which can only be demonstrated on an inferior view of the two maxillae. The two palatine processes form the anterior portion of the roof of the mouth, called the hard or bony palate. The two palatine processes are solidly united in the midline to form a synarthrodial joint. A common congenital defect called a cleft palate is an opening left between the palatine processes, caused by an incomplete joining of the two bones.

The posterior part of the hard palate is formed by the horizontal portions of two other facial bones, the **palatine bones.** Note that the posterior part of the hard palate is formed by the palatine bones, while the anterior part of the hard palate is formed by the palatine processes of the two maxillary bones.

The most inferior portions of the sphenoid bone of the cranium are also shown on the inferior view of the hard palate in *Fig. 11-5*. These two processes, the **pterygoid hamuli,** are likened to the outstretched legs of a bat (Chapter 10).

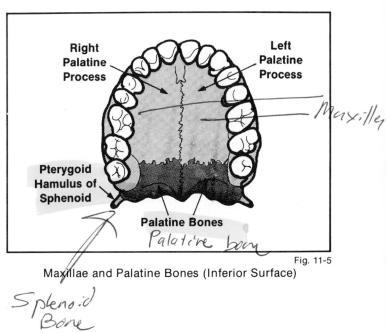

Maxillae and Palatine Bones (Inferior Surface)

Fig. 11-5

Zygomatic (Malar) Bone

One **zygomatic bone,** or **malar bone,** is located lateral to the zygomatic process of each maxilla. These bones form the prominence of the cheek and make up the lower outer portion of each orbit. The malar bone articulates with the frontal, sphenoid and temporal bones of the cranium. Projecting posteriorly from the zygomatic bone is a slender process connecting with the zygomatic process of the temporal bone to form the **zygomatic arch.** The zygomatic arch is a fairly delicate structure and is sometimes fractured or "caved in" by a blow to the cheek. Note that the zygomatic arch is formed in part by the zygomatic or malar bone, and in part by the temporal bone.

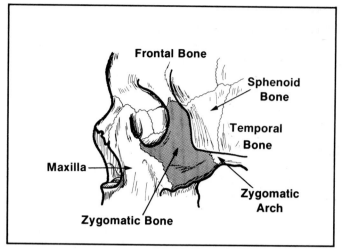

Zygomatic (Malar) Bone   Fig. 11-6

Nasal and Lacrimal Bones

The **lacrimal** and **nasal** bones are the thinnest and most fragile bones in the entire body. The two very delicate lacrimal bones lie anteriorly on the medial side of each orbit. Lacrimal, derived from a word meaning tear, is appropriate since the lacrimal bones are closely associated with the tear ducts.

The two nasal bones form the bridge of the nose and are somewhat variable in size. Some persons have very prominent nasal bones, while others are quite small. Much of the nose is made up of cartilage, but the upper portion at the bridge of the nose is formed by the two nasal bones.

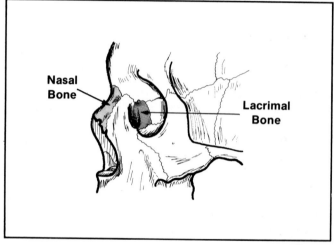

Nasal and Lacrimal Bones   Fig. 11-7

The two **nasal bones** join in the midline to form a suture or synarthrodial joint. The point of junction of the two nasal bones with the frontal bone is a positioning landmark termed the **nasion.** The **frontal process of each maxilla** extends upward on each side to lie between one nasal bone and the lacrimal bone.

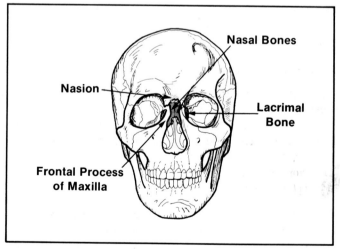

Nasal and Lacrimal Bones   Fig. 11-8

214

Inferior Nasal Conchae

Within the nasal cavity are two thin, curved or scroll-shaped facial bones termed the **inferior nasal conchae** or **turbinates.** These two bones project from the lateral walls of the nasal cavity on each side and extend medially. The **superior** and **middle nasal conchae** or turbinates are similar scroll-like projections that extend from the ethmoid bone into the nasal cavities.

In summary, there are three pairs of nasal conchae or turbinates. The superior and middle pair are parts of the ethmoid bone, while the inferior pair are separate facial bones. The effect of the three pair of turbinates is to divide the nasal cavities into various departments. These irregular compartments tend to break up or mix the flow of air coming into the nasal cavities before it reaches the lungs. In this way the incoming air is somewhat warmed and cleaned before reaching the lungs.

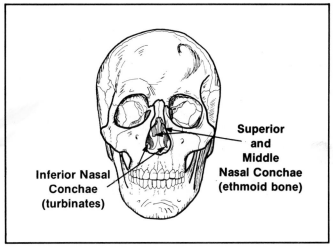

Inferior Nasal Conchae

Fig. 11-9

Inferior Nasal Conchae and Palatine Bones

The relationship between the various nasal conchae and the lateral wall of one nasal cavity is illustrated in *Fig. 11-10.* In this illustration, the midline structures making up the nasal septum have been removed so that the lateral portion of the right nasal cavity can be seen. Note that the **superior** and **middle conchae** are part of the ethmoid bone, and the **inferior nasal conchae** are separate facial bones. The **cribriform plate** and the **crista galli** of the ethmoid bone help to separate the cranium from the facial bone mass.

The two palatine bones are difficult to visualize when studying a dry skeleton because they are located internally and are not visible from the outside. Each palatine bone is roughly L-shaped. The vertical portion of the L extends upward between one maxilla and one pterygoid plate of the sphenoid bone. The horizontal portion of each L helps to make up the posterior portion of the hard palate.

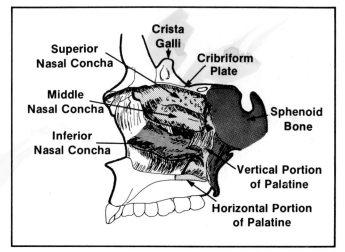

Inferior Nasal Conchae and Palatine Bones

Fig. 11-10

Bony Nasal Septum

The midline structures of the nasal cavity, including the **bony nasal septum,** are shown in *Fig. 11-11.* The bony nasal septum is formed by two bones, the **ethmoid** and the **vomer.** It is formed superiorly by the **perpendicular plate** of the ethmoid bone and inferiorly by the single vomer bone. Anteriorly, the nasal septum is cartilaginous and is termed the **septal cartilage.**

The bony nasal septum is thus formed by the perpendicular plate of the ethmoid bone and the vomer bone, and becomes important radiographically in severe trauma to the nasal bone area. The septum may get pushed to one side, away from the midline. This injury would be termed a deviated nasal septum.

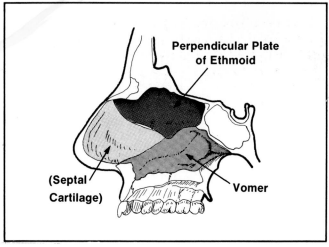

Bony Nasal Septum

Fig. 11-11

Labeled Photographs of Facial Bones

Certain anatomical parts of the facial bones are identified on the photograph of a dry skull in *Fig. 11-12*. Part **A** is the body of the right maxilla; **B** is the frontal process of the right maxilla; **C** is the right nasal bone; **D** is the zygomatic process of left maxilla; and **E** is the alveolar process of the left maxilla.

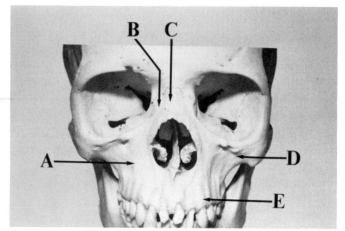

Facial Bones

Fig. 11-12

Those parts labeled in *Fig. 11-13* are: **(A)** vomer, **(B)** perpendicular plate of the ethmoid bone, **(C)** nasion, **(D)** inferior nasal concha, and **(E)** anterior nasal spine.

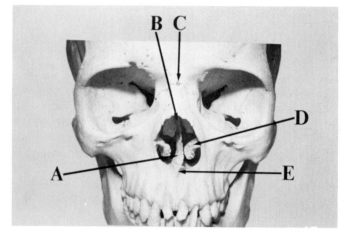

Facial Bones

Fig. 11-13

The lateral view of a dry skull in *Fig. 11-14* identifies the following: **(A)** the zygomatic arch formed by the processes from the temporal bone and the malar or zygomatic bone, **(B)** the right zygomatic or malar bone, **(C)** the right nasal bone, **(D)** the frontal process of the right maxilla, and **(E)** the anterior nasal spine.

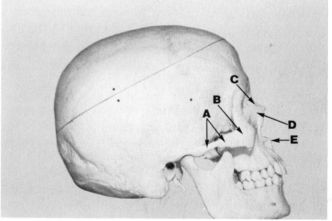

Facial Bones

Fig. 11-14

216

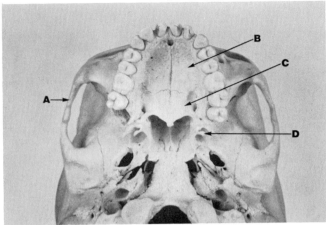

The photograph in *Fig. 11-15* illustrates a dry skull from the inferior aspect with the mandible removed. Part **A** is the right zygomatic arch; **B** is the palatine process of the left maxilla; **C** is the horizontal portion of the left palatine bone; and **D** is the left pterygoid hamulus of the sphenoid bone.

Facial Bones   Fig. 11-15

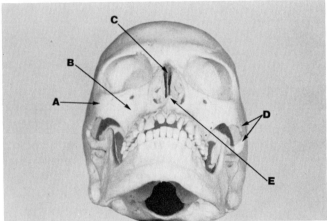

When radiographing the facial bone area, the most common position utilized is the Waters' position. The head is tilted back so that the facial anatomy is projected as shown in the photograph in *Fig. 11-16*. **A** is the right zygomatic or malar bone; **B** is the body of the right maxilla; **C** is the bony nasal septum; **D** is the left zygomatic arch; and **E** is the anterior nasal spine.

Facial Bones (Waters' position)   Fig. 11-16

Orbits

The complex anatomy of the 14 facial bones helps to form several facial cavities. Those cavities formed in total or in part by the facial bones are the mouth or oral cavity, the nasal cavities and the bilateral orbits. The mouth and nasal cavities are primarily passageways and, as such, are not often radiographed specifically; however, the **orbits** containing the vital organs of sight and associated nerves and blood vessels, are often radiographed. The structure and shape of the orbits are illustrated in *Fig. 11-17*. Each orbit is a **cone-shaped,** bony-walled structure composed of parts of seven bones. The rim of the orbit, corresponding to the circular portion of the cone, is called the **base.** The base of the orbit is seldom a true circle, however, and may even look like a figure with four definite sides. The most posterior portion of the cone, the **apex,** corresponds to the **optic foramen** through which the optic nerve passes.

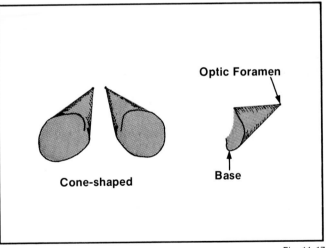

Orbits   Fig. 11-17

The simplified drawing in *Fig. 11-18* illustrates that the orbits project both upward and toward the midline. If one's head were placed in an upright A.P. or lateral position with the orbitomeatal line adjusted parallel to the floor, each orbit would project upward or superiorly at an angle of **30 degrees,** and toward the midsagittal plane at an angle of **37 degrees.** These two important angles are used during radiographic positioning of the optic foramina. Remember that each optic foramen is located at the apex of its respective orbit. In order to radiograph either optic foramen it is necessary to both extend the patient's chin by 30 degrees and rotate the head 37 degrees. The central ray is then projected through the center of the base of the orbit and along the long axis of the cone-shaped orbit.

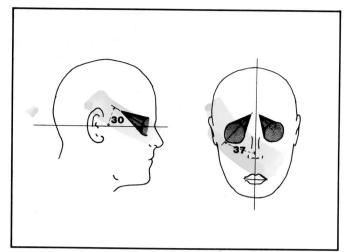

Orbits   Fig. 11-18

Bony Orbit

Each orbit is composed of parts of seven bones. The circumference or circular base of each orbit is composed of parts of three bones, the **frontal bone (orbital plate)** from the cranium, and the **maxilla** and **zygomatic bones** from the facial mass. Inside each orbital cavity are a roof, a floor and two walls, parts of which are also formed by these three bones. The orbital plate of the frontal bone forms most of the roof of the orbit. The zygomatic bone forms much of the lateral wall and some of the floor of the orbit, while a portion of the maxilla helps to form the floor.

FMZ

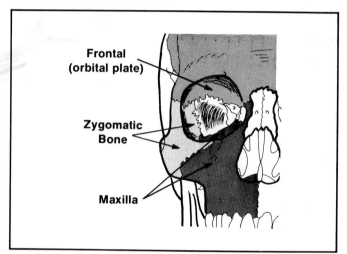

Base of Orbit   Fig. 11-19

All seven bones that form each orbit are shown in *Fig. 11-20.* The **frontal bone, zygomatic bone** and **maxilla** make up the base of the orbit. Some of the medial wall of the orbit is formed by the thin **lacrimal bone.** The **sphenoid** and **ethmoid** bones make up most of the posterior orbit, while only a small bit of the **palatine** bone contributes to the very posterior portion of the floor of each orbit.

In summary, the seven bones making up each orbit include three cranial bones — the frontal, sphenoid and ethmoid; and four facial bones — the maxilla, zygomatic, lacrimal and palatine.

F2M

Many People Let Someone Else Fail Zoology

Poping Zits May Lead from Severe eating

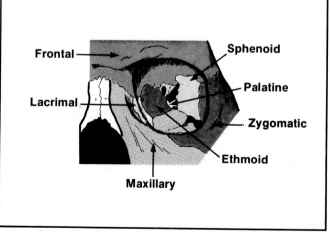

Orbit (7 bones)   Fig. 11-20

Openings in Posterior Orbit

Each orbit also contains three holes or openings in the posterior portion of the orbit, as demonstrated in *Fig. 11-21*. The **optic foramen** is a small hole in the sphenoid bone, located posteriorly at the apex of the cone-shaped orbit. The **superior orbital fissure** is a cleft or opening between the greater and lesser wings of the sphenoid bone, located lateral to the optic foramen. A third opening is the **inferior orbital fissure,** located between the maxilla, zygomatic bone and greater wing of the sphenoid.

The small root of bone separating the superior orbital fissure and the optic canal is known as the **sphenoid strut.** The optic canal is a small canal into which the optic foramen opens. Therefore, any abnormal enlargement of the optic nerve could cause erosion of the sphenoid strut, which is actually a portion of the lateral wall of the optic canal.

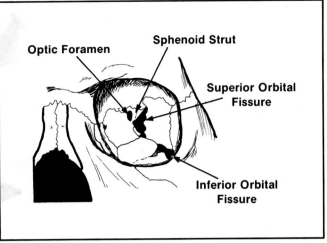

Orbit (Posterior openings)   Fig. 11-21

Orbital Fractures

Due to the unique construction of the orbit (a closed cone) and to the fact that the orbit is filled with structures containing large amounts of water (water does not compress), certain fractures are common to the orbit. One type of fracture is called a **"blow-out" fracture.** If the front of the orbit is struck solidly, such as with a ball or a fist, the contents of the cavity have no place to go. Since the bone along the floor of the orbit is quite thin, the orbital contents "blow-out" in that direction. Since the orbital contents involve vision, diagnosis of this type of fracture must be made early in treatment.

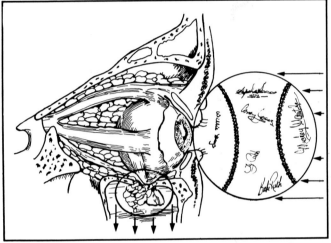

"Blow-out" Fracture   Fig. 11-22

Another unique fracture of the facial bone area is called the **"tripod" fracture.** This fracture essentially involves the zygomatic bone and its three connections. If fractures were to occur at the three points of attachment with the maxilla, temporal and frontal bones, as might result from a direct blow to the cheek, then the result is a free-floating zygomatic bone or a "tripod" fracture. The bones in this area of the body are highly vascular. Healing is quite rapid, which can be both good and bad. If either a "blow-out" or "tripod" fracture is not diagnosed early, the fracture may heal out of place and cause additional problems. The fracture might even have to be rebroken to be set properly.

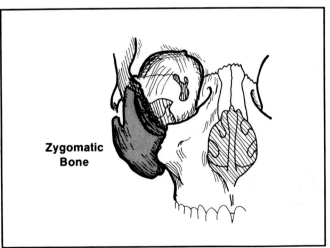

Zygomatic Bone

"Tripod" Fracture   Fig. 11-23

Orbit

Seven bones comprising the left orbit are illustrated in *Fig 11-24*. Part **A** is the frontal bone; **B** is the sphenoid bone; **C** is a very small portion of the palatine bone; **D** is the zygomatic bone; **E** is the maxillary bone; **F** is the ethmoid bone; and **G** is the lacrimal bone.

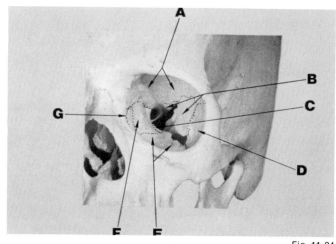

Orbit   Fig. 11-24

Those structures labeled on the photograph in *Fig. 11-25* are: **(A)** optic foramen, **(B)** sphenoid strut, **(C)** superior orbital fissure, and **(D)** inferior orbital fissure.

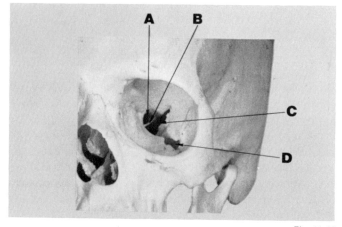

Orbit   Fig. 11-25

Anatomical Relationships

The two radiographs illustrated in *Fig. 11-26* are a P.A. and lateral skull. The P.A. skull on the left was taken with no tube angulation and with the O.M.L. perpendicular to the plane of the film. No angulation was used as indicated by the fact that the orbits appear totally filled by the petrous ridges. Drawn on both radiographs is a line through the roof of the orbits and through the petrous ridges. With the orbits superimposed by the petrous pyramids, very little facial bone detail can be demonstrated radiographically.

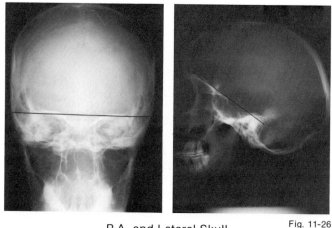

P.A. and Lateral Skull   Fig. 11-26

In order to better visualize the facial bone mass, it is necessary to project the petrous pyramids inferiorly. The petrous pyramids are such dense, bony structures that they must be removed from the facial bone area of interest, either by tube angulation or by extending the neck. The two radiographs in *Fig. 11-27* demonstrate how this can be accomplished. The roof of the orbit and the petrous ridge are now separated by the distance marked A. The radiograph on the left is the Waters' position, which, if done correctly, will project the petrous pyramids just below the maxillary sinuses.

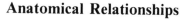

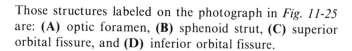

Waters' and Lateral Skull   Fig. 11-27

Part II. Radiographic Positioning
Facial Bones, Zygomatic Arches and Optic Foramina

Basic and Optional Projections/Positions

Certain basic and optional projections or positions for facial bones, zygomatic arches and optic foramina are demonstrated and described on the following pages. **Basic projections** are those projections commonly taken on average helpful patients. It should be noted that departmental routines (basic projections) vary in different hospitals or departments. **Optional projections** include those more common projections taken as extra or additional projections for better demonstration of specific body parts or pathologic conditions.

Many of the basic principles studied in Chapter 10, concerning positioning of the cranium, will be utilized in basic positions of the bones of the facial skeleton. Certain alternative methods are presented that may be helpful when radiographing the uncooperative or difficult patient.

Facial Bones
Basic
- Parietoacanthial (Waters')
- Lateral
Optional
- Modified Parietoacanthial (Mod. Waters')

Facial Bones
Trauma
- Lateral - Horizontal Beam
- Acanthioparietal
Optional
- Modified Acanthioparietal

Nasal Bones
Basic
- Lateral (Both)
- Parietoacanthial (Waters') or P.A. (Caldwell)
Optional
- Superoinferior (Axial)

Zygomatic Arch
Basic
- Lateral
- Parietoacanthial (Waters')
- Basilar
Optional
- Semiaxial A.P. (Towne)
- Oblique Axial

Optic Foramina
Basic
- Parieto-orbital (Bilateral)

Facial Bones
Basic
- **Parietoacanthial** (Waters')
- Lateral

Optional
- Modified Parietoacanthial (Mod. Waters')

• **Parietoacanthial Projection**
Waters' Position

Film Size:
>   10 x 12 in. (24 x 30 cm.)
>   **or**
>   8 x 10 in. (18 x 24 cm.)

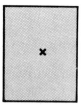

Bucky:
- Moving or stationary grid.

Patient Position:
- Prone or upright.

Part Position:
- No rotation or tilt.
- Midsagittal plane perpendicular to table.
- Rest on chin.
- O.M.L. forms **37°** angle with plane of film.
- Closely collimate.
- Immobilize if necessary.
- Tip of nose off table .5 to 1.5 cm.

Central Ray:
- C.R. enters at posterior sagittal suture and exits at acanthion.
- C.R. parallel to mentomeatal line.
- 40 in. (102 cm.) F.F.D.

NOTE: • Petrous ridges should visualize at inferior margin of maxillary sinuses.

Structures Best Shown:
Orbits, zygomatic bones, zygomatic arches, maxillae and maxillary sinuses.

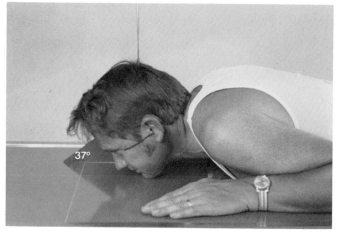

Parietoacanthial Projection (Waters')   Fig. 11-28

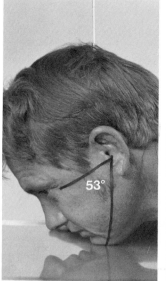
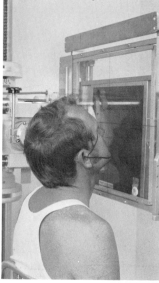

Parietoacanthial Projection (Waters')   Fig. 11-29

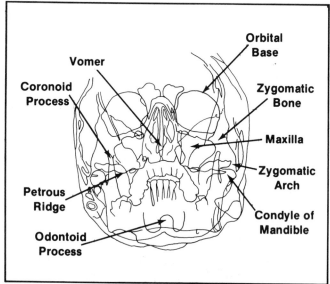

Fig. 11-31   Parietoacanthial Projection (Waters')

Orbital Base

Vomer

Coronoid Process

Zygomatic Bone

Maxilla

Zygomatic Arch

Petrous Ridge

Condyle of Mandible

Odontoid Process

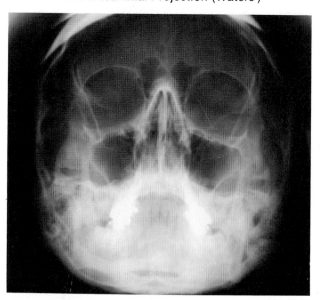

Parietoacanthial Projection (Waters')   Fig. 11-30

Facial Bones

- **Lateral Position**

Facial Bones
Basic
- Parietoacanthial (Waters')
- **Lateral**

Optional
- Modified Parietoacanthial
  (Mod. Waters')

Film Size:

    8 x 10 in. (18 x 24 cm.)

Bucky:

- Moving or stationary grid.

Patient Position:

- Semiprone or upright with head turned to lateral position.

Part Position:

- Head must be in true lateral position.
- Interpupillary line perpendicular to film.
- Midsagittal plane parallel to table.
- I.O.M.L. perpendicular to front edge of cassette.
- Closely collimate.

Central Ray:

- C.R. perpendicular to film and passes through prominence of zygomatic bone.
- 40 in. (102 cm.) F.F.D.

Structures Best Shown

Facial bones with both sides superimposed.

NOTE: • Similar to lateral skull and lateral paranasal sinuses except for centering point.

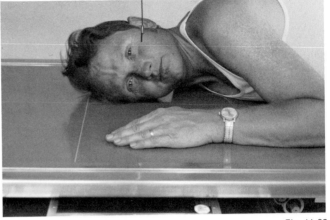

Right Lateral Position   Fig. 11-32

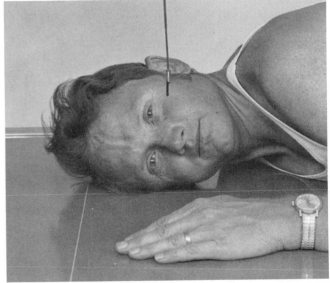

Right Lateral Position   Fig. 11-33

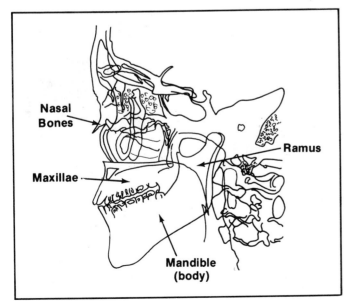

Fig. 11-35   Lateral Position

Nasal Bones

Ramus

Maxillae

Mandible (body)

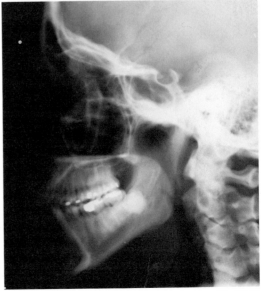

Lateral Position   Fig. 11-34

Facial Bones
Basic
- Parietoacanthial (Waters')
- Lateral

Optional
- **Modified Parietoacanthial**
(Mod. Waters')

• **Modified Parietoacanthial Projection**
Modified Waters' Position

Film Size:
8 x 10 in. (18 x 24 cm.)

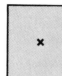

Bucky:
- Moving or stationary grid.

Patient Position:
- Prone or upright.

Part Position:
- No rotation or tilt.
- Midsagittal plane perpendicular to table.
- Rest on chin and nose.
- O.M.L. forms an angle of **55°** with plane of film.
- Closely collimate.
- Immobilize if necessary.

Central Ray:
- C.R. enters at posterior sagittal suture and exits at acanthion.
- C.R. perpendicular to film holder.
- 40 in. (102 cm.) F.F.D.

NOTE: • Petrous ridges projected into maxillary sinuses just inferior to infraorbital margin. • Excellent position for possible "blow-out" fracture.

Structures Best Shown:
Floor of orbit.

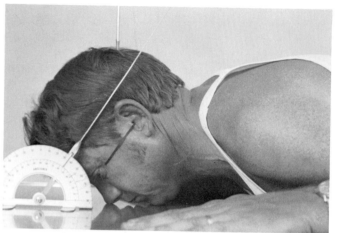

Modified Parietoacanthial Projection   Fig. 11-36
(Mod. Waters')

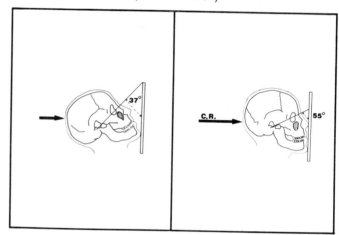

Parietoacanthial Projection   Fig. 11-37
(Waters')   (Mod. Waters')

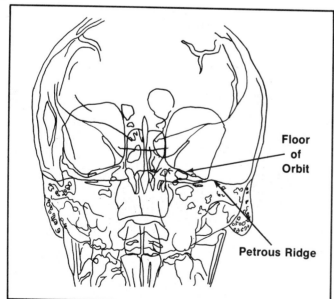

Fig. 11-39
Modified Parietoacanthial Projection
(Mod. Water's)

**Floor
of
Orbit**

Petrous Ridge

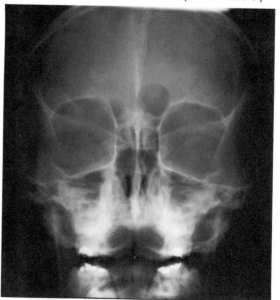

Modified Parietoacanthial Projection   Fig. 11-38
(Mod. Waters')

Facial Bones

• **Trauma Series**

Facial Bones
Trauma
• **Lateral** - Horizontal Beam
• **Acanthioparietal**
Optional
• **Modified Acanthioparietal**

Film Size:

    10 x 12 in. (24 x 30 cm.)
        or
    8 x 10 in. (18 x 24 cm.)

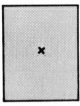

Bucky:

- Moving or stationary grid.

Patient Position:

- Supine.

Part Position:

Acanthioparietal

- No rotation or tilt.
- Midsagittal plane perpendicular to table.
- If **NO** spinal injury, chin up until mentomeatal line is vertical.
- If spinal injury is questionable, angle tube cephalad so central ray parallels mentomeatal line.
- Closely collimate.
- Immobilize if necessary.
- C.R. passes through acanthion.

Modified Acanthioparietal

- Same as acanthioparietal, except O.M.L. and plane of film form 55° angle.

Lateral

- Head in true lateral.
- Use grid cassette placed vertically.
- Side of injury closest to film.
- Center to prominence of zygomatic bone.

NOTE: • Rule out cervical spine fracture or dislocation before attempting facial bone trauma series. • The reverse Waters' is a poor substitute for the basic parietoacanthial projection.

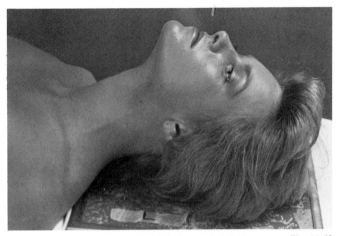

Acanthioparietal Projection
(C.R. parallel to mentomeatal line)
    Fig. 11-40

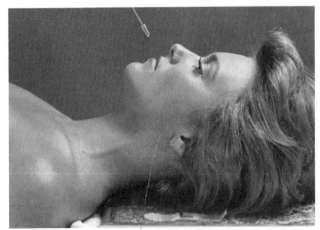

Acanthioparietal Projection
(Cephalic angulation of C.R.)
    Fig. 11-41

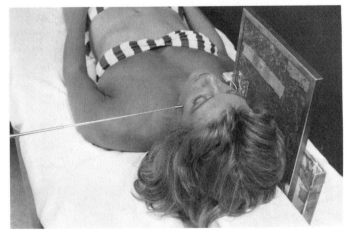

Fig. 11-43

Lateral - Horizontal Beam

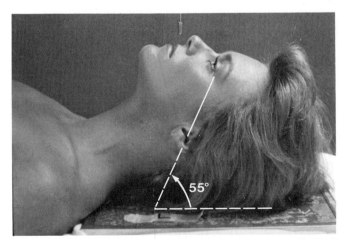

Mod. Acanthioparietal Projection
(C.R. vertical, 55° angle O.M.L. and film)
    Fig. 11-42

Nasal Bones
Basic
- **Lateral** (Both)
- Parietoacanthial (Waters')
  or P.A. (Caldwell)

Optional
- Superoinferior (Axial)

Nasal Bones

- **Lateral Position**

Film Size:
    8 x 10 in. (18 x 24 cm.)
    - Half for each side.

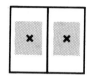

Non-Bucky:
- Detail screen or CBH.

Patient Position:
- Semiprone or upright with head turned to lateral position.

Part Position:
- Head true lateral.
- Interpupillary line perpendicular to film.
- Midsagittal plane parallel to film.
- Closely collimate.

Central Ray:
- C.R. perpendicular to film and centered to bridge of nose.
- 40 in. (102 cm.) F.F.D.

NOTE: • Both laterals are done. • Nasal bone closest to film shows best.

Structures Best Shown:
Nasal bones and soft tissues of the nose.

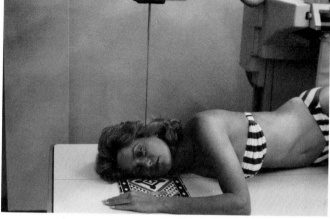

Lateral   Fig. 11-44

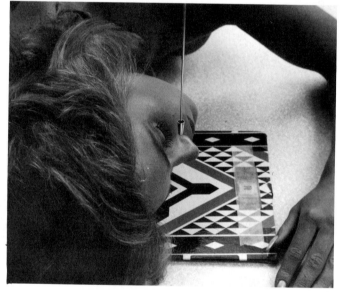

Lateral   Fig. 11-45

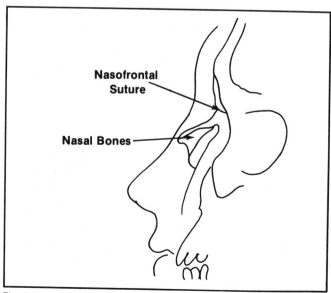

Fig. 11-47

Lateral

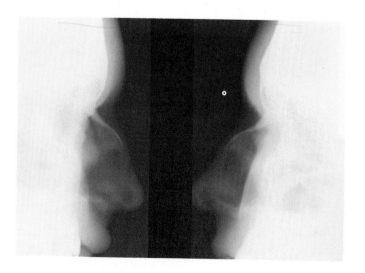

Lateral (R. and L.)   Fig. 11-46

Nasofrontal Suture

Nasal Bones

Nasal Bones

- **Parietoacanthial Projection** (Waters')
- **Posteroanterior Projection** (Caldwell)

Nasal Bones

Basic
- Lateral (Both)
- **Parietoacanthial** (Waters')
  or **P.A.** (Caldwell)

Optional
- Superoinferior (Axial)

Film Size:
   8 x 10 in. (18 x 24 cm.)

Bucky:
- Moving or stationary grid.

Patient Position:
- Prone or upright.

Part Position:
Waters'
- No rotation or tilt.
- Midsagittal plane perpendicular to table.
- Rest on chin.
- O.M.L. forms **37° angle** with plane of film.
- Closely collimate.
- Immobilize if necessary.
- C.R. passes through **acanthion.**

Caldwell
- No rotation or tilt.
- O.M.L. perpendicular to plane of film.
- Midsagittal plane perpendicular to table.
- Closely collimate.
- Immobilize if necessary.
- Angle 15° **caudad.**
- Center to **nasion.**
- 40 in. (102 cm.) F.F.D.

NOTE: • Will demonstrate deviated bony nasal septum.

Structures Best Shown:
Bony nasal septum.

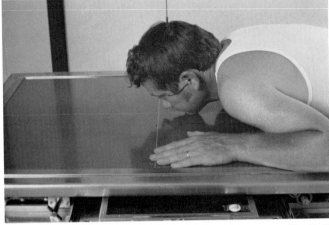

Parietoacanthial Projection (Waters')   Fig. 11-48

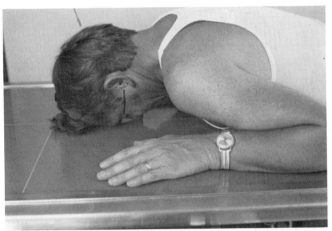

P.A. Projection (Caldwell)   Fig. 11-49

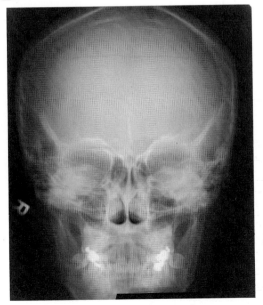

Fig. 11-51   P.A. Projection (Caldwell)

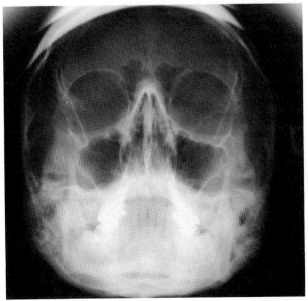

Parietoacanthial Projection (Waters')   Fig. 11-50

Nasal Bones

• Superoinferior Projection
Axial Position

Nasal Bones
Basic
• Lateral (Both)
• Parietoacanthial (Waters')
or P.A. (Caldwell)
Optional
• **Superoinferior** (Axial)

Film Size:
Occlusal film packet
or
5 x 7 in. (13 x 18 cm.) CBH

Non-Bucky:
- Occlusal film or CBH.

Patient Position:
- Supine, prone or upright.

Part Position:

Supine
- Head elevated.
- Occlusal film packet extending from mouth, or CBH beneath chin.

Prone or Upright
- Chin extended, similar to verticosubmental projection.
- Film packet extending from mouth, or CBH beneath chin.

Central Ray:
- Should skim glabella and upper front teeth.
- C.R. same as glabelloalveolar line, which is perpendicular to film.
- 40 in. (102 cm.) F.F.D.

NOTE: • Best to use occlusal film packet. • Any combination of prominent forehead, small nose or protruding front incisors may make visualization of the nasal bones impossible.

Structures Best Shown:
Both nasal bones.

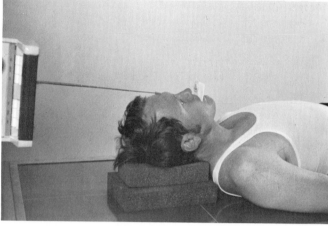

Superoinferior Projection (Axial position)   Fig. 11-52

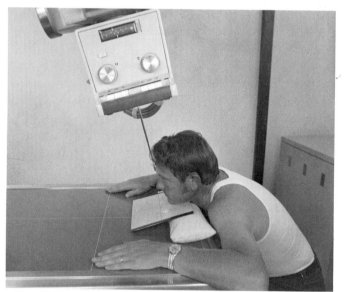

Superoinferior Projection (Axial position)   Fig. 11-53

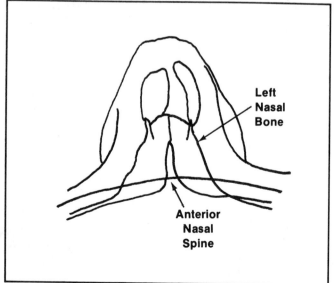

Left Nasal Bone

Anterior Nasal Spine

Fig. 11-55   Superoinferior Projection

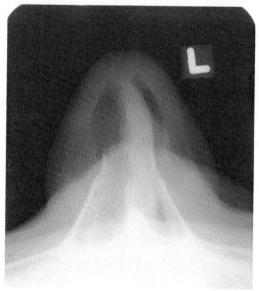

Superoinferior Projection   Fig. 11-54

Zygomatic Arch

- ● **Lateral Position**
- ● **Parietoacanthial Projection** (Waters')
- ● **Basilar Position**

Zygomatic Arch

Basic
- ● **Lateral**
- ● **Parietoacanthial** (Waters')
- ● **Basilar**

Optional
- ● Semiaxial A.P. (Towne)
- ● Oblique Axial

Film Size:

8 x 10 in. (18 x 24 cm.)
Crosswise.

Bucky:

- Moving or stationary grid.

Patient Position:

- Recumbent or upright.

Part Position:

Lateral

- Head true lateral (same as for facial bones).
- C.R. to prominence of zygomatic bone, perpendicular to film.

Parietoacanthial

- O.M.L. forms 37° angle with plane of film (same as for facial bones).
- C.R. exits at acanthion, perpendicular to film.

Basilar

- I.O.M.L. parallel to plane of film (same as for basilar of cranium).
- Decrease exposure factors compared to basilar for cranium (25% of original mAs).
- C.R. enters inferior to chin and exits at vertex.
- 40 in. (102 cm.) F.F.D.

NOTE: ● The optional positions visualize the zygomatic arches free from superimposition.

Structures Best Shown:

Zygomatic arches (bilateral).

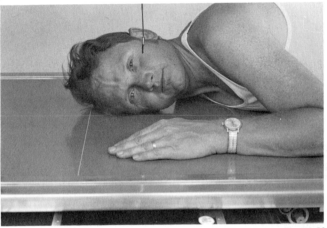

Right Lateral Position

Fig. 11-56

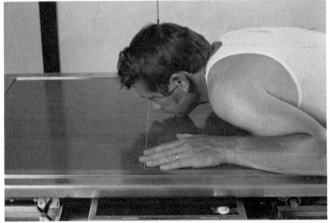

Parietoacanthial Projection

Fig. 11-57

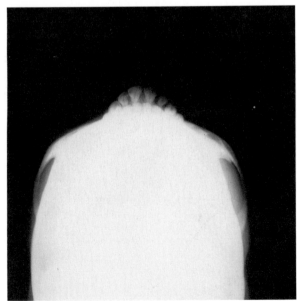

Fig. 11-59

Basilar Position

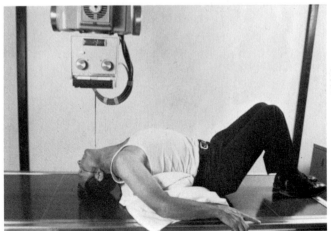

Basilar Position

Fig. 11-58

• Semiaxial Anteroposterior Projection
Towne Position

Zygomatic Arch
Basic
- Lateral
- Parietoacanthial (Waters')
- Basilar

Optional
- **Semiaxial A.P.** (Towne)
- Oblique Axial

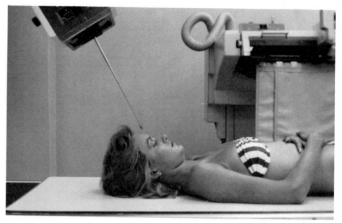
Semiaxial A.P. Projection
(Towne)
Fig. 11-60

Film Size:
   8 x 10 in. (18 x 24 cm.)
   Crosswise.

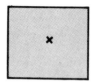

Bucky:
- Moving or stationary grid.

Patient Position:
- Supine or upright.

Part Position:
- O.M.L. perpendicular to table.
- No rotation or tilt.
- Midsagittal plane perpendicular to table.
- Closely collimate and immobilize.
- Center film to gonion.

Central Ray:
- Tube angled **30°** caudad.
- C.R. enters at glabella.

NOTE: • Decrease exposure factors compared to semi-axial A.P. of cranium (50% of original mAs).

Structures Best Shown:
Zygomatic arches (bilateral).

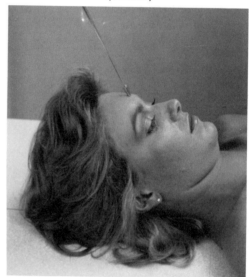
Semiaxial A.P. Projection
(Towne)
Fig. 11-61

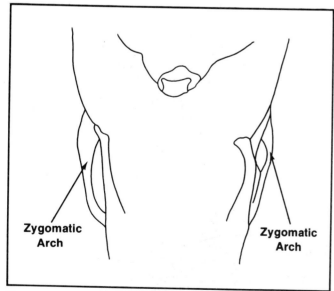
Fig. 11-63
Semiaxial A.P. Projection
(Towne)

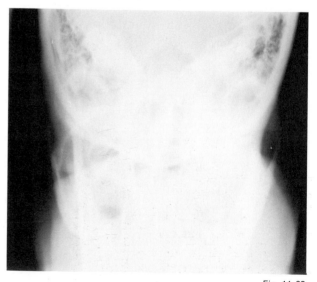
Semiaxial A.P. Projection
(Towne)
Fig. 11-62

Zygomatic Arch
Basic
- Lateral
- Parietoacanthial (Waters')
- Basilar

Optional
- Semiaxial A.P. (Towne)
- **Oblique Axial**

Zygomatic Arch
• Oblique Axial Position

Film Size:

8 x 10 in. (18 x 24 cm.)
Crosswise.

Bucky:

- Moving or stationary grid.

Patient Position:

- Supine or upright.

Part Position:

- Similar to basilar position of cranium.
- I.O.M.L. parallel to plane of film.
- Tilt head 15° toward side to be examined.
- Immobilize and closely collimate.

Central Ray:

- I.O.M.L. perpendicular to C.R.
- C.R. skims parietal eminence and body of mandible.

NOTE: • Both sides are radiographed for comparison.
• Decrease exposure factors compared to basilar of cranium (25% of original mAs).

Structures Best Shown:

One zygomatic arch per exposure free from bony super-imposition.

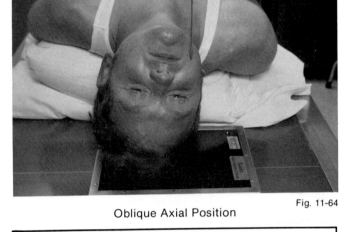

Oblique Axial Position

Fig. 11-64

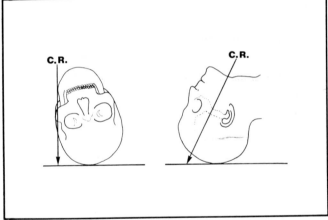

Oblique Axial Position

Fig. 11-65

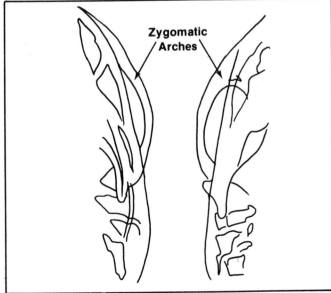

Fig. 11-67

Oblique Axial Position

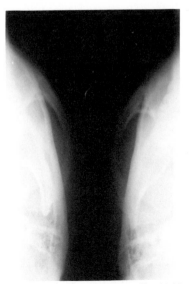

Fig. 11-66

Oblique Axial Position

Optic Foramina
Basic
• **Parieto-orbital** (Bilateral)

Optic Foramina

• Parieto-orbital Projection

Rhese Position

"Three-point Landing" Position

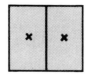

Film Size:

8 x 10 in. (18 x 24 cm.)
Crosswise.
Divided in half.

Bucky:

- Moving or stationary grid.

Patient Position:

- Prone or upright.

Part Position:

- Head rests on **chin, cheek** and **nose**.
- Acanthiomeatal line perpendicular to plane of film.
- Head rotated **37°** from true P.A.
- Midsagittal plane and tabletop form angle of 53°.
- Center to orbit next to table.
- Forehead should **NOT** touch table.

Central Ray:

- C.R. exits at center of orbit, nearest the table.

NOTE: • When performed correctly, optic foramen should be projected into the **lower, outer** quadrant of the orbit examined.

Structures Best Shown:

Cross section of each optic canal.

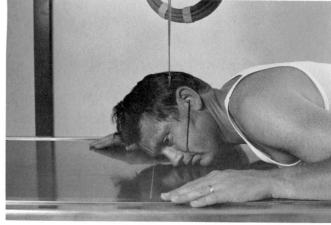

Parieto-orbital Projection

Fig. 11-68

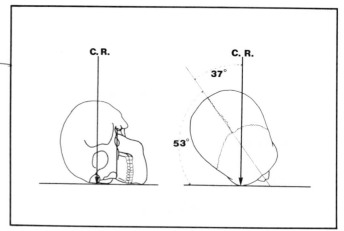

Parieto-orbital Projection

Fig. 11-69

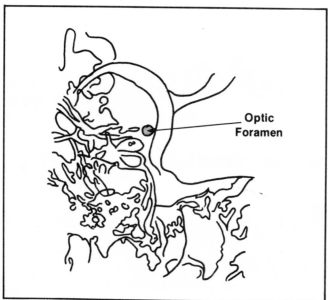

Fig. 11-71

Parieto-orbital Projection

Optic
Foramen

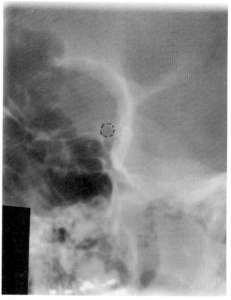

Parieto-orbital Projection

Fig. 11-70

CHAPTER 12

Radiographic Anatomy and Positioning of the
Mandible, Temporomandibular Joints, Sinuses and Temporal Bone

Part I. Radiographic Anatomy
Mandible, Temporomandibular Joints, Sinuses and Temporal Bone

Radiographic anatomy of most of the cranium and facial bones is described in Chapters 10 and 11. Three notable exceptions are addressed in this chapter. These exceptions include (1) the **mandible,** (2) the **paranasal sinuses,** and (3) the **temporal bone.** The mandible is the largest of the fourteen facial bones and is the only movable bone in the entire skull. The paranasal sinuses are air-containing cavities within the facial and cranial bones. The delicate organs of hearing and equilibrium are housed within the temporal bones.

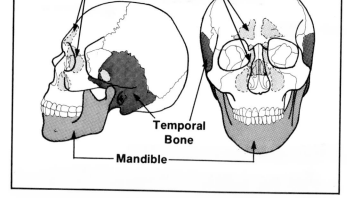

Mandible, Sinuses, Temporal Bone   Fig. 12-1

Mandible

The lower jaw or **mandible,** a single bone in the adult, actually originates as two separate bones. These two bones in the infant join to become one bone at approximately one year of age. The external aspect of the left half of the adult mandible is shown in *Fig. 12-2*. The **gonion** or **angle** of the mandible divides each half of the mandible into two main parts. That area anterior to the gonion is termed the **body** of the mandible, while that area superior to the gonion is termed the **ramus.** Since the mandible is a single bone, the body actually extends from the left gonion around to the right gonion. The lower teeth are rooted in the mandible; therefore, an **alveolar process** or ridge extends along the superior portion of the body of the mandible.

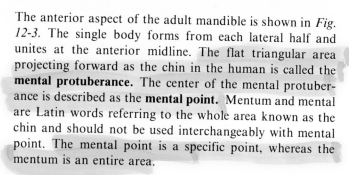

Mandible, left side   Fig. 12-2

The anterior aspect of the adult mandible is shown in *Fig. 12-3*. The single body forms from each lateral half and unites at the anterior midline. The flat triangular area projecting forward as the chin in the human is called the **mental protuberance.** The center of the mental protuberance is described as the **mental point.** Mentum and mental are Latin words referring to the whole area known as the chin and should not be used interchangeably with mental point. The mental point is a specific point, whereas the mentum is an entire area.

Located on each half of the body of the mandible are the **mental foramina.** These foramina serve as passageways for nerves and blood vessels. The area of fusion of the two halves of the mandible is termed the **symphysis** of the mandible or **symphysis menti.** This area of fusion is just superior to the mental protuberance and extends upward to the alveolar border.

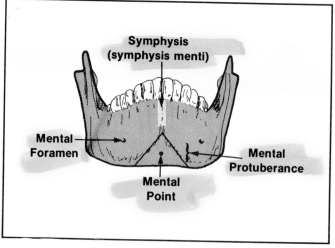

Mandible, anterior   Fig. 12-3

234

Ramus

The upper portion of each **ramus** terminates in a U-shaped notch termed the **mandibular notch.** At each end of the mandibular notch is a process. The process at the anterior end of the mandibular notch is termed the **coronoid process.** The coronoid process does not articulate with another bone and cannot be easily palpated since it lies beneath the zygomatic arch.

The **coronoid process** of the mandible must not be confused with the **coronoid process** of the proximal ulna of the forearm, or the **coracoid process** of the scapula. One way to remember these terms is to associate the **a** in coracoid with the **a**'s in scapula, and the **n** in coronoid with the **n**'s in ulna and in mandible.

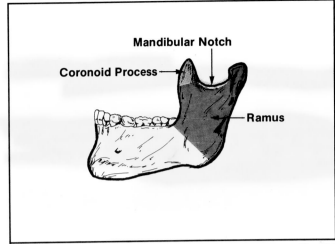

Mandible, left side   Fig. 12-4

Temporomandibular Joint (T.M.J.)

The posterior process of the upper ramus is termed the **condyloid process** and consists of two parts. The rounded end of the condyloid process is called the **condyle** or **head**, while the constricted area directly below the condyle is the **neck.** The condyle of the condyloid process fits into the temporomandibular fossa of the temporal bone to form the **temporomandibular joint** or **T.M.J.**

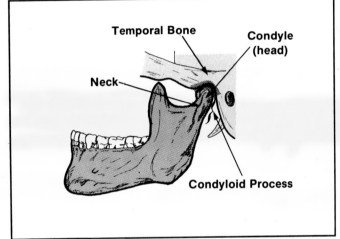

Temporomandibular Joint (T.M.J.)   Fig. 12-5

Axiolateral Position. The mandible, as illustrated in *Fig. 12-6,* is tilted so that the left half of the mandible is projected above the right half. This is called an axiolateral or oblique position. Since both sides of the mandible would be superimposed on a true lateral, part of the routine mandible positioning series calls for tilting the mandible to show primarily one side, as seen in this illustration. The opposite axiolateral position shows the other side in the same way. These tilted lateral positions clearly demonstrate the **body** and entire **ramus,** including the **coronoid process,** the **condyle** and the **condyloid process.**

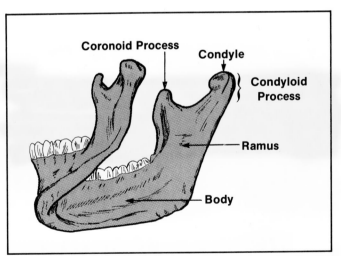

Mandible   Fig. 12-6

Submentovertex Projection. The horseshoe shape of the mandible is well visualized on a **submentovertex** projection, as seen in *Fig. 12-7.* Note that the mandible is a fairly thin structure, which explains why it is susceptible to fractures. The area of the chin or **mentum** is well demonstrated as are the **body** and **rami** of the mandible. The relative positions of the upper ramus and its associated **coronoid process** and **condyle** are also demonstrated.

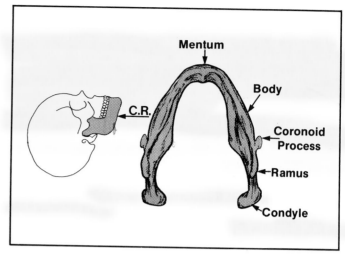

Submentovertex Projection of Mandible   Fig. 12-7

Mandible

The photograph of a mandible in *Fig. 12-8* identifies the following labeled parts: **(A)** one coronoid process, **(B)** the mandibular notch, **(C)** the neck, **(D)** the condyle, **(E)** the condyloid process, **(F)** the ramus, **(G)** the gonion or angle of the jaw, **(H)** the body, and **(I)** the alveolar process.

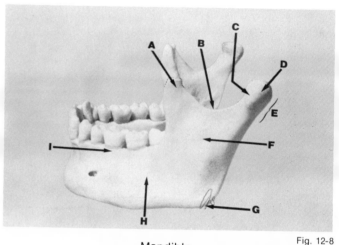

Mandible   Fig. 12-8

Temporomandibular Joint (T.M.J.). A photograph of one temporomandibular joint is illustrated in *Fig. 12-9.* The T.M.J. is a diarthrodial or freely movable joint. Each T.M.J. is formed by the **condyle** or head of the condyloid process of the mandible fitting into the **temporomandibular fossa** of the temporal bone. Note that the T.M.J. is located just anterior to the **external auditory meatus** or **E.A.M.**

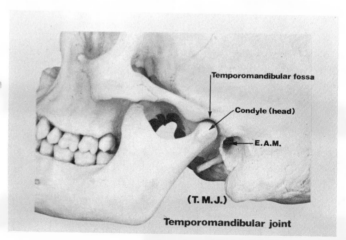

Temporomandibular Joint   Fig. 12-9

T.M.J. Motion: The temporomandibular fossa is not a deep fossa. It allows a large range of motion at the T.M.J. as evidenced by the drawings of the joint in *Fig. 12-10*. These drawings illustrate the T.M.J. in both an **open** and a **closed mouth** position. When one opens the mouth widely, the condyle moves forward to the front edge of the fossa. If the condyle slips too far anteriorly, the temporomandibular joint may dislocate. If the T.M.J. dislocates, either by force or by jaw motion, it may be difficult or even impossible to close the mouth, which returns the condyle to its normal position.

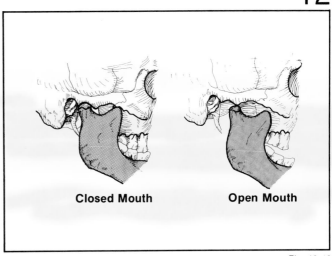

Closed Mouth Open Mouth

T.M.J. Motion

Fig. 12-10

Paranasal Sinuses

The large, air-filled cavities of the paranasal sinuses are sometimes called the accessory nasal sinuses. These sinuses are divided into four groups as follows:

- **Maxillary** (2)
- **Frontal** (usually 2)
- **Ethmoid** (many)
- **Sphenoid** (1 or 2)

Maxillary Sinuses

The large **maxillary sinuses** are paired structures, one being located within the body of each maxillary bone. An older term for maxillary sinus is antrum, an abbreviation of "antrum of Highmore." Each maxillary sinus is shaped somewhat like a pyramid, as illustrated in *Fig. 12-11*.

The bony walls of the maxillary sinuses are thin. The floor of each maxillary sinus is approximately at the same level as the floor of each nasal fossa. The maxillary sinuses are the largest of the paranasal sinuses, although the two sinuses are variable in size from one person to another and from one side to the other.

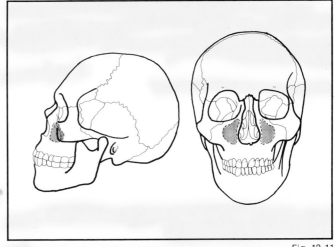

Maxillary Sinuses

Fig. 12-11

The paranasal sinus cavities communicate with the **nasal fossae** or **cavities.** In the case of the maxillary sinuses, this site of communication is located somewhat superior to or above the sinus cavity itself, as demonstrated in *Fig. 12-12*. Therefore, when a person is erect, any mucus or fluid trapped within the sinus will tend to stay there and layer out, forming an air-fluid level. Radiographic positioning of the paranasal sinuses should be accomplished with the patient in the erect position to demonstrate any possible air-fluid levels.

Projecting into the floor of each maxillary sinus are several conical elevations relating to roots of the maxillary teeth. Occasionally, infections originating in the teeth, particularly the molars and premolars, may travel upward into the maxillary sinus.

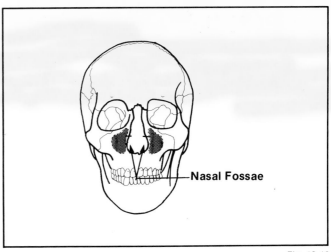

Nasal Fossae

Maxillary Sinuses

Fig. 12-12

Frontal Sinuses

The **frontal sinuses** are located between the inner and outer tables of the skull, posterior to the glabella. Whereas the maxillary sinuses are always paired and are usually fairly symmetrical in size and shape, the frontal sinuses are rarely symmetrical. The frontal sinuses may form one single cavity, although there are usually two. If there are two, there may be a wide variation in their sizes and shapes. The maxillary sinuses usually have some air in them at birth, but the frontals rarely become aerated before age six.

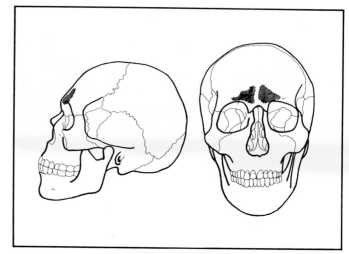

Frontal Sinuses   Fig. 12-13

Ethmoid Sinuses

The **ethmoid sinuses** are made up of many air cells contained within the lateral masses or labyrinths of the ethmoid bone. These air cells are grouped into anterior, middle and posterior collections, but they all intercommunicate. These cells also communicate with the nasal cavities via a single passageway from each side. As seen from the side, it would appear that the ethmoid sinuses fill the orbits. These sinuses are medial to the orbits, however, and are contained in the lateral masses of the ethmoid bone, which help to form the medial wall of each orbit.

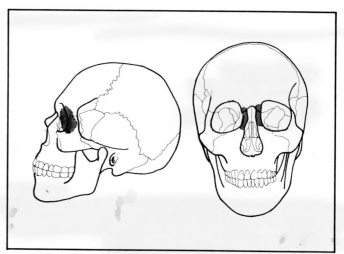

Ethmoid Sinuses   Fig. 12-14

Sphenoid Sinus

The **sphenoid sinus** lies in the body of the sphenoid bone, directly below the sella turcica. Usually there is only one sphenoid cavity, but occasionally there are two. Since the sphenoid sinus is so close to the base or floor of the cranium, sometimes a pathologic process makes its presence known by its effect on the sphenoid sinus. An example of this occurrence is the demonstration of an air-fluid level within the sphenoid sinus following skull trauma. This demonstration could be the only radiographic proof obtainable that the patient has a basal skull fracture, and that either blood or cerebrospinal fluid is leaking through the fracture into the sphenoid sinus.

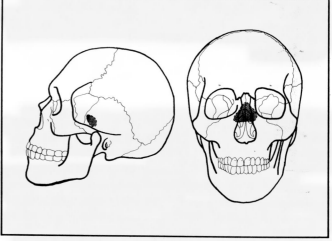

Sphenoid Sinus   Fig. 12-15

Paranasal Sinus Groups: The relative positions of the four paranasal sinus groups are shown in *Fig. 12-16.* Note that in the frontal position the sphenoid sinus is located behind the lower ethmoid sinuses. If the chin were raised, as in a Waters' position, the sphenoid sinus would then be projected below the ethmoids. If the patient's mouth is opened in the Waters' position, the sphenoid sinus is fairly well visualized. However, portions of both the sphenoid and the ethmoid sinuses are superimposed by the nasal cavities and other structures in the area. These somewhat schematic drawings show the various sinuses with definite and fairly visible borders; however, the various borders are not nearly so definite in actual radiographs. The ethmoid and sphenoid sinuses, in particular, are difficult to visualize on any frontal projection.

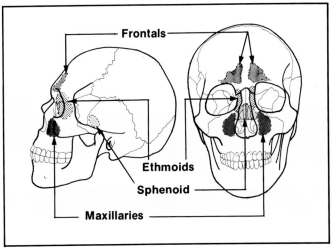

Paranasal Sinuses

Fig. 12-16

Temporal Bones

Each **temporal bone** is divided into three main portions. The thin upper portion forming part of the wall of the skull is the **squamous portion.** The area posterior to the external auditory meatus is the **mastoid portion,** with its prominent mastoid process or tip. The third main portion is the dense **petrous portion,** also called the **petrous pyramid** or **pars petrosa.** Without resorting to body-section radiography or computed tomography, the temporal bone is probably the most difficult part of the entire body to radiograph with consistently high quality.

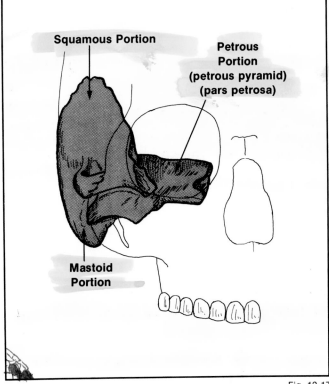

Temporal Bone

Fig. 12-17

Ear

The organs of hearing and equilibrium are the main structures found within the petrous portion of the temporal bones. These small, delicate structures are difficult to visualize radiographically, due not only to their small size, but also to the increased density of the temporal bones surrounding them. The internal structures of the temporal bone, including the three important divisions of the ear (the external, middle and internal portions) are illustrated in *Fig. 12-18*. The **external ear** begins outside the head with the **auricle** or **pinna,** which channels sound waves into a tubelike opening, the **external auditory meatus.** This tubelike meatus ends at the eardrum, which is properly called the **tympanic membrane.** The **middle ear,** located between the tympanic membrane and the inner ear, contains the **three** small bones called **ossicles.** These small bones transmit sound vibrations from the tympanic membrane to the sensory apparatus of hearing in the **internal ear.** Certain nerves and blood vessels pass through the **internal auditory meatus** to connect the inner ear with the brain.

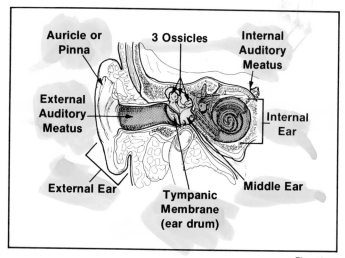

Ear

Fig. 12-18

External Ear. As previously described, the **external ear** begins with the **auricle** or **pinna** on each side of the head. The **tragus** is part of this external structure. It is the small liplike structure located anterior to the E.A.M., acting as a partial shield to the ear opening. The canal of the external ear is termed the **external auditory meatus.** Some references refer to the external opening as the external auditory meatus, and refer to the canal as the external auditory canal. In this text the entire canal is referred to as the external auditory meatus. The meatus is about 2.5 centimeters long, half of which is bony in structure and half of which is cartilaginous. The **mastoid tip** of the temporal bone is posterior to the external auditory meatus, while the **styloid process** is slightly anterior. The meatus narrows somewhat as it meets the tympanic membrane. The eardrum is situated at an oblique angle, forming a depression or well at the lower medial end of the meatus.

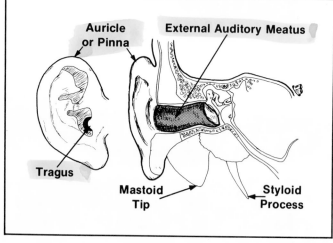

External Ear

Fig. 12-19

Middle Ear. The middle ear is an irregularly shaped, air-containing cavity located between the external and the internal ear portions. The three main components of the middle ear are the **tympanic membrane,** the **three** small bones called **auditory ossicles,** and the **tympanic cavity.** The tympanic membrane is considered part of the middle ear even though it serves as a partition between the external and middle ears. The tympanic cavity is further divided into two parts. The larger cavity opposite the eardrum is called the **tympanic cavity proper.** The area above the level of the external auditory meatus and the eardrum is called the **attic** or the **epitympanic recess.** A structure important radiographically is the **drum crest** or **spur.** The tympanic membrane is attached to this sharp, bony projection. The drum crest or spur separates the external auditory meatus from the epitympanic recess. The tympanic cavity communicates anteriorly with the nasopharynx by way of the Eustachian tube or the auditory tube.

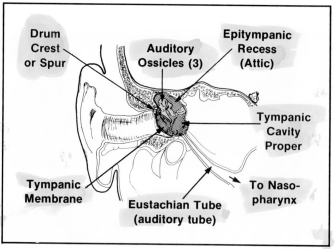

Middle Ear

Fig. 12-20

The frontal drawing in *Fig. 12-21* illustrates the general relationships of the **external auditory meatus** and Eustachian tube to the external features. The passageway between the middle ear and the **nasopharynx** is labeled as the **Eustachian** or **auditory tube.** This tube is about 4 centimeters long and serves to equalize the pressure within the middle ear to the outside atmospheric air pressure through the nasopharynx. The sensation of one's ears popping is caused by the pressure being adjusted internally in the middle ear to prevent damage to the eardrum. A problem associated with this direct communication between the middle ear and the nasopharynx is that disease organisms have a direct passageway from the throat to the middle ear. Therefore, ear infections often accompany sore throats.

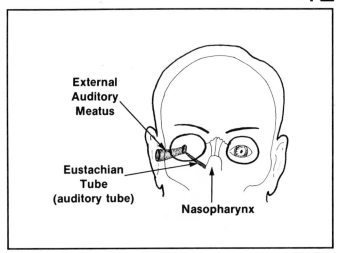

Middle Ear Fig. 12-21

Internal Auditory Meatus: The drawing in *Fig. 12-22* demonstrates the ear structures as they would appear in a modified P.A. projection (Caldwell position). A 10-degree caudal angle to the orbitomeatal line will project the petrous ridges to the midorbital level. The result is a special transorbital view taken to demonstrate the **internal auditory meatus.** The opening to the internal auditory meatus is an oblique aperture, smaller in diameter than the opening to the external auditory meatus. Certain auditory and facial nerves, as well as blood vessels, pass through the internal auditory meatus. Note that in the modified Caldwell position the internal auditory meatus is projected into the orbital shadow slightly below the petrous ridge, allowing it to be visualized on radiographs taken in this position. Remember that the lateral portions of the petrous ridges are at approximately the level of the **T.E.A.** (top of ear attachment). These external relationships to the internal structures are important to remember.

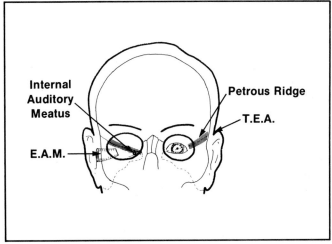

Modified Caldwell (10°) Fig. 12-22

Mastoids: A second direct communication into the middle ear occurs posteriorly from the **mastoid air cells.** The schematic drawing in *Fig. 12-23* is a sagittal section showing the relationship of the mastoid air cells to the **attic** or **epitympanic recess** and the **tympanic cavity proper.** The **aditus** is the opening between the epitympanic recess and the mastoid portion of the temporal bone. The aditus connects directly to a large chamber within the mastoid portion termed the **antrum.** The antrum then connects to the various mastoid air cells. This communication allows infection in the middle ear, which may have originated in the throat, to pass into the mastoid area. Once within the mastoid area, infection is separated from brain tissue by only thin bone. Before the common use of effective antibiotics, this was often a pathway for a serious infection of the brain, termed encephalitis. The thin plate of bone forming the roof of the antrum, aditus and attic area of the tympanic cavity is called the **tegman tympani.**

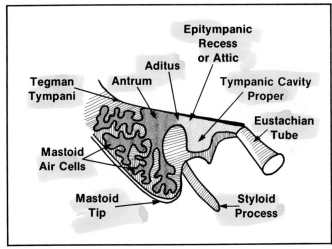

Mastoid Connection Fig. 12-23

Auditory Ossicles. The **auditory ossicles** are three small bones that are prominent structures within the middle ear. The drawing in *Fig. 12-24* demonstrates that these three small bones are articulated to permit vibratory motion. The three auditory ossicles are located partly in the attic or epitympanic recess, and partly in the tympanic cavity proper. These delicate bones bridge the middle ear cavity to transmit sound vibrations from the **tympanic membrane** to the internal ear. Vibrations are first picked up by the **malleus,** meaning hammer, which is attached directly to the inside surface of the tympanic membrane. The head of the malleus articulates with the central ossicle, the **incus.** The incus receives its name from a supposed resemblance to an anvil, but it actually looks more like a premolar tooth with a body and two roots. The incus then connects to the stirrup-shaped **stapes,** which is the smallest of the three auditory ossicles. The foot plate of the stapes is then attached to another membrane called the **oval window** leading into the inner ear.

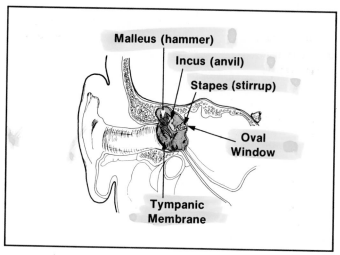

Auditory Ossicles   Fig. 12-24

The drawings in *Fig. 12-25* illustrate the relationship of the **auditory ossicles** to one another in both a frontal view and a lateral view. As seen from the front, the most lateral of the three bones is the **malleus,** while the most medial of the three bones is the **stapes.** The lateral-view drawing demonstrates how the ossicles would appear if one looked through the **external auditory meatus** to see the bony ossicles of the middle ear. Note that the malleus, with its attachment to the eardrum, is located slightly anterior to the other two bones. The resemblance of the **incus** to a premolar tooth with a body and two roots is well visualized in the lateral drawing. One root of the incus then connects to the stapes, which in turn connects to the oval window.

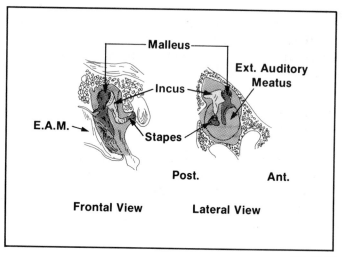

Auditory Ossicles   Fig. 12-25

Internal Ear
The following is a summary outline of the internal ear structures.
Internal Ear (labyrinth)
- Osseous Labyrinth
  - Cochlea
  - Vestibule
  - Semicircular Canals
- Membranous Labyrinth
  (inside osseous labyrinth)
  - Endolymphatic Duct

Internal Ear. The very complex **internal ear** contains the essential sensory apparatus of both hearing and equilibrium. Lying within the densest portion of the petrous pyramid, it can be divided into two main parts, the **osseous** or **bony labyrinth,** important radiographically, and the **membranous labyrinth.** The osseous labyrinth is a bony chamber housing the membranous labyrinth, a series of intercommunicating ducts and sacs. One such duct is the **endolymphatic duct,** a blind pouch or closed duct contained in a small canallike, bony structure. The canal of the endolymphatic duct arises from the medial wall of the vestibule and extends to the posterior wall of the petrous pyramid, located both posterior and lateral to the **internal auditory meatus.**

The osseous labyrinth is divided into three distinctly shaped parts, the **cochlea** (meaning snail shell), the **vestibule** and the **semicircular canals.** The osseous labyrinth completely surrounds and encloses the ducts and sacs of the membranous labyrinth. As illustrated in *Fig. 12-26,* the snail-shaped, bony cochlea houses a long tubelike duct of the membranous labyrinth. The cochlea is the most anterior of the three parts of the osseous labyrinth. The vestibule is the central portion of the bony labyrinth and contains the **oval window,** sometimes called the vestibular window. The three semicircular canals are located posterior to the other inner ear structures.

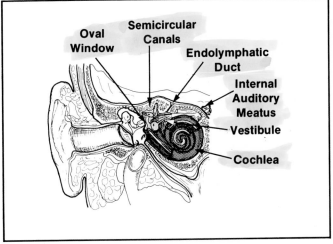

Internal Ear

Fig. 12-26

Osseous Labyrinth: A lateral view of the **osseous labyrinth** is shown in *Fig. 12-27.* Included are the three main divisions of the osseous or bony labyrinth: the cochlea, vestibule and semicircular canals. The three semicircular canals are named according to their position, thus they are called the **superior, posterior** and **lateral semicircular canals.** Observe that each is located at right angles to the other two, allowing a sense of equilibrium as well as a sense of direction. It is important to remember that the semicircular canals relate to the sense of direction or equilibrium, and the cochlea relates to the sense of hearing.

The two openings into the inner ear are covered by membranes. These are termed the **oval** or **vestibular window,** and the **round** or **cochlear window.** The oval or vestibular window receives vibrations from the external ear through the foot plate of the stapes of the middle ear, and transmits these vibrations into the **vestibule** of the internal ear. The round or cochlear window is located at the base of the first coil of the cochlea. The round window is a membrane that allows movement of fluid within the closed duct system of the membranous labyrinth. As the oval window moves slightly inward with a vibration, the round window moves outward since this is a closed system and fluid does not compress.

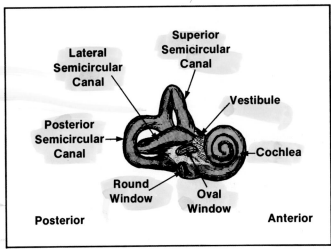

Osseous Labyrinth

Fig. 12-27

Tomography or body section radiography is usually required to adequately visualize the delicate structures of the middle and internal ear. Tomography requires a good understanding of not only the specific anatomy, but also of distances between various structures. Certain structures labeled **A** through **I** are identified in *Fig. 12-28*. Distances and relationships between these structures should be noted. Part **A** is the cochlea; **B** is the Eustachian or auditory tube; **C** is the bony ossicles in the tympanic cavity of the middle ear; **D** is the external auditory meatus; **E** is the antrum; **F** are the semicircular canals; **G** is the endolymphatic duct; **H** is the vestibule; and **I** is the internal auditory meatus.

It is important to note that almost all of the structures of the ear are located between the cochlea (toward the anterior) and the antrum (toward the posterior) in a distance of approximately 1 centimeter or 10 millimeters. The distance from the back of the head to the center of the external auditory meatus is approximately 10 centimeters.

Average distances between structures are based on the average-shaped skull with the O.M.L. perpendicular to the tabletop, and they will vary with the shape and size of the skull. If the O.M.L. were not kept perpendicular to the tabletop, these distances would also vary. Generally speaking, however, the most important structures of the middle and internal ear can be located in the 1 centimeter distance between 9.5 cm. and 10.5 cm. from the tabletop.

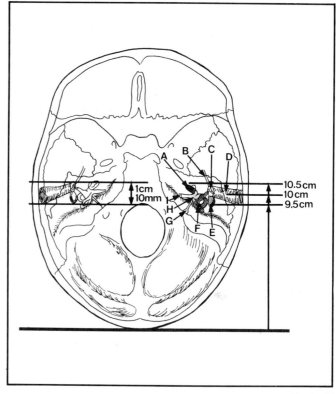

Ear Structures

Fig. 12-28

Figure 12-29 gives a top view of the head with the patient in a lateral position. The various ear structures are again shown with important distances identified. From the table top, the average distance to the midline is 7 centimeters, and to the internal auditory meatus, 9 centimeters. The internal auditory meatus extends 1 centimeter or 10 millimeters toward the inner ear. The inner ear extends another 1 centimeter and the middle ear extends approximately 5 millimeters farther. The distance from the tympanic membrane to the external auditory opening is 2.5 centimeters or 25 millimeters. These figures demonstrate that the distance from the external opening of the external auditory meatus to the internal auditory meatus is approximately 5 centimeters in the average-shaped skull. The interrelationships between the various structures of the middle and internal ear, as well as the various distances from the table top, are most important in tomography or body section radiography of these various structures.

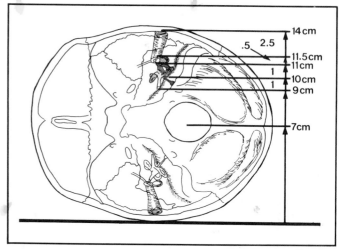

Ear Structures

Fig. 12-29

Part II. Radiographic Positioning
Mandible, Temporomandibular Joints, Sinuses and Temporal Bone

Basic and Optional Projections/Positions

Certain basic and optional projections or positions for the mandible, temporomandibular joints, paranasal sinuses and temporal bone are demonstrated and described on the following pages. **Basic projections** are those projections commonly taken on average helpful patients. It should be noted that departmental routines (basic projections) vary in different hospitals or departments. **Optional** projections include those more common projections taken as extra or additional projections for better visualization of specific anatomy or pathologic conditions.

Positioning of the mandible, paranasal sinuses and delicate structures of the temporal bone requires exacting techniques. Double angles are utilized in many of these positions. Not only will the head be rotated from P.A., A.P., or lateral, but tube angles will also be utilized.

Comparison radiographs of both right and left sides are required on lateral positions for the mandible, T.M.J.'s, mastoids and petrous pyramids. In addition, the lateral T.M.J.'s require both mouth-open and mouth-closed positions.

Descriptive terms for projections are used rather than the proper nouns for these radiographic examinations. The most common names, however, such as Waters' and Caldwell, are also listed.

Mandible
Basic
- P.A.
- Axiolateral (Oblique)

Optional
- Semiaxial A.P.
- Superoinferior (Extraoral)
- Submentovertex

T.M.J.'s
Basic
- Semiaxial Transcranial
  or
- Lateral Transcranial

Paranasal Sinuses
Basic
- Parietoacanthial (Waters')
- P.A. (Caldwell)
- Lateral

Optional
- Submentovertex (Basilar Position)
- Semiaxial Transoral (Open-mouth Waters')

Temporal Bone
Survey
- Submentovertex
- Semiaxial A.P.

Mastoids
Basic
- Lateral Transcranial
- Posterior Profile

Petrous Pyramids
Basic
- Semiaxial Oblique
- Anterior Profile

Mandible
Basic
- **P.A.**
- Axiolateral (Oblique)

Optional
- Semiaxial A.P.
- Superoinferior (Extraoral)
- Submentovertex

Mandible
• Posteroanterior Projection

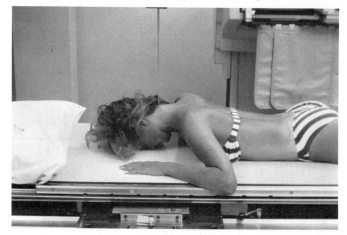

P.A.   Fig. 12-30

Film Size:
    8 x 10 in. (18 x 24 cm.)

Bucky:
- Moving or stationary grid.

Patient Position:
- Prone or upright.

Part Position:
- O.M.L. perpendicular to table.
- Forehead and nose touching table.
- No rotation or tilt.
- Midsagittal plane perpendicular to table.
- Center to junction of lips.

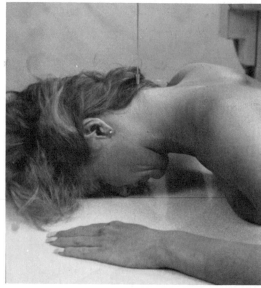

P.A.   Fig. 12-31

Central Ray:
- C.R. perpendicular to film holder, passing between upper and lower lips.
- 40 in. (102 cm.) F.F.D.

NOTE: • Mid body and mentum obscured by cervical spine.

Structures Best Shown:
Mandibular rami and lateral portions of the body.

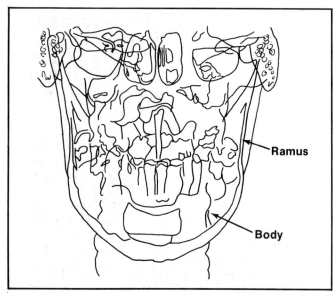

Fig. 12-33   P.A.

Ramus

Body

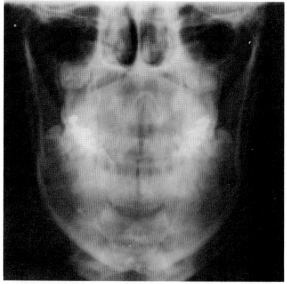

P.A.   Fig. 12-32

Mandible

• Axiolateral (Oblique) Position

Mandible
Basic
- P.A.
- Axiolateral (Oblique)

Optional
- Semiaxial A.P.
- Superoinferior (Extraoral)
- Submentovertex

Film Size:

8 x 10 in. (18 x 24 cm.)
Crosswise.

Bucky:
- Moving or stationary grid.

Patient Position:
- Upright or supine.

Part Position:
- Head lateral; extend chin.
  Three part positions are possible, depending on which portion of the mandible is to be best visualized.
  - Head in true lateral best shows ramus.
  - Chin turned toward film 30° best shows body.
  - Chin turned toward film 45° best shows mentum.

Central Ray:
- C.R. directed between mandibular angles, 35° cephalic.
- Always maintain 55° angle between midsagittal plane and C.R.
- 40 in. (102 cm.) F.F.D.

NOTE: • Upright position easiest for patient. • Extend chin so there will be no superimposition on cervical spine. • Area of interest always placed parallel to film.

Structures Best Shown:
Half of mandible closest to film, with ramus, body or mentum best visualized depending on head rotation.

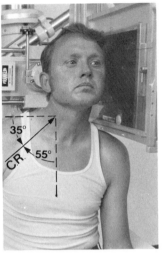
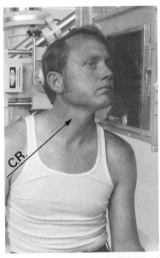

Axiolateral (Oblique) Position   Fig. 12-34

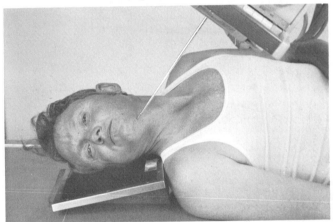

Axiolateral (Oblique) Position   Fig. 12-35

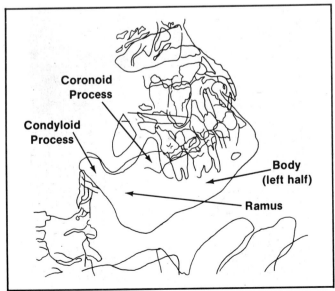

Coronoid Process

Condyloid Process

Body (left half)

Ramus

Fig. 12-37   Axiolateral (Oblique) Position

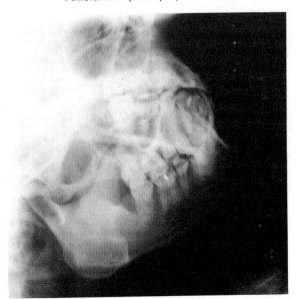

Axiolateral (Oblique) Position   Fig. 12-36

Mandible
Basic
● P.A.
● Axiolateral (Oblique)
Optional
● **Semiaxial A.P.**
● Superoinferior (Extraoral)
● Submentovertex

Mandible

● **Semiaxial Anteroposterior Projection**

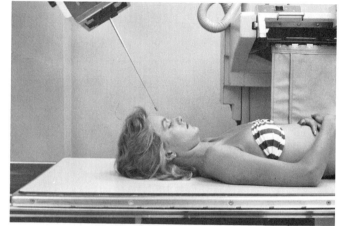

Semiaxial A.P.   Fig. 12-38

Film Size:

8 x 10 in. (18 x 24 cm.)

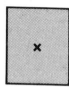

Bucky:

- Moving or stationary grid.

Patient Position:

- Supine or upright.

Part Position:

- O.M.L. perpendicular to table.
- No rotation or tilt.
- Midsagittal plane perpendicular to table.
- Closely collimate and immobilize.

Central Ray:

- Tube angled 30° caudad.
- C.R. passes through a point slightly caudad to T.M.J.'s.
- 40 in. (102 cm.) F.F.D.

NOTE: ● Similar to semiaxial A.P. projection of cranium, except C.R. more caudal.

Structures Best Shown:

Condyloid processes of mandible and temporomandibular fossae.

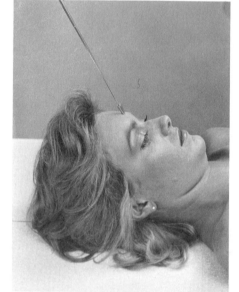

Semiaxial A.P.   Fig. 12-39

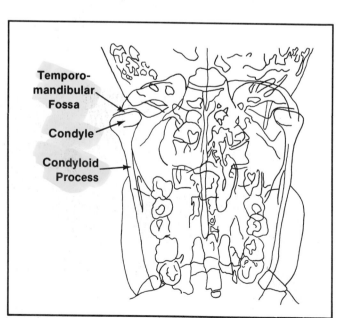

Temporo-
mandibular
Fossa

Condyle

Condyloid
Process

Fig. 12-41

Semiaxial A.P.

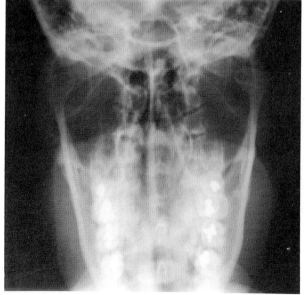

Semiaxial A.P.   Fig. 12-40

Mandible
Basic
- P.A.
- Axiolateral (Oblique)

Optional
- Semiaxial A.P.
- **Superoinferior (Extraoral)**
- Submentovertex

Mandible (Mentum)

- **Superoinferior Projection (Extraoral)**

Film Size:
Occlusal Film Packet

or

5 x 7 in. (13 x 18 cm.) CBH

Non-Bucky:
- Occlusal film or CBH.

Patient Position:
- Seated at end of table, or supine.

Part Position:
Seated
- Extend and place chin in close contact with film holder.
- Elevate film holder.

Supine
- Back of head rests on table.
- Adjust film holder parallel with inferior border of mandible.
- Patient holds film holder in position.

Central Ray:
- C.R. is angled 45° to plane of film to pass through mentum.
- 40 in. (102 cm.) F.F.D.

NOTE: • Fractures of the mentum and symphysis menti can be best demonstrated on this projection.

Structures Best Shown:
Mandibular mentum and symphysis menti.

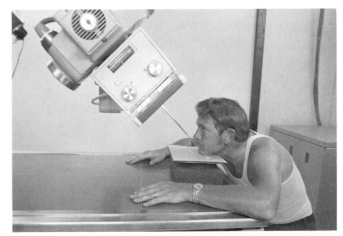

Superoinferior Projection (Extraoral)   Fig. 12-42

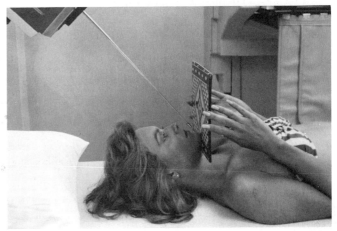

Superoinferior Projection (Extraoral)   Fig. 12-43

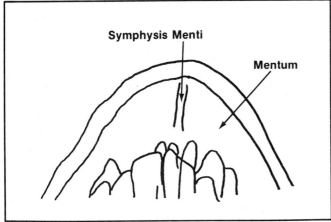

Fig. 12-45
Superoinferior Projection (Extraoral)

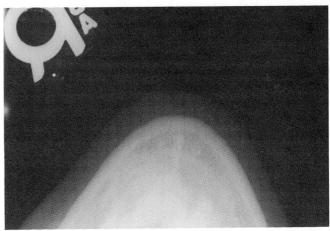

Superoinferior Projection (Extraoral)   Fig. 12-44

• **Submentovertex Projection**

Film Size:

   8 x 10 in. (18 x 24 cm.)
   Crosswise.

Bucky:

- Moving or stationary grid.

Patient Position:

- Supine (supports under back, knees flexed) or upright.

Part Position:

- I.O.M.L. **parallel** to table.
- Midsagittal plane perpendicular to table.
- Head rests on vertex.
- Neck hyperextended.

Central Ray:

- C.R. must be **perpendicular to I.O.M.L.**
- C.R. enters midway between angles of mandible.
- 40 in. (102 cm.) F.F.D.

NOTE: • Mandibular condyles are projected anterior to petrous pyramids.

Structures Best Shown:

U-shaped outline of mandible, coronoid and condyloid processes.

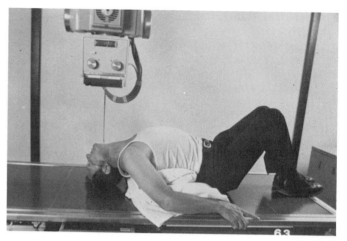

Submentovertex Projection   Fig. 12-46

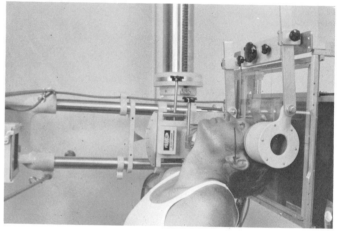

Submentovertex Projection   Fig. 12-47

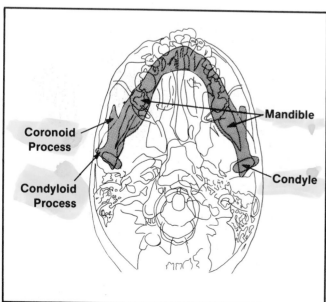

Mandible

Coronoid Process

Condyloid Process

Condyle

Fig. 12-49

Submentovertex Projection

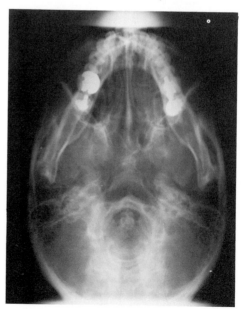

Submentovertex Projection   Fig. 12-48

T.M.J.'s
Basic
- **Semiaxial Transcranial**
  or
- **Lateral Transcranial**

T.M.J.'s

- **Semiaxial Transcranial Projection**
Schuller Position

Film Size:
  8 x 10 in. (18 x 24 cm.)
  Divide in half, crosswise.

open   closed

Bucky:
- Moving or stationary grid.

Patient Position:
- Semiprone or upright with head turned to lateral position.

Part Position:
- Head in true lateral.
- Closely collimate and immobilize.
- Side of interest closest to film.

Central Ray:
- Angle C.R. 25° caudad.
- Center to T.M.J. closest to film (1 cm. anterior to E.A.M.)
- 40 in. (102 cm.) F.F.D.

NOTE: • Need to rule out fracture of mandible before doing T.M.J.'s. • Both laterals are taken, each with the mouth closed and open. • Both sides are needed for comparison. • Tomography, with the patient in a true lateral position, is an optional procedure to visualize the T.M.J.'s.

Structures Best Shown:
Temporomandibular joint closest to film, demonstrating anterior movement when the mouth is opened.

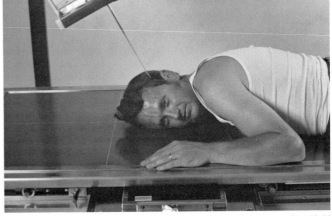

T.M.J.   Fig. 12-50

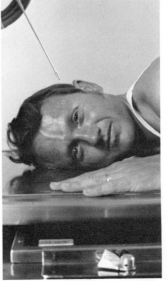

T.M.J.   Fig. 12-51

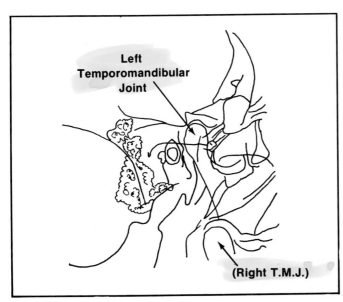

Left Temporomandibular Joint

(Right T.M.J.)

Fig. 12-53   T.M.J.

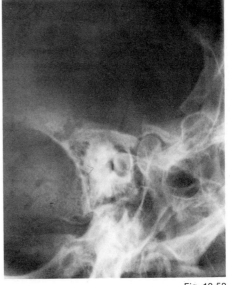

T.M.J.   Fig. 12-52

The Law made Schullers dife difficult
Droped his face 15° + Made him return alateral
home

<table><tr><td>**T.M.J.'s**
Basic
• Semiaxial Transcranial
or
• **Lateral Transcranial**</td></tr></table>

T.M.J.'s

• **Lateral Transcranial Projection**
Law Position

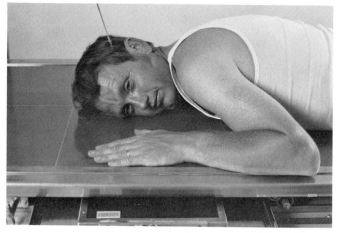

T.M.J. (right)

Fig. 12-54

Film Size:
8 x 10 in. (18 x 24 cm.)
Divide in half, crosswise.

open   closed

Bucky:
- Moving or stationary grid.

Patient Position:
- Semiprone or upright with head turned to lateral position.

Part Position:
- Place head in true lateral, then rotate face toward table 15°.
- Do not allow chin to sag.
- Interpupillary line perpendicular to table.
- Closely collimate and immobilize.
- Side of interest closest to film.

Central Ray:
- Angle C.R. 15° caudad.
- Center to downside T.M.J. (1 cm. anterior to E.A.M.).
- 40 in. (102 cm.) F.F.D.

NOTE: • Need to rule out fracture of mandible before doing T.M.J.'s. • Both laterals are taken, each with the mouth closed and open. • Both sides are done for comparison.

Structures Best Shown:
Temporomandibular joint closest to film, demonstrating anterior movement when the mouth is opened.

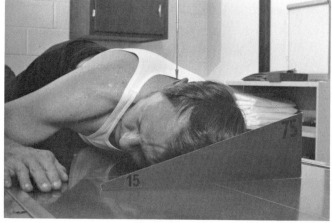

T.M.J. (left)

Fig. 12-55

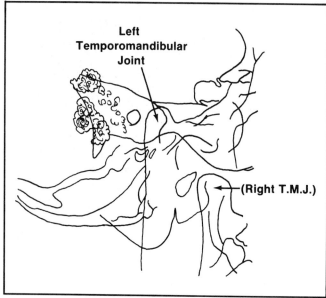

Left Temporomandibular Joint

(Right T.M.J.)

Fig. 12-57

T.M.J.

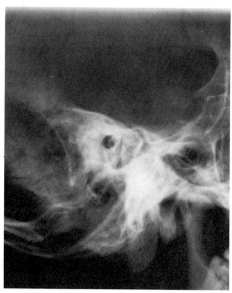

T.M.J.

Fig. 12-56

Paranasal Sinuses
Basic
- **Parietoacanthial**
  (Waters')
- P.A. (Caldwell)
- Lateral

Optional
- Submentovertex
- Semiaxial Transoral

Paranasal Sinuses

- **Parietoacanthial Projection**
Waters' Position

Film Size:
 8 x 10 in. (18 x 24 cm.)

Bucky:
- Moving or stationary grid.

Patient Position:
- Upright.

Part Position:
- No rotation or tilt.
- Midsagittal plane perpendicular to table.
- Rest head on chin.
- O.M.L. forms 37° angle with plane of film.
- Closely collimate.
- Immobilize, if necessary.
- Tip of nose is approximately 1 cm. from table.

Central Ray:
- C.R. enters at posterior sagittal suture and exits at acanthion.
- C.R. parallel to mentomeatal line and perpendicular to film holder.
- 40 in. (102 cm.) F.F.D.

NOTE: • Must be upright in order to show air-fluid levels.

Structures Best Shown:
Maxillary sinuses above petrous pyramids.

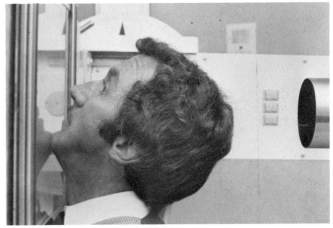

Parietoacanthial Projection
Fig. 12-58

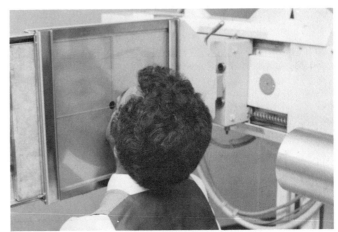

Parietoacanthial Projection
Fig. 12-59

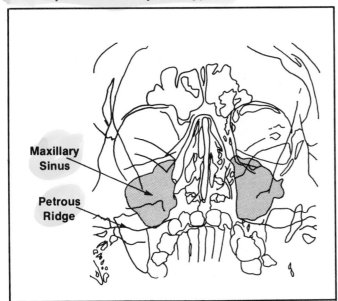

Maxillary Sinus

Petrous Ridge

Fig. 12-61
Parietoacanthial Projection

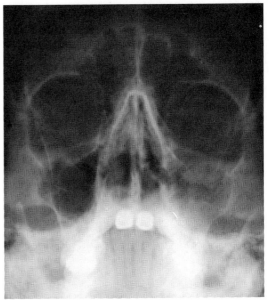

Parietoacanthial Projection
Fig. 12-60

Paranasal Sinuses
Basic
- Parietoacanthial
  (Waters')
- **P.A.** (Caldwell)
- Lateral
Optional
- Submentovertex
- Semiaxial Transoral

Paranasal Sinuses

- **Posteroanterior Projection**
  Caldwell Position

Film Size:
  8 x 10 in. (18 x 24 cm.)

Bucky:
- Moving or stationary grid.

Patient Position:
- Upright.

Part Position:
- O.M.L. perpendicular to table.
- Forehead and nose touch table.
- No rotation or tilt.
- Midsagittal plane perpendicular to table.
- Closely collimate and immobilize.
- Beam should be horizontal.

Central Ray:
- C.R. horizontal.
- Table or film holder angled 15°.
- C.R. passes through nasion.
- O.M.L. perpendicular to plane of film.
- 40 in. (102 cm.) F.F.D.

Angle tube 15° Caudad

NOTE: • Beam must be horizontal and patient must be upright to demonstrate air-fluid levels.

Structures Best Shown:
Frontal and ethmoid sinuses.

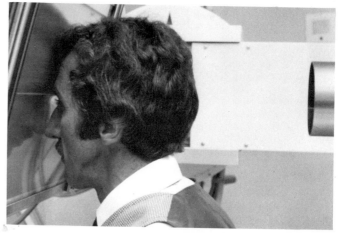

P.A.   Fig. 12-62

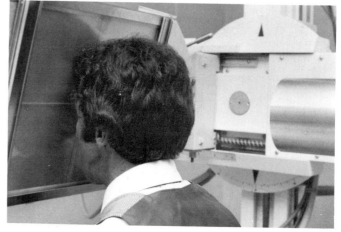

P.A.   Fig. 12-63

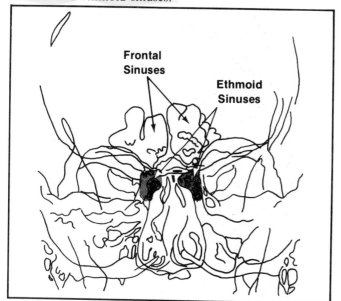

Frontal Sinuses

Ethmoid Sinuses

Fig. 12-65

P.A.

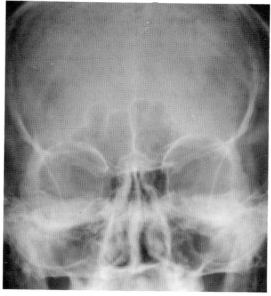

P.A.   Fig. 12-64

Paranasal Sinuses

• Lateral Position

Paranasal Sinuses
Basic
- Parietoacanthial
  (Waters')
- P.A. (Caldwell)
- **Lateral**
Optional
- Submentovertex
- Semiaxial Transoral

Film Size:
   8 x 10 in. (18 x 24 cm.)

Bucky:
- Moving or stationary grid.

Patient Position:
- Upright.

Part Position:
- Head in true lateral.
- Interpupillary line perpendicular to film.
- Midsagittal plane parallel to table.
- I.O.M.L. perpendicular to front edge of cassette.
- Closely collimate and immobilize.

Central Ray:
- C.R. perpendicular to film holder.
- C.R. exits at outer canthus.
- 40 in. (102 cm.) F.F.D.

NOTE: • Lateral cranium, lateral facial bones and lateral paranasal sinuses are all similar except for centering point.
• Patient must be upright and beam horizontal.

Structures Best Shown:
Sphenoid sinus. Other sinuses shown, but superimposed.

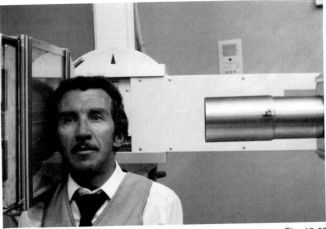

Lateral Position   Fig. 12-66

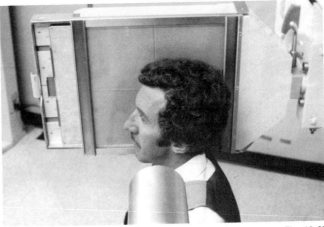

Lateral Position   Fig. 12-67

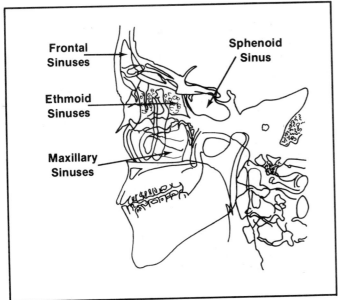

Frontal
Sinuses

Sphenoid
Sinus

Ethmoid
Sinuses

Maxillary
Sinuses

Fig. 12-69   Lateral Position

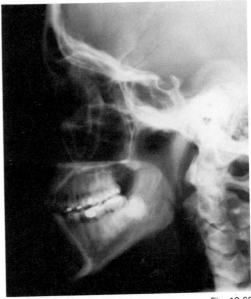

Lateral Position   Fig. 12-68

- **Submentovertex Projection**
Basilar Position

Film Size:

   8 x 10 in. (18 x 24 cm.)

Bucky:

- Moving or stationary grid.

Patient Position:

- Upright.

Part Position:

- I.O.M.L. parallel to table.
- Midsagittal plane perpendicular to table.
- Head contacts table at vertex.
- Neck hyperextended.
- Closely collimate and immobilize.

Central Ray:

- C.R. must be perpendicular to I.O.M.L.
- C.R. enters midway between gonia, exits at vertex, and passes through sella turcica.
- 40 in. (102 cm.) F.F.D.

NOTE: • Area of interest is anterior to foramen magnum.

Structures Best Shown:

Sphenoid sinus. Other structures shown are ethmoid sinuses and nasal fossae.

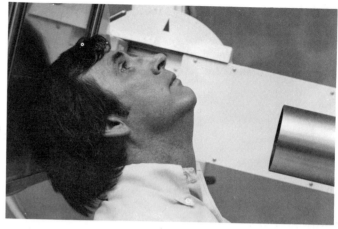

Submentovertex Projection   Fig. 12-70

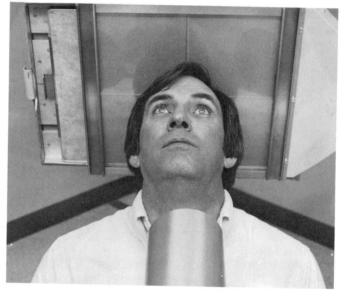

Submentovertex Projection   Fig. 12-71

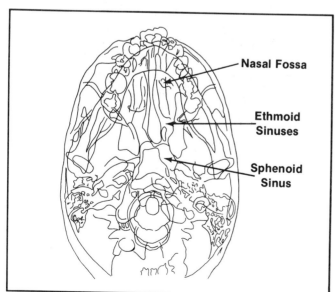

Fig. 12-73

Submentovertex Projection

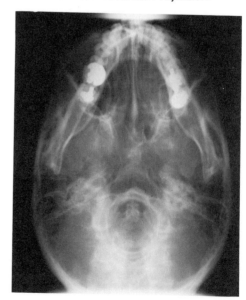

Nasal Fossa

Ethmoid Sinuses

Sphenoid Sinus

Submentovertex Projection   Fig. 12-72

Paranasal Sinuses
Basic
- Parietoacanthial (Waters')
- P.A. (Caldwell)
- Lateral

Optional
- Submentovertex
- **Semiaxial Transoral**

Paranasal Sinuses

• Semiaxial Transoral Position
Open-mouth Waters' Position

Film Size:
>   8 x 10 in. (18 x 24 cm.)

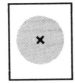

Bucky:
- Moving or stationary grid.

Patient Position:
- Upright.

Part Position:
- Mouth fully open.
- Patient rests on chin and nose.
- Midsagittal plane perpendicular to table.
- Immobilize and reduce field size with extension cylinder.

Central Ray:
- C.R. perpendicular to film holder.
- C.R. passes through sella turcica to exit at center of open mouth.
- 40 in. (102 cm.) F.F.D.

NOTE: • Sphenoid sinus will be visualized within shadow of open mouth.

Structures Best Shown:
Sphenoid sinus. Other structures shown are maxillary sinuses and nasal fossae.

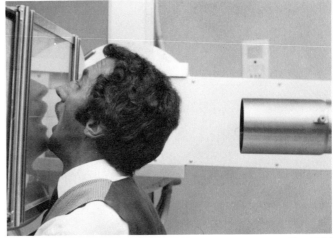

Semiaxial Transoral Position

Fig. 12-74

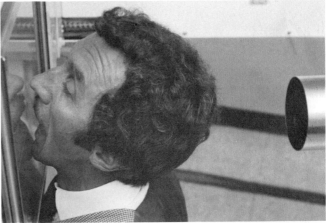

Semiaxial Transoral Position

Fig. 12-75

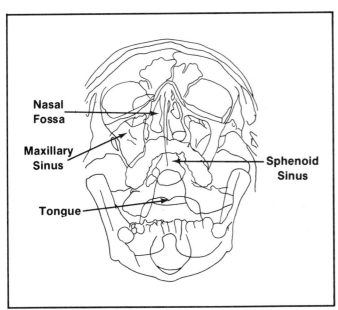

Fig. 12-77

Semiaxial Transoral Position

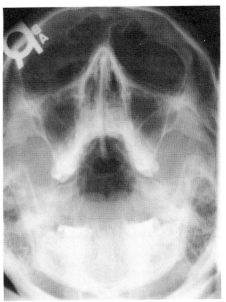

Semiaxial Transoral Position

Fig. 12-76

Temporal Bone — Survey
• Submentovertex Projection
• Semiaxial Anteroposterior Projection

Film Size:
>   10 x 12 in. (24 x 30 cm.)

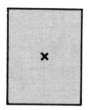

Bucky:
- Moving or stationary grid.

Patient Position:
- Upright or supine.

Part Position:
Submentovertex Projection
- I.O.M.L. parallel to film.
- Midsagittal plane perpendicular to table.
- Head rests on vertex.
- Neck hyperextended.
- C.R. perpendicular to I.O.M.L.
- C.R. passes through sella turcica.

Semiaxial A.P. Projection
- O.M.L. perpendicular to table.
- No rotation or tilt.
- Midsagittal plane perpendicular to table.
- Closely collimate and immobilize.
- C.R. 30° caudad and passes through line connecting E.A.M.'s.
- 40 in. (102 cm.) F.F.D.

NOTE: • Positioning is the same as for similar projections of the cranium.

Structures Best Shown:
Petrous pyramids, including bilateral internal auditory canals, bony labyrinths and tympanic cavities.

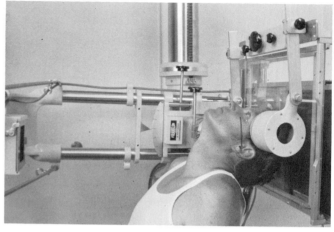

Submentovertex Projection   Fig. 12-78

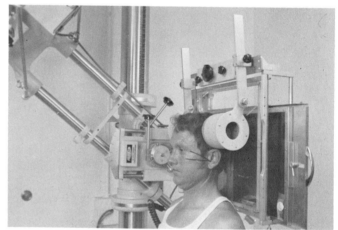

Semiaxial A.P. Projection   Fig. 12-79

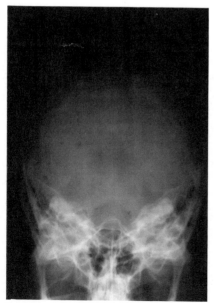

Fig. 12-81   Semiaxial
A.P. Projection

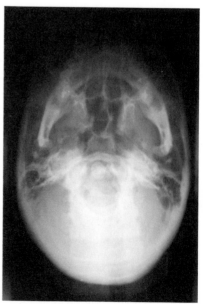

Submentovertex Fig. 12-80
Projection

Mastoids
Basic
• Lateral Transcranial
• Posterior Profile

Mastoids

• Lateral Transcranial Position
Law Position

Film Size:
  8 x 10 in. (18 x 24 cm.)
  Divide in half, crosswise.

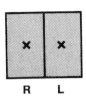

Bucky:
- Moving or stationary grid.

Patient Position:
- Semiprone or upright with head turned to lateral position.

Part Position:
- Place head in true lateral, then rotate face toward table 15°.
- Do not allow chin to sag.
- Interpupillary line perpendicular to table.
- Side of interest closest to film.
- Closely collimate and immobilize.
- Tape auricle forward.

Central Ray:
- Angle C.R. 15° caudad.
- Center 1 in. (2.5 cm.) posterior to E.A.M. closest to film.
- 40 in. (102 cm.) F.F.D.

NOTE: • Both sides are examined for comparison.

Structures Best Shown:
Mastoid air cells.

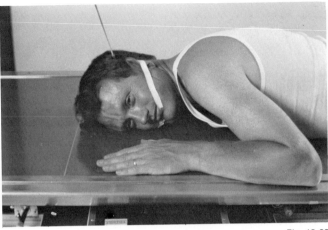
Lateral Transcranial Position (right)   Fig. 12-82

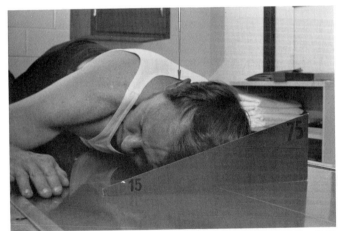
Lateral Transcranial Position (left)   Fig. 12-83

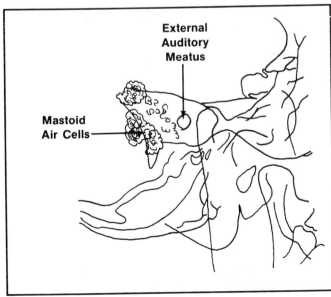
Fig. 12-85
Lateral Transcranial Position

External
Auditory
Meatus

Mastoid
Air Cells

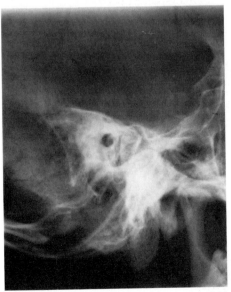
Lateral Transcranial   Fig. 12-84
Position

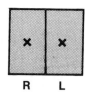

Mastoids
Basic
- Lateral Transcranial
- **Posterior Profile**

Mastoids

• **Posterior Profile Position**
Stenvers' Position

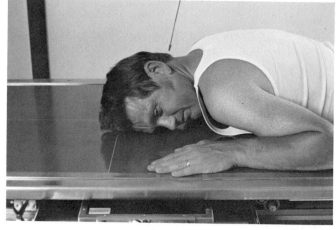
Posterior Profile Position   Fig. 12-86

Film Size:
    8 x 10 in. (18 x 24 cm.)
    Divide in half, crosswise.

Bucky:
- Moving or stationary grid.

Patient Position:
- Prone or upright.

Part Position:
- Head rotated 45°.
- Head rests on forehead, nose and cheek.
- I.O.M.L. perpendicular to front edge of film.
- Side of interest is the side closest to film.
- Side of interest is parallel to film.
- Tape auricle forward.
- Closely collimate and immobilize.

Central Ray:
- C.R. angled 12° cephalad and passes through a point 1 in. (2.5 cm.) anterior to downside E.A.M.
- 40 in. (102 cm.) F.F.D.

NOTE: • Side of interest is parallel to film. • Both sides examined for comparison. • Posterior and anterior profile positions give similar results.

Structures Best Shown:
Mastoid process, petrous ridge, tympanic cavity, bony labyrinth and internal auditory meatus.

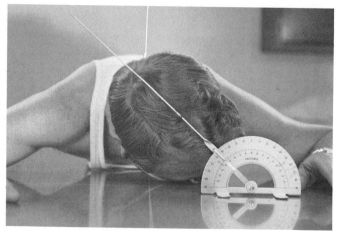
Posterior Profile Position   Fig. 12-87

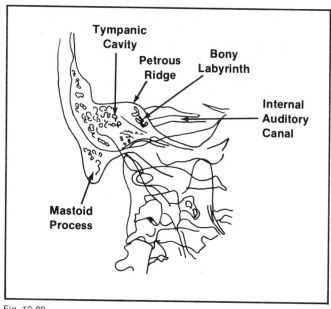
Fig. 12-89
Posterior Profile Position

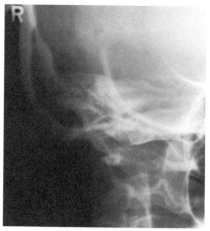
Posterior Profile Position   Fig. 12-88

Petrous Pyramids
Basic
- **Semiaxial Oblique**
- Anterior Profile

Petrous Pyramids

- **Semiaxial Oblique Position**

Owen Modification of Mayer Position

Film Size:
8 x 10 in. (18 x 24 cm.)
Divide in half, crosswise.

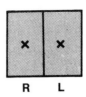

R L

Bucky:
- Moving or stationary grid.

Patient Position:
- Supine or upright.

Part Position:
- Head rotated 30° up from lateral.
- I.O.M.L. perpendicular to front edge of film.
- Interpupillary line perpendicular to plane of film.
- Closely collimate and immobilize.
- Tape auricle forward.

Central Ray:
- Angle C.R. 30° caudad.
- C.R. passes through downside E.A.M.
- 40 in. (102 cm.) F.F.D.

NOTE: • Side of interest is closest to film. • Both sides examined for comparison.

Structures Best Shown:
Tympanic cavity and ossicles, attic, aditus, antrum and E.A.M.

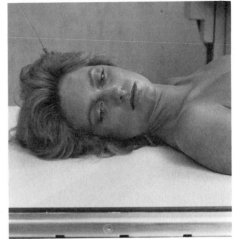

Semiaxial
Oblique Position

Fig. 12-90

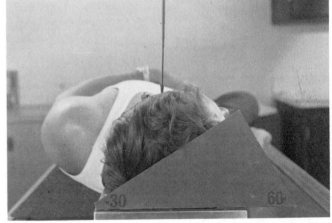

Semiaxial Oblique Position

Fig. 12-91

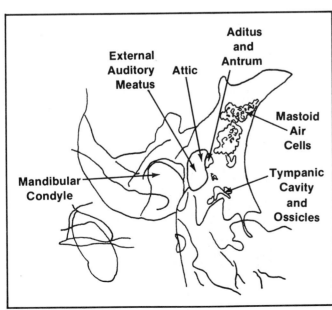

Fig. 12-93

Semiaxial Oblique Position

External
Auditory
Meatus

Attic

Aditus
and
Antrum

Mastoid
Air
Cells

Tympanic
Cavity
and
Ossicles

Mandibular
Condyle

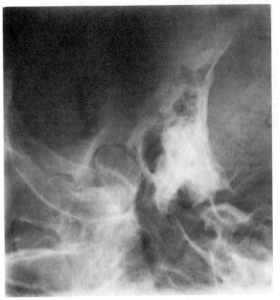

Semiaxial Oblique Position

Fig. 12-92

Petrous Pyramids
Basic
- Semiaxial Oblique
- **Anterior Profile**

Petrous Pyramids
• **Anterior Profile Position**
Arcelin or Reverse Stenvers' Position

Film Size:

    8 x 10 in. (18 x 24 cm.)
    Divide in half, crosswise.

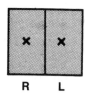

Bucky:

- Moving or stationary grid.

Patient Position:

- Supine or upright.

Part Position:

- Head rotated 45°.
- I.O.M.L. perpendicular to front edge of film.
- Side of interest is upside.
- Side of interest is parallel to film.
- Closely collimate and immobilize.

Central Ray:

- C.R. angled 12° caudad and passes through a point 1 in. (2.5 cm.) anterior to the upside T.E.A.
- 40 in. (102 cm.) F.F.D.

NOTE: • Side of interest is away from film (upside), which is parallel to film. • This position increases magnification slightly when compared to Stenvers' position. • Anterior and posterior profile positions give similar results. • Both sides examined for comparison.

Structures Best Shown:

Mastoid process, petrous ridge, tympanic cavity, bony labyrinth and internal auditory meatus.

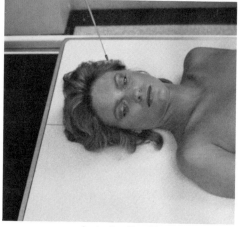

Anterior Profile Projection   Fig. 12-94

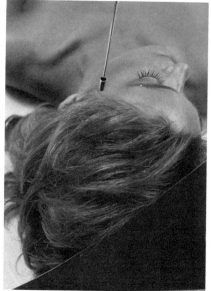

Anterior Profile Projection   Fig. 12-95

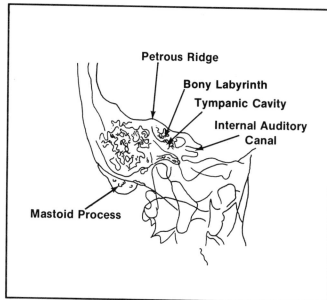

Petrous Ridge

Bony Labyrinth

Tympanic Cavity

Internal Auditory Canal

Mastoid Process

Fig. 12-97

Anterior Profile Projection

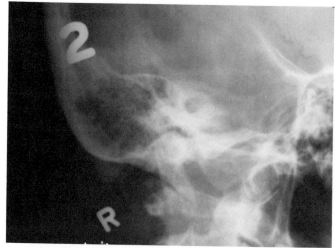

Anterior Profile Projection   Fig. 12-96

CHAPTER 13

Radiographic Anatomy and Positioning
of the
Coccyx, Sacrum and Lumbar Spine

Part I. Radiographic Anatomy
Coccyx, Sacrum and Lumbar Spine

Vertebral Column

The vertebral column, a complex succession of many bones, encloses and protects the spinal cord. This column is located in the midsagittal plane and forms the posterior or dorsal aspect of the bony trunk of the body. The entire column is divided by regions into five groups. The vertebrae of the neck region are termed **cervical;** the upper back vertebrae are termed **thoracic;** and the lower back vertebrae are referred to as **lumbar** vertebrae. The most inferior portion of the column consists of several fused segments termed the **sacrum** and the **coccyx.**

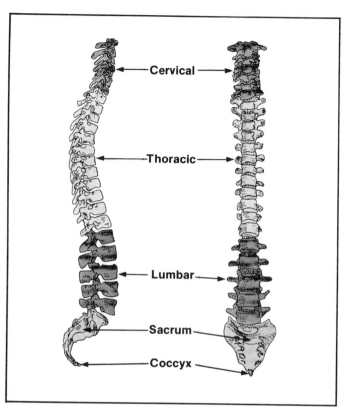

Vertebral Column   Fig. 13-1

Cervical, Thoracic, Lumbar Vertebrae, Sacrum and Coccyx

Within each of the five regions there are a certain number of vertebrae that have distinctive characteristics of that particular region. The **first seven** have similarities that group them as **cervical vertebrae.** While there may be a slight variation in the height of each vertebra from one individual to another, every human has seven cervical vertebrae. In fact, another mammal, the long-necked giraffe, also has only seven cervical vertebrae, but each of his averages 9 to 10 inches in height.

The next twelve vertebrae each connect to a pair of ribs. Since there are twelve pairs of ribs, there are **twelve thoracic vertebrae.** An older and incorrect term for the thoracic vertebrae is dorsal vertebrae. However, all of the vertebrae, being located on the posterior or dorsal aspect of the body, could correctly be called dorsal vertebrae; therefore, the twelve vertebrae of the upper back should correctly be called thoracic vertebrae.

The largest individual vertebrae are the **five lumbar vertebrae.** Each of the vertebrae in the cervical, thoracic and lumbar regions forms as a separate vertebra in the child, and is retained as a separate bone in the adult. The sacrum and coccyx, however, are different. In children there are **five** separate **sacral segments** and from **three** to **five coccygeal segments.** The sacrum and the coccyx tend to fuse into two single bones in the adult. Counting the sacrum and coccyx as single bones, the adult vertebral column is composed of **26 separate bones.**

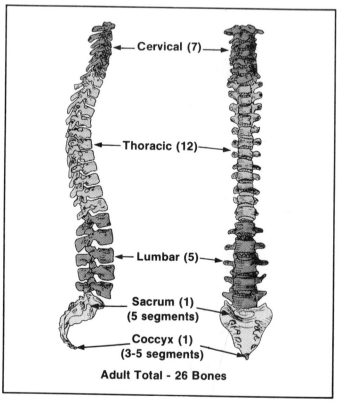

Vertebral Column   Fig. 13-2

Spinal Curvatures

The vertebral column forms a series of anteroposterior curves. These curves, as viewed from the side or on a lateral radiograph, are illustrated in *Fig. 13-3*. Only the **thoracic and sacral curves** are present when a child is born. These two curves are **concave forward** early in life and remain concave forward in the adult. When a child begins to raise his head and look around, and later when the child sits up, a compensatory curve forms in the opposite direction in the cervical region. Although this **cervical curve** is the least pronounced of the four curves, it is described as a **convex forward** curve.

The final curve to form is the **lumbar curvature**, also **convex forward.** This lumbar curvature develops when the child learns to walk. Both the lumbar and sacral curvatures are usually more pronounced in the female than they are in the male.

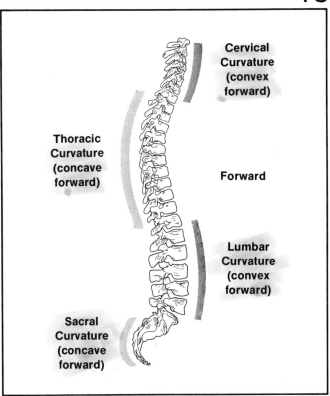

Normal Adult Curvatures

Fig. 13-3

Lordosis

The compensatory curves in the lumbar and cervical regions, which develop after birth, are termed lordotic curvatures. Any convex forward curve may be described as a lordosis, or a lordotic curvature.

Kyphosis

A kyphosis is a greater than normal curvature that sometimes develops in the thoracic region. Kyphosis refers to any accentuated thoracic curvature or humpback type of deformity.

In summary, the usual type of curvature found in the cervical or lumbar regions (convex forward) is termed a lordosis, while the abnormal, humpback type of curvature found in the thoracic region (concave forward) is termed kyphosis.

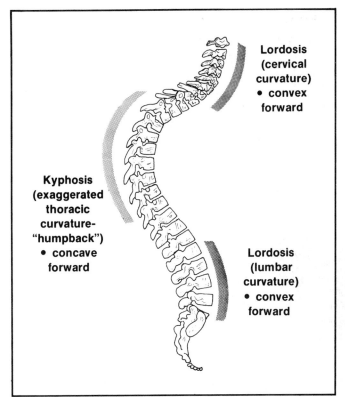

Lordosis - Kyphosis

Fig. 13-4

Scoliosis

An abnormal sideways or lateral curvature is called scoliosis. If the spine is viewed from the front, as on an A.P. radiograph (illustrated in *Fig. 13-5)*, the vertebral column is usually straight and has no lateral curvature. Occasionally, there is a slight lateral curvature in the upper thoracic region of a healthy adult. This curvature is usually associated with the dominant extremity, so the curvature is convex to the right in a right-handed person and convex to the left in a left-handed person. A more serious type of problem occurs when there is a pronounced S-shaped lateral curvature. This deformity, which may be congenital, is termed scoliosis and may cause severe deformity of the entire thorax.

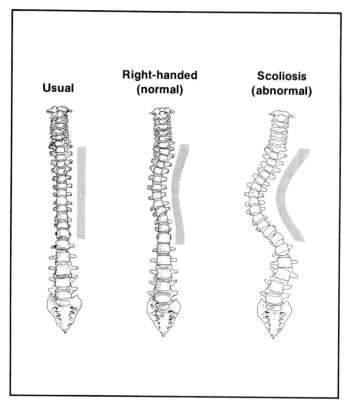

Usual **Right-handed (normal)** **Scoliosis (abnormal)**

Lateral Curvature

Fig. 13-5

Typical Vertebra

A typical vertebra is composed of two main parts. Anteriorly, a large mass of bone called the **body** is roughly cylindrical in shape. Extending posteriorly from the body is a ring of bone called the **vertebral arch.** With the body in front, and the vertebral arch on the sides and in the back, a circular opening called the **vertebral foramen** is formed. When several vertebrae are stacked, as they are in the normal articulated vertebral column, the succession of vertebral foramina forms a tubelike opening along the complete length of the spine. This opening, called the spinal canal, encloses the spinal cord.

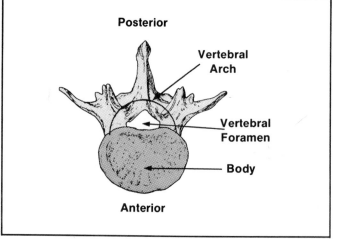

Posterior

Vertebral Arch

Vertebral Foramen

Body

Anterior

Typical Vertebra

Fig. 13-6

Typical Vertebra (superior view)

Part of the vertebral arch is formed by two projections, termed **pedicles,** that extend posteriorly from either side of the body. Pedicle is a Latin term meaning "little foot." The pedicles form most of the sides of the vertebral arch. The posterior part of the vertebral arch is formed by two flat layers of bone termed laminae. Each **lamina** extends posteriorly from each pedicle to unite in the midline.

Extending laterally from approximately the junction of each pedicle and lamina is a projection termed the **transverse process.** At the midline junction of the two laminae, extending posteriorly, is another process called the **spinous process.** The spinous processes are the most posterior extensions of the vertebrae and can often be palpated along the dorsal surface of the neck and back.

In summary, the typical vertebra has two pedicles and two laminae that form the vertebral arch and enclose the vertebral foramen, two transverse processes extending laterally, and one spinous process extending posteriorly.

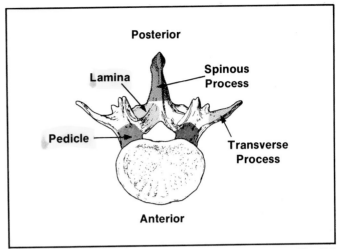

Typical Vertebra   Fig. 13-7

Typical Vertebra (lateral view)

A typical vertebra as seen from the side is illustrated in *Fig. 13-8.* The large **body** is most anterior and the **spinous process** is most posterior. Extending posteriorly from the body is one **pedicle,** which terminates in the area of the **transverse process.** Continuing posteriorly from the origin of the transverse process is one **lamina.**

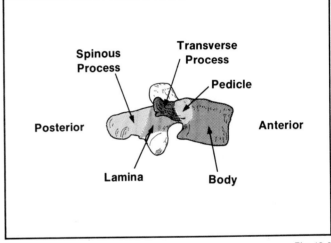

Typical Vertebra   Fig. 13-8

Each typical vertebra has four articular processes projecting from approximately the area of the junction of the pedicles and laminae. As seen from the side in *Fig. 13-9,* the process projecting upward is termed the **superior articular process** and the process projecting downward is termed the **inferior articular process.** Two similar processes are also found on the opposite side of the typical vertebra. The importance of these processes becomes apparent when vertebrae are stacked together to form the vertebral column. The two superior articular processes of one vertebra articulate with the two inferior articular processes of the vertebra above, forming joints called apophysial joints.

Along the upper surface of each pedicle is a notch termed the **superior vertebral notch,** and along the lower surface of each pedicle is another notch termed the **inferior vertebral notch.**

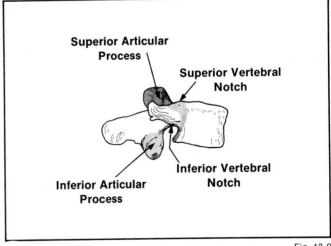

Typical Vertebra   Fig. 13-9

Apophysial Joints and Intervertebral Foramina

In the articulated vertebral column, the inferior vertebral notches of the vertebra above and the superior vertebral notches of the vertebra below form the important openings, the **intervertebral foramina.** Between every two vertebrae there are two intervertebral foramina, one on each side. It is through these intervertebral foramina that spinal nerves and blood vessels are transmitted.

A portion of the joint formed by the superior inferior articular processes is shown in *Fig. 13-10.* These upward-pointing **superior articular processes** form a joint with the downward-projecting **inferior articular processes** of the vertebra above. Each of these joints is termed an **apophysial joint.** Since there are two superior and two inferior articular processes on each vertebra, there are also two apophysial joints between any two vertebrae, one on each side. It is often necessary to demonstrate these apophysial joints on certain radiographs of the vertebral column.

The term facet is sometimes used interchangeably with the term apophysial joint; however, this is incorrect because the facet is actually only the articulating surface, not the entire superior or inferior articular process.

The intervertebral foramina and apophysial joints must be demonstrated radiographically by the appropriate position or projection in each of the three major portions of the vertebral column. Correct positioning is summarized in Chapter 14, *Radiographic Anatomy and Positioning of the Thoracic Spine and Cervical Spine.*

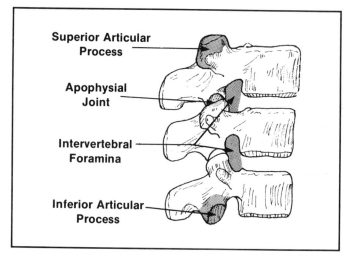

Apophysial Joints
and Intervertebral Foramina

Fig. 13-10

Intervertebral Disc

Intervertebral discs are found between the bodies of any two vertebrae. These discs provide a resilient cushion between the vertebrae, helping to absorb shock. The vertebral column would be rigidly immovable without the intervertebral discs and apophysial joints. Each disc consists of an outer fibrous portion termed the **annulus fibrosus** and a soft, semigelatinous inner part called the **nucleus pulposus.** Each intervertebral disc is similar to a donut, with the outer part being the annulus fibrosus and the hole of the donut, when filled, being similar to the nucleus pulposus. If, due to injury, the soft inner part protrudes to press on the spinal cord or spinal nerves, the condition is termed a "slipped disc" or, much more properly, herniated nucleus pulposus (H.N.P.).

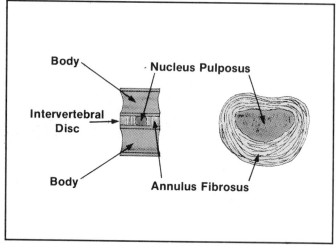

Intervertebral Disc

Fig. 13-11

Vertebral Column Joints

The joints of the vertebral column between cervical vertebra number 2 and the sacrum are of two types. The **intervertebral joints** between the bodies of any two vertebrae allow only a slight amount of motion and are termed **amphiarthrodial** joints. The **apophysial joints** between the superior and inferior articular processes allow more freedom of motion and are termed **diarthrodial** joints of the **gliding** type. While there is not a great deal of motion between any two vertebrae, the combined effect of all the vertebrae in the column allows a considerable range of motion.

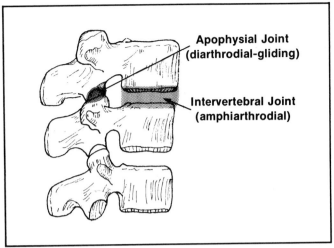

Joints   Fig. 13-12

Coccyx

Anterior Coccyx

The most distal portion of the vertebral column is the coccyx. The anterior surface of the "tailbone" or coccyx is illustrated in *Fig. 13-13*. This portion of the vertebral column has greatly regressed in the human so there remains little resemblance to vertebrae. Three to five segments (an average of four) have fused in the adult to form the single coccyx. The most superior segment is the largest and broadest of the four sections and even has two lateral projections that are small **transverse processes.** The distal pointed tip of the coccyx is termed the **apex**, while the broader, superior portion is termed the **base.** Occasionally the second segment does not fuse solidly with the larger first segment; however, the coccyx usually is one, small, fairly insignificant end of the vertebral column.

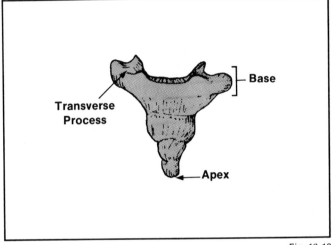

Coccyx, anterior   Fig. 13-13

Posterior Coccyx

The posterior aspect of an actual coccyx is pictured in *Fig. 13-14* along with a common U.S. postage stamp to allow a size comparison of the two. (Note that there is a small piece of bone missing on the right upper surface of the transverse process.) Ordinarily the coccyx curves forward, so the apex points toward the symphysis pubis of the anterior pelvis. This forward curvature is more pronounced in males and less pronounced, or straighter, in females. The coccyx projects into the birth canal in the female and, if angled excessively forward, it can impede the birth process.

The most common injury associated with the coccyx results from a direct blow to the lower vertebral column when a person is in a sitting position. A wild ride on a toboggan might provide the type of force required to angulate the coccyx more forward than normal and make sitting down an action to be avoided for a period of time.

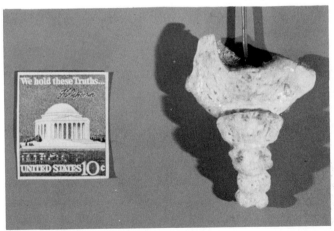

Coccyx, actual size   Fig. 13-14

Sacrum

Anterior Sacrum

The anterior surface of a sacrum is illustrated in *Fig. 13-15*. The bodies of the original five segments can be seen, but they have fused into a single bone in the adult. The sacrum is shaped somewhat like a shovel, with the **apex** the most inferior portion. Four sets of foramina or holes are shown on the anterior surface. These foramina serve to transmit nerves and blood vessels. The holes on the anterior surface are termed the **anterior sacral foramina.**

The large masses of bone lateral to the **body** of the first sacral segment are called the **alae** or wings of the sacrum. The upper surface of the sacrum closely resembles the last lumbar vertebra with which it articulates. Each **superior articular process** of the sacrum forms an apophysial joint with the inferior articular process of the fifth lumbar vertebra. The anterior edge of the body of the first sacral segment helps to form the inlet of the true pelvis and is termed the **promontory** of the sacrum.

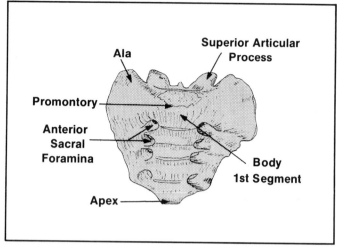

Sacrum, anterior   Fig. 13-15

Lateral Sacrum and Coccyx

A lateral drawing of both the sacrum and the coccyx in *Fig. 13-16* clearly illustrates the dominant curve of the sacrum and the forward projection of the coccyx. These curves determine how the central ray must be angled for a true A.P. projection of the sacrum or the coccyx.

The **sacral promontory** is the most anterior portion of the sacrum. The sacral promontory is seen anterior to the body of the first sacral segment. As seen in *Fig. 13-15,* the posterior surface of the sacrum is much rougher and more irregular than the smooth anterior surface.

The sacrum articulates with the ilium of the pelvis on the **articular surface** of the upper lateral sacrum to form the **sacroiliac joint.**

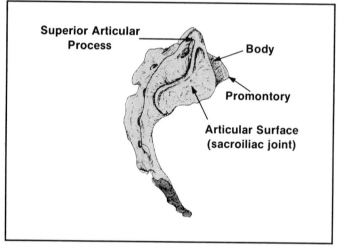

Sacrum and Coccyx, lateral   Fig. 13-16

Posterior Sacrum

Figure 13-17 is a photograph of an actual sacrum as seen from the posterior aspect. The large, wedge-shaped articular surface for the sacroiliac joints can be seen only on this posterior view. Each sacroiliac joint opens obliquely backward at an angle of 30 degrees, indicating why the articulating surface cannot be seen on an anterior view, but only from the side or from the posterior aspect.

The articulating surfaces or facets of the superior articular processes also open to the rear and are shown on this photograph. There are eight posterior sacral foramina, corresponding to the same number of anterior sacral foramina.

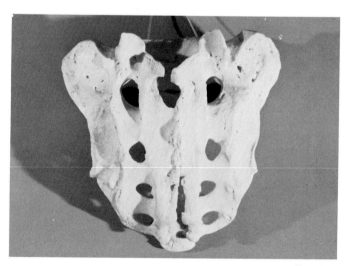

Sacrum, posterior   Fig. 13-17

Lumbar Vertebrae

Lateral Lumbar Vertebra

A typical lumbar vertebra as seen from the side is illustrated in *Fig. 13-18*. The **bodies** of the lumbar vertebrae are large in comparison to the vertebral bodies in the thoracic and cervical regions, with the last body, L-5, being largest of all. The **transverse processes** are fairly small, while the posteriorly projecting **spinous process** is quite large and blunt. The palpable lower tip of each lumbar spinous process lies at the level of the intervertebral disc space inferior to each vertebral body.

The **intervertebral foramina** are well seen from the side and are best visualized on a true lateral of the lumbar spine. The intervertebral foramina are shown in black on the drawing to demonstrate the area where they are located. They, of course, are not actually part of the lumbar vertebrae.

The **superior** and the **inferior articular processes** are shown. These processes form the apophysial joints when several vertebrae are stacked on top of each other.

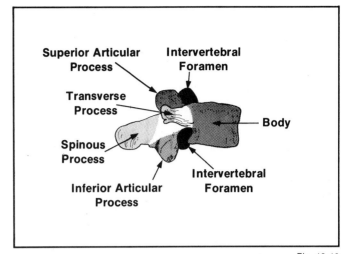

Lumbar Vertebra, lateral
Fig. 13-18

Superior Lumbar Vertebra

A typical lumbar vertebra as seen from above is illustrated in *Fig. 13-19*. The **laminae** are large sturdy structures in a lumbar vertebra. The portion of each lamina lying between the two articular processes has a special name, the **pars interarticularis.** Occasionally the pars interarticularis fails to unite the front and back of an individual vertebra. This condition allows the front part of one vertebra to slip forward on the vertebral body below it, a condition known as **spondylolisthesis.**

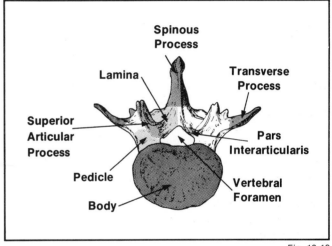

Lumbar Vertebra, top
Fig. 13-19

Posterior Lumbar Vertebra

The posterior aspect of a lumbar vertebra is illustrated in *Fig. 13-20*. This is the general appearance of a lumbar vertebra as seen on an A.P. radiograph of the lumbar spine. Since the **spinous process** is being seen on end, just the outline of this process shows through the **body** on an A.P. radiograph. The **transverse processes** extending to each side are well shown on this view. The **superior** and **inferior articular processes** are also visualized; however, the actual apophysial joint is best seen on an oblique radiograph of the lumbar vertebral column. The **pars interarticularis** is seen as that part of the **lamina** lying between the two articular processes.

A common defect, most often seen in the fifth lumbar vertebra, is the failure of two lamina to unite, leaving a space or opening where the spinous process is usually found. This condition, termed **spina bifida,** usually causes no problems as long as the structures within the vertebral canal remain in place. However, sometimes the soft tissues of the spinal cord coverings herniate posteriorly through this opening.

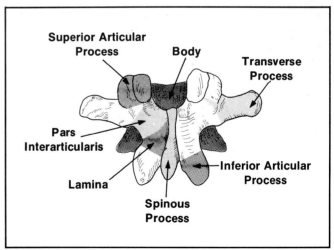

Lumbar Vertebra, posterior
Fig. 13-20

Lumbosacral Spine Radiographs

Superoinferior Lumbar Vertebra. Certain parts on the superoinferior projection of a lumbar vertebra are labeled in *Fig. 13-21*. These labeled parts are: **(A)** the spinous process, **(B)** the lamina, **(C)** the pedicle, **(D)** the vertebral foramen, **(E)** the body, and **(F)** the transverse process.

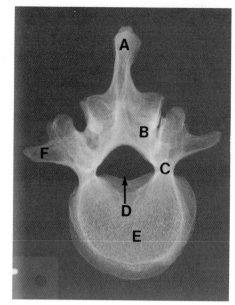

Lumbar Vertebra, superoinferior   Fig. 13-21

Lateral Lumbar Vertebra

Parts labeled A through F on the lateral view of a lumbar vertebra in *Fig. 13-22* are as follows: **(A)** body, **(B)** inferior vertebral notch, **(C)** area of the articulating facet of the inferior articular process, **(D)** spinous process, **(E)** superior articular process, and **(F)** pedicle.

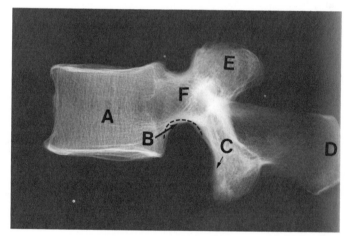

Lumbar Vertebra, lateral   Fig. 13-22

A.P. Lumbar Spine

Individual structures are more difficult to identify when the vertebrae are superimposed by the soft tissues of the abdomen. The A.P. lumbar spine radiograph shown in *Fig. 13-23* illustrates this principle. Those structures labeled A through E are: **(A)** the transverse process of L-5, **(B)** the lower lateral portion of the body of L-4, **(C)** the lower part of the spinous process of L-4 as visualized on end, **(D)** one inferior articular process of L-3, and **(E)** the superior articular process of L-4. The facets of the inferior and superior articular processes **(D** and **E)** make up one apophysial joint.

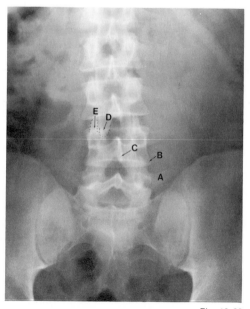

Lumbar Spine, A.P.   Fig. 13-23

272

Appearance of "Scotty Dog" (45° oblique)

Any bone and its parts, when seen in an oblique position, are more difficult to recognize than the same bone seen in the conventional frontal or lateral view. A vertebra is no exception; however, imagination can help us in the case of the lumbar vertebrae. A good 45-degree oblique will project the various structures in such a way that a "Scotty dog" seems to appear. The drawing in *Fig. 13-24* shows the various components of the "Scotty dog." The head and neck of the dog are probably the easiest features to recognize. The neck is one **pars interarticularis.** The **ear** of the dog is one **superior articular process,** while the **eye** is formed by one **pedicle.** One **transverse process** forms the **nose.** The **front legs** are formed by one **inferior articular process.**

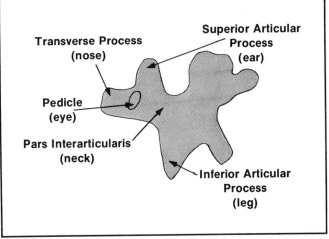

The "Scotty Dog"   Fig. 13-24

Oblique Lumbar Vertebrae

The radiograph in *Fig. 13-25* shows the "Scotty dog" appearance that should be visible on a good oblique radiograph of the lumbar spine. Part **A** is the nose of the "Scotty dog," formed by one transverse process. Part **B** appears to be an eye and is one pedicle seen on end. Part **C** (with the dotted lines added) appears to be a collar around the neck of the dog. This is the area of the pars interarticularis. Part **D,** which looks like the front leg of the animal, is formed by one inferior articular process. Part **E,** which looks like a pointed ear, is actually one of the superior articular processes. Each of the five lumbar vertebrae should assume a similar "Scotty dog" appearance on a good oblique radiograph. Examine the "Scotty dog" in the vertebra below the one enhanced with dotted lines.

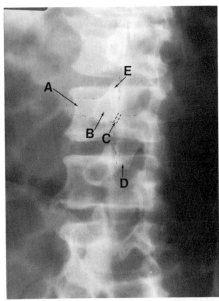

The "Scotty Dog"   Fig. 13-25

Lumbosacral Joint

Walking on two legs as humans do places a great deal of stress and strain on the last movable joint of the vertebral column. This joint is the lumbosacral junction, commonly called the L-5 — S-1 joint. Due to the lordotic curvature of the lumbar spine, an additional problem in that area results from the fact that the L-5 — S-1 joint sits at an angle when a person is standing. This lumbosacral angle is greater in a female, being approximately 35 degrees, while in the male the same angle averages about 30 degrees. These specific angles become important when radiographing the lumbosacral joint.

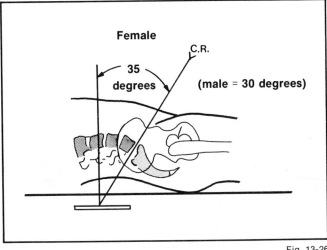

L-5 — S-1 Joint   Fig. 13-26

Lateral Lumbosacral Joint

A well-collimated radiograph of the lumbosacral articulation in the lateral position is shown in *Fig. 13-27*. Part **A** is the body of the fourth lumbar vertebra; **B** is the body of L-5; **C** is the area of interest on this radiograph and is the L-5 — S-1 joint or intervertebral disc; and **D** is the first segment of the sacrum.

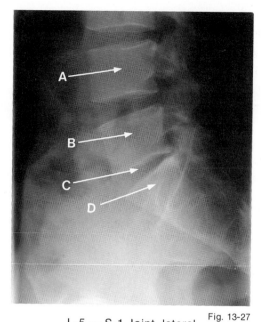

L-5 — S-1 Joint, lateral   Fig. 13-27

Lateral Lumbosacral Spine

A radiograph of the entire lumbosacral spine in the lateral position is shown in *Fig. 13-28*. Part **A** is the body of the first lumbar vertebra. (The body of the fifth lumbar vertebra is usually the easiest to identify; therefore, one should begin at L-5 and count upward until the first lumbar vertebra is located.) Part **B** is the body of the third lumbar vertebra. Part **C** locates the area of the intervertebral disc between the fourth and fifth lumbar vertebral bodies. **D** is the body of the fifth lumbar vertebra; **E** is the spinous process of L-4; and **F** indicates the superimposed intervertebral foramina between the second and third lumbar vertebrae. The intervertebral foramina in the lumbar spine are best seen in the lateral position.

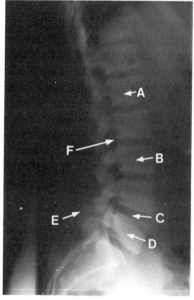

Fig. 13-28
Lumbar Spine,
lateral

A.P. Lumbosacral Spine

An anteroposterior projection of the lumbosacral spine is shown in *Fig. 13-29*. Normally, the contents of the abdomen overlie the lumbosacral spine and make easy visualization somewhat difficult.

Part **A** is the last thoracic vertebra. (Whereas the fifth lumbar is the easiest to locate on a lateral radiograph, T-12 is probably the easiest to locate on an A.P. because short ribs can be seen attached to the last thoracic vertebra.) Part **B**, directly below T-12, has no ribs, identifying it as L-1. Part **C** is the third lumbar vertebra, while part **D** is the final lumbar vertebra, number 5. (The upper portion of the sacrum often resembles L-5, and care must be taken before deciding which area is which.) Part **E** is the sacrum and **F** is the small coccyx.

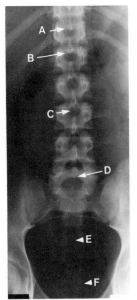

Lumbosacral   Fig. 13-29
Spine, A.P.

Certain smaller parts are labeled A through D on the A.P. lumbosacral spine radiograph in *Fig. 13-30*. Part **A** is the laterally extending, transverse process of L-1; **B** is the spinous process of L-1, seen on end; **C** is the disc space between L-3 and L-4; and **D** is the sacroiliac joint on the patient's left side.

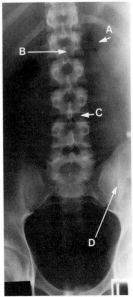

Lumbosacral   Fig. 13-30
Spine, A.P.

Topographical Landmarks: Various bony topographical landmarks, used to position the individual sections of the vertebral column or to locate the level of any one specific vertebra, are summarized by drawings and model photographs in Chapter 14.

Part II. Radiographic Positioning
Coccyx, Sacrum and Lumbar Spine

Basic and Optional Projections/Positions

Basic and optional projections or positions for the lower vertebral column are demonstrated and described on the following pages. Basic projections are those commonly taken on average helpful patients. It should be noted that departmental routines (basic projections) may vary in different hospitals or departments. The single optional projection presented in this chapter is the A.P. L-5 — S-1 joint.

Coccyx
Basic
- Angled A.P.
- Lateral

Sacrum
Basic
- Angled A.P.
- Lateral

Lumbar
Basic
- A.P.
- Lateral
- Obliques (Both)
- Lat. L-5 — S-1
Optional
- A.P. L-5 — S-1

Coccyx
Basic
- **Angled A.P.**
- Lateral

Coccyx
• Angled Anteroposterior Projection

Film Size:
   8 x 10 in. (18 x 24 cm.)

Bucky:
- Moving or stationary grid.

Patient Position:
- Supine.

Part Position:
- Align midsagittal plane to midline of table.
- No rotation of pelvis.
- Closely collimate.
- Suspend breathing on expiration.

Central Ray:
- C.R. 10° caudad to enter 2 in. (5 cm.) superior to symphysis pubis.
- 40 in. (102 cm.) F.F.D.

NOTE: • For comfort, place support under knees. • May be done prone, if necessary (angled 10° cephalad). • Rectosigmoid contents may obscure coccyx.

Structures Best Shown:
Coccyx free of self-superimposition and superimposition of symphysis pubis.

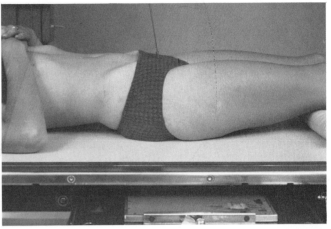

A.P. - 10° caudad   Fig. 13-31

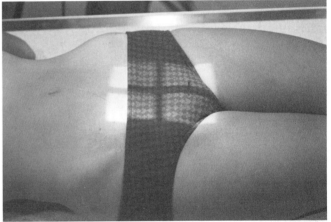

A.P. - 10° caudad   Fig. 13-32

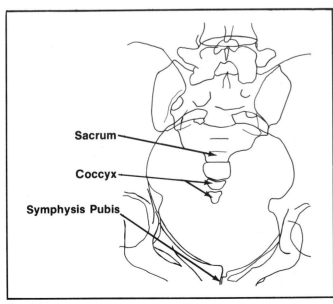

Fig. 13-34

A.P. - 10° caudad

Sacrum

Coccyx

Symphysis Pubis

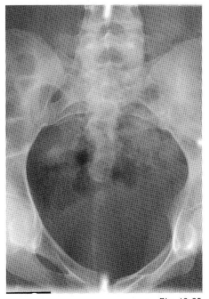

A.P. - 10° caudad   Fig. 13-33

Coccyx
Basic
• Angled A.P.
• **Lateral**

Coccyx

• **Lateral Position**

Film Size:
   8 x 10 in. (18 x 24 cm.)

Bucky:
- Moving or stationary grid.

Patient Position:
- Lateral recumbent; usually left lateral.

Part Position:
- Flex hips and knees.
- Support under small of waist, and between knees and ankles.
- Plane through long axis of coccyx coincides with midline of table.
- Closely collimate.
- Suspend breathing on expiration.

Central Ray:
- C.R. perpendicular to film holder.
- Center 1/2 in. (1 cm.) superior to tip of coccyx.
- 40 in. (102 cm.) F.F.D.

NOTE: • Coccyx easier to palpate with patient in left lateral position. • Do not overexpose (requires less exposure than lateral sacrum).

Structures Best Shown:
Coccyx (forward angulation is best demonstrated in this position).

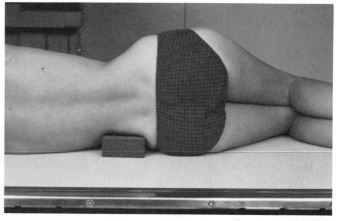
Lateral   Fig. 13-35

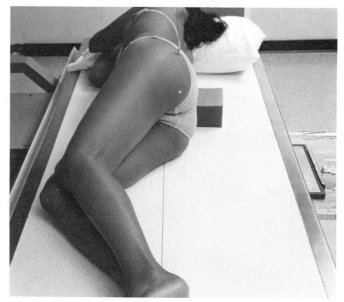
Lateral   Fig. 13-36

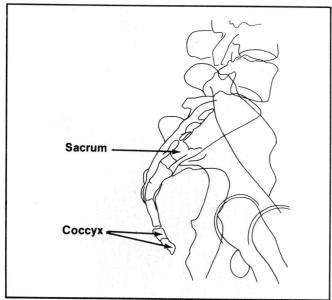
Sacrum

Coccyx

Fig. 13-38   Lateral

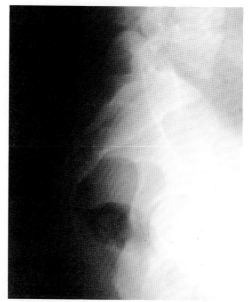
Lateral   Fig. 13-37

Sacrum
• Angled Anteroposterior Projection

Film Size:
    10 x 12 in. (24 x 30 cm.)

Bucky:
- Moving or stationary grid.

Patient Position:
- Supine.

Part Position:
- Align midsagittal plane to midline of table.
- No rotation of pelvis.
- Closely collimate.
- Make patient comfortable.
- Suspend breathing on expiration.

Central Ray:
- C.R. 15° cephalad, to enter midway between symphysis pubis and a line connecting the two A.S.I.S.'s.
- 40 in. (102 cm.) F.F.D.

NOTE: • Rectosigmoid contents may obscure sacrum.

Structures Best Shown:
Sacrum (not foreshortened), S.I. joints, ilia of pelvis and sacral foramina.

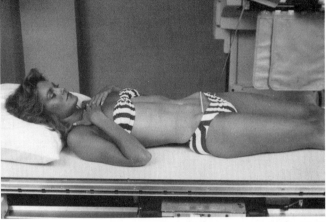

A.P. - 15° cephalad
Fig. 13-39

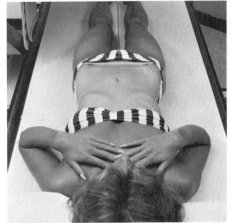

A.P. - 15° cephalad
Fig. 13-40

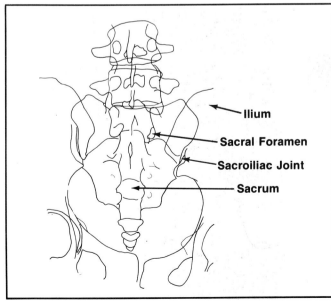

Fig. 13-42
    A.P. - 15° cephalad

Labels: Ilium, Sacral Foramen, Sacroiliac Joint, Sacrum

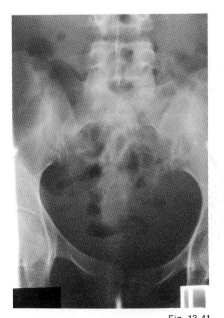

A.P. - 15° cephalad
Fig. 13-41

Sacrum
• Lateral Position

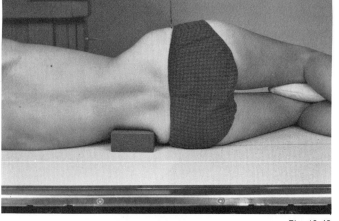

Lateral   Fig. 13-43

Film Size:
> 10 x 12 in. (24 x 30 cm.)

Bucky:
- Moving or stationary grid.

Patient Position:
- Lateral recumbent; usually left lateral.

Part Position:
- Flex hips and knees.
- Support under small of waist, and between knees and ankles.
- Pelvis and entire body true lateral.
- Closely collimate.
- Suspend breathing on expiration.

Central Ray:
- C.R. perpendicular to film holder.
- Center longitudinally to A.S.I.S. (S-2) and 2 in. (5 cm.) anterior to posterior sacral surface.
- 40 in. (102 cm.) F.F.D.

NOTE: • Sacrum easier to palpate with patient in left lateral position.

Structures Best Shown:
Sacrum and L-5 — S-1 joint.

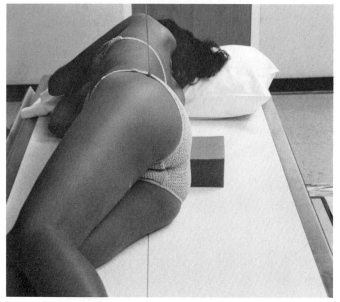

Lateral   Fig. 13-44

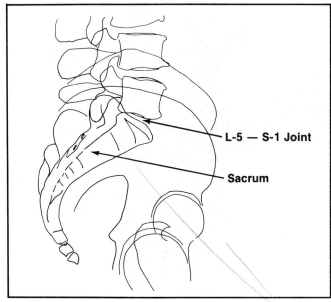

Fig. 13-46

L-5 — S-1 Joint

Sacrum

Lateral

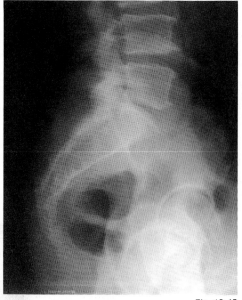

Lateral   Fig. 13-45

Lumbar Spine
• Anteroposterior Projection

Lumbar
Basic
- **A.P.**
- Lateral
- Obliques (Both)
- Lat. L-5 — S-1

Optional
- A.P. L-5 — S-1

Film Size:
14 x 17 in. (35 x 43 cm.)

Bucky:
- Moving or stationary grid.

Patient Position:
- Supine with hips and knees flexed, and head on adequate pillow.

Part Position:
- Align midsagittal plane to midline of table.
- Closely collimate, especially on lateral margins.
- Utilize gonadal shield.
- Arms comfortable and out of field.
- No pelvic rotation.
- Suspend breathing on expiration.

Central Ray:
- Center to level of iliac crest (L-4 — L-5), perpendicular to film holder.
- This centering will include lumbar vertebrae, sacrum and coccyx.
- 40 in. (102 cm.) F.F.D.

NOTE: • Supine with legs extended closes up intervertebral joint spaces; therefore, flex hips and knees. • May be taken prone since a P.A. projection will open up intervertebral joint spaces better than A.P. • Can be obtained upright, if patient cannot lie down.

Structures Best Shown:
Lumbar vertebral bodies, intervertebral joint spaces, spinous and transverse processes, laminae, S.I. joints and alae of sacrum.

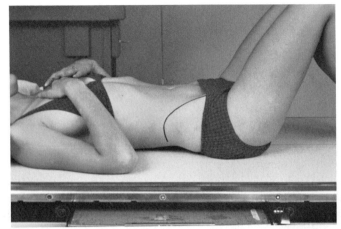
A.P.
Fig. 13-47

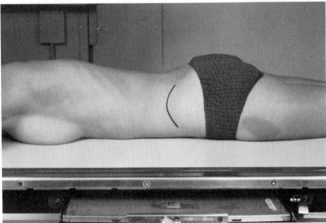
P.A.
Fig. 13-48

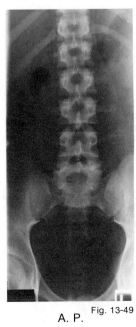
A. P.
Fig. 13-49

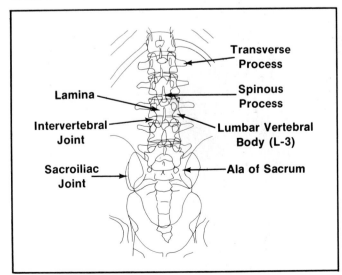
Fig. 13-50
A.P.

Lumbar Spine

• Lateral Position

Lumbar
Basic
- A.P.
- **Lateral**
- Obliques (Both)
- Lat. L-5 — S-1

Optional
- A.P. L-5 — S-1

Film Size:
   14 x 17 in. (35 x 43 cm.)

Bucky:
- Moving or stationary grid.

Patient Position:
- Lateral recumbent; usually left lateral.

Part Position:
- Align midaxillary plane to midline of table or film.
- Flex hips and knees.
- Radiolucent support under small of waist, and supports between knees and ankles.
- Pelvis and trunk true lateral.
- Legs and, especially, knees superimposed.
- Closely collimate.
- Suspend breathing on expiration.

Central Ray:
- Center to iliac crest (L-4 — L-5), perpendicular to film holder.
- This centering will include lumbar vertebrae, sacrum and coccyx.
- 40 in. (102 cm.) F.F.D.

NOTE: • Support patient so that line connecting spinous processes is parallel to film. • A slight sag may actually open up more intervertebral joints than the parallel situation.

Structures Best Shown:
Lumbar bodies, intervertebral joints, spinous processes, L-5 — S-1 joint and sacrum. First four intervertebral foramina shown.

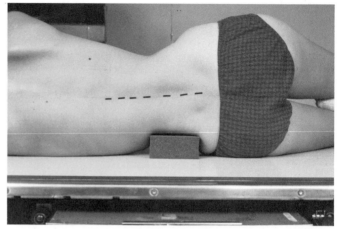

Lateral (Female)   Fig. 13-51

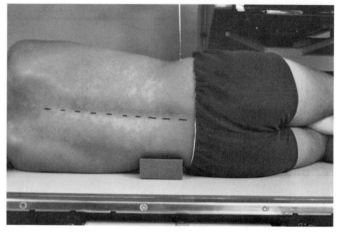

Lateral (Male)   Fig. 13-52

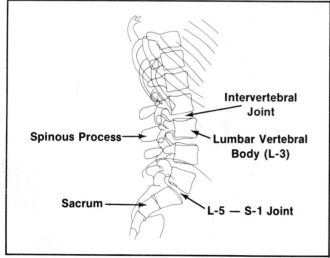

Fig. 13-54

Lateral

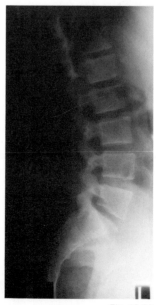

Fig. 13-53

Lateral

Lumbar Spine

• Oblique Position

Lumbar
Basic
- A.P.
- Lateral
- **Obliques (Both)**
- Lat. L-5 — S-1

Optional
- A.P. L-5 — S-1

Film Size:
10 x 12 in. (24 x 30 cm.)

Bucky:
- Moving or stationary grid.

Patient Position:
- Semisupine or semiprone.

Part Position:
- Rotate body 45°.
- Hand should grasp table edge (don't pinch fingers).
- Support back, pelvis and knees.
- Make comfortable.
- Closely collimate.
- Suspend breathing on expiration.

Central Ray:
- Center to L-3 (inferior rib margin), perpendicular to film holder.
- Center 2 in. (5 cm.) toward the midline from the spinous process of L-3.
- 40 in. (102 cm.) F.F.D.

NOTE: • A 30° oblique may be necessary to best visualize the apophysial joints at L-5 — S-1. • Both anterior **or** both posterior obliques must be done.

Structures Best Shown:
Apophysial joints, R.P.O. and L.P.O. show downside. R.A.O. and L.A.O. show upside. Good oblique will visualize "Scotty dogs."

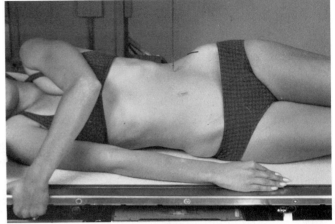

R.P.O - Semisupine   Fig. 13-55

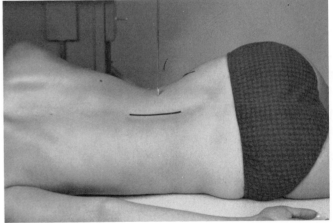

L.A.O. - Semiprone   Fig. 13-56

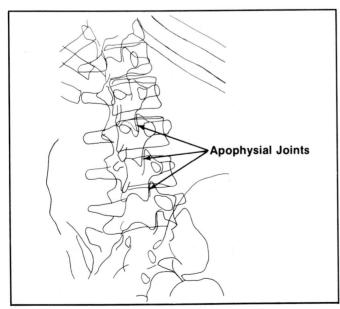

Apophysial Joints

Fig. 13-58
Oblique

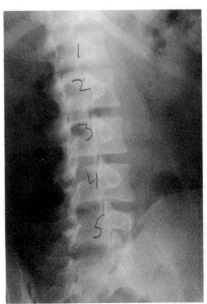

Fig. 13-57
Oblique

Lumbar Spine
• Lateral L-5 — S-1

Lumbar
Basic
- A.P.
- Lateral
- Obliques (Both)
- **Lat. L-5 — S-1**
Optional
- A.P. L-5 — S-1

Film Size:
  8 x 10 in. (18 x 24 cm.)

Bucky:
- Moving or stationary grid.

Patient Position:
- Lateral recumbent; usually left lateral.

Part Position:
- Flex hips and knees.
- Radiolucent support under small of waist, and supports between knees and ankles.
- Pelvis and trunk true lateral.
- Legs and, especially, knees superimposed.
- Closely collimate.
- Suspend breathing on expiration.

Central Ray:
- No angle, C.R. perpendicular to film holder.
- Center 1½ in. inferior to iliac crest and 1½ in. anterior to the bony posterior surface.
- 40 in. (102 cm.) F.F.D.

NOTE: • If waist is not properly supported, resulting in a sagging of the lumbar spine, then angle 5 to 8° caudal, as shown in *Figs. 13-59* and *13-60.*

Structures Best Shown:
Lumbosacral joint space.

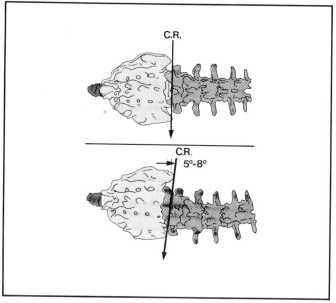

Lateral L-5 — S-1   Fig. 13-59

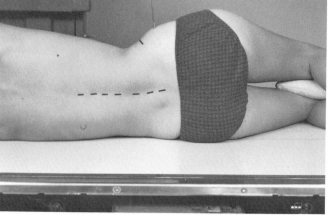

Lateral L-5 — S-1 (with angle)   Fig. 13-60

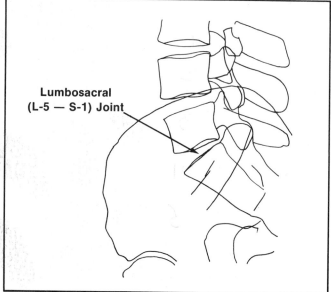

**Lumbosacral
(L-5 — S-1) Joint**

Fig. 13-62

Lateral L-5 — S-1

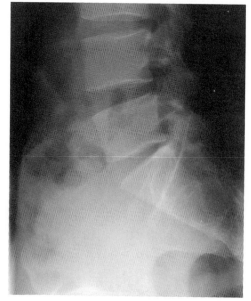

Lateral L-5 — S-1   Fig. 13-61

Lumbar Spine
• Angled Anteroposterior Projection
• Frontal L-5 — S-1 Position

Lumbar
Basic
- A.P.
- Lateral
- Obliques (Both)
- Lat. L-5 — S-1

Optional
- **A.P. L-5 — S-1**

Film Size:
   8 x 10 in. (18 x 24 cm.)

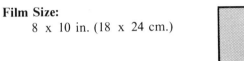

Bucky:
- Moving or stationary grid.

Patient Position:
- Supine with legs extended.

Part Position:
- Align midsagittal plane to midline of table.
- Closely collimate.
- No pelvic rotation.
- Suspend breathing on expiration.

Central Ray:
- Angle C.R. 30° (males) to 35° (females) cephalad.
- C.R. should enter at the A.S.I.S. level and pass through a plane midway between iliac crest and A.S.I.S.
- 40 in. (102 cm.) F.F.D.

NOTE: • Angled A.P. projection opens up L-5 — S-1 joint. • Collimated lateral is more informative than is the A.P. projection.

Structures Best Shown:
L-5 — S-1 and S.I. joints.

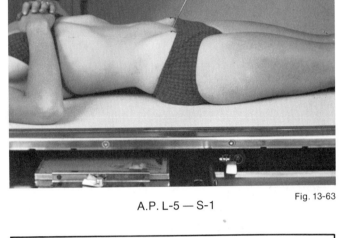

A.P. L-5 — S-1   Fig. 13-63

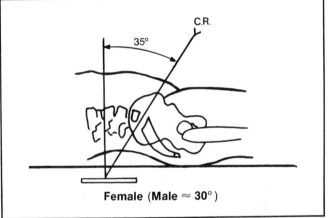

Female (Male ≈ 30°)

A.P. L-5 — S-1   Fig. 13-64

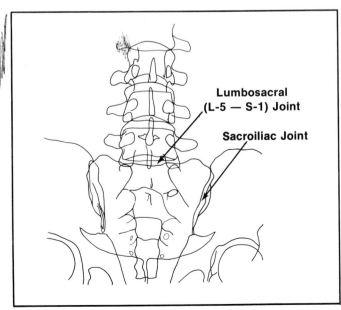

Lumbosacral
(L-5 — S-1) Joint

Sacroiliac Joint

Fig. 13-66   A.P. L-5 — S-1

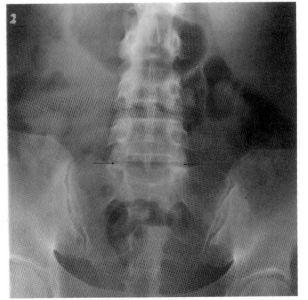

A.P. L-5 — S-1   Fig. 13-65

CHAPTER 14

Radiographic Anatomy and Positioning of the Thoracic Spine and Cervical Spine

Part I. Radiographic Anatomy
Thoracic Spine and Cervical Spine

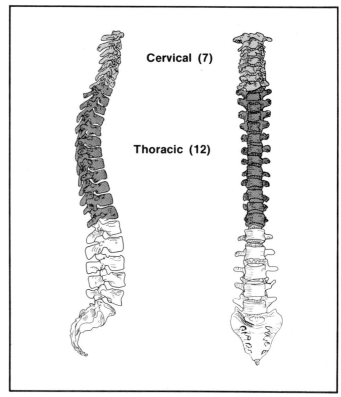

Upper Vertebral Column

Fig. 14-1

Cervical and Thoracic Vertebrae

The upper or cephalic portion of the vertebral column is divided into two portions, the **thoracic vertebrae** and the **cervical vertebrae.** Typically, there are 12 thoracic vertebrae and 7 cervical vertebrae.

Thoracic Vertebrae

The lumbar vertebrae, presented in Chapter 13, most closely resemble typical vertebrae. As one progresses further up the vertebral column, there are greater and greater differences compared to the lumbar vertebrae. The middle four thoracic vertebrae, numbers 5, 6, 7 and 8, are considered typical thoracic vertebrae. The lower four assume some of the characteristics of the lumbar vertebrae, while the upper four gradually assume features of the cervical region.

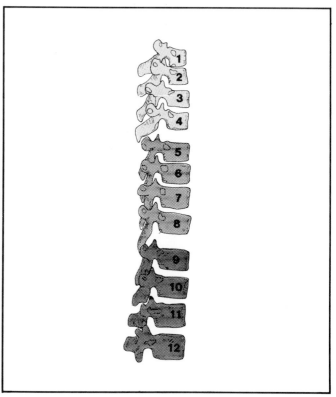

Thoracic Vertebrae

Fig. 14-2

Rib Articulations

The one feature of all thoracic vertebrae that serves to distinguish them from all others is that all thoracic vertebrae have facets for articulation with ribs. Each thoracic vertebra is closely associated with one pair of ribs. Since there are 12 pairs of ribs, there are also 12 thoracic vertebrae.

All 12 vertebrae have either a full **facet** or two partial facets, termed **demifacets,** on each side of the body. Each facet or combination of two demifacets accepts the head of a rib to form a **costovertebral joint.** In addition, each of the first ten thoracic vertebrae have facets (one on each transverse process) that articulate with the tubercles of ribs 1 through 10. These articulations are termed **costotransverse joints.**

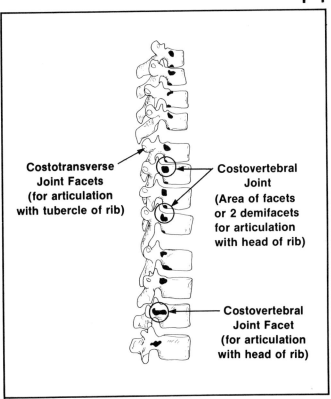

Fig. 14-3

Thoracic Vertebrae
(rib articulations)

Costovertebral and Costotransverse Joints: The costovertebral joint and costotransverse joint of one rib are shown in *Fig. 14-4.* Those vertebrae with two demifacets share the heads of two ribs on each side. The demifacet on the bottom of one vertebra articulates with the superior portion of the head of a particular rib, while the demifacet near the top of the next vertebra articulates with the inferior part of the same head. The combination of the **head** of one **rib** and two **demifacets** comprise a **costovertebral joint.** Vertebrae 10, 11 and 12 have a single costal facet on each side. The combination of the heads of these ribs and one full facet forms costovertebral joints on these vertebrae.

As the first ten pairs of ribs flare out away from the upper ten vertebrae, the **tubercle** of each **rib** articulates with one transverse process to form a **costotransverse joint.**

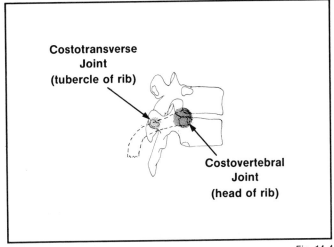

Fig. 14-4

Costovertebral and
Costotransverse Joints

Typical Thoracic Vertebrae

A side view of two typical thoracic vertebrae is shown in *Fig. 14-5.* As the thoracic vertebrae progress upward from twelve to one, they look less and less like typical lumbar vertebrae. The thoracic vertebrae are smallest near T-1 and largest near T-12.

Each thoracic vertebra possesses the seven processes of the typical lumbar vertebra. The large **spinous process** of each thoracic vertebra is longer and points more downward compared to the thick, blunt lumbar spinous process. The two **transverse processes** of each thoracic vertebra are unique in that each presents a facet near its end. The **superior articular processes** and the **inferior articular processes** serve to connect the successive thoracic vertebrae.

On each side, between any two thoracic vertebrae, is an **intervertebral foramen.** The intervertebral foramina of the thoracic region are well seen on a direct lateral view such as *Fig. 14-5.* The main distinguishing characteristic of the thoracic vertebrae, however, is the fact that each thoracic vertebra possesses facets for rib articulation.

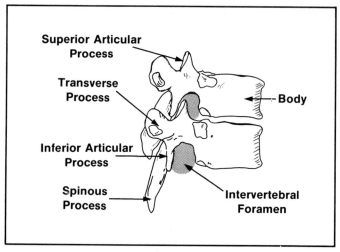

Typical Thoracic Vertebra
(side view)

Fig. 14-5

Superior View

A typical thoracic vertebra as seen from above is illustrated in *Fig. 14-6.* The usual features of a typical vertebra plus the distinguishing characteristics of the **facets** are well shown. The **body** is the most anterior structure, while the **spinous process** is the most posterior structure. The spinous process seems fairly short when viewed in this direction, but remember that it is projected primarily downward. The vertebral arch is composed of the two **pedicles** projecting from the body and the two **laminae.** Each **transverse process** projects from the junction of the pedicle and the lamina on each side. A single **rib** is shown in position to demonstrate the **costovertebral joint** and the **costotransverse joint** on one side.

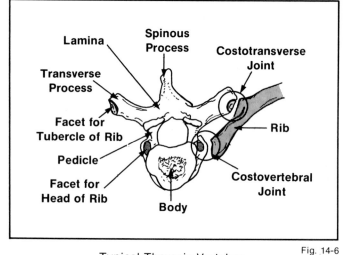

Typical Thoracic Vertebra
(superior view)

Fig. 14-6

Cervical Vertebrae

Typical Cervical Vertebrae

The typical cervical vertebra resembles a typical lumbar vertebra even less than a thoracic vertebra resembles a lumbar vertebra. In fact, the upper two cervical vertebrae, C-1 and C-2, are quite unusual. **C-1** is often termed the **atlas**, a name derived from the Greek god who bore the world upon his shoulders. The **second cervical** is called the **axis**, since much of the rotation of the head occurs between C-1 and C-2.

The third through sixth cervical vertebrae are typical cervical vertebrae. The last or **seventh cervical vertebra** assumes many of the features of the thoracic vertebrae, including an extra long spinous process that gives C-7 its special name, the **vertebra prominens.**

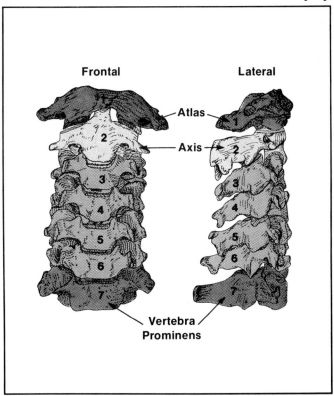

Cervical Spine

Fig. 14-7

Superior View

Figure 14-8 shows a typical cervical vertebra as viewed from above. While the parts forming the vertebral arch are all present and the vertebra has the usual seven processes, they are somewhat different from those of the typical lumbar vertebra. The **transverse processes**, for instance, are quite small and arise from both the **pedicle** and the **body**, rather than from the pedicle-lamina junction. In addition, there is a hole in each transverse process termed a **transverse foramen**. Important blood vessels and nerves pass through these successive transverse foramina. The **spinous process** is fairly short and usually ends in two tips rather than only one. This double or forked tip is termed a **bifid tip.**

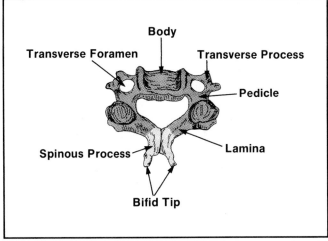

Typical Cervical Vertebra
(superior view)

Fig. 14-8

Lateral View

A typical cervical vertebra as viewed from the side is illustrated in *Fig. 14-9*. The **body** is the most anterior structure and the **spinous process** is the most posterior structure. Located behind the transverse process at the junction of the pedicle and the lamina is a short column of bone that is much more supportive than the similar area in the rest of the spinal column. This column of bone is termed the **articular pillar,** sometimes shortened to just pillar. Located on the top of each pillar is the **superior articular process.** On the bottom is found the **inferior articular process.** Each cervical vertebra and vertebral body continues to get smaller, progressing up from the seventh cervical to the third cervical vertebra.

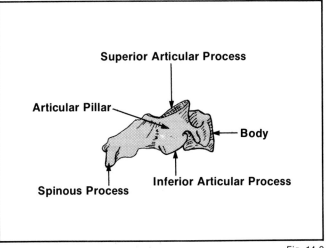

Typical Cervical Vertebra
(side view)

Fig. 14-9

Axis (C-2)

The most distinctive feature of the second cervical vertebra, the axis, is the strong conical process projecting from the upper surface of the **body**. This radiographically important projection is termed the **odontoid process,** sometimes referred to as the **dens.**

Rotation of the head primarily occurs between C-1 and C-2, with the odontoid process making this type of motion possible. The **superior articular processes** are large flat surfaces assisting in rotation of the head. Severe stress as the possible result of a forced flexion-hyperextension type of injury may cause a fracture of the odontoid process. Any fracture of the vertebral column at this level could result in serious damage to the spinal cord as well. The **inferior articular process** for articulation with C-3 lies inferior to the **lamina.** Below the superior articular process is the transverse process with its **transverse foramen.** The blunt **spinous process** extends posteriorly.

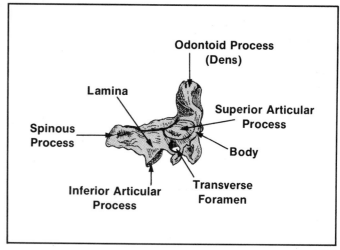

Axis (side view)   Fig. 14-10

Atlas (C-1)

The first cervical vertebra, C-1, as seen from above, is illustrated in *Fig. 14-11.* C-1, or the atlas, least resembles a typical vertebra. Anteriorly, there is no body, but simply an arch of bone termed the **anterior arch.** The odontoid process is actually the body of C-1, but embryologically the C-1 body fuses to C-2 and becomes the odontoid process. Therefore, in an adult, the odontoid process of C-2 projects up through the large central opening of C-1.

Posteriorly, another arch of bone, the **posterior arch,** may bear a small tubercle at the midline. This tubercle is all that remains of a spinous process. Each **superior articular process** presents a large depressed surface for articulation with the respective occipital condyle of the skull. The **transverse processes** are smaller, but still contain the **transverse foramina** distinctive of all cervical vertebrae. Lateral to the arches, on each side of C-1, is a large area of bone termed the **lateral mass.**

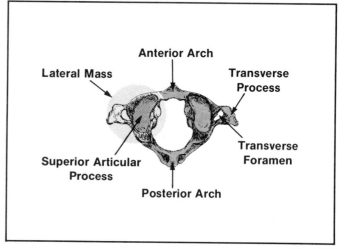

Atlas (superior view)   Fig. 14-11

Relationship of C-1 and C-2

The relationship of C-2, with its odontoid process, to C-1, and the relationship of C-1 to the base of the skull, are highly important. *Fig. 14-12* illustrates the important structural relationship of these three areas. This is the type of view seen on a radiograph of the upper cervical spine taken with the mouth wide open. The anterior arch of C-1, which lies in front of the odontoid process, is not visible on this frontal view because it is a fairly thin piece of bone and is not well visualized on a frontal radiograph.

Normally, the various articulations between C-2 and C-1, and between C-1 and the skull, are perfectly symmetrical. Accordingly, the relationship of the **odontoid process** to C-1 must also be perfectly symmetrical. Both injury and improper positioning can render these areas asymmetrical. For this reason, a perfectly positioned radiograph of this area can be of utmost importance.

The **lateral masses** of C-1 are well demonstrated on this view, with their inferior articular processes on the lower borders. The joint between the **inferior** and the **superior articular processes** is called an **apophysial joint.** The **apophysial joint space** between C-1 and C-2 must be well visualized on this view. Extending laterally from each lateral mass of C-1 are the **transverse processes** of C-1.

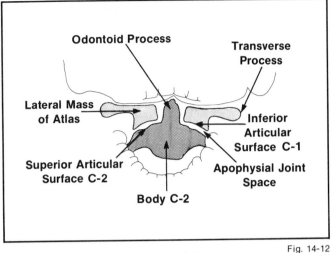

Fig. 14-12

Atlas and Axis
(open-mouth position)

Cervical Spine Radiographs

The radiograph in *Fig. 14-13* illustrates the first two cervical vertebrae, C-1 and C-2, in the **A.P. open-mouth position.** This particular radiograph gives an exceptional view of C-1 and C-2 because this patient has no teeth. Unless positioning is perfect, teeth usually tend to superimpose portions of the vertebrae.

This radiograph should look similar to the drawing in *Fig. 14-12.* Part **A** is the odontoid process or dens of C-2; **B** is one lateral mass of C-1; **C** is the left apophysial joint; **D** is the body of C-2, or the axis; and **E** is one transverse process of C-1.

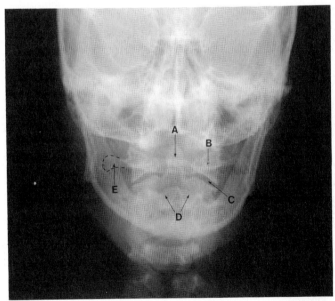

Fig. 14-13

Radiograph of C-1 and C-2
(open-mouth position)

A **conventional A.P. radiograph** of the cervical spine is illustrated in *Fig. 14-14*. Usually, the first two or three thoracic vertebrae, as well as C-7 up to C-3, are seen well on this projection. Identifying specific vertebrae can be difficult, but T-1 is probably the easiest to find. T-1 should have the first pair of ribs attached to it. Therefore, to localize T-1, locate the most superior ribs and find the vertebra to which they appear to connect. After locating T-1, the visible cervical vertebrae can be identified by starting at C-7 and counting upward.

Part **A** on this radiograph is the first thoracic vertebra, determined by discovering that part **B** is the first rib on the patient's right side. Part **C** is the fourth cervical vertebra. Part **D** is the articular pillar of C-3. The white area at the top of the radiograph is created by the combined shadows of the base of the skull and the mandible. These structures effectively cover up the first two cervical vertebrae on this type of radiograph. Part **E** is the spinous process of C-3 seen on end.

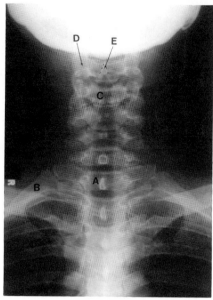

Radiograph
of Cervical Spine (A.P.)

Fig. 14-14

The single most important radiograph in any cervical spine series is **a good lateral.** An excellent lateral cervical spine radiograph is demonstrated in *Fig. 14-15*. Radiographers must always try to show all seven cervical vertebrae on any lateral cervical spine radiograph. At times this is difficult on those patients with thick shoulders and a short neck. In order to determine if all seven cervical vertebrae are being shown, locate the atlas, or C-1, and count downward. In *Fig. 14-15,* the seventh cervical vertebra is marked with an X.

Part **A** is the odontoid process, enhanced with dotted lines on this visual. Part **B** is the posterior arch of the atlas. Part **C** is the body of C-3; **D** is the apophysial joint between C-4 and C-5; and **E** is the spinous process of C-6. The lower anterior margins of the last four or five cervical vertebral bodies have a slight lipped appearance which, along with the general shape of the bodies, requires that the central ray be angled approximately 20 degrees toward the head to "open up" these lower intervertebral spaces.

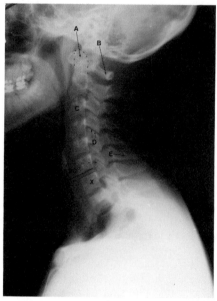

Radiograph
of Cervical Spine (Lat.)

Fig. 14-15

A good **oblique cervical spine** radiograph is shown in *Fig. 14-16*. The primary purpose of the oblique position is to show the **intervertebral foramina.** Spinal nerves to and from the spinal cord are transmitted through these intervertebral foramina.

Part **A** is the posterior arch of C-1; **B** is the intervertebral foramen between the fourth and fifth cervical vertebrae; **C** is the pedicle of C-6; and **D** is the body of C-7.

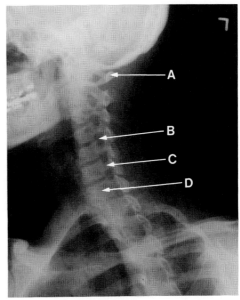

Radiograph
of Cervical Spine (Obli.)

Fig. 14-16

Topographical Landmarks

The most reliable topographical landmarks for the spine are the various palpable bony prominences that are fairly constant from one person to another. However, it should be emphasized that the landmarks presented in the following sections refer to a healthy, erect, normally developed adult male or female. These landmarks will vary in subjects with anatomical and, especially, skeletal anomalies. The very young and the very old will also have slightly different features than the average adult.

Sternum

The sternum provides some useful landmarks for locating various levels of the thoracic spine. The sternum is divided into three basic sections. The upper section is called the **manubrium.** The very top part of the manubrium, the **suprasternal notch,** can be easily felt. The central portion of the sternum is called the **body.** The manubrium and body connect at a slight, easily located angle termed the **sternal angle.** The most inferior end of the sternum is called the **xiphoid process.** It takes some pressure to locate the xiphoid process on a patient.

With careful palpation or probing of these topographic landmarks, certain anatomical structures and relationships between structures can be determined. For example, the level of specific thoracic vertebrae can be determined from these three sternal landmarks — the suprasternal notch, the sternal angle and the xiphoid process. Both the sternal angle and the xiphoid process can be palpated, although they are not as easy to locate as the suprasternal notch.

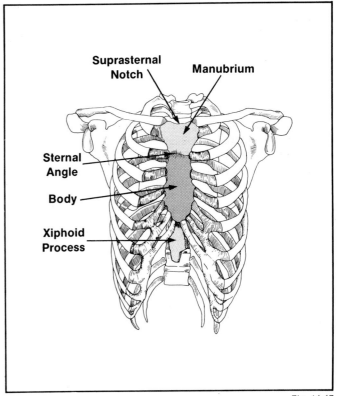

Sternum

Fig. 14-17

Lower Spine Landmarks

The drawing in *Fig. 14-18* illustrates various landmarks relative to the lower vertebral column. Level **A** corresponds to the easily palpable superior margin of the **symphysis pubis**, which is at the same level as the **coccyx**. Although the coccyx may be palpated directly, it is not always convenient to do so. The **anterior superior iliac spine** (A.S.I.S.) is at the same level **(B)** as the **second sacral segment**. Level **C** is the most superior portion of the **iliac crest** and is at approximately the same level as the junction of the **fourth** and **fifth lumbar vertebrae**. The lowest margin of the ribs or **lower costal margin (D)** is at the approximate level of **L-3**.

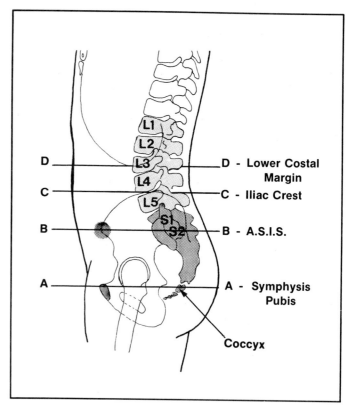

Lower Spine Landmarks   Fig. 14-18

The lower vertebral column landmarks are illustrated on the model in *Fig. 14-19*. One should be able to relate the various topographical landmarks to their corresponding vertebral level. **A** is the level of the symphysis pubis anteriorly, corresponding to the level of the coccyx posteriorly. **B** is the anterior superior iliac spine anteriorly, located at the level of S-2, the second segment of the sacrum. Landmark **C** is the iliac crest, at the same level as the disc space between L-4 and L-5. **D** corresponds to the lower part of the rib cage, usually at the level of L-3.

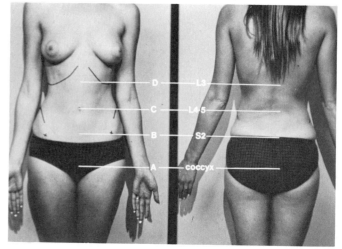

Lower Spine Landmarks   Fig. 14-19

Thoracic Spine Landmarks

The bottom part of the xiphoid process, the **xiphoid tip,** is at the level of the **tenth thoracic vertebra** as indicated by line **A** in *Fig. 14-20*. The sternal angle is most easily located if one first locates the suprasternal notch and then follows the manubrium down 5 centimeters until a slight bump is felt. The slight bump on the surface of the sternum should be the sternal angle. The **sternal angle** (line **C**) locates the **junction of T-4 and T-5.** Line **B** locates T-7 at a level 3 inches or 7.5 centimeters below the sternal angle, the approximate center of the thoracic portion of the vertebral column. The seventh thoracic vertebra is the center of the 12 thoracic vertebrae since the lower thoracic vertebrae are larger in size than are the upper thoracic vertebrae.

The suprasternal notch, sometimes called the sternal notch, is identified by line **D.** The **suprasternal notch** is at the same level as the **disc space between T-2 and T-3.** Often, on a prepared skeleton, the suprasternal notch is closer to T-1, but this is not true on a person standing upright. On an average, standing adult, T-1 is located 1.5 inches or 3.75 centimeters above the suprasternal notch, marked as Line **E.**

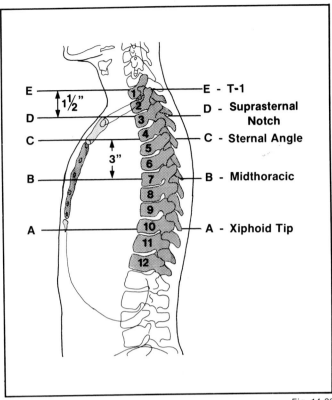

Thoracic Spine Landmarks

Fig. 14-20

The standard landmarks for the thoracic spine are illustrated on the model in *Fig. 14-21*. Line **A** is at the level of the xiphoid tip, which locates thoracic vertebra number 10. Line **B** is about 3 inches or 7.5 centimeters below the sternal angle and is at the level of T-7. Line **C** is at the sternal angle and corresponds to the disc space between T-4 and T-5. The suprasternal notch corresponds to line **D** and is the easiest of these landmarks to palpate. The suprasternal notch corresponds to the level of the junction between T-2 and T-3. Line **E** corresponds to T-1 and is about 1.5 inches or 3.75 centimeters above the suprasternal notch.

These anterior landmarks, utilizing the sternum as a reference, can be used to locate any specific thoracic vertebra. The use of these landmarks becomes necessary when well-collimated radiographs are required of specific thoracic vertebrae. When the patient is supine rather than erect, the rib cage and sternum will be at a slightly more cephalic level. This fact must be remembered when using the sternum as a topographical landmark on a recumbent patient.

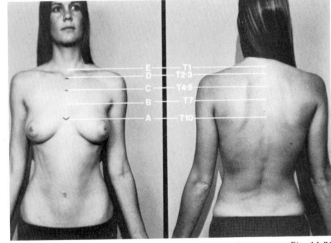

Thoracic Spine Landmarks

Fig. 14-21

Cervical Spine Landmarks

The prominent topographical landmarks of the cervical region are illustrated in *Fig. 14-22*. The last cervical vertebra, **C-7** (vertebra prominens), is at about the same level **(A)** as the **top of the shoulders.** The shoulders occasionally superimpose the last cervical vertebra on a lateral cervical spine radiograph. When this problem occurs, the shoulders must be depressed as much as possible.

The most prominent part of the larynx, the **thyroid cartilage** or "Adam's apple" **(B)**, is at the level of **C-5**. With the head in a neutral position, the angle of the jaw or **gonion (C)** is at the same level as the **third cervical vertebra.** The **mastoid tip (D)** corresponds to the level of C-1. The external auditory meatus **(E)** is easy to locate on any person; however, the E.A.M. is above any portion of the vertebral column.

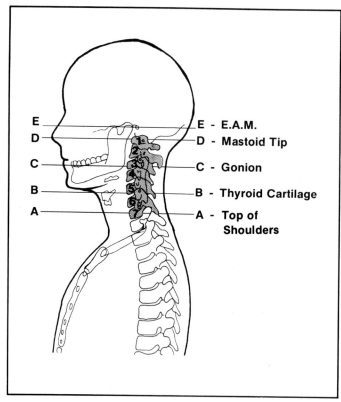

E - E.A.M.
D - Mastoid Tip
C - Gonion
B - Thyroid Cartilage
A - Top of Shoulders

Cervical Spine Landmarks   Fig. 14-22

Cervical spine landmarks are identified on the model pictured in *Fig. 14-23*. The tops of the shoulders on an average adult are located at about the same level as C-7. This landmark does vary on different people, however, since on a very thin patient the shoulders may go down to T-2 or T-3, while on a very husky male there may be very little visible neck. Since the spinous process of C-7 is very prominent, it can be used to help locate cervical vertebra number 7.

The thyroid cartilage of the larynx or "Adam's apple" localizes C-5. The gonion or angle of the mandible is at the level of the third cervical vertebra when the head is in a neutral position. The top of the cervical spine or C-1 is at the level of the mastoid tip. The mastoid tip can also be used to find the most inferior level of the base of the skull. The occipital condyles and foramen magnum are basal skull structures in line with the mastoid tip.

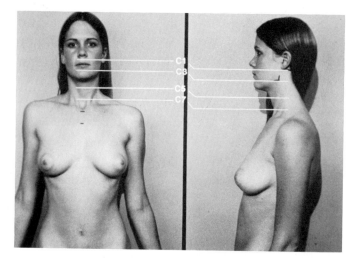

Cervical Spine Landmarks   Fig. 14-23

Intervertebral Foramina vs. Apophysial Joints

Cervical Spine

Two anatomical areas that must be demonstrated by the proper radiographs are the intervertebral foramina and the apophysial joints. The physician gains important information concerning the relationship of consecutive vertebrae by studying these two areas on the appropriate radiograph. To complicate matters, however, depending on the part of the spine to be radiographed (cervical, thoracic, or lumbar), a different body position is required to best show each anatomical area.

Two photographs of the cervical spine are shown in *Fig. 14-24*. On the left is a cervical section of the vertebral column in a left lateral position, while to the right is a 45-degree left posterior oblique position (L.P.O.). On the lateral position on the left, the apophysial joints visualize well. On the right, the posterior oblique with a 45-degree rotation shows that the intervertebral foramina are well opened. It is important to know that the left posterior oblique position opens up the foramina on the right side. Therefore, on a posterior oblique cervical spine radiograph, the upside is the side on which the intervertebral foramina are opened well.

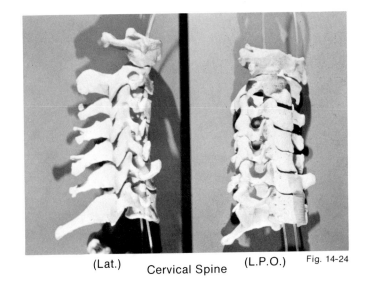

(Lat.)   Cervical Spine   (L.P.O.)   Fig. 14-24

The two radiographs of the cervical spine in *Fig. 14-25* illustrate the same anatomy in the same two positions as shown on the previous illustration, *Fig. 14-24*. The lateral position on the left best shows the apophysial joints. The joint on each side is superimposed upon the joint on the opposite side. One should remember that the apophysial joints are located between the articular pillars of each vertebra. The small x marks C-7, which must be shown on a good lateral radiograph of the cervical spine.

The oblique cervical spine radiograph on the right shows the circular intervertebral foramina well opened. In each oblique radiograph only one set of foramina are opened, while the ones on the opposite side are closed. Since this position is a left posterior oblique, the right intervertebral foramina are being shown. It is important to remember that the L.P.O. will show the same anatomy as the R.A.O. Therefore, if the patient is placed in an anterior oblique position, the foramina closest to the film will be shown. In either case, L.P.O. or R.A.O., the right intervertebral foramina will be visualized.

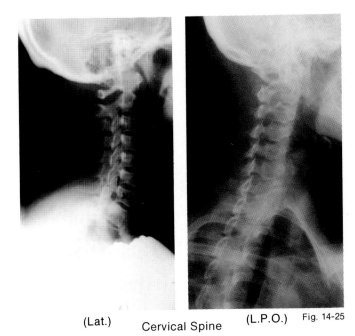

(Lat.)   Cervical Spine   (L.P.O.)   Fig. 14-25

Thoracic Spine

Two photographs of the thoracic spine are shown in *Fig. 14-26*. To the left is the thoracic spine in a lateral position, while to the right is an oblique. A 70-degree oblique is necessary to open up the apophysial joints on the thoracic spine, while it is the lateral position of the thoracic spine that best shows the intervertebral foramina. The oblique position on the right shows the apophysial joint on the upside.

It is important to remember that the cervical and thoracic vertebrae differ in the anatomy demonstrated in specific positions. The intervertebral foramina are best shown in the oblique cervical spine and in the lateral thoracic spine. The apophysial joints are best shown in the lateral cervical spine and in the 70-degree oblique thoracic spine.

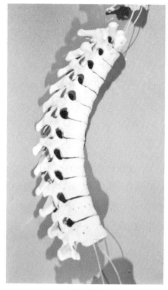
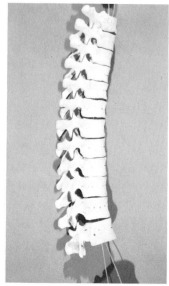

(Lat.)   Thoracic Spine   (Obli.)   Fig. 14-26

Radiographs of the thoracic spine in the lateral position (left) and in the 70-degree oblique position (right) are shown in *Fig. 14-27*. Observe that the holes or superimposed intervertebral foramina are best visualized on the lateral radiograph on the left. The apophysial joints are best visualized on the oblique radiograph on the right. The oblique radiograph is in a 70-degree R.P.O. position, which should best visualize the apophysial joints on the upside or those farthest away from the film. The R.P.O. position best shows the left apophysial joints.

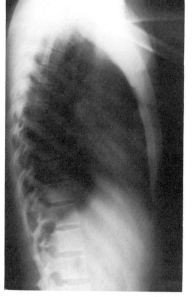
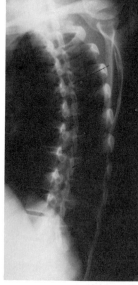

(Lat.)   Thoracic Spine   (R.P.O.)   Fig. 14-27

Lumbar Spine

Figure 14-28 shows two photographs of the lumbar spine. The lumbar spine lateral is on the left and a 45-degree oblique is on the right. The oblique of the lumbar spine is viewed from the posterior, however, so the position visualized is a left anterior oblique position. The lateral position on the left best shows the superimposed intervertebral foramina. Therefore, both the lateral thoracic position and the lateral lumbar position best show the intervertebral foramina.

The apophysial joints are best seen when the lumbar spine is in an oblique position. In the 45-degree oblique, the lower joints (L-3, L-4 and L-5) are the joints opened best. The joints on the upside, those farthest away from the film, show best. Therefore, radiographs of a patient in an anterior oblique position will best demonstrate the joints farthest from the film or those nearest the x-ray tube. In this R.A.O. position, the left apophysial joints are best visualized.

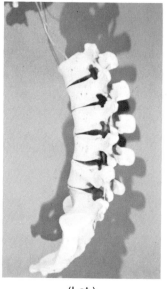
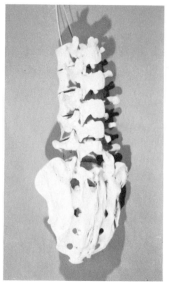

(Lat.)   Lumbar Spine   (Obli.)   Fig. 14-28

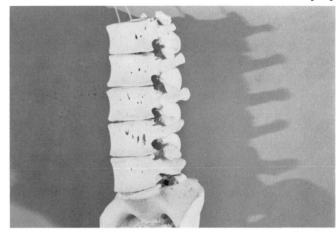

Fig. 14-29

Lumbar Spine (Posterior Oblique)

A 45-degree posterior oblique of the lumbar spine is shown in *Fig. 14-29*. The apophysial joints are not visible on this photograph because, in a posterior oblique position, these joints are nearest the film or underneath the skeleton. Radiographically, these important joints can be visualized, however, as demonstrated on the posterior oblique lumbar spine radiograph in *Fig. 14-31*.

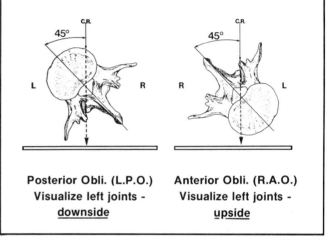

Posterior Obli. (L.P.O.) Visualize left joints - <u>downside</u>

Anterior Obli. (R.A.O.) Visualize left joints - <u>upside</u>

Fig. 14-30

Lumbar Spine

The drawings in *Fig. 14-30* compare both anterior and posterior lumbar obliques. On the left is a posterior oblique in the 45-degree L.P.O. position, best visualizing the down-side or left apophysial joints. On the right is an anterior oblique (R.A.O.) position that best visualizes the upside apophysial joints. Therefore, both the L.P.O. and the R.A.O. will visualize the left apophysial joints.

A lateral lumbar spine radiograph and an oblique lumbar spine radiograph are shown in *Fig. 14-31*. On the lateral to the left, the large intervertebral foramina are clearly shown. The right posterior oblique position to the right clearly shows the ears of the "Scotty dogs", the superior articular processes which help to form the apophysial joints. Since this is a posterior oblique position, the downside joints are best shown. The right posterior oblique position best shows the right apophysial joints.

One way to remember which anatomy shows best on posterior obliques, upside or downside, is to associate the **upper** part of the body (cervical and thoracic) with the **up** side, while the bottom part or **downside** of the body (lumbar) shows the **down** side best.

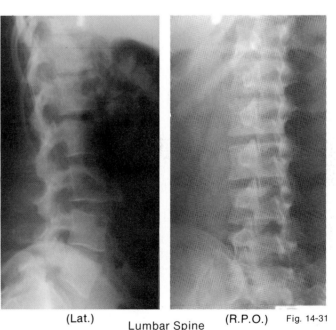

(Lat.)   Lumbar Spine   (R.P.O.)   Fig. 14-31

Summary of Intervertebral Foramina and Apophysial Joints

The chart in *Fig. 14-32* summarizes which position of each region of the spine best visualizes either the intervertebral foramina or the apophysial joints. The intervertebral foramina are best shown on the oblique cervical, and on the lateral thoracic or lumbar.

The apophysial joints are best seen on the lateral cervical, the near lateral thoracic and the 45-degree oblique lumbar. The upper body, the cervical and thoracic regions, show the upside best, while the lower body shows the downside best when radiographed anterior to posterior.

	Cervical	Thoracic	Lumbar
Intervertebral foramina	• Oblique 45° • Upside (L.P.O. or R.P.O.)	• Lateral	• Lateral
Apophysial joints	• Lateral	• Oblique - 70° • Upside (L.P.O. or R.P.O.)	• Oblique - 45° • Down side (L.P.O. or R.P.O.)

Summary   Fig. 14-32

Part II. Radiographic Positioning
Thoracic Spine and Cervical Spine

Basic and Optional Projections/Positions

Certain basic and optional projections or positions for the thoracic and cervical spine are demonstrated and described on the following pages. **Basic projections,** sometimes referred to as routine projections, are those projections commonly taken on average helpful patients. It should be noted that departmental routines or basic projections vary in different hospitals or departments. **Optional projections** include those more common projections taken as extra or additional projections to better demonstrate specific anatomical parts or certain pathological conditions.

Generally, basic projections or positions for a routine thoracic spine include an A.P. and a lateral. Optional positions include the swimmer's lateral or both obliques. Basic positioning for the cervical spine usually includes a lateral, an A.P. and both obliques. Optional positions include the open-mouth odontoid, the A.P. chewing, plus flexion and hyperextension in the lateral position.

Thoracic Spine
Basic
- A.P.
- Lateral

Optional
- Swimmer's Lateral
- Obliques (Both)

Cervical Spine
Basic
- Lateral
- A.P.
- Obliques (Both)

Optional
- Lateral - Flexion
- Lateral - Hyperextension
- Odontoid - Open-mouth
- A.P. - Chewing

Thoracic Spine

• Anteroposterior Projection

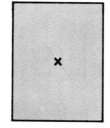

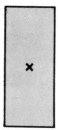

Film Size:
>   14 x 17 in. (35 x 43 cm.)
>   **or**
>   7 x 17 in. (18 x 43 cm.)

Bucky:
- Moving or stationary grid.

Patient Position:
- Supine.

Part Position:
- Align midsagittal plane to midline of table.
- Flex knees and hips.
- No rotation of the body.
- Arms beside body.
- Head on tabletop or thin pillow.
- Collimate closely, especially on lateral margins.
- Suspend breathing on inspiration.

Central Ray:
- C.R. perpendicular to film holder.
- Center to T-7 (3 in. or 7.5 cm. below the sternal angle).
- 40 in. (102 cm.) F.F.D.

NOTE: • T-7 is center of thoracic spine since lower vertebrae are larger. • Top of film should be slightly above level of shoulders.

Structures Best Shown:
Thoracic vertebral bodies, intervertebral joint spaces, distance between pedicles, spinous and transverse processes, posterior ribs and costovertebral articulations.

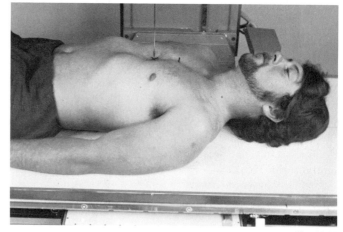

A.P.   Fig. 14-33

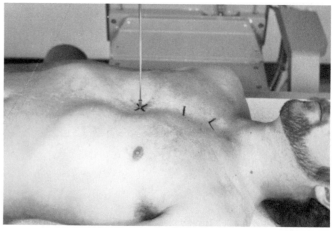

A.P.   Fig. 14-34

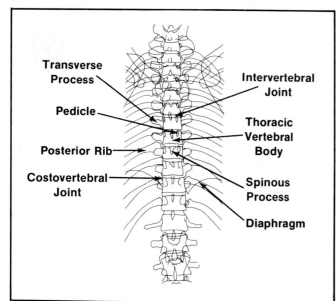

Transverse Process

Intervertebral Joint

Pedicle

Thoracic Vertebral Body

Posterior Rib

Costovertebral Joint

Spinous Process

Diaphragm

Fig. 14-36
                     A.P.

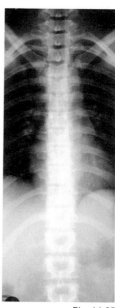

Fig. 14-35
A.P.

Thoracic Spine

• Lateral Position

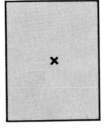

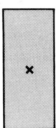

Film Size:
14 x 17 in. (35 x 43 cm.)
or
7 x 17 in. (18 x 43 cm.)

Bucky:
- Moving or stationary grid.

Patient Position:
- Left lateral recumbent.

Part Position:
- Align midaxillary plane to midline of table.
- Flex hips and knees.
- Arms well forward and up.
- Head on pillow and waist supported so entire spine is parallel to table.
- Collimate closely.
- Use breathing techniques (shallow, even breaths during exposure).

Central Ray:
- C.R. perpendicular to film holder. **(See NOTE).**
- Center to T-7 (3 in. or 7.5 cm. below the sternal angle).
- 40 in. (102 cm.) F.F.D.

NOTE: • If entire spine is not parallel to table, it may be necessary to angle slightly cephalad. • Top of film should be slightly above level of shoulders.

Structures Best Shown:
Thoracic vertebral bodies, intervertebral joint spaces and intervertebral foramina. Upper 3 or 4 vertebrae are not well visualized.

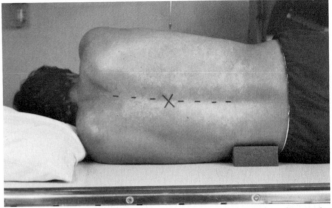

Lateral   Fig. 14-37

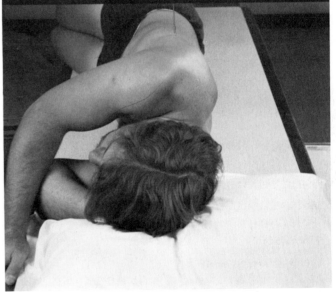

Lateral   Fig. 14-38

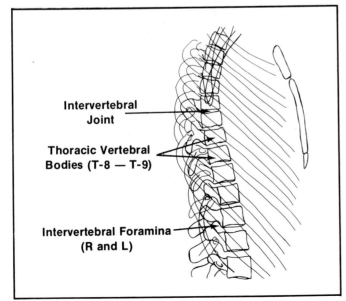

Intervertebral Joint

Thoracic Vertebral Bodies (T-8 — T-9)

Intervertebral Foramina (R and L)

Fig. 14-40
Lateral

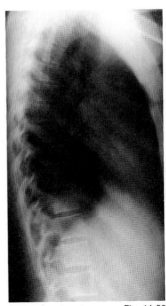

Lateral   Fig. 14-39

Thoracic
Basic
- A.P.
- Lateral

Optional
- **Swimmer's Lateral**
- Obliques (Both)

Thoracic Spine
• **Lateral Position for Cervicothoracic Region**
Swimmer's Lateral

Film Size:
    10 x 12 in. (24 x 30 cm.)

Bucky:
- Moving or stationary grid.

Patient Position:
- Lateral recumbent or upright.

Part Position:
- Align midaxillary plane to midline of table.
- Flex hips and knees (recumbent).
- Arm and shoulder nearest film up and forward, with hand on or near patient's head.
- Arm and shoulder nearest x-ray tube down and posterior.
- Cervical and thoracic vertebral column should be as lateral as possible.
- Collimate closely.
- Suspend breathing on inspiration.

Central Ray:
- C.R. perpendicular to film holder **(See NOTE)**.
- Center to T-2 (¾ in. or 2 cm. above suprasternal notch).
- 40 in. (102 cm.) F.F.D.

NOTE: • A caudal angulation of 5° may be necessary to help separate the two shoulders. • May be done supine on trauma patients.

Structures Best Shown:
Lower cervical and upper thoracic vertebral bodies and intervertebral disc spaces projected between the shoulders.

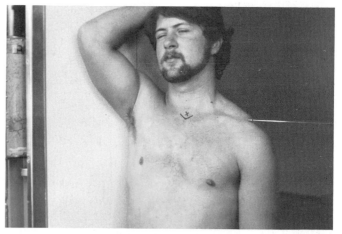

Swimmer's Lateral   Fig. 14-41

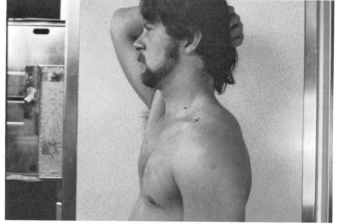

Swimmer's Lateral   Fig. 14-42

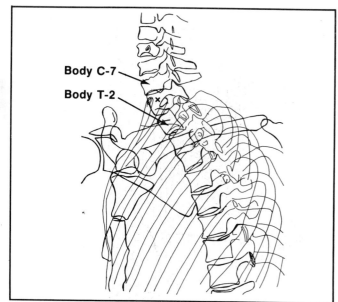

Body C-7
Body T-2

Fig. 14-44
    Swimmer's Lateral

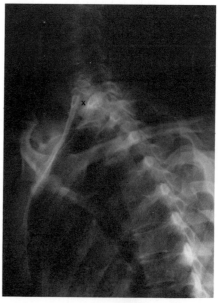

Swimmer's Lateral   Fig. 14-43

Thoracic Spine
• Oblique Position (70°)

Thoracic
Basic
- A.P.
- Lateral

Optional
- Swimmer's Lateral
- **Obliques (Both)**

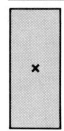

Film Size:

14 x 17 in. (35 x 43 cm.)
or
7 x 17 in. (18 x 43 cm.)

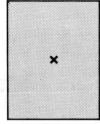

Bucky:
- Moving or stationary grid.

Patient Position:
- Lateral recumbent.

Part Position:
- Align midaxillary plane to midline of table.
- Flex hips and knees.
- For posterior oblique, arm nearest table up and forward; arm nearest x-ray tube down and posterior.
- For anterior oblique, arm nearest table down and posterior; arm nearest x-ray tube up and forward.
- Body rotated 20° from true lateral.
- Closely collimate.
- Suspend breathing on inspiration.

Central Ray:
- C.R. perpendicular to film holder.
- Center to T-7 (3 in. or 7.5 cm. below the sternal angle).
- 40 in. (102 cm.) F.F.D.

NOTE: • Body is almost lateral for each oblique. • Rotate 20° from the true lateral position. • May take as posterior or anterior obliques.

Structures Best Shown:
Apophysial joints. R.P.O. and L.P.O. show upside. R.A.O. and L.A.O. show downside.

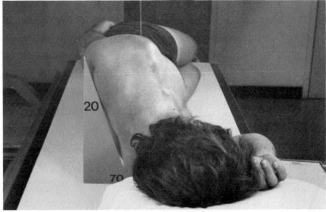

Oblique (R.P.O.)   Fig. 14-45

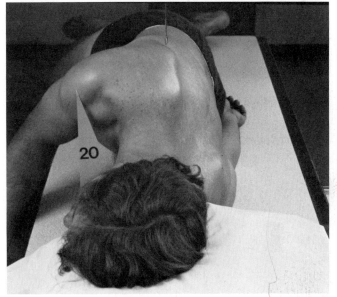

Oblique (L.A.O.)   Fig. 14-46

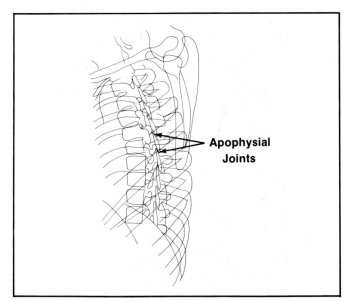

Apophysial Joints

Fig. 14-48

Oblique

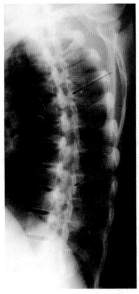

Fig. 14-47

Oblique

Cervical Spine

● Lateral Position (Recumbent)
Cross Table Lateral Position
(Trauma Routine)

Cervical
Basic
- **Lateral**
- A.P.
- Obliques (Both)

Optional
- Lateral - Flexion
- Lateral - Hyperextension
- Odontoid - Open-mouth
- A.P. - Chewing

Film Size:

> 10 x 12 in. (24 x 30 cm.)
> Lengthwise to patient.

Bucky:
- Stationary grid.

Patient Position:
- Supine, do **NOT** move patient.

Part Position:
- Do **NOT** manipulate neck.
- Place cassette vertically near shoulder.
- Top of cassette is about 2 in. (5 cm.) above E.A.M.
- Shoulders must be depressed.
- Traction on arms can be applied by assistant.
- Closely collimate.
- Suspend breathing on **expiration.**

Central Ray:
- C.R. directed horizontally to C-4, perpendicular to film holder.
- 72 in. (183 cm.) F.F.D.

NOTE: ● Good lateral showing **all 7** cervical vertebrae must be checked by physician before remainder of series can be done. ● A good lateral is the single most important position when the patient has experienced injury or trauma to the neck. ● Any bony injury must be ruled out before the head and neck are moved.

Structures Best Shown:
Cervical vertebral bodies, intervertebral joint spaces, articular pillars, spinous processes and apophysial joints.

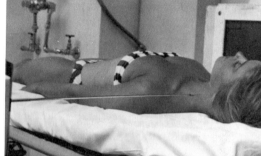

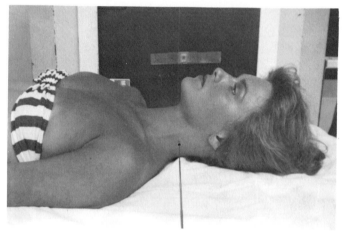

Lateral (Recumbent)   Fig. 14-49

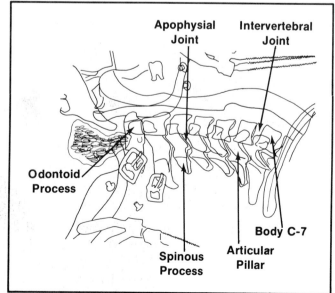

Lateral (Recumbent)   Fig. 14-50

Fig. 14-52
Lateral (Recumbent)

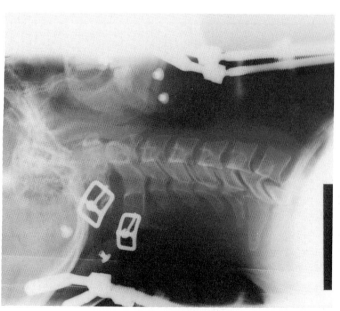

Lateral (Recumbent)   Fig. 14-51

Apophysial Joint   Intervertebral Joint

Odontoid Process

Spinous Process   Articular Pillar   Body C-7

Cervical Spine
• Lateral Position (Upright)
(Nontrauma Routine)

Cervical
Basic
- **Lateral**
- A.P.
- Obliques (Both)

Optional
- Lateral - Flexion
- Lateral - Hyperextension
- Odontoid - Open-mouth
- A.P. - Chewing

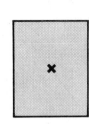

Film Size:
> 10 x 12 in. (24 x 30 cm.)
> or
> 8 x 10 in. (18 x 24 cm.)

Bucky:
- Moving or stationary grid.

Patient Position:
- Upright lateral, either sitting or standing.

Part Position:
- Shoulder against vertical cassette.
- Top of cassette about 2 in. (5 cm.) above E.A.M.
- Shoulders must be depressed (hold weights in hands).
- Relax and drop shoulders as much as possible.
- Jut chin forward.
- Closely collimate.
- Suspend breathing on **expiration.**

Central Ray:
- C.R. directed horizontally to C-4, perpendicular to film holder.
- 72 in. (183 cm.) F.F.D.

NOTE: • 7th cervical vertebra **must be shown.**

Structures Best Shown:
Cervical vertebral bodies, intervertebral joint spaces, articular pillars, apophysial joints and spinous processes.

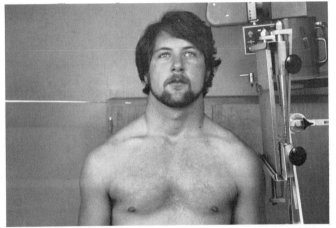

Lateral (Upright)

Fig. 14-53

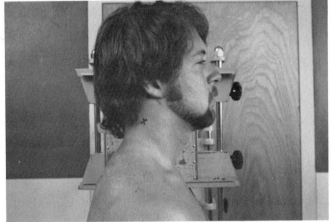

Lateral (Upright)

Fig. 14-54

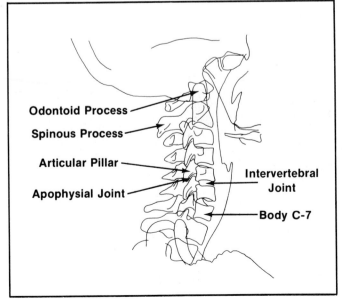

Odontoid Process
Spinous Process
Articular Pillar
Apophysial Joint
Intervertebral Joint
Body C-7

Fig. 14-56

Lateral

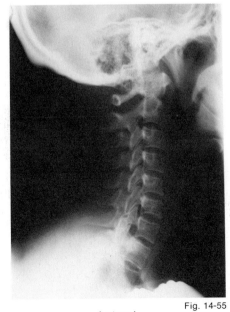

Lateral

Fig. 14-55

Cervical Spine
- **Anteroposterior Projection**

Film Size:
   8 x 10 in. (18 x 24 cm.)

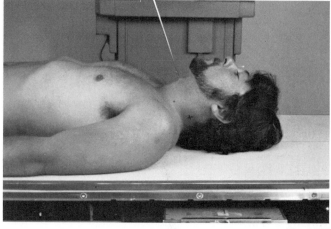

A.P.   Fig. 14-57

Bucky:
- Moving or stationary grid.

Patient Position:
- Supine or upright.

Part Position:
- Align midsagittal plane to midline of table.
- Arms beside body.
- Head against table.
- Line up bottom of front incisors and base of skull perpendicular to film.
- Immobilize head and closely collimate.
- Suspend respiration and do not swallow during exposure.

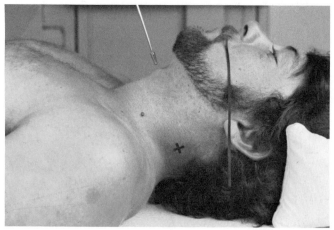

A.P.   Fig. 14-58

Central Ray:
- C.R. angled 20° cephalad to enter at level of thyroid cartilage.
- Film will be centered to C-4.
- 40 in. (102 cm.) F.F.D.

NOTE: • Cephalad angulation will open up intervertebral disc spaces and displace mandible superiorly.

Structures Best Shown:
Cervical vertebrae 3 through 7 to include vertebral bodies, space between pedicles, intervertebral disc spaces and spinous processes.

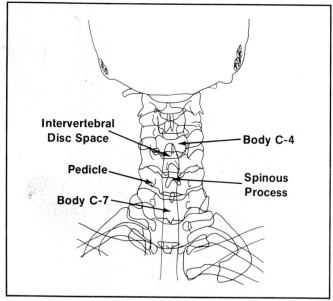

Intervertebral Disc Space — Body C-4 — Pedicle — Spinous Process — Body C-7

Fig. 14-60   A.P.

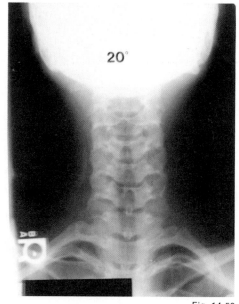

20°

A.P.   Fig. 14-59

Cervical Spine

• Oblique Positions

Film Size:

> 8 x 10 in. (18 x 24 cm.)
>   **or**
> 10 x 12 in. (24 x 30 cm.)

Bucky:

- Moving or stationary grid.

Patient Position:

- Semiprone, semisupine or upright oblique.

Part Position:

R.A.O. or L.A.O.

- Spine centered to midline of table.
- Body and head rotated 45° and supported.
- Arms comfortable.
- Chin jutted.
- Closely collimate.

L.P.O. or R.P.O.

- Spine centered to midline of table.
- Body and head rotated 45° and supported.
- Arms comfortable.
- Chin jutted.
- Closely collimate.

Central Ray:

- Anterior Obliques — 15° caudad to C-4.
- Posterior Obliques — 15° cephalad to C-4.
- 40 in. (102 cm.) F.F.D.

NOTE: • Both obliques must be taken. • Some routines allow the head to be turned to a true lateral position.

Structures Best Shown:

Anterior Obliques — Intervertebral foramina and pedicles closest to film.

Posterior Obliques — Intervertebral foramina and pedicles remote from film.

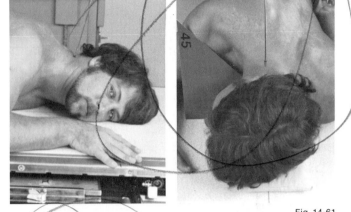

L.A.O.   L.A.O.

Fig. 14-61

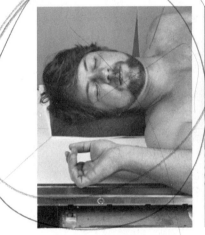

R.P.O.   L.P.O. (upright)

Fig. 14-62

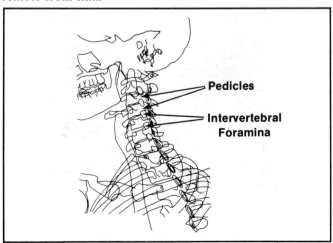

Pedicles

Intervertebral Foramina

Fig. 14-64

Oblique

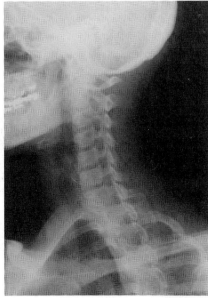

Oblique   Fig. 14-63

Cervical Spine

• Lateral Position with Flexion

Cervical
Basic
- Lateral
- A.P.
- Obliques (Both)

Optional
- **Lateral - Flexion**
- Lateral - Hyperextension
- Odontoid - Open-mouth
- A.P. - Chewing

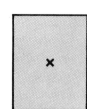

Film Size:
    10 x 12 in. (24 x 30 cm.)
        or
    8 x 10 in. (18 x 24 cm.)

Bucky:
- Moving or stationary grid.

Patient Position:
- Upright lateral, either sitting or standing.

Part Position:
- Shoulder against vertical cassette.
- Top of cassette about 2 in. (5 cm.) above E.A.M.
- Shoulders must be depressed.
- Chin depressed onto chest.
- Back should remain perpendicular to floor.
- Closely collimate.
- Suspend breathing on **expiration.**

Central Ray:
- C.R. directed to C-4, perpendicular to film holder.
- 72 in. (183 cm.) F.F.D.

NOTE: • Patient should remain in position no longer than necessary.

Structures Best Shown:
Functional study to demonstrate motion or lack of motion of cervical vertebrae.

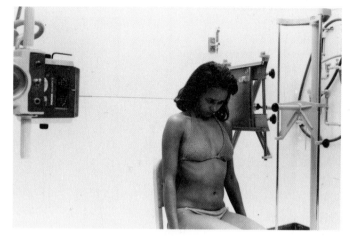

Lateral - Flexion   Fig. 14-65

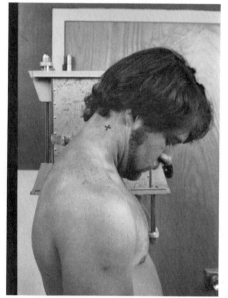

Lateral - Flexion   Fig. 14-66

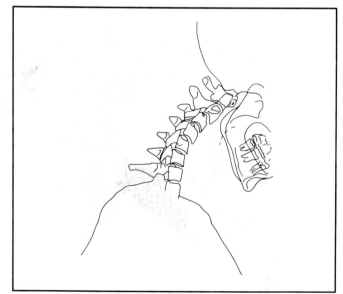

Fig. 14-68

Lateral - Flexion

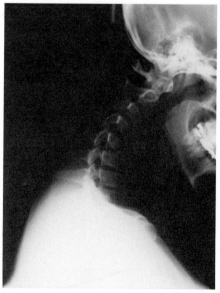

Lateral - Flexion   Fig. 14-67

Cervical Spine

• Lateral Position with Hyperextension

Cervical
Basic
- Lateral
- A.P.
- Obliques (Both)

Optional
- Lateral - Flexion
- **Lateral - Hyperextension**
- Odontoid - Open-mouth
- A.P. - Chewing

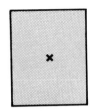

Film Size:
> 10 x 12 in. (24 x 30 cm.)
> **or**
> 8 x 10 in. (18 x 24 cm.)

Bucky:
- Moving or stationary grid.

Patient Position:
- Upright lateral, either sitting or standing.

Part Position:
- Shoulder against vertical cassette.
- Top of cassette about 2 in. (5 cm.) above E.A.M.
- Shoulders must be depressed.
- Chin elevated as much as possible.
- Back should remain perpendicular to floor.
- Closely collimate.
- Suspend breathing on **expiration.**

Central Ray:
- C.R. directed to C-4, perpendicular to film holder.
- 72 in. (183 cm.) F.F.D.

NOTE: • Patient should remain in position no longer than necessary.

Structures Best Shown:
Functional study to demonstrate motion or lack of motion of cervical vertebrae.

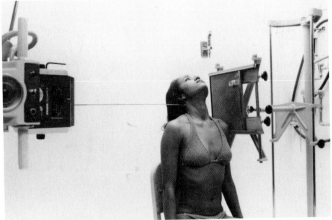

Lateral - Hyperextension

Fig. 14-69

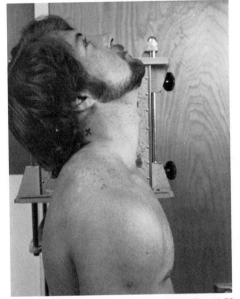

Lateral - Hyperextension

Fig. 14-70

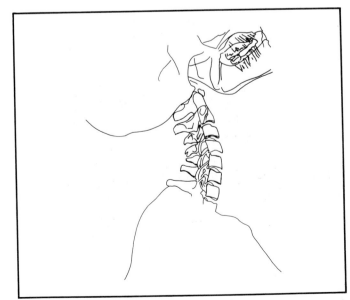

Fig. 14-72

Lateral - Hyperextension

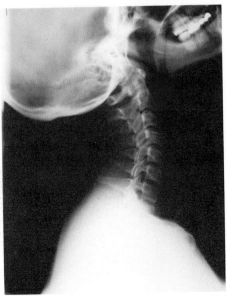

Fig. 14-71

Lateral - Hyperextension

Cervical Spine

• A.P. Projection of Atlas and Axis

Cervical
Basic
• Lateral
• A.P.
• Obliques (Both)
Optional
• Lateral - Flexion
• Lateral - Hyperextension
• **Odontoid - Open-mouth**
• A.P. - Chewing

Film Size:
  8 x 10 in. (18 x 24 cm.)

Bucky:
- Moving or stationary grid.

Patient Position:
- Supine.

Part Position:
- Align midsagittal plane to midline of table.
- Arms beside body.
- Head against table and securely immobilized.
- Line up bottom of front incisors and base of skull (mastoid tip) perpendicular to film.
- Closely collimate.
- Mouth open wide during exposure.

Central Ray:
- C.R. through center of open mouth, perpendicular to film holder.
- 40 in. (102 cm.) F.F.D.

NOTE: • Teeth obscure odontoid if head is not tipped up enough. • Base of skull obscures odontoid if head is tipped up too far.

Structures Best Shown:
Odontoid process and vertebral body of C-2, lateral masses of C-1, and apophysial joints between C-1 and C-2.

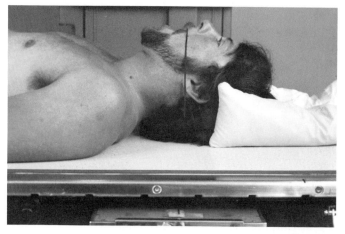

Open-mouth Odontoid   Fig. 14-73

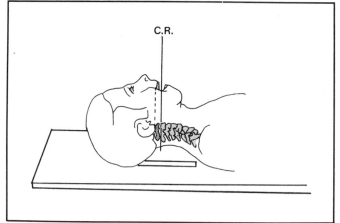

Open-mouth Odontoid   Fig. 14-74

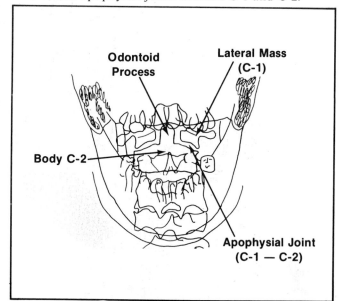

Fig. 14-76
Open-mouth Odontoid

Odontoid Process

Lateral Mass (C-1)

Body C-2

Apophysial Joint (C-1 — C-2)

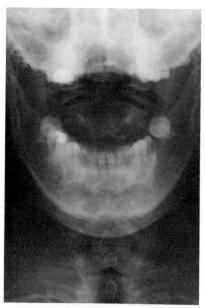

Open-mouth Odontoid   Fig. 14-75

Cervical Spine

• Anteroposterior Projection (Chewing)

Cervical
Basic
- Lateral
- A.P.
- Obliques (Both)

Optional
- Lateral - Flexion
- Lateral - Hyperextension
- Odontoid - Open-mouth
- **A.P. - Chewing**

Film Size:
 8 x 10 in. (18 x 24 cm.)

Bucky:
- Moving or stationary grid.

Patient Position:
- Supine.

Part Position:
- Align midsagittal plane to midline of table.
- Arms beside body.
- Head against table and securely immobilized.
- Line up bottom of front incisors and base of skull perpendicular to film.
- Closely collimate.
- Use long exposure.
- Mandible must be in continuous motion during exposure.
- Make certain that only the mandible is in motion; the rest of the skull, including the upper teeth, must not move.

Central Ray:
- C.R. centered to C-4, perpendicular to film holder.
- 40 in. (102 cm.) F.F.D.

NOTE: • Practice with patient before actual exposure.

Structures Best Shown:
Entire cervical spine with mandible blurred.

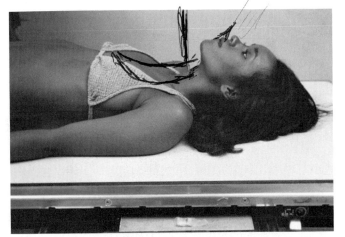

A.P. - Chewing　　　　　Fig. 14-77

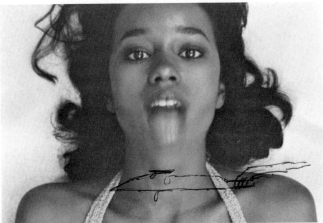

A.P. - Chewing　　　　　Fig. 14-78

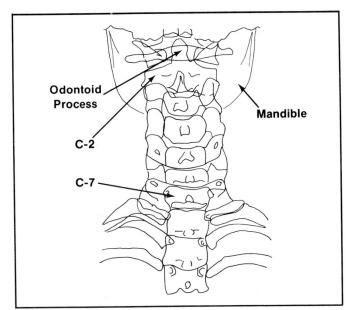

**Odontoid
Process**

Mandible

C-2

C-7

Fig. 14-80

A.P. - Chewing

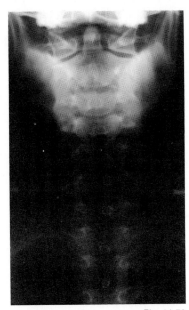

A.P. - Chewing　　Fig. 14-79

CHAPTER 15

Radiographic Anatomy and Positioning of the Bony Thorax and Soft Tissues of the Chest (Sternum, Ribs and Mammary Glands)

Part I. Radiographic Anatomy
Bony Thorax (Sternum and Ribs)

The bony thorax consists of the **sternum** anteriorly, the **thoracic vertebrae** posteriorly, and the **12 pairs of ribs** connecting the sternum to the vertebral column. The bony thorax serves to protect important organs of the respiratory system and vital structures within the mediastinum such as the heart and great vessels.

Sternum

An average sternum or breastbone is shown both from the front and from the side in *Fig. 15-1*. The sternum is a thin, narrow, flat bone with three divisions. The upper portion is termed the **manubrium,** which is from the Latin meaning handle. The manubrium averages 2 inches or 5 centimeters in length.

The longest part of the sternum is the **body,** which is about 4 inches or 10 centimeters long. The Latin word for body is **corpus.** Another, but older, term for the body is **gladiolus,** which means sword. Of the three names that can be used for the middle portion of the sternum, either body or corpus is preferable.

The most distal portion of the sternum is the **xiphoid process,** which can also be called the **ensiform process.** The xiphoid process is usually rather small; although it can be quite variable in size, shape, and degree of ossification, sometimes remaining totally cartilaginous.

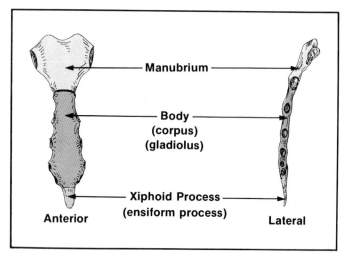

Sternum

Fig. 15-1

The uppermost border of the manubrium is an important external landmark that is very easy to palpate. This border is termed the **suprasternal notch.** Other names for this area are **manubrial notch** or **jugular notch.** All three terms describe the area between the two clavicles along the upper border of the sternum. The suprasternal notch is at the same level as the disc space between the second and third thoracic vertebrae.

Each **clavicle** joins the manubrium lateral to the suprasternal notch on each side. The joint formed is called the **sternoclavicular joint.** The only bony connection between each upper limb and the bony thorax is at the sternoclavicular joint.

The lower end of the manubrium joins the body or corpus to form a palpable angle, the **sternal angle.** The sternal angle is at the level of the disc space between the fourth and fifth thoracic vertebrae in an average-shaped, upright adult.

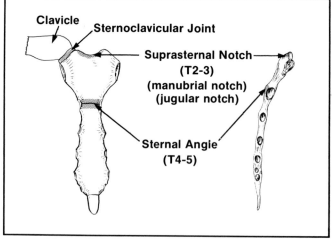

Sternum

Fig. 15-2

318

Sternal Articulations

The **clavicles** and the **cartilages** of the **first seven pairs of ribs** connect directly to the sternum. Below each sternoclavicular joint is a depression or **facet** for articulation with the cartilage of the first rib. The drawing in *Fig. 15-3* illustrates that the ribs do not unite directly with the sternum, but do so with a short piece of cartilage termed **costocartilage.** The costocartilages and ribs have been added to one side of this drawing to show this relationship.

The second costocartilage connects to the sternum at the level of the sternal angle. An easy way to locate the anterior end of the second rib is to locate the sternal angle first, then feel laterally along the cartilage and the bone of the rib. The third through the seventh costocartilages connect directly to the body of the sternum.

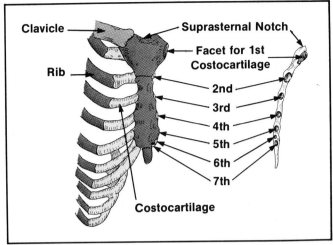

Sternal Articulations   Fig. 15-3

Bony Thorax

The remainder of the bony thorax has been added to the drawing in *Fig. 15-4* to show the relationship of the sternum to the 12 pairs of ribs and 12 thoracic vertebrae. The ribs that attach to the sternum do so by costocartilage and do not attach directly. The costocartilages of the first pair of ribs and the upper part of the second pair of ribs connect to the **manubrium.** The costocartilages of the lower part of the second ribs and the third through the seventh ribs all connect to the **body.** Ribs 8, 9 and 10 also possess costocartilage, but these cartilages connect to the number 7 costocartilages, which then connect to the sternum.

As demonstrated in *Fig. 15-4*, the thin sternum superimposes the thicker, denser thoracic spine in a direct frontal position. An A.P. or P.A. projection radiograph would show the thoracic spine well, but would show the sternum only faintly, if at all.

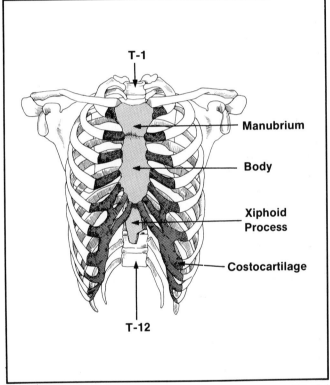

Bony Thorax   Fig. 15-4

Ribs

Each rib is numbered according to the thoracic vertebra to which it attaches; therefore, the ribs are numbered from the top down. The first seven pairs of ribs are considered **true ribs.** Each true rib attaches directly to the sternum by its own costocartilage. The term **false ribs** applies to the last five pairs of ribs, numbered 8, 9, 10, 11 and 12.

The drawing in *Fig. 15-5* shows that, although ribs 8 through 10 have costocartilages, they connect to the costocartilage of the seventh rib. The last two pairs of false ribs are unique in that they do not possess costocartilage. The term **floating ribs** can be used to designate these last two pairs of ribs. Therefore, the last two pairs of ribs, in addition to being false ribs, can also be called floating ribs.

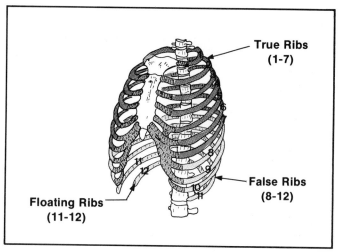

Ribs

Fig. 15-5

Typical Rib

A typical rib viewed from its inferior surface is illustrated in *Fig. 15-6*. A central rib is used to show the common characteristics of a typical rib. Each rib has two ends, a posterior or **vertebral end,** and an anterior or **sternal end.** Between the two ends is the body or **shaft** of the rib.

The vertebral end consists of a **head,** which articulates with one or two thoracic vertebral bodies, and a flattened **neck.** Lateral to the neck is an elevated **tubercle** that articulates with the transverse process of a vertebra and allows for attachment of a ligament. The shaft extends laterally from the tubercle, then angles forward and downward. The area of forward angulation is termed the **angle** of the rib.

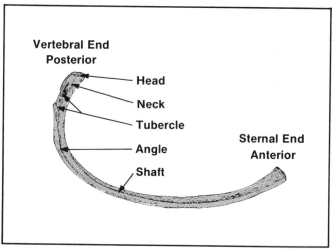

Typical Rib (inferior)

Fig. 15-6

As viewed from the back or posterior, a typical rib appears as illustrated in *Fig. 15-7*. Seen are the **head, neck** and **tubercle** at the vertebral end of the rib. Progressing laterally, the **angle** of the rib is where the shaft bends forward and downward toward the sternal end. The posterior or vertebral end of a typical rib is 3 to 5 inches or 7.5 to 12.5 centimeters **higher** than the anterior or sternal end. Therefore, when viewing a radiograph of a chest or ribs, one must remember that the part of a rib most superior is the posterior end or the end nearest the vertebrae. The anterior end or end near the sternum is more inferior.

The lower inside margin of each rib protects an **artery,** a **vein** and a **nerve**; therefore, rib injuries are very painful and may be associated with substantial hemorrhage. This inside margin, containing the blood vessels and nerves, is termed the **costal groove.**

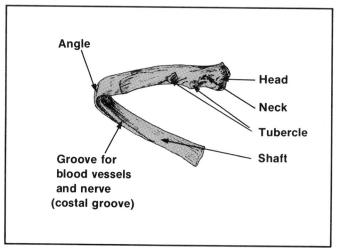

Typical Rib (posterior)

Fig. 15-7

Rib Cage

The drawing in *Fig. 15-8* illustrates the bony thorax with the sternum and costocartilages removed. The fifth ribs have been shaded to better illustrate the downward angulation of the ribs.

Not all ribs have the same appearance. The first ribs are short and broad, and are the most vertical of all the ribs. Counting downward from the short first pair, the ribs get longer and longer down to the seventh ribs. From the seventh ribs down they get shorter and shorter through the fairly short twelfth or last pair of ribs.

Most of the ribs have a gentle curve from back to front. The first ribs are the most sharply curved of all ribs. The bony thorax is **widest** at the lateral margins of the **eighth** or **ninth ribs.**

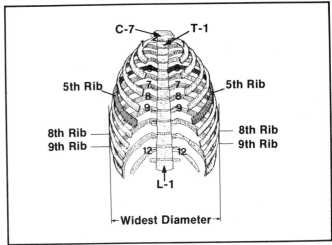

Rib Cage   Fig. 15-8

Sternum

The sternum is both difficult to radiograph and difficult to study anatomically on the finished radiograph. The parts of the sternum listed A through F on the photograph of an actual sternum in *Fig. 15-9* are: **(A)** the suprasternal notch, **(B)** the facet for the costocartilage of the first rib, **(C)** the manubrium, **(D)** the sternal angle, **(E)** the body or corpus, and **(F)** the area of the xiphoid process.

Part **B** is not the area of articulation of the clavicle to the sternum. Remember that the clavicle articulates just lateral to the suprasternal notch and just above the articulation of the cartilage of the first rib. Also, on this particular sternum the xiphoid process has not ossified, but **F** is the area where it would normally be found if it were cartilaginous or osseous.

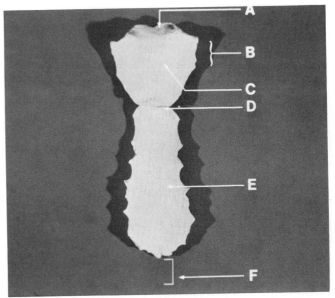

Sternum   Fig. 15-9

Sternum Radiographs

A radiograph of the sternum in the frontal position is illustrated in *Fig. 15-10*. This is a conventional frontal radiograph of the sternum taken in a slight right anterior oblique position. The slight degree of obliquity tends to project the thoracic vertebrae to one side of the sternum.

The various parts of the sternum are difficult to visualize on radiographs of the sternum, so parts of this radiograph have been enhanced. The labeled parts are: **(A)** the sternal end of one clavicle, **(B)** the suprasternal notch, **(C)** the manubrium, **(D)** the sternal angle, **(E)** the body, and **(F)** the area of the xiphoid process.

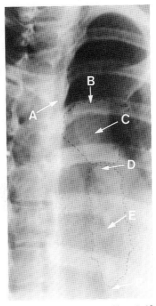

Fig. 15-10
R.A.O. Sternum

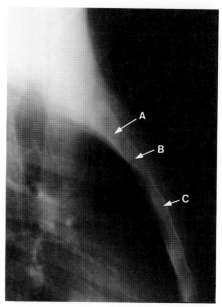

A radiograph of the sternum in the lateral position is illustrated in *Fig. 15-11.* Part **A** is the upper part of the sternum or the manubrium; and **B** is the sternal angle, while **C** is the body.

Lateral Sternum   Fig. 15-II

Typical Rib

A photograph of a typical rib as viewed from the undersurface is illustrated in *Fig. 15-12.* **A, B,** and **C** are structures at the posterior or vertebral end of the rib. **A** is the head, **B** is the neck, and **C** is the tubercle of this rib. Part **D** is the angle of the rib, and **E** is a portion of the costal groove.

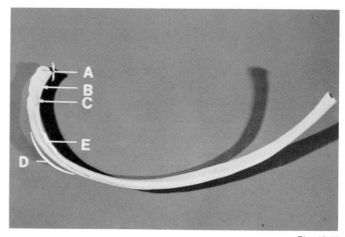

Typical Rib   Fig. 15-12

Thoracic Cage Articulations

The front of an articulated thorax is illustrated in *Fig. 15-13*. This photograph summarizes the names of the joints and the types of motion allowed along the anterior bony thorax.

Part **A** is the joint between costocartilage and the sternal end of the fourth rib, and is called a **costochondral joint** or junction. These joints, permitting no actual motion, are termed synarthrodial joints.

Part **B** is one **sternoclavicular joint.** The sternoclavicular joints permit a gliding motion and are, therefore, diarthrodial joints.

Part **C** is the **sternocostal joint** of the first rib. The cartilage of the first rib attaches directly to the manubrium with no capsule and allows no motion, making this a synarthrodial joint.

Part **D** is the fourth sternocostal joint, typical of the second through the seventh joints between costocartilage and sternum. These joints allow a slight gliding motion, making them diarthrodial joints.

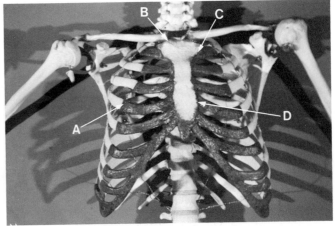

Articulated Thorax

Fig. 15-13

The remaining types of joints (posterior articulations) in the bony thorax are illustrated in *Fig. 15-14*. The joints between the ribs and the vertebral column, the costotransverse joints and the costovertebral joints, allow a gliding motion, which classifies them as diarthrodial.

Two other joints involving the bony thorax are those between any two thoracic vertebrae. The apophysial joints between the superior and inferior articular processes have a gliding motion, which makes them diarthrodial joints. The joints between the bodies of any two thoracic vertebrae have a more restricted type of motion and are termed amphiarthrodial joints. Although no one joint in the entire thorax moves very much, the combined actions of many joints do allow quite a range of motion for the thorax as a whole.

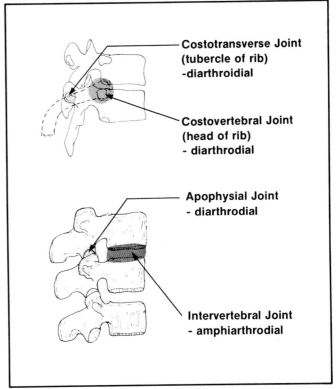

Costotransverse Joint (tubercle of rib) -diarthroidial

Costovertebral Joint (head of rib) - diarthrodial

Apophysial Joint - diarthrodial

Intervertebral Joint - amphiarthrodial

Posterior Articulations

Fig. 15-14

Part II. Radiographic Positioning
Bony Thorax (Sternum and Ribs)

Basic and Optional Projections/Positions

Certain basic projections or positions for the sternum and ribs are demonstrated and described on the following pages. Basic projections, sometimes referred to as routine projections, are those projections commonly taken on average, helpful patients. It should be noted that department routines or basic projections vary in different hospitals or departments.

Optional projections include those more common projections taken as extra or additional projections to better demonstrate specific anatomical parts or certain pathological conditions. No optional positions or projections are actually demonstrated in this section, although the opposite oblique or spot radiographs of certain ribs are sometimes requested.

Generally, basic projections or positions for a routine sternum include a slight R.A.O. and a lateral. Basic positioning for the ribs usually includes a routine P.A. chest, an A.P. of the ribs utilizing either above-the-diaphragm or below-the-diaphragm technique, and one oblique of the ribs. Since the dome or central portion of each half of the diaphragm is the most superior part of the diaphragm, it is the dome of the diaphragm that is used to determine the degree of inspiration on chest radiographs. On a full inspiration, the dome of the diaphragm should be at the level of the tenth posterior ribs. Since injuries to the ribs may be quite painful, the patient may not be able to take a full inspiration. In order to properly radiograph those ribs near the diaphragm, it is necessary to know the degree of inspiration or expiration in relationship to the ribs of interest. If the ribs to be radiographed will be projected below the diaphragm, then exposure factors will need to be increased compared to exposure factors for ribs projected above the diaphragm. Therefore, below-the-diaphragm technique is usually necessary on rib injuries below the eighth posterior rib.

Sternum	**Ribs**
Basic	Basic
• R.A.O.	• P.A. Chest
• Lateral	• A.P. Ribs
	(A.D. or B.D.)
	• Oblique Ribs

Sternum

● **Right Anterior Oblique Position**

Film Size:
  10 x 12 in. (24 x 30 cm.)

Bucky:
- Moving or stationary grid.

Patient Position:
- Semiprone (15 to 20° R.A.O.).

Part Position:
- Long axis of sternum centered to film.
- Sternum should be superimposed on heart shadow (providing homogeneous background to better visualize sternum).
- Slight oblique (15 to 20°) shifts vertebral column to right of sternum.
- **Right** anterior oblique will superimpose sternum and heart shadow.
- Closely collimate.

Central Ray:
- C.R. perpendicular to film holder.
- C.R. enters slightly left of the vertebral column and is centered midway between suprasternal notch and xiphoid process.
- Less than 40 in. (102 cm.) F.F.D., if possible **(See NOTE).**

NOTE: ● Short F.F.D. will help to blur out posterior ribs. ● Shallow breathing with long exposure (3 to 4 sec.) will help to blur out pulmonary markings. ● Low kVp (58 to 60) will provide added contrast.

Structures Best Shown:
Sternum with pulmonary markings and posterior ribs somewhat blurred.

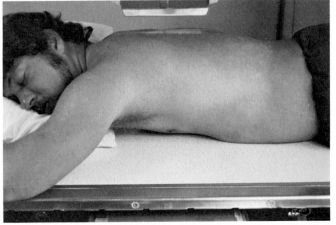

Right Anterior Oblique   Fig. 15-15

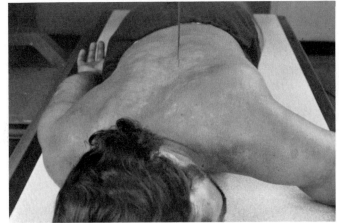

Right Anterior Oblique   Fig. 15-16

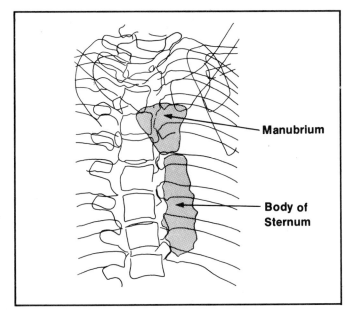

Manubrium

Body of
Sternum

Fig. 15-18   R.A.O.

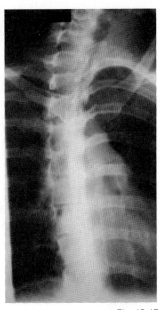

R.A.O.   Fig. 15-17

Sternum
Basic
• R.A.O.
• Lateral

Sternum

• **Lateral Position**

15

Bony Thorax
(Sternum and Ribs)

Film Size:
10 x 12 in. (24 x 30 cm.)

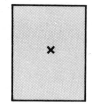

Bucky:
- Moving or stationary grid.

Patient Position:
- Upright or lateral recumbent, or dorsal recumbent.

Part Position:
- Upright — standing or seated with shoulders and arms well back.
- Lateral recumbent — arms forward and well above head.
- Dorsal recumbent — patient supine with arms at sides and cassette placed vertically (used if patient cannot be moved due to severity of injuries).
- Body and sternum must be true lateral.

Central Ray:
- C.R. perpendicular to film holder.
- Midsternum (top of cassette 1½ in. or 4 cm. above suprasternal notch).
- 40 in. (102 cm.) F.F.D.

NOTE: • Low kVp (70) with suspended inspiration provides added contrast. • Lateral chest radiograph does not visualize sternum adequately.

Structures Best Shown:
Sternum (fractures especially well visualized).

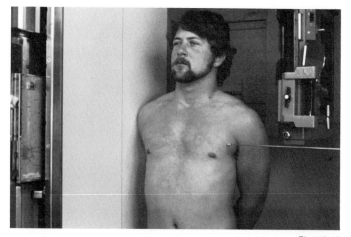

Lateral — upright   Fig. 15-19

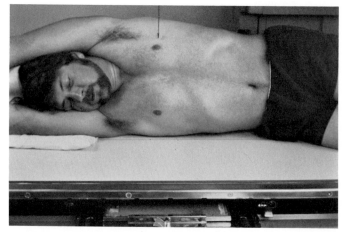

Lateral — recumbent   Fig. 15-20

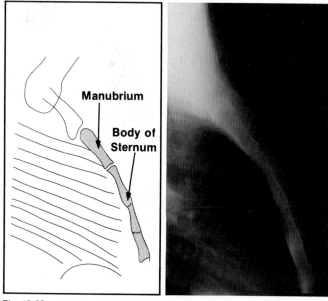

Fig. 15-22

Manubrium

Body of Sternum

Lateral

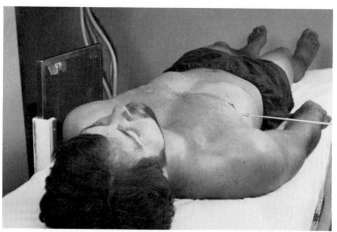

Lateral — dorsal decubitus   Fig. 15-21

Ribs
Basic
- **P.A. Chest**
- A.P. Ribs
  (A.D. or B.D.)
- Oblique Ribs

Ribs
● **Posteroanterior Projection (Upright Chest)**

Film Size:
    14 x 17 in. (35 x 43 cm.)

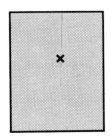

Bucky:
- Moving or stationary grid.

Patient Position:
- Upright (supine or semiupright, if upright is not possible).

Part Position:
- Midsagittal plane of body must coincide with midline of film.
- Rotate scapulae from lung fields by rolling shoulders forward.
- Usually expose on suspended inspiration (expiration will best visualize a small pneumothorax).
- Chin up, head forward.
- Closely collimate.

Central Ray:
- C.R. should pass through T-4 (2 in. or 5 cm. above film center) and be perpendicular to film holder.
- 72 in. (183 cm.) F.F.D.

NOTE: ● Upright chest is the most important radiograph of rib series. ● Upright is necessary to show fluid levels, such as hemothorax. ● Pneumothorax or hemothorax may be life-threatening.

Structures Best Shown:
Thoracic viscera, including lungs and mediastinal structures.

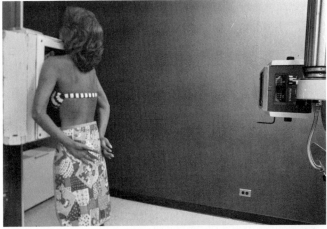
P.A. Projection
Fig. 15-23

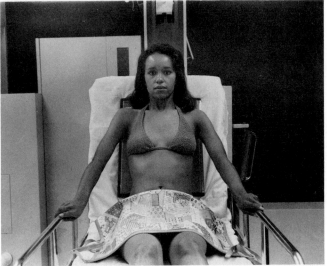
A.P. (upright)
Fig. 15-24

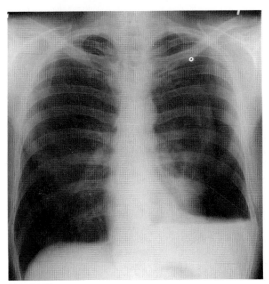
Fig. 15-26
Hemopneumothorax (left side)

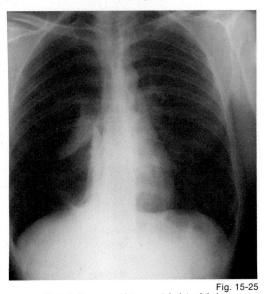
Total Pneumothorax (right side)
Fig. 15-25

Ribs
Basic
- P.A. Chest
- **A.P. Ribs**
  (A.D. or B.D.)
- Oblique Ribs

Ribs

- **Anteroposterior Projection**
(Above Diaphragm, A.D.)

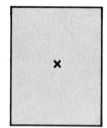

Film Size:
    14 x 17 in. (35 x 43 cm.)

Bucky:
- Moving or stationary grid.

Patient Position:
- Supine or upright.

Part Position:
- Midsagittal plane of body coincides with midline of film.
- Arms at sides.
- Internally rotate arms to remove scapulae from lung fields.
- Collimate closely.
- Expose on **full inspiration.**

Central Ray:
- C.R. perpendicular to center of film at T-7 level to show ribs above the diaphragm.
- 40 in. (102 cm.) F.F.D.

NOTE: • Avoid unnecessary movement of the patient since rib injuries are very painful.

Structures Best Shown:
Ribs above the diaphragm, especially the posterior part of each rib.

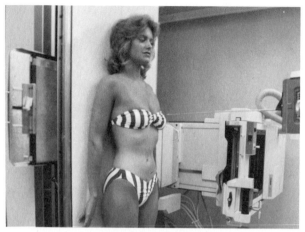

A.P. Projection (A.D.)   Fig. 15-27

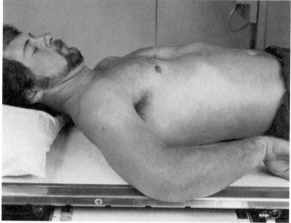

A.P. Projection (A.D.)   Fig. 15-28

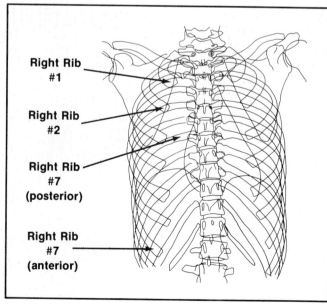

Right Rib #1

Right Rib #2

Right Rib #7 (posterior)

Right Rib #7 (anterior)

Fig. 15-30

A.P. Projection (A.D.)

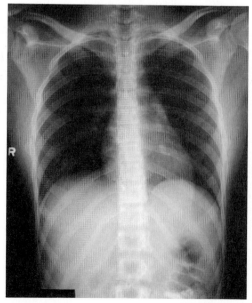

A.P. Projection (A.D.)   Fig. 15-29

Ribs
Basic
- P.A. Chest
- **A.P. Ribs**
  (A.D. or **B.D.**)
- Oblique Ribs

Ribs
• Anteroposterior Projection
(Below Diaphragm, B.D.)

Film Size:
14 x 17 in. (35 x 43 cm.)
Crosswise.

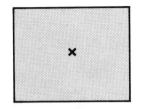

Bucky:
- Moving or stationary grid.

Patient Position:
- Supine or upright.

Part Position:
- Midsagittal pla..e of body coincides with midline of film.
- Arms at sides or across upper chest.
- Collimate closely.
- Expose on **full exhalation.**

Central Ray:
- C.R. perpendicular to film holder at T-12 level to best show lower four pairs of ribs.
- T-12 level is about 3 in. (7.5 cm.) below xiphoid tip.
- 40 in. (102 cm.) F.F.D.

NOTE: • Iₙ pain ' below level of xiphoid tip, use B.D. technique. • Cassette must be crosswise because rib cage is widest at 8th or 9th rib.

Structures Best Shown:
Ribs below the diaphragm (9, 10, 11 and 12).

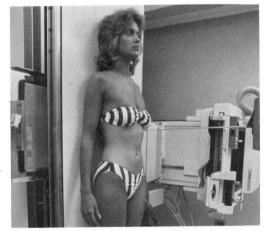

A.P. Projection (B.D.)

Fig. 15-31

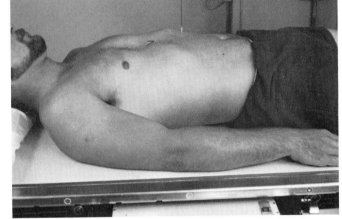

A.P. Projection (B.D.)

Fig. 15-32

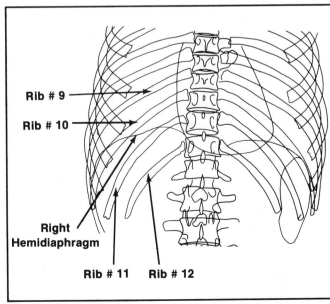

Rib # 9
Rib # 10
Right Hemidiaphragm
Rib # 11   Rib # 12

Fig. 15-34   A.P. Projection (B.D.)

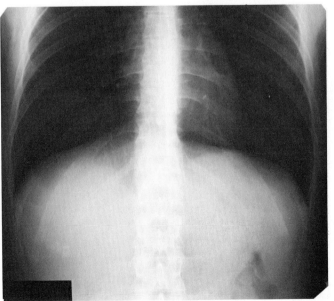

A.P. Projection (B.D.)

Fig. 15-33

Ribs
Basic
- P.A. Chest
- A.P. Ribs
  (A.D. or B.D.)
- **Oblique Ribs**

Ribs

- **Oblique Position**

Film Size:
14 x 17 in. (35 x 43 cm.)

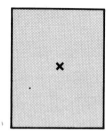

Bucky:
- Moving or stationary grid.

Patient Position:
- Semisupine or semiprone, or upright with body rotated 45°.

Part Position:
- Rotate body 45°.
- Spine must always be rotated away from ribs of interest.
- Injury to the right side would require R.P.O. or L.A.O.
- Injury to the left side would require L.P.O. or R.A.O.
- Collimate closely.

Central Ray:
- C.R. perpendicular to center of film holder at T-7 level for ribs above the diaphragm, and at T-12 for ribs below the diaphragm.

NOTE: • To avoid confusion, many routines call for only posterior obliques. • Posterior obliques are always done with the injured side closest to the film, while anterior obliques are always done with the injured side away from the film.

Structures Best Shown:
Axillary margin of ribs on the side of interest.

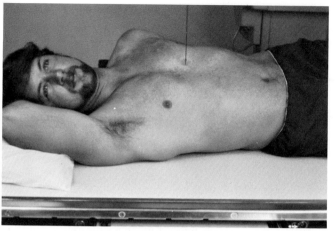

Right Posterior Oblique
(injury along right margin)

Fig. 15-35

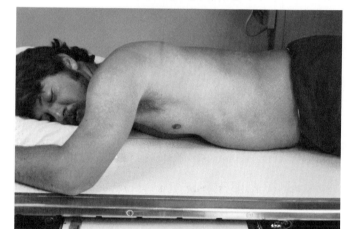

Right Anterior Oblique
(injury along left margin)

Fig. 15-36

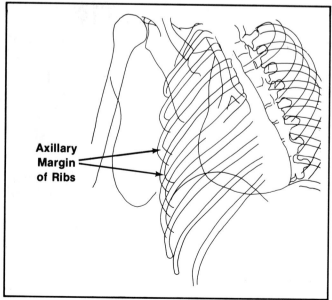

Axillary Margin of Ribs

Fig. 15-38

R.P.O.

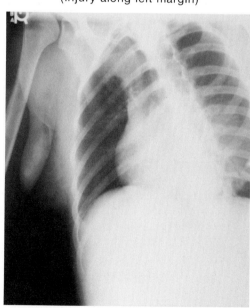

R.P.O.

Fig. 15-37

Part III. Radiographic Anatomy
Soft Tissues (Mammary Glands)

Anatomy of the Breast

In the adult female, each of the mammary glands or breasts is a conical or hemispherical eminence located on the anterior and lateral chest wall. There is a great deal of variation in breast size from one individual to another, and even in the same woman, depending on her age and the influence of various hormones; however, the usual breast extends from the anterior portion of the **second rib** down to the **sixth or seventh rib** and from the lateral border of the sternum well into the axilla.

The surface anatomy includes the **nipple**, a small projection containing a collection of duct openings from the secretory glands within the breast tissue. The pigmented area surrounding the nipple is termed the **areola,** defined as a circular area of a different color surrounding a central point. The junction of the inferior part of the breast with the anterior chest wall is called the **inframammary crease.**

Surface anatomy of the mammary gland, as seen from the front, is shown in *Fig. 15-40.* The previously described **nipple, areola,** and **inframammary crease** are shown. The width of the average breast is usually greater than is the measurement from top to bottom. The top to bottom measurement, which may be described as the craniocaudad diameter, averages from 12 to 15 centimeters at the chest wall.

The radiographer must realize that there is more breast tissue than the tissue that extends obviously from the chest. There is mammary tissue overlying the costocartilages near the sternum and breast tissue extending well up into the axilla. The breast tissue extending into the axilla is called the **tail of the breast** or the **axillary prolongation** of the breast.

Methods of Localization

Two methods are commonly used to subdivide the breast into smaller areas for localization purposes. The quadrant system, shown on the left in *Fig. 15-41,* is easiest to use. Four quadrants can be described by using the nipple as the center. These quadrants are the U.O.Q. (upper outer quadrant), the U.I.Q. (upper inner quadrant), the L.O.Q. (lower outer quadrant), and the L.I.Q. (lower inner quadrant).

A second method, shown on the right in *Fig. 15-41,* compares the surface of the breast to the face of a clock. A problem with the clock method arises when a medial or lateral portion of either breast is described. What is described at 3 o'clock in the right breast has to be described at 9 o'clock in the left breast. If either the referring physician or the patient has felt a mass or any suspicious area in either breast, one of these methods is used to describe the area of special interest to radiology personnel.

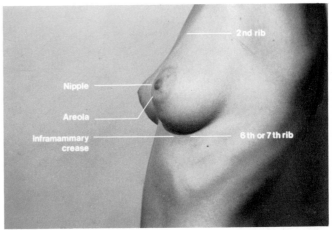
Surface Anatomy

Fig. 15-39

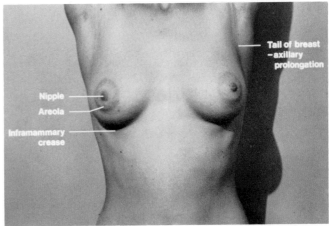
Surface Anatomy

Fig. 15-40

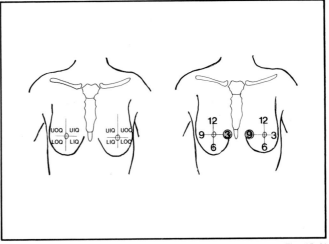
Breast Localization

Fig. 15-41

Breast (sagittal section)

A sagittal section through a mature breast is illustrated in *Fig. 15-42,* showing the relationship of the mammary gland to the underlying structures of the chest wall. On this drawing the **inframammary crease** is at the level of the seventh rib, but a great deal of variation does exist among individuals.

The large **pectoralis major muscle** is seen overlying the bony thorax. A sheet of fibrous tissues surrounds the breast below the skin surface. A similar sheet of tissue covers the pectoralis major muscle. These two fibrous sheets connect in an area termed the **retromammary space.** This retromammary space must be demonstrated on at least one projection during the radiographic study of the mammary gland. Since the connections within the retromammary space are fairly loose, the normal breast exhibits considerable mobility on the chest wall.

The relative position of glandular tissue versus adipose tissue is illustrated in *Fig. 15-43.* The central portion of the breast is primarily **glandular tissue.** Varying amounts of **adipose** or **fatty tissue** surround the glandular tissue. Size variation from individual to individual is due primarily to the amount of fatty tissue in the breast. The amount of glandular tissue is fairly constant from one female to another. Since the primary function of the mammary gland is lactation, or the secretion of milk, size of the female breast has no bearing on the functional ability of the gland.

The glandular tissue is divided into 15 or 20 lobes arranged like the spokes of a wheel surrounding the nipple. Each of these major lobes branches like a tree into smaller and smaller subdivisions. The smallest subdivisions are stimulated during pregnancy to prepare for lactation and, following birth, to actually produce milk. The **skin** covering the breast is seen to be uniform in thickness, except in the area of the nipple.

Breast (Frontal)

A frontal drawing with portions of the breast removed is illustrated in *Fig. 15-44.* This drawing clearly shows the radial arrangement of the glandular tissue. The glandular lobes are not clearly separated, but they do drain by individual ducts. Each duct enlarges into a small reservoir or **ampulla** just prior to terminating in a tiny opening on the surface of the **nipple.**

While most of the **adipose tissue** appears to lie peripherally, smaller amounts are usually found in between the **glandular tissues.** Bands of **connective tissue** pass through the substance of the breast, connecting fibrous tissue in the retromammary space to the skin. These fibrous bands are known as **suspensory ligaments** of the breast or **Cooper's ligaments,** and function to provide support for the mammary glands. Later in life these ligaments lose some of their supportive capability and the breast becomes pendulous. A popular phrase denoting this condition is "Cooper's Droop."

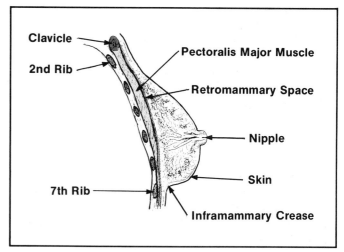

Breast, sagittal section   Fig. 15-42

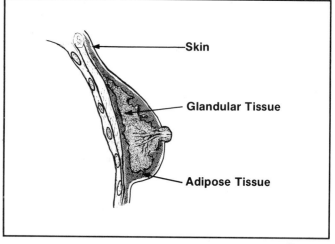

Breast, sagittal section   Fig. 15-43

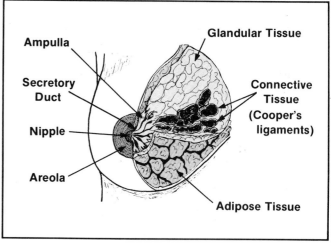

Breast, anterior   Fig. 15-44

Each breast is abundantly supplied by blood vessels, nerves and lymphatic vessels. The veins of the mammary gland are usually larger than the arteries, and are located more peripherally. Some of the larger **veins** usually can be seen distinctly on a mammogram, a radiographic study of the breast. The term trabeculae is used by radiologists to describe various small structures seen on the finished radiograph. The various small blood vessels, fibrous connective tissues, ducts and other small structures that cannot be differentiated are collectively termed trabeculae.

Breast Tissue Types

One of the major problems in radiography of the breast is that the various tissues are of similar density. Breast tissue can be divided into three main types of tissues: **fibrous** or **connective, glandular** and **adipose.** Since these tissues are all "soft tissues," there is no bone or air-filled tissue to provide contrast. The fibrous and glandular tissues are of similar density — that is, radiation is absorbed by these two tissues in a similar fashion.

The major difference in the breast tissues is the fact that adipose tissue is less dense than either the fibrous or glandular tissue. Since there is this difference in density between the fatty tissue and the remaining tissues, a photographic difference is apparent on the finished radiograph.

Summary of Breast Tissues

Three Types of Breast Tissue
(soft tissues)

1. Fibrous or Connective ⎫
2. Glandular ⎬ similar density
3. Adipose ———————— less dense

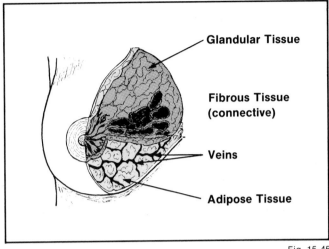

Breast, anterior   Fig. 15-45

Breast Classifications

Technical radiographic factors for any one part of the body are determined mainly by the thickness of that particular part. A large elbow will require greater exposure factors than a small elbow. However, in mammography, the actual measurement of the breast contributes only minimally to the technique selection. The relative density of the breast tissue is far more important. This relative density of the breast is primarily affected by the patient's age and the number of pregnancies. The mammary gland undergoes cyclic changes associated with the rise and fall of hormonal secretions during the menstrual cycle, and permanent changes during pregnancy and lactation. Generally speaking, however, breasts can be classified into three broad categories, depending on the relative amounts of fibroglandular tissue versus fatty tissue.

Fibro-Glandular Breast

The first category is the Fibro-Glandular breast. The younger breast is usually quite dense, since it contains relatively little fatty tissue. The common age grouping for the Fibro-Glandular category is postpuberty to about age thirty. However, those females over the age of 30 who have never given birth to a live infant will probably also be in this general grouping. Pregnant or lactating females of any age are also placed in this grouping because they possess a very dense type of breast.

1. Fibro-Glandular Breast

- **Common age group - 15-30 years**
- **Radiographically dense**
- **Very little fat**
- **Childless females over age 30**
- **Pregnant or lactating females**

Fibro-Glandular Breast   Fig. 15-46

Fibro-Fatty Breast

A second general category is the Fibro-Fatty breast. As the female ages and more changes occur in the breast tissues, there is a gradual shift from scant amounts of fatty tissue to a more equal distribution. Therefore, in the 30- to 50-year-old group the breast is not quite so dense as in the younger group.

Radiographically, this breast is of average density and requires less exposure than the Fibro-Glandular type of breast. Several pregnancies early in a woman's reproductive life will accelerate her breast development toward this Fibro-Fatty category.

2. Fibro-Fatty Breast

- **Common age group - 30 to 50 years**
- **Radiographically average**
- **50% fat - 50% fibroglandular**
- **Young women with 3 or more pregnancies**

Fibro-Fatty Breast   Fig. 15-47

Fatty Breast

A third and final grouping is the Fatty breast that occurs following menopause. Following a female's reproductive life, most of the glandular breast tissue atrophies and is converted to fatty tissue. Even less exposure is required on this type of breast than is required on the first two types of breasts.

The breasts of children and most males contain mostly fat in small proportions and, therefore, fall into this category also. While most mammograms are performed on the female patient, it is well to realize that between one and two percent of all breast cancer is found in the male; therefore, mammograms will occasionally be performed on a male.

Summary: In summary, the average density of the tissues of the breast, rather than size, will determine exposure factors. The most dense breast is the Fibro-Glandular type. The least dense is the Fatty type, and the breast with equal amounts of fatty and fibroglandular tissue is termed Fibro-Fatty.

3. Fatty Breast

- **Common age group - 50 years and up**
- **Post menopausal**
- **Minimal density, radiographically**
- **Atrophic**
- **Breasts of children**
- **Most male breasts**

Fatty Breast   Fig. 15-48

334

Part IV. Radiographic Positioning
Soft Tissues (Mammary Glands)

Breast Positioning

In mammography, the great variability of the breast, with respect to the proportion of fatty tissue to fibroglandular tissue, presents certain technical difficulties. In producing a superior quality mammogram, the shape and contour of the normal breast poses additional problems to the radiographer.

The **base** of the breast is that portion near the chest wall, while the area near the nipple is termed the **apex.** In either the craniocaudad or the mediolateral projection, the base of the breast is much thicker and contains much denser tissues than the apex. To overcome this anatomical difference, the central ray is directed to pass through the base of the breast, while the less intense divergent beam passes through the outer periphery of the breast. Correct positioning for the craniocaudad projection is illustrated in *Fig. 15-49.*

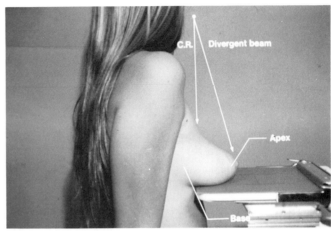

Correct Positioning

Fig. 15-49

Imaging Modalities

Various imaging modalities for studying the tissues of the breast have been postulated. Since the breast anatomy is purely soft tissue, the inherent radiographic contrast is very low. Other difficulties encountered in breast imaging relate to the lack of a discrete internal structure (the fatty and fibroglandular tissues are interspersed), the low physiologic activity of the breast and the complex blood supply to this area.

Film Mammography

Early mammographic techniques utilized extremely fine-grain, nonscreen-type industrial film to record the minute structures of the breast. Mammograms must clearly show structures a hundred times smaller than those structures demonstrated on routine radiographs of many other parts of the body. Trabeculae the size of spiders' webs and micro-calcifications associated with early breast cancer in the 25 to 50 micron size range must be depicted on the finished mammogram.

The conventional film-type mammogram requires very low kVp values (20 to 30), minimal filtration (less than 1 millimeter aluminum equivalent), and high mAs settings (several hundred). A film-type mammogram is shown in *Fig. 15-50.* The major drawback to the fine-grain film method of mammography is the large radiation exposure to the patient.

Film-screen Combination: A method designed to reduce radiation dosage and still retain the film-type mammogram is a film-screen combination. A single emulsion film and a single screen packaged in a vacuum bag does decrease radiation exposure, but may also decrease resolution. Supporters of this technique point out that decreased patient motion results from shorter exposure times; therefore, overall resolution is improved.

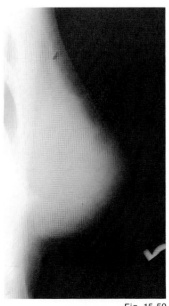

Fig. 15-50

Film
Mammogram

Xeroradiography

Another mammographic procedure that has been widely accepted is xeroradiography. X-radiation is used to produce the image, but a photoelectric recording method is used rather than fine-grain film. A simplified explanation of this system appears in *Fig. 15-51*. The xeroradiographic plate has an aluminum base with a thin layer of vitreous selenium, as shown in the upper drawing in *Fig. 15-51*. The construction of the plate allows an electrical charge to be placed and held in the selenium layer.

Step I of this process involves charging the plate in a special conditioning device. The selenium on the plate is termed a photoconductor. Electrical charges are neutralized by x-radiation passing through the breast, forming a latent image of the pattern of the breast tissues. This step (Step II) is demonstrated on the center drawing, showing the x-ray exposure.

Step III is carried out in a special processor. In the processor the latent image is first sprayed by a blue, finely divided, charged powder, producing a visible image on the surface of the plate. Using a heat transfer, the image on the plate is then transferred to a plastic coated paper.

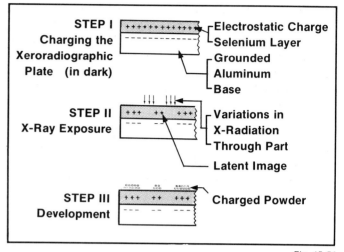

The Xeroradiographic Process   Fig. 15-51

An example of a xeroradiograph is shown in *Fig. 15-52*. In actual practice xeroradiographs are various shades of blue rather than black, gray and white. However, since this illustration was produced with a black and white film rather than a color film, the blue color is not shown. On the original xeroradiograph the dark gray areas were dark blue and the light gray areas were a lighter shade of blue.

In addition, xeroradiographs are usually positives rather than negatives. The thick parts of the breast appear dark blue, while the thin parts appear as a lighter blue. It is a simple matter, however, to produce a negative that would be similar to the film-type mammograph.

Supporters of xeroradiography point to the excellent visualization of fine detail and the advantages of faster exposure times and higher kVp techniques, both resulting in less radiation exposure to the patient. The border between any two density regions shows up much better using electroradiographic methods than do the same borders on a film mammogram. This concept is known as edge enhancement and serves to accentuate the small differences in breast tissues.

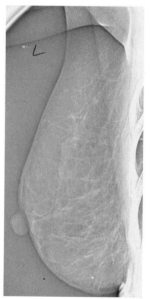

Fig. 15-52

Xeroradiograph

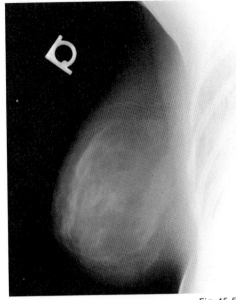

Ionography (Electron Radiography)

An alternate electrostatic method in use is ionography or electron radiography. An x-ray beam is passed through the breast and the remnant radiation is collected in a high-pressure gas chamber. Photoelectric interaction within the gas results in a collection of electrons that forms a latent image. Special methods are used to produce a visible image on a polyester sheet.

Ionography produces an image with high resolution and variable edge enhancement. The process is very sensitive, but it does require complex mechanics. An example of an ionographic mammogram is shown in *Fig. 15-53*.

Fig. 15-53

Ionograph

Ultrasonography

Ultrasonic imaging of the breast requires that the breast be suspended in a water bath and that the scanning take place from below. The patient lies prone on a special couch, similar to the one shown in *Fig. 15-54*. A typical ultrasound transducer cannot be held directly against the skin surface as other sonograms can because the underlying tissues would move and the results would be meaningless.

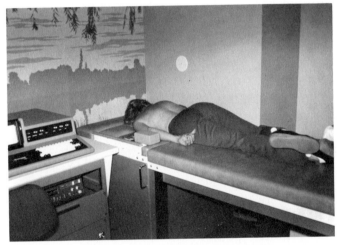

Fig. 15-54

Breast Ultrasound with Water Bath

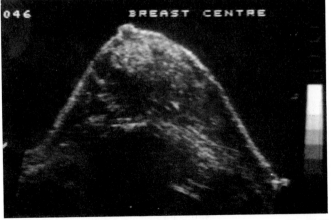

Advantages of ultrasound are that no radiation exposure is necessary and that the examination can be repeated frequently. These advantages may allow ultrasonography of the breast to be used as a screening device to indicate the need for other methods of imaging. An example of a B-mode ultrasound scan taken within a water bath is shown in *Fig. 15-55*. Ultrasonic images of the breast lack the fine resolution produced using other systems, but they can differentiate solids from cystic lesions quite well.

Fig. 15-55

Breast Ultrasonogram

Thermography

Infrared thermography is a method of visualizing heat patterns emitted at the skin surface. The heat patterns can be displayed as thermograms. In order to detect a disease process using this method, the process must change the temperature of the superficial tissues through modification of the subcutaneous blood supply. Generally, a malignant growth is associated with a higher skin temperature than normal. The temperature difference can often be detected on multiple thermograms of both breasts. Thermography is not used by itself, but in conjunction with other imaging modalities. A frontal thermogram is shown in *Fig. 15-56*.

Summary

The various techniques of imaging the mammary glands are used in conjunction with self-examination, and physician consultation and palpation. Breast cancer is the number one type of carcinoma found in the female; however, through the combined use of available imaging methods, breast carcinoma can be easily detected and successfully treated.

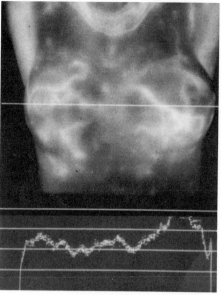

Thermogram   Fig. 15-56

Basic Projections/Positions

Three basic projections or positions are demonstrated and described on the following pages. Some departments or hospitals will omit the axillary position as a routine and only include it when it is determined to be necessary. A minimum examination includes the craniocaudad and mediolateral projections. These three projections/positions are illustrated using a film holder as the recording medium. Positioning for various electrostatic recording methods is similar.

> **Breast**
> Basic
> - Craniocaudad
> - Mediolateral
> - Axillary

Mammary Gland

• Craniocaudad Projection

Film Size:

   8 x 10 in. (18 x 24 cm.)

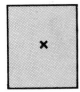

Non-Bucky:
- Film or photoelectric imaging.

Patient Position:
- Seated upright.

Part Position:
- Remove all clothing and artifacts from breast and axilla.
- Table height must be at level of inframammary crease.
- Breast in firm contact with film holder.
- Smooth out any wrinkles or skin folds.
- Place nipple in exact profile.
- Patient sits in military posture with back straight.
- Head turned away from side being examined.
- Closely collimate.

Central Ray:
- C.R. passes through center of base of breast, perpendicular to film holder.

NOTE: • Markers placed facing tube and toward axilla. • Patient must be relaxed and comfortable. • Suspend respiration during exposure.

Structures Best Shown:

As much breast tissue as possible, demonstrating both glandular and fatty tissue with nipple in profile.

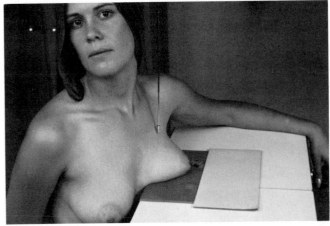

Craniocaudad Projection

Fig. 15-57

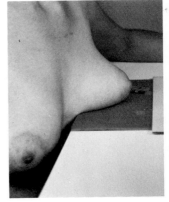
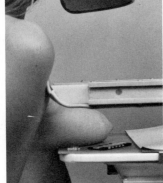

Craniocaudad Projection

Fig. 15-58

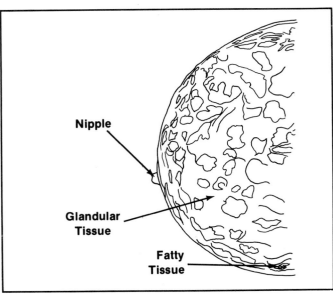

Nipple

Glandular Tissue

Fatty Tissue

Fig. 15-60

Craniocaudad Projection

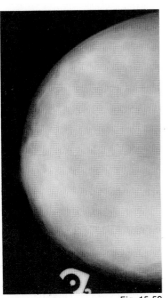

Fig. 15-59

Craniocaudad Projection

Breast
Basic
- Craniocaudad
- **Mediolateral**
- Axillary

Mammary Gland

• **Mediolateral Projection**

Film Size:
   8 x 10 in. (18 x 24 cm.)

Non-Bucky:
- Film or photoelectric imaging.

Patient Position:
- Recumbent; possibly erect.

Part Position:
- Entire breast supported by film holder.
- Smooth out any wrinkles or skin folds.
- Patient rotates far enough to place breast in lateral position with nipple in exact profile.
- Arm on side being examined must be at 90° angle to body.
- Opposite breast is retracted.
- Closely collimate.

Central Ray:
- C.R. passes through center of base of breast, perpendicular to film holder.

NOTE: • Retromammary space must be visualized. • Markers placed facing tube and toward axilla. • Suspend respiration during exposure.

Structures Best Shown:
A maximum amount of breast tissue, including glandular and fatty tissue and retromammary space with nipple in profile.

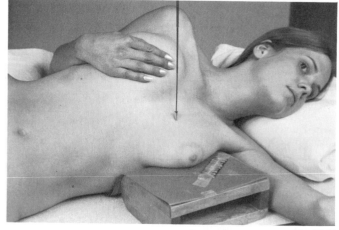

Mediolateral Projection   Fig. 15-61

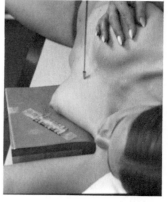
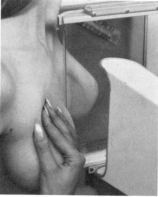

Mediolateral Projection   Fig. 15-62

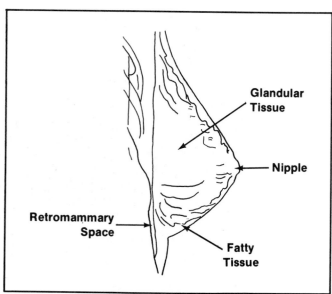

Fig. 15-64
Mediolateral Projection

Glandular Tissue

Nipple

Retromammary Space

Fatty Tissue

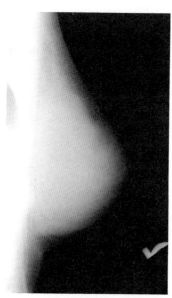

Mediolateral Projection   Fig. 15-63

Mammary Gland

• **Axillary Position**

Film Size:

    8 x 10 in. (18 x 24 cm.)

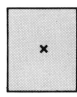

Non-Bucky:

- Film or photoelectric imaging.

Patient Position:

- Recumbent; possibly erect.

Part Position:

- Remove all clothing and artifacts from breast and axilla.
- Breast is allowed to hang pendent.
- Arm on side being examined **must** be at 90° angle to body.
- Body rotated 15 to 30°; rib margins and scapula must be perpendicular to film holder.
- Closely collimate.

Central Ray:

- C.R. should skim bony thorax and be centered 2 in. (5 cm.) below apex of axilla, perpendicular to film holder.

NOTE: • Higher kVp needed for this position. • Markers placed facing tube and toward the axilla. • Suspend respiration during exposure.

Structures Best Shown:

Axillary prolongation or tail of breast, and structures in the upper outer quadrant.

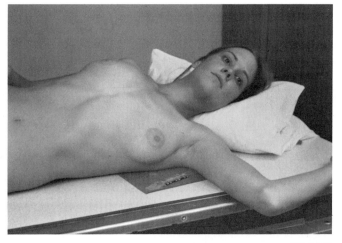

Axillary Position   Fig. 15-65

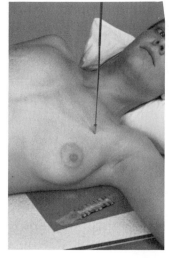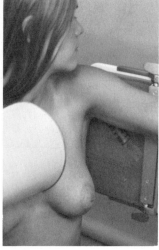

Axillary Position   Fig. 15-66

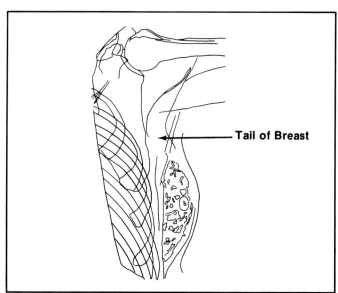

Tail of Breast

Fig. 15-68

Axillary Position

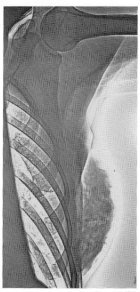

Fig. 15-67

Axillary Position

CHAPTER 16

Radiographic Anatomy and Positioning Cerebral Pneumography

Part I. Radiographic Anatomy
Cerebral Pneumography

Anatomy of the Central Nervous System

Anatomy of the central nervous system and, specifically, the ventricular system of the brain is complex, but it must be understood in order to appreciate the various positions used during cerebral pneumography.

The central nervous system can be divided into two main divisions: (1) the **brain** or **encephalon,** which occupies the cavity of the cranium, and (2) the **spinal cord** or **medulla spinalis,** which extends inferiorly from the brain and is protected by the bony vertebral column. The spinal cord terminates at the interspace of L-1 and L-2 with a tapered area called the **conus medullaris.**

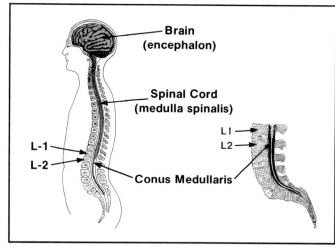

Central Nervous System

Fig. 16-1

Brain (Encephalon)

The brain can be divided into three general areas: (1) the **forebrain,** (2) the **midbrain,** and (3) the **hindbrain.** These three divisions of the brain are further divided into specific areas and structures. Understanding relationships between the structures in each of these three divisions helps in understanding the anatomy of the brain.

The forebrain consists primarily of the **cerebrum** and involves two smaller portions called the **thalamus** and the **hypothalamus.** The hindbrain consists primarily of the **cerebellum** and includes the **pons** and **medulla.** The midbrain connects the forebrain to the hindbrain. The combination of midbrain, pons and medulla is termed the **brain stem.**

Brain Divisions

1. Forebrain
    - Cerebrum
    - Thalamus
    - Hypothalamus

2. Midbrain —— Midbrain

3. Hindbrain
    - Pons
    - Medulla
    - Cerebellum

Brain Stem

Forebrain. The forebrain in humans is quite large and is located superiorly with the major portion being the cerebrum. The remainder of the forebrain is composed of structures located near the midline of the brain, including the thalamus and hypothalamus. Only the general areas of the thalamus and hypothalamus are demonstrated in *Fig. 16-2.* More detail on these portions of the brain is given later in this chapter.

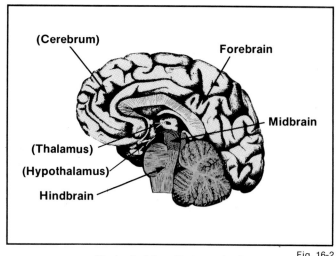

Brain (midsagittal section)

Fig. 16-2

344

Midbrain. The midbrain is a short, constricted portion of the brain stem connecting the forebrain to the hindbrain.

Brain Stem and Hindbrain. The hindbrain consists of the **cerebellum, pons** and **medulla.** As seen in the drawing in *Fig. 16-3,* the cerebellum is the largest portion of the hindbrain and the second largest portion of the entire brain.

In addition to the pons and medulla, the brain stem includes the **midbrain.** The pons is a prominent swelling inferior to the midbrain. The medulla is the final portion of the brain stem, located at the level of the foramen magnum, the opening at the base of the skull. Thus, the brain stem is composed of midbrain, pons and medulla, and serves to connect the forebrain to the spinal cord.

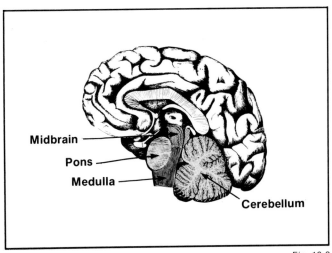

Brain Stem and Hindbrain   Fig. 16-3

Cerebrum

A sagittal section through the head and neck leaving the brain and upper spinal cord intact is demonstrated in *Fig. 16-4,* showing the relative size of the various structures. The cerebrum occupies the majority of the cranial cavity. The cerebellum lies inferior to the cerebrum and posterior to the brain stem. The spinal cord is continuous with the brain stem and is located inferior to the foramen magnum, the opening at the base of the skull.

Five Lobes of Each Cerebral Hemisphere. Each side of the cerebrum is termed a cerebral hemisphere and is divided into five lobes. The four lobes seen in *Fig. 16-4* lie beneath the cranial bones of the same name. The frontal lobe lies under the frontal bone and the parietal lobe under the parietal bone. Similarly, the occipital lobe and the temporal lobe lie under their respective cranial bones. The fifth lobe is more centrally located and cannot be seen on a lateral view. The fifth lobe is termed the insula or central lobe.

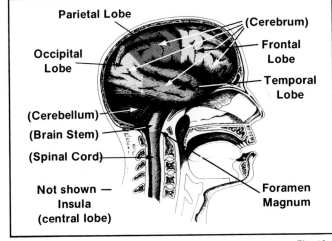

Brain and Upper Spinal Cord   Fig. 16-4

Cerebral Hemispheres

The top of the brain is shown in *Fig. 16-5.* The cerebrum is partially separated by a deep **longitudinal fissure** in the midsagittal plane. This fissure divides the cerebrum into a right and a left cerebral hemisphere. Parts of the **frontal, parietal** and **occipital lobes** are visualized.

The surface of each cerebral hemisphere is marked by numerous grooves and convolutions. Each convolution or raised area is termed a gyrus. Two such gyri, the **anterior central gyrus** and the **posterior central gyrus,** are shown in *Fig. 16-5.* Between any two gyri is either a shallow groove termed a sulcus or a deeper groove termed a fissure. An example of a sulcus is the shallow groove labeled **central sulcus.** The deeper separation between the two hemispheres, the longitudinal fissure, is an example of a fissure.

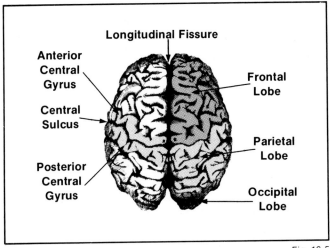

Brain (right half)   Fig. 16-5

Right Half of Brain. A midsagittal section of the brain shown in *Fig. 16-6* reveals the large **right cerebral hemisphere.** The **corpus callosum** is white brain tissue connecting the two cerebral hemispheres. The **thalamus** and **hypothalamus** are located centrally, beneath the cerebrum and corpus callosum.

Also shown on this midsaggital section of the brain are the three portions of the hindbrain: the **cerebellum, pons** and **medulla.**

Two important midline structures are demonstrated in *Fig. 16-6.* The **pituitary gland** is located just inferior to the hypothalamus, and the **pineal gland** is superior to the cerebellum.

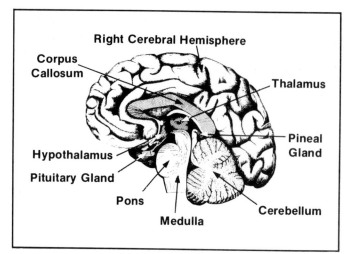

Brain (midsagittal section)   Fig. 16-6

Frontal Section of Brain. A frontal or coronal section through the brain and spinal cord shows a different orientation to the brain structures. As seen in *Fig. 16-7,* the large cerebral hemispheres fill the major portion of the cranial vault. The **cerebellum** is located inferior to the cerebrum and is posterior to this coronal section. The **pons, medulla** and **spinal cord** connect to higher centers of the brain. The deep **longitudinal fissure** terminates at the **corpus callosum,** which interconnects the right and left cerebral hemispheres. The **thalamus** is demonstrated surrounding the **third ventricle,** an important fluid-filled structure which will be described in detail later in this chapter.

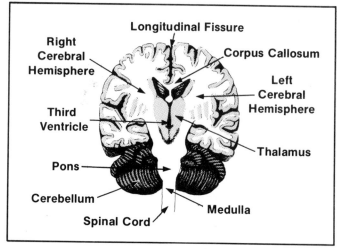

Brain (frontal section)   Fig. 16-7

Brain Coverings — Meninges

Both the brain and spinal cord are enclosed by three protective coverings or membranes termed meninges. The innermost of these membranes is the **pia mater,** literally meaning "tender mother." This membrane is very thin and highly vascular and lies next to the brain and spinal cord. It encloses the entire surface of the brain, dipping into each of the fissures and sulci.

The outermost membrane is the **dura mater** which means "hard" or "tough mother." This strong fibrous brain covering has an inner and an outer layer. The outer layer is tightly fused to the inner layer, except for spaces that are provided for large venous blood channels called **venous sinuses.** The outer layer closely adheres to the inner table of the **cranium** or skull.

Between the pia mater and dura mater is a delicate avascular membrane resembling a spider web and called the **arachnoid.** Delicate threads attach the arachnoid to the pia mater.

Meningeal Spaces. Immediately exterior to each meningeal layer is a space or potential space. Exterior to the dura mater, between the dura and the inner table of the skull, is a potential space termed the **epidural space.** Beneath the dura

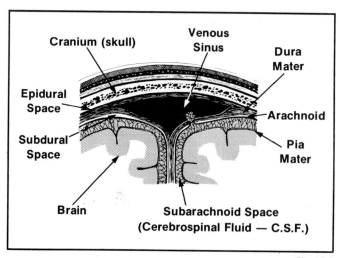

Meninges and Meningeal Spaces   Fig. 16-8

mater, between the dura and the arachnoid, is a narrow space called the **subdural space** which contains a thin film of fluid. Both the epidural and the subdural space are potential sites for hemorrhage following trauma to the head.

Beneath the arachnoid, between the arachnoid and the pia mater, is a comparatively wide space termed the **subarachnoid space.** The subarachnoid space is normally filled with cerebrospinal fluid (C.S.F.).

Cerebral Ventricles

Thorough understanding of the cerebral ventricles is important for cerebral pneumography and cranial computed tomography. The ventricular system of the brain is connected to the subarachnoid space. There are four cavities in the ventricular system. These four cavities are filled with cerebrospinal fluid and interconnect through small tubes. The lateral drawing of the ventricular system in *Fig. 16-9* demonstrates the **right and left lateral ventricles,** the **third ventricle** and the **fourth ventricle.** The two lateral ventricles are located within the right and left cerebral hemispheres, while the third and fourth ventricles are midline structures.

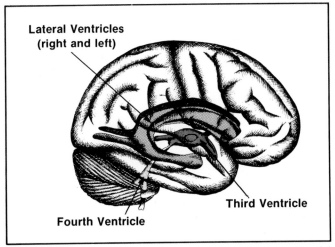

Cerebral Ventricles   Fig. 16-9

Lateral Ventricles

Each lateral ventricle is composed of four parts. The superior and lateral views in *Fig. 16-10* demonstrate that each of the lateral ventricles has a centrally located **body** and three projections or horns extending from the body. The **anterior** or **frontal horn** is toward the front. The **posterior** or **occipital horn** is toward the back, and the **inferior** or **temporal horn** extends inferiorly.

The two lateral ventricles are located on each side of the midsagittal plane within the cerebral hemispheres and are mirror images of each other. A space-occupying lesion or "mass lesion" would alter the symmetrical appearance of the ventricular system.

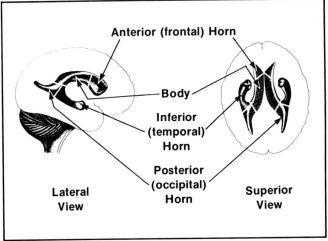

Lateral Ventricles   Fig. 16-10

Third Ventricle

Each of the lateral ventricles connects to the third ventricle through an **interventricular foramen** or **foramen of Monro.** The **third ventricle** is located in the midline and is roughly four-sided in shape. It lies just below the level of the bodies of the two lateral ventricles. The **pineal gland** is located just posterior to the third ventricle and causes a recess in the posterior part of the ventricle.

Fourth Ventricle

The cavity of the third ventricle connects posteroinferiorly with the **fourth ventricle** through a passage known as the **cerebral aqueduct** or **aqueduct of Sylvius.** The diamond-shaped, fourth ventricle connects with a wide portion of the subarachnoid space called the **cisterna magna.** On each side of the fourth ventricle is a lateral extension termed the **lateral recess,** which also connects with the subarachnoid space through an opening or foramen.

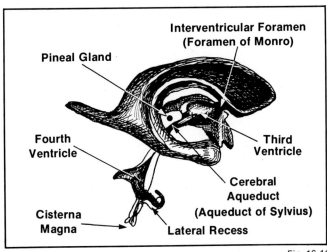

Ventricles (lateral view)   Fig. 16-11

Superior View of Ventricles. A superior view of the ventricles is shown in *Fig. 16-12*. This view demonstrates the relationship of the **third** and **fourth ventricles** to the two **lateral ventricles.** The third ventricle is a narrow, slitlike structure lying in the midline between and below the bodies of the lateral ventricles. The **cerebral aqueduct** is clearly shown connecting the third ventricle to the fourth ventricle.

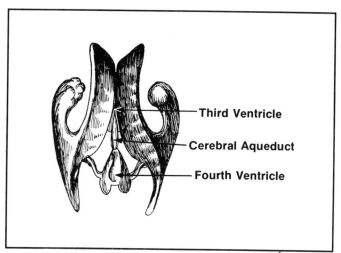

Ventricles (superior view)   Fig. 16-12

Anterior View of Ventricles. An anterior view of the ventricles with the outline of the brain in place is shown in *Fig. 16-13*. The **interventricular foramina** connect the body of each lateral ventricle to the third ventricle. This view emphasizes the fact that the **third** and the **fourth ventricles** are midline structures. The **anterior horn, body** and **inferior horn** of each lateral ventricle are shown on this drawing as they would appear on a frontal projection of a cerebral pneumogram.

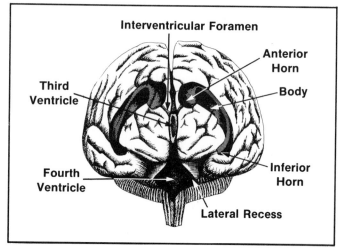

Ventricles (anterior view)   Fig. 16-13

Subarachnoid Cisterns

Cerebrospinal fluid is normally manufactured within each ventricle. After cerebrospinal fluid leaves the **fourth ventricle,** it completely surrounds the brain and spinal cord by filling the subarachnoid space, as shown by the shaded area in *Fig. 16-14.* Any blockage along the pathway leading from the ventricles to the subarachnoid space may cause excessive accumulation of cerebrospinal fluid within the ventricles, a condition known as hydrocephalus.

There are several larger areas within the subarachnoid space or system called cisterns, the largest being the **cisterna magna.** These cisterns are usually named according to their locations. An example is the **cisterna pontis,** located just anterior to the **pons.**

Additional anatomy of the brain is described and illustrated in Chapter 18, Cranial Computed Tomography.

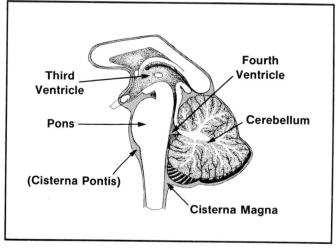

Subarachnoid Cisterns   Fig. 16-14

Part II. Radiographic Procedure and Positioning

Cerebral Pneumography

Cerebral pneumography refers to the **radiographic examination of the brain following an injection of a negative contrast medium such as air, carbon dioxide or oxygen into the ventricular system.** Brain tissue and the fluid-filled ventricular system possess similar radiographic densities. An injection of a gaseous contrast medium is one method utilized to study the normal and abnormal anatomy of the intracranial structures. The lateral skull radiograph in *Fig. 16-15* shows nothing of the ventricular system, while the lateral pneumoencephalogram shows distinct differentiation between the brain and the air-filled ventricular system.

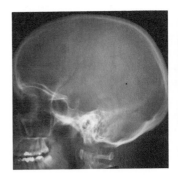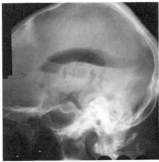

Lateral Skull Radiograph   Pneumoencephalogram

Fig. 16-15

Pneumoencephalography

Injection of air or another gaseous medium into the ventricular system of the brain may be accomplished by a direct or an indirect method. **Pneumoencephalography** is cerebral pneumography following an **indirect** injection of a gaseous contrast medium, usually via lumbar puncture. This method is termed indirect since the air is injected inferior to the ventricular system and allowed to ascend to the ventricles.

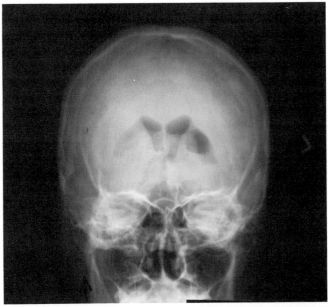

Pneumoencephalogram

Fig. 16-16

Pneumoventriculography

Pneumoventriculography is cerebral pneumography following a **direct** injection of a gaseous contrast medium into the ventricular system via surgical burr holes. This procedure is usually begun in surgery with the neurosurgeon placing a needle or catheter through burr holes, across the brain tissue, and directly into the cerebral ventricular system. The air is usually injected directly into the ventricles in surgery before the patient is transported to the radiology department. Pneumoventriculography generally includes both a forward somersault and a backward somersault movement during the examination in order to shift air into various portions of the ventricular system.

Pneumoencephalography is more common than pneumoventriculography and will be described in more detail in this chapter.

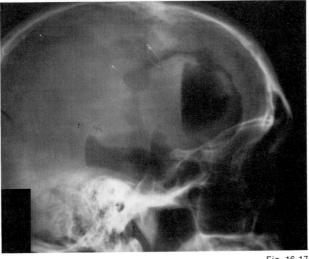

Pneumoventriculogram

Fig. 16-17

Pneumoencephalography Procedure

Indications for Cerebral Pneumography

Both cranial computed tomography and selective angiography of the brain's vascular system have greatly reduced the value and necessity of pneumoencephalography. The prime indication for pneumoventriculography is blockage of the ventricular system leading to hydrocephalus and increased intracranial pressure. Small mass lesions in the area of the third or fourth ventricles, the aqueduct of Sylvius, the hypothalamus or the visual centers of the brain may need to be studied further through pneumoencephalography. Computed tomography, however, can be used to visualize enlarged ventricles much easier and quicker than can cerebral pneumography.

Contraindications

Certain patient conditions cannot be studied with cerebral pneumography. Contraindications to air studies include acute infection, active hemorrhage and recent craniocerebral trauma.

Patient Preparation

The patient is usually examined under mild sedation to allow the patient to relax, yet be able to cooperate during the procedure. Patients should be N.P.O. prior to the examination because the addition of air to the ventricular system often causes vomiting.

Pneumo Tray

A sterile pneumo tray must be available with the following items: (1) spinal needles with stylets, (2) syringes, (3) syringe and needle for local anesthetic, (4) gauze squares or cotton balls, (5) medicine glasses, (6) a fenestrated sheet and towels for draping, (7) cotton-tipped applicators, and (8) a sponge forceps. In addition, sterile gloves are provided for the physician and, in some cases, a sterile mask and gown are also provided.

Spinal Puncture or Spinal Tap

Spinal puncture and spinal tap are general terms for the surgical procedure in which a long needle is inserted into the subarachnoid space to withdraw cerebrospinal fluid. The most common site for needle placement is the lower lumbar area between L-3 and L-4. This site is preferred since it is below the termination of the spinal cord.

Withdrawal of Cerebrospinal Fluid and Injection of Air

After the puncture site has been prepared and properly scrubbed with an antiseptic solution, local anesthetic is injected to numb the area of needle placement. *Figure 16-19* shows a spinal needle properly placed with the tip in the subarachnoid space ready for the withdrawal of a small amount of cerebrospinal fluid.

As the procedure continues, small amounts of air are injected for each increment of cerebrospinal fluid withdrawn. This withdrawal of cerebrospinal fluid is done slowly and in small amounts. This procedure can be painful and trying for the patient, so it is important to communicate with the patient and carefully observe any changes, such as a rise or fall in pulse rate or blood pressure. A well-equipped emergency cart should be readily available.

Possible Complications

The major complication associated with pneumoencephalography results from the disturbance of cerebrospinal fluid circulation. The throbbing headache that often follows spinal puncture can be minimized by having the patient remain as flat as possible in bed for at least 24 hours. Any attempt at an upright position will increase the severity of the headache.

Other possible complications include a transient meningeal inflammation; a sharp increase, or rarely, a sharp decrease in blood pressure; various intracranial hemorrhages and/or herniation of a portion of the brain through the foramen magnum.

Contrast Media

Occasionally iodized oils or the water-soluble, metrizamide compounds are used in place of air for examinations of the basal cisterns. On very rare occasions the ventricular system is studied with opaque media, either from below or by direct injection. A major problem associated with the use of iodized oils is the adequate removal of the contrast medium. Oils are very slowly absorbed by the human system and remain in the ventricles or the base of the brain for long periods of time. This problem is not encountered with the water-soluble media.

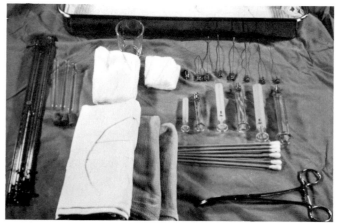

Pneumo Tray

Fig. 16-18

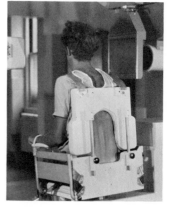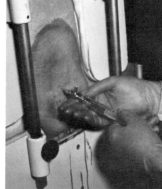

Spinal Puncture or Tap

Fig. 16-19

Equipment

Pneumoencephalography can be performed with relatively simple radiographic equipment, such as a head unit, grid cassettes and a folding chair, but many problems can result. The opposite extreme is a specialized room, shown in *Fig. 16-20,* which includes a special pneumo chair along with a single radiographic tube.

This unit is also equipped with an image intensifier and a television monitor, as well as a Bucky device shown moved in front of the image intensifier ready for general radiography.

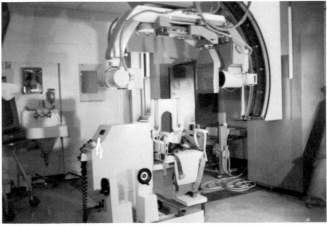

Pneumoencephalographic Room

Fig. 16-20

Pneumo Chair

The pneumo chair enables the radiologist to rotate the patient either forward or backward through a 360-degree somersault. This somersault motion is best accomplished by a motor-driven mechanism.

When small amounts of air are added to the ventricular system, it is necessary to distribute the air to various parts of the system by patient positioning and manipulation. By strapping the patient securely into the pneumo chair, the patient can be moved into any position with a minimal amount of effort. The patient's head may be immobilized, if necessary. Straps are placed across the legs, across the lap and across the chest to hold the patient firmly in place. The arms are also strapped and padded at the wrist joints.

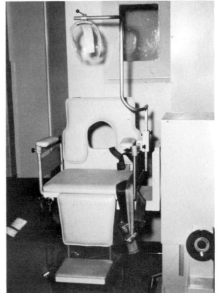

Pneumo Chair

Fig. 16-21

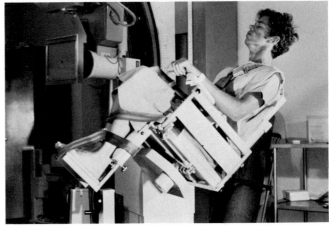

Pneumo Chair

Fig. 16-22

351

Pneumoencephalography Positioning Routine

Positioning Lines

Positioning routines for pneumoencephalography require a thorough knowledge of basic skull positioning, and associated landmarks and lines. Important positioning lines are the **orbitomeatal line** (O.M.L.) and the **interpupillary line.** All positions in this examination require that the **midsagittal plane** of the patient always be either parallel or perpendicular to the plane of the film.

Two more positioning lines necessary for this procedure are the auricular line and the anthropologic base line. The **anthropologic base line** is similar to the familiar infraorbitomeatal line, except that the superior border of the external auditory meatus is used rather than the center. The orbitomeatal line and the anthropologic base line form an angle of 10 degrees. The **auricular line** is perpendicular to the anthropologic base line and passes through the external auditory meatus.

An important positioning point, termed the **concentric point,** is 3 to 4 centimeters above the external auditory meatus (E.A.M.) on the auricular line. The concentric point lies just above the auricle and is the center of the cranium.

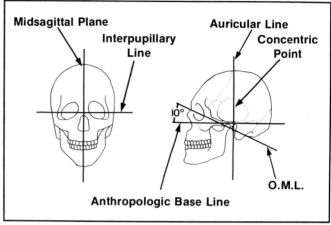

Positioning Lines   Fig. 16-23

Positioning Landmarks

In the lateral position, with the midsagittal plane parallel to the plane of the film and the interpupillary line perpendicular to the plane of the film, there are four different centering points used. Determination of which centering point to use depends on the area of interest. If the entire cranium is to be centered, the **concentric point** (3 to 4 centimeters above the E.A.M.) is used. Most of the laterals will be centered to this point. Early in the exam it may be necessary to center to the foramen magnum, in which case the **mastoid process** is used as the centering point.

To center to the **fourth ventricle** requires centering 1 centimeter superior and 2 centimeters posterior to the external auditory meatus. If it is necessary to center to the basal cisterns, center to the area of the **sella turcica,** 2 centimeters anterior and superior to the E.A.M.

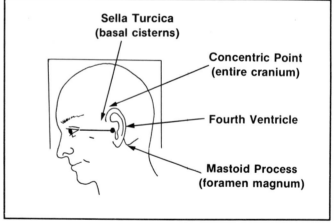

Positioning Landmarks   Fig. 16-24

Five Basic Projections/Positions

There are basically five projections or positions that may be used each time there is a major change in the position of the head during pneumoencephalography. Two or more of these projections or positions are necessary each time the head position is changed, because of a redistribution of available air which always rises to the highest available space. These five projections or positions are as follows: (1) **true lateral** position with different centering points depending on the area of interest, (2) **0-degree Caldwell** position, (3) **25- to 30-degree semiaxial A.P. or P.A.** projection, (4) **15-degree modified semiaxial A.P. or P.A.** projection, (5) **25-degree cephalic angle transorbital A.P.** projection.

All frontal projections are based on the orbitomeatal line being perpendicular to the plane of the film. The first series of radiographs and maneuvers in a standard pneumoencephalogram will be described as Series I and includes four positioning sets. Each of these positioning sets includes two or more projections or positions.

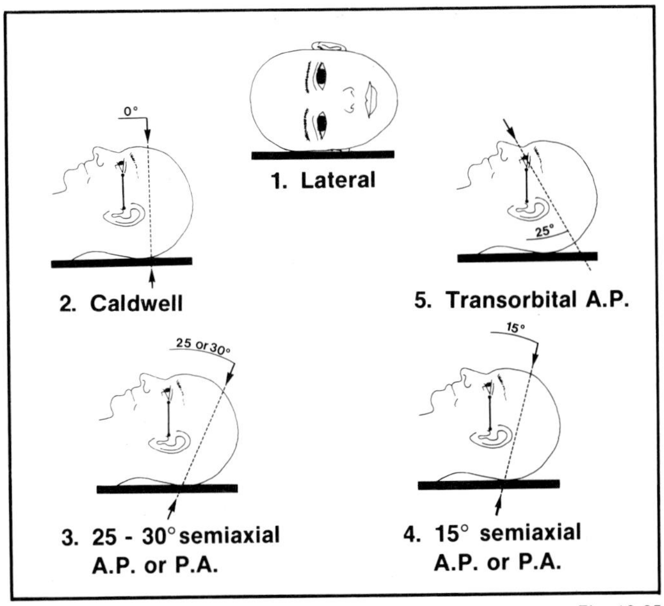

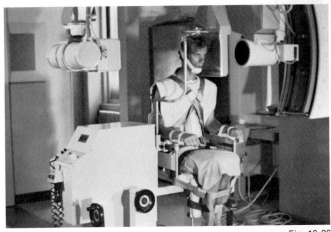

1. Lateral
2. Caldwell
3. 25 - 30° semiaxial A.P. or P.A.
4. 15° semiaxial A.P. or P.A.
5. Transorbital A.P.

Fig. 16-25

Five Basic Projections/Positions

Series I
(Four Positioning Sets)

1. Starting Position Set (P.A. and Lateral Scouts)

The procedure begins with the patient sitting in an upright position with the orbitomeatal line parallel to the floor. After removal of 3 cc's of C.S.F., and after manometer readings but before any air is injected, a P.A. 0-degree Caldwell projection and a true lateral of the entire cranium are taken. These two scout radiographs are taken to check technical factors and positioning of the skull. It is essential that there be no rotation or tilt on these radiographs.

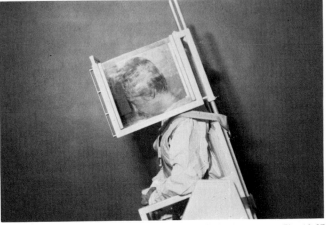

Starting Position

Fig. 16-26

2. Filling Position Set (Posterior Fossa Study)

Procedure. The filling position requires a 30-degree forward rotation of the pneumo chair. This rotation causes the head to be tilted down 30 degrees (orbitomeatal line 30 degrees from horizontal), as demonstrated in *Fig. 16-27*.

Without removing any more C.S.F., 5 cc's of air are injected and a lateral scout or filling radiograph centered to the mastoid process is obtained to check for any herniation of the brain stem or cerebellum through the foramen magnum. After checking the scout radiograph and assuring that there are no herniations, the remaining 10 cc's of air are injected and the five radiographs are taken.

Filling Position

Fig. 16-27

Five Projections/Positions. The following radiographs are taken in the filling position: (1) a **lateral** centered to the posterior fossa (fourth ventricle), (2) a **lateral autotomogram** of the same area, (3) a **30-degree semiaxial P.A.,** (4) a **15-degree modified semiaxial P.A.,** (5) a **0-degree Caldwell.** The central ray for these frontal projections should pass midway between the concentric points and project to the center of the film holder. The lateral should be centered to the fourth ventricle or 1 cm. superior and 2 cm. posterior to the E.A.M.

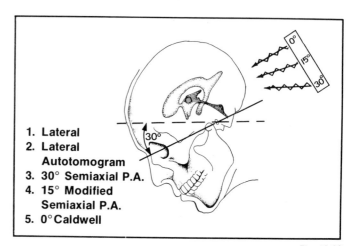

1. Lateral
2. Lateral Autotomogram
3. 30° Semiaxial P.A.
4. 15° Modified Semiaxial P.A.
5. 0° Caldwell

Filling Position Set

Fig. 16-28

Lateral Autotomogram. The lateral autotomogram is used to better visualize the area of the fourth ventricle, a midline structure. Ordinarily the mastoid processes of the temporal bones overlie the fourth ventricle, making visualization difficult. By gently rocking the patient's head in an arc of approximately 10 degrees as if shaking the head "no," laterally placed structures can be blurred out, as shown on the radiographs in *Fig. 16-30.* If the patient is not able to perform the autotomographic movements of the head, a sling device may be used to rotate the patient's head. In some cases the pneumo chair is moved into the tomographic room for selected tomograms, instead of obtaining an autotomogram.

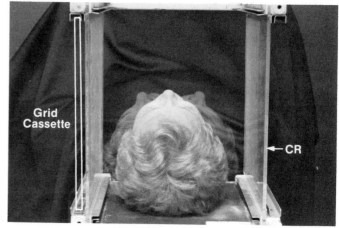

Grid Cassette

CR

Lateral Autotomogram

Fig. 16-29

Structures Best Shown. The filling position set of radiographs, taken in the 30-degree forward tilt position, best demonstrates the third and fourth ventricles, the aqueduct of Sylvius and some basal cisterns.

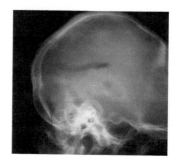 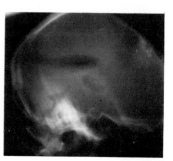

Lateral Pneumogram

Lateral Autotomogram

Fig. 16-30

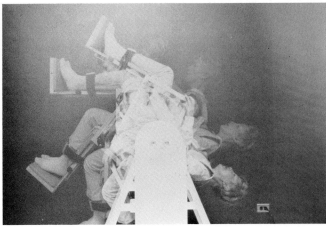

Fig. 16-31

Hanging-head Position

3. Hanging-head Position Set

Procedure. The third positioning set of Series I is the hanging-head position, which involves rotating the pneumo chair backward through an arc of **150 degrees,** as shown in *Fig. 16-31.* This position fills the frontal horns and the anterior portion of the third ventricle with air. A gentle rocking of the head may be necessary to distribute the gas equally into each lateral ventricle. Any major chair movement, such as that movement shown in *Fig. 16-31,* must be done slowly while carefully observing the patient.

Five Possible Projections/Positions. Radiographs in the hanging-head position may include: (1) a **lateral** centered to the sella turcica, (2) an **autotomogram lateral** of the same area, (3) a **0-degree Caldwell,** (4) a **15-degree modified semiaxial A.P. or P.A.** and, if possible, (5) a **30-degree semiaxial A.P. or P.A.**

Structures Best Shown. The hanging-head position best demonstrates the frontal horns of the lateral ventricles and the anterior portion of the third ventricle.

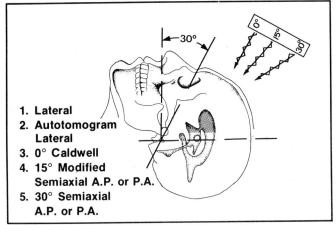

1. Lateral
2. Autotomogram Lateral
3. 0° Caldwell
4. 15° Modified Semiaxial A.P. or P.A.
5. 30° Semiaxial A.P. or P.A.

Fig. 16-32

Hanging-head Position Set

4. Brow-up Position Set

Procedure. The final position set for this series is the brow-up position, which entails rotating the patient upward into a horizontal position. This is an easier and more comfortable position for the patient. Air distribution is similar to that of the hanging-head position.

Three Projections/Positions. At least three radiographs are taken in the brow-up position, including (1) a **lateral,** (2) a **0-degree Caldwell** and (3) a **15-degree modified semiaxial P.A. or A.P.**

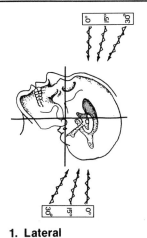
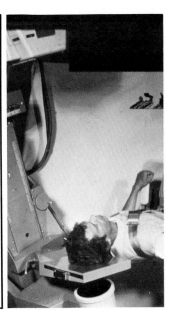

1. Lateral
2. 0° Caldwell
3. 15° Modified Semiaxial P.A. or A.P.

Fig. 16-33

Brow-up Position Set

Structures Best Shown. The brow-up position best demonstrates the frontal horns of the lateral ventricles and the anterior portion of the third ventricle, as shown on the radiographs in *Fig. 16-34*.

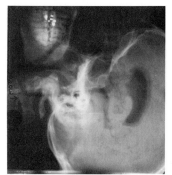
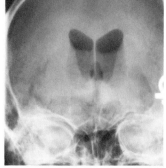

Lateral   0° P.A.   Fig. 16-34
                  Caldwell

Summary of Series I

1. **Starting Position Set** (erect, no rotation)
   - P.A. 0° Caldwell scout
   - Lateral scout

2. **Filling Position Set** (30° forward rotation)
   - Lateral
   - Autotomogram lateral
   - 30° P.A. semiaxial
   - 15° modified P.A. semiaxial
   - 0° P.A. Caldwell

   Structures Best Shown. Third ventricle, fourth ventricle, aqueduct of Sylvius and certain basal cisterns.

3. **Hanging-head Position Set** (150° backward rotation)
   - Lateral
   - Autotomogram lateral
   - 0° Caldwell
   - 15° semiaxial A.P. or P.A.
   - 30° semiaxial A.P. or P.A.

   Structures Best Shown. Frontal horns and anterior third ventricle.

4. **Brow-up Position Set**
   - Lateral
   - 0° Caldwell
   - 15° semiaxial A.P. or P.A.

   Structures Best Shown. Frontal horns and anterior third ventricle.

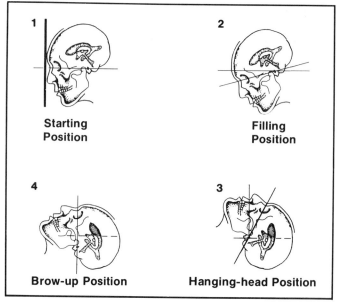

Series I
(Four Positioning Sets)

Fig. 16-35

Series II
(Four Positioning Sets)

After the first series of radiographs have been taken, the neuroradiologist assesses the amount of ventricular filling present. Depending on the amount of air already injected and how well the ventricular system is being visualized, the physician may inject up to 15 cc's more air. Additional air injected at this stage is preceded by the removal of an equal amount of cerebrospinal fluid.

The second series includes four more sets of radiographs in each of four stops of the pneumo chair, as shown in *Fig. 16-36*. The major maneuver in this series is the forward somersault, which traps air in the temporal horns of the lateral ventricles.

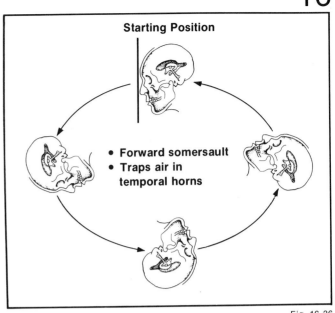

Starting Position

- Forward somersault
- Traps air in temporal horns

Series II

Fig. 16-36

1. Starting Position Set (Upright Filling Position)

Procedure. The first positioning set of Series II is the starting position set, taken in the upright or starting position. The orbitomeatal line in this position is horizontal. This positioning step may also be called the filling position, which occasionally is omitted from the routine if adequate air is present from the first series.

The photograph on the right in *Fig. 16-37* demonstrates the patient in position for this set of radiographs. A glass model of the ventricles, filled with a dark fluid, is being held behind the patient's head. The glass model demonstrates how air rises in this position to fill the uppermost portions of the ventricles, resulting in the visualization of the bodies of the lateral ventricles on radiographs.

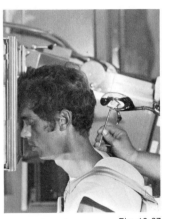

1. Lateral
2. 0° Caldwell
3. 15° Modified Semiaxial P.A.

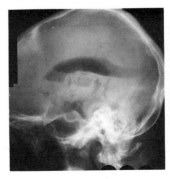

Series II Starting Position Set
(upright)

Fig. 16-37

Three Projections/Positions. The projections/positions for this set include (1) a **lateral**, (2) a **0-degree P.A. Caldwell**, and (3) a **15-degree modified semiaxial P.A.**

Structures Best Shown. The structures best visualized in this set are the bodies or main portions of the two lateral ventricles, as demonstrated on the radiographs in *Fig. 16-38*.

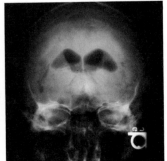

Lateral   Upright   0° Caldwell

Fig. 16-38

2. Brow-down Positioning Set

Procedure. The second positioning set for Series II is the brow-down position. The patient is rotated forward into the brow-down position, placing the orbitomeatal line perpendicular to the floor.

Three Projections/Positions. The three projections or positions in this positioning set include (1) a **lateral,** (2) a **0-degree P.A. Caldwell,** and (3) a **15-degree modified semiaxial P.A.**

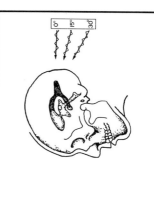
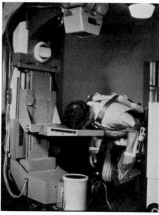

1. Lateral
2. 0° P.A. Caldwell
3. 15° Modified Semiaxial P.A.

Series II
Brow-down Positioning Set

Fig. 16-39

Structures Best Shown. The posterior or occipital horns of the lateral ventricles are best visualized in this position. The radiographs in *Fig. 16-40* demonstrate air visualized in these structures.

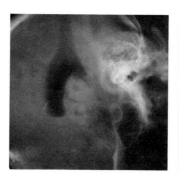

Lateral   15° Semiaxial
Brow-down

Fig. 16-40

3. Inverted Positioning Set (Upside-down Position)

Procedure. The third positioning set of Series II is the inverted or upside-down position. The patient is rotated slowly from the previous brow-down position into a completely inverted position. This is obviously an extremely uncomfortable position, therefore speed is essential in making the two radiographs.

Two Projections/Positions. The two radiographs taken in this position include (1) a **lateral,** and (2) a **0-degree P.A. Caldwell.**

Structures Best Shown. The **temporal horns** of the ventricles have not been demonstrated so far in this series. The somersaulted, inverted position fills these structures with air. This maneuver completely distends the temporal horns and isolates them from the remainder of the ventricular system, which is filled with fluid.

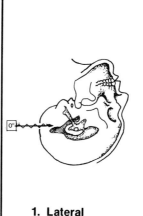
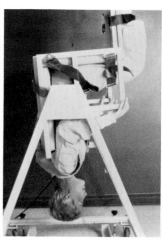

1. Lateral
2. 0° P.A. Caldwell

Inverted Positioning Set

Fig. 16-41

4. Brow-up Position Set

Procedure. The fourth and final positioning set of Series II is the return to the brow-up position. Beginning with the upright position, the patient now has been completely somersaulted, resulting in some air being trapped in the temporal horns. Therefore, this final positioning set includes one special projection for the temporal horns. This projection is a 25-degree transorbital A.P. projection, which projects the temporal horns through the orbits. This position is shown in *Fig. 16-42.*

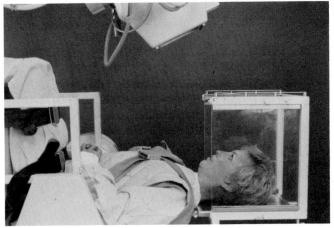

Brow-up
25° Transorbital A.P.

Fig. 16-42

Five Projections/Positions. The five projections or positions for the final brow-up positioning set include: (1) a **25-degree transorbital A.P.** projection with the central ray angled toward the head, (2) a **0-degree Caldwell**, (3) a **15-degree semiaxial A.P.**, (4) a **30-degree semiaxial A.P.**, and (5) a **lateral** position, which may be ordered as a stereo pair.

Structures Best Shown. The structures best demonstrated in this brow-up position after the somersaulting motion are the **temporal horns,** demonstrated only in the inverted and brow-up positions. The temporal lobes of the brain are second in size and neoplasia site frequency only to the frontal lobes. This fact makes it extremely important to fill the temporal horns with air, which can only be accomplished adequately by the somersaulting motion. The **anterior horns** are also visualized in this position.

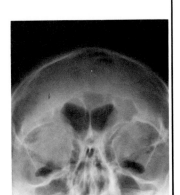

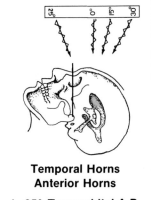

**Temporal Horns
Anterior Horns**

1. **25° Transorbital A.P.**
2. **0° Caldwell**
3. **15° Semiaxial A.P.**
4. **30° Semiaxial A.P.**
5. **Lateral (stereo)**

Brow-up Positioning Set

Fig. 16-43

Summary of Series II

1. **Starting Position Set** (Upright Filling Position)
   - Lateral
   - 0° P.A. Caldwell
   - 15° semiaxial P.A.

   Structures Best Shown. Body of lateral ventricles.

2. **Brow-down Position Set**
   - Lateral
   - 0° P.A. Caldwell
   - 15° semiaxial P.A.

   Structures Best Shown. Posterior or occipital horns.

3. **Inverted Position Set** (Upside-down Position)
   - Lateral
   - 0° P.A. Caldwell
   Structures Best Shown. Temporal horns.

4. **Brow-up Position Set**
   - 25° transorbital A.P.
   - 0° Caldwell
   - 15° semiaxial A.P.
   - 30° semiaxial A.P.
   - Lateral (stereo)

   Structures Best Shown. Temporal horns and anterior horns.

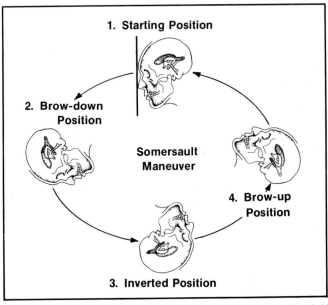

Series II
(Four Positioning Sets)

Fig. 16-44

359

CHAPTER 17

Radiographic Anatomy and Positioning Cerebral Angiography

Part I. Radiographic Anatomy
Cerebral Angiography

Cranial Circulatory System

Cerebral Angiography

Cerebral angiography refers to the radiographic examination of the blood vessels of the brain following injection of a positive contrast medium. Since the brain and cranial vasculature possess similar radiographic densities, a positive contrast medium must be added in order to study normal and abnormal distribution of the cranial circulatory system. The routine lateral skull radiograph in *Fig. 17-1* demonstrates none of the vessels of the cranial circulatory system, while the lateral carotid arteriogram clearly differentiates between brain and blood vessels.

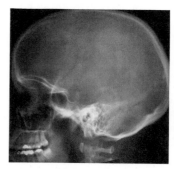 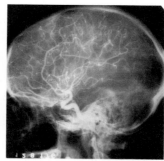

Lateral Skull
Radiograph

Lateral Carotid Fig. 17-1
Arteriogram

Systemic Circulation

The circulatory or cardiovascular system consists of an efficient pump — the heart, and a closed system of vessels termed arteries, veins and capillaries. Blood flow from the left ventricle of the heart, through blood vessels in all parts of the body, and back to the right atrium of the heart is termed systemic circulation.

Arteries are the major vessels leading away from the heart. Major arteries distribute blood to various organs, such as the brain. Each major artery branches and rebranches to form smaller and smaller arteries. The smallest arteries are termed **arterioles.** The arterioles branch to form extremely small vessels called **capillaries.** The capillaries gradually unite to form vessels of increasing size. The very small capillaries unite to form **venules.** Small venules unite to form larger **veins.** Eventually the veins become quite large and function to return blood to the heart, completing the systemic circulation.

Pulmonary Circulation

A second blood and blood vessel circuit is the **pulmonary circulation.** Venous blood passes from the right ventricle to the lungs and back to the left atrium to form the pulmonary circulation.

Arteriograms and Venograms. In any angiographic series, such as the cerebral angiogram, the initial radiographs are termed arteriograms and will visualize the arterial phase of circulation. A capillary phase follows. The final radiographs of the series, known as venograms, visualize the veins.

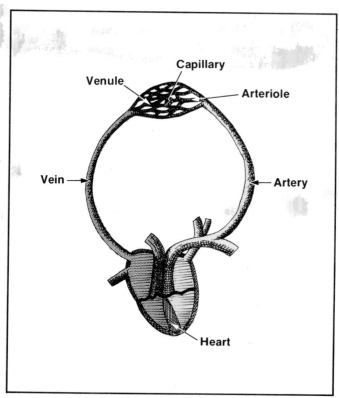

Systemic Circulation   Fig. 17-2

362

Arteries

Blood Supply to the Brain

The brain is supplied with blood by major arteries of the systemic circulation. The four major arteries supplying the brain are (1) the **right common carotid artery,** (2) the **left common carotid artery,** (3) the **right vertebral artery,** and (4) the **left vertebral artery.** Major branches of the two common carotids supply the anterior circulation of the brain, while the two vertebrals supply the posterior circulation. Radiographic examination of the neck vessels and entire brain circulation is referred to as a "four-vessel angiogram" since these four vessels are collectively and selectively injected with contrast medium. Another common series is the "three-vessel angiogram" in which the two carotids and only one vertebral artery are studied.

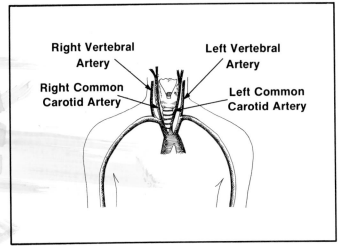

Blood Supply to Brain   Fig. 17-3

Branches of the Aortic Arch

The aorta is the major artery leaving the left ventricle of the heart. There are three major branches arising from the **arch** of the **aorta.** These are (1) the **brachiocephalic artery,** (2) the **left common carotid artery,** and (3) the **left subclavian artery.** The brachiocephalic trunk is a short vessel which bifurcates into the right common carotid artery and the **right subclavian artery.** The right and left vertebral arteries are branches of the subclavian arteries on each side. Since the left common carotid artery rises directly from the arch of the aorta, it is slightly longer than the right common carotid artery.

In the cervical region, the two common carotids resemble one another. Each common carotid artery passes cephalad from its origin along either side of the trachea and larynx to the level of the upper border of the thyroid cartilage. Here, each common carotid artery divides into **external** and **internal carotid arteries.** The level of bifurcation of each common carotid is the level of the fourth cervical vertebra.

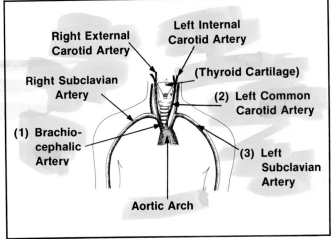

Branches of Aortic Arch   Fig. 17-4

Neck and Head Arteries

The major arteries supplying the head, as seen from the right side of the neck, are shown in *Fig. 17-5.* The **brachiocephalic trunk artery** bifurcates into the **right common carotid artery** and the **right subclavian artery.** The right common carotid artery ascends to the level of the fourth cervical vertebra to branch into the **external carotid artery** and the **internal carotid artery.** Each external carotid artery primarily supplies the anterior neck, the face and the greater part of the scalp and meninges (brain coverings). Each internal carotid artery supplies the anterior portion of the brain.

The **right vertebral artery** arises from the right subclavian artery to pass through the transverse foramina of C-6 through C-1. Each vertebral artery passes posteriorly along the superior border of C-1 before angling upward through the foramen magnum to enter the cranium.

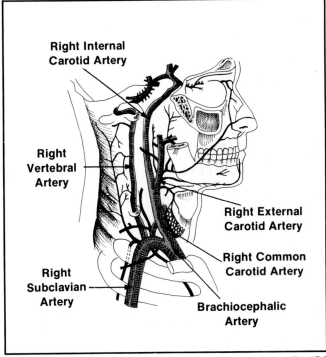

Neck and Head Arteries (right side)   Fig. 17-5

External Carotid Artery Branches

The four major branches of the external carotid artery are shown in *Fig. 17-6.* These are (1) the **facial artery,** (2) the **maxillary artery,** (3) the **superficial temporal artery,** and (4) the **occipital artery.** The most important branch of the maxillary artery is the **middle meningeal artery,** which has an **anterior** and a **posterior** branch. This middle meningeal artery enters the cranial cavity and produces a groove along the inner table of the cranium. Trauma to the squamous portion of the temporal bone, sufficient to fracture the bone, may lead to a laceration of the middle meningeal artery and a subsequent epidural hemorrhage.

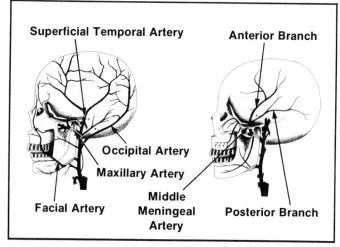

External Carotid Artery Branches

Fig. 17-6

Internal Carotid Artery

Each internal carotid artery ascends to enter the carotid canal in the petrous portion of the temporal bone. Within the petrous pyramid the artery curves forward and medialward. Before supplying the cerebral hemispheres, each internal carotid artery passes through a collection of venous channels around the sella turcica. Each internal carotid artery passes through the dura mater, medial to each anterior clinoid process, to bifurcate into the cerebral branches. The S-shaped portion of each internal carotid artery is termed the **carotid siphon** and is studied carefully by the neuroradiologist.

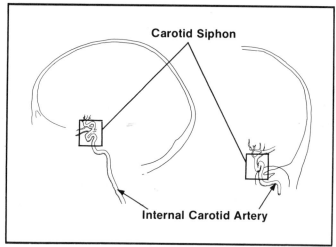

Internal Carotid Artery

Fig. 17-7

Anterior Cerebral Artery

The two end branches of each **internal carotid artery** are the **anterior cerebral** and the **middle cerebral arteries.** Each anterior cerebral artery and its branches supply much of the forebrain near the midline. The anterior cerebral arteries curve around the corpus callosum, giving off several branches to each cerebral hemisphere. Each anterior cerebral artery connects to the opposite one, as well as to the posterior brain circulation.

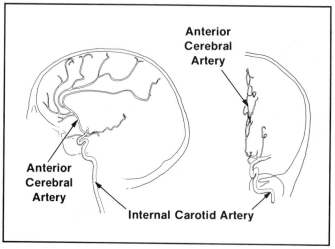

Anterior Cerebral Artery

Fig. 17-8

364

Middle Cerebral Artery

The middle cerebral artery is the largest branch of each internal carotid artery. This artery supplies the lateral aspects of the anterior cerebral circulation. As the middle cerebral artery courses toward the periphery of the brain, branches extend upward along the lateral portion of the **insula** or **central lobe** of the brain. These small branches supply brain tissue deep within the brain.

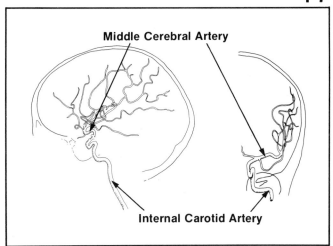

Middle Cerebral Artery

Fig. 17-9

Internal Carotid Arteriogram

When one internal carotid artery is injected with contrast medium, both the anterior cerebral artery and the middle cerebral artery fill. The arterial phase of a cerebral carotid angiogram is similar to the drawings in *Fig. 17-10*. In the anteroposterior projection there is little superimposition of the two vessels, since the anterior cerebral courses toward the midline and the middle cerebral extends laterally. In the lateral position there obviously is some superimposition. Note that the internal carotid artery supplies primarily the anterior portion of the brain.

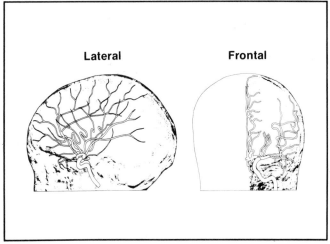

Internal Carotid Arteriogram

Fig. 17-10

Vertebrobasilar Arteries

The two **vertebral arteries** enter the cranium through the foramen magnum and unite to form the single **basilar artery.** The vertebral arteries and basilar artery and their branches form the vertebrobasilar system. By omitting much of the occipital bone in *Fig. 17-11*, these arteries are shown along the base of the skull. Several arteries arise from each vertebral artery prior to their point of convergence to form the basilar artery. These branches supply the spinal cord and the hindbrain. The basilar artery rests upon the **clivus,** the portion of the occipital bone anterior to the foramen magnum.

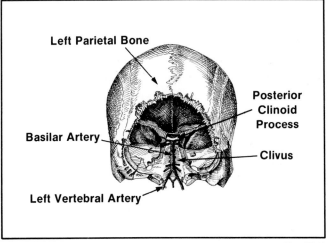

Vertebrobasilar Arteries

Fig. 17-11

Circle of Willis

The posterior brain circulation communicates with the anterior circulation along the base of the brain in the arterial circle, or circle of Willis. Not only are the anterior and posterior circulations connected, but also both sides connect across the midline. Therefore, an elaborate anastomosis interconnects the entire arterial supply to the brain. As the **basilar artery** courses forward toward the circle of Willis, it gives off several branches to the hindbrain and posterior cerebrum. The **posterior cerebral arteries** are two of the larger branches.

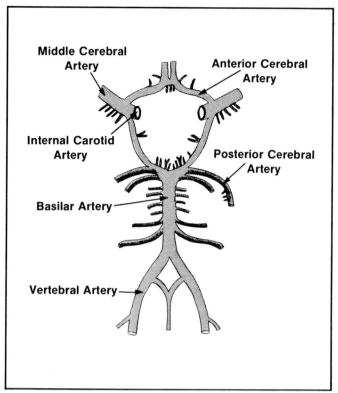

Circle of Willis

Fig. 17-12

Vertebrobasilar Arteriogram

A standard vertebrobasilar arteriogram appears similar to the simplified drawing in *Fig. 17-13*. The vertebral arteries, basilar artery and posterior cerebral arteries can be seen. The several branches to the cerebellum have not been labeled on this drawing.

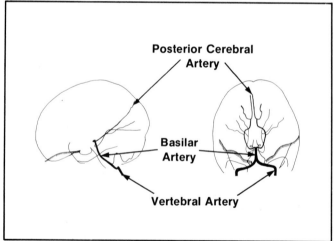

Vertebrobasilar Arteriogram

Fig. 17-13

Veins

Great Veins of the Neck

The great veins of the neck drain blood from the head, face and cervical regions. Each **internal jugular vein** drains the cranial and orbital cavities. In addition, many smaller veins join each internal jugular vein as it passes caudad to connect to the **brachiocephalic vein** on each side. The right and left brachiocephalic veins join to form the superior vena cava, which returns blood to the right heart.

The **external jugular veins** are more superficial trunks that drain the scalp and much of the face and neck. Each external jugular vein joins the respective **subclavian vein.** The **vertebral veins** form outside the cranium and drain the upper neck and occipital region. Each vertebral vein enters the transverse foramen of C-1, descends to C-6 and then enters the subclavian vein.

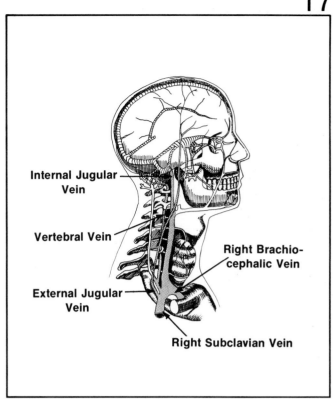

Great Veins of Neck   Fig. 17-14

Dura Mater Sinuses

The sinuses of the dura mater are venous channels that drain blood from the brain. The sinuses are situated between the two layers of the dura mater. The **falx cerebri** is a strong membranous portion of the dura mater extending down into the longitudinal fissure between the two cerebral hemispheres. A space between the two layers of the dura, along the superior portion of the longitudinal fissure, contains the **superior sagittal sinus.** The **inferior sagittal sinus** flows posteriorly to drain into the **straight sinus.** The straight sinus and the superior sagittal sinus empty into opposite transverse sinuses. Each **transverse sinus** curves medially to occupy a groove along the mastoid portion of the temporal bone. The sinus in this region is termed the **sigmoid sinus.** Each sigmoid sinus then curves caudad to continue as the **internal jugular vein** at the jugular foramen. The **occipital sinus** courses posteriorly from the foramen magnum to join the superior sagittal sinus, straight sinus and transverse sinuses at their confluence. The **confluence of sinuses** is located near the internal occipital protuberance. Other major dura mater sinuses drain the area on either side of the sphenoid bone and sella turcica.

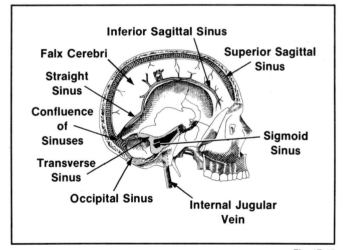

Dura Mater Sinuses   Fig. 17-15

Cranial Venous System

The major veins of the entire cranial venous system are shown in *Fig. 17-16*. Only the most prominent veins are identified. One group not individually named are the external cerebral veins, which drain the outer surfaces of the cerebral hemispheres. Like all veins of the brain, the external cerebral veins possess no valves and are extremely thin since they have no muscle tissue. Another important group are the deep cerebral veins that drain into the straight sinus along with the inferior sagittal sinus. These deep cerebral veins drain the area of the midbrain.

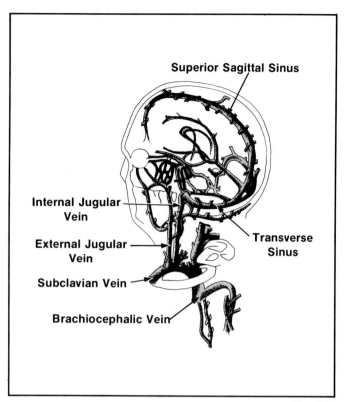

Cranial Venous System   Fig. 17-16

Part II. Radiographic Procedure and Positioning

Cerebral Angiography

Purpose

Cerebral angiography is the **radiographic examination of the blood vessels of the brain following injection of a positive contrast medium.** The primary purpose of cerebral angiography is to provide an exact vascular road map, enabling involved physicians to satisfactorily localize and diagnose certain abnormalities.

Indications

Cerebral angiography is indicated whenever surgical treatment is under strong consideration, and when other imaging modalities and nonradiographic studies have not provided a precise diagnosis. Cranial computed tomography is often performed prior to the angiographic study and, in many instances, provides sufficient information for diagnosis. Vascular lesions, including arterial occlusions, aneurysms and arteriovenous malformations, are best visualized by cerebral angiography.

Contraindications

There are few strict contraindications to cerebral angiography, although certain conditions make the examination more difficult for the neuroradiologist. These conditions include the young and the aged, advanced arteriosclerosis, and especially atherosclerosis, severe hypertension and severe cardiac decompensation. A history of anaphylactoid reaction to iodinated contrast media will cause some concern, as will a strong history of thromboembolism. One absolute contraindication to use of the femoral approach is lack of pulsation of either femoral artery. Serious illness exists in most cases requiring cerebral angiography; therefore, the procedure will be attempted in spite of most contraindications.

Seldinger Technique

Early cerebral angiography was accomplished utilizing direct needle puncture of the carotid or the vertebral artery supplying that portion of the brain to be studied. Other methods utilizing arteries of the arm or shoulder followed. Currently, the most accepted method involves placement of a catheter into the femoral artery, using the basic Seldinger technique.

The Seldinger catheterization technique allows the radiologist to perform selective angiographic procedures with reduced amounts of contrast medium. The Seldinger technique requires the use of long catheters and guide wires, as demonstrated in *Fig. 17-17.* These devices are threaded from the puncture site in the femoral artery in the groin, up the aorta to the specific cranial artery. The catheters have different shapes at the distal end to permit easier access to the various cranial vessels. The radiographer must be familiar with the various dimensions, types, construction, tip design and radiopacity of the catheters and guide wires in use in the radiology department.

Patient Preparation

Patient preparation for cerebral angiography depends on patient condition, which dictates the amount of time available before the examination. The patient will be hospitalized and, ideally, should be N.P.O. to prevent problems associated with premature evacuation of the stomach contents. Mild sedatives are generally prescribed so that the patient is relaxed, but able to fully cooperate. Adequate sedation lessens the intensity of burning pain felt along the pathway of the rapidly injected contrast medium. Certain patients may require general anesthesia or heavy sedation.

The patient must also be psychologically prepared to undergo the examination. Ideally, the neuroradiologist should visit the patient on the day prior to the examination to explain most of what will be done. This explanation must be done in language that the patient understands.

Consent Form. At the time of the neuroradiologist's visit, informed consent for the procedure is obtained from the patient or other legally authorized person. The examination is verbally described to the patient, and any complications that may occur are discussed. A printed sheet outlining relative risks and describing the procedure is presented to the patient for his signature. This informed consent sheet is then signed by the neuroradiologist, witnessed by an appropriate person and is placed in the patient's chart.

Contrast Media

Contrast media for cerebral angiography are various salts of organic iodide compounds. Cerebral angiography is usually performed using 100 percent meglumine salts at 60 percent weight-to-volume concentrations. Injectable meglumine salts tend to be less toxic than the sodium salts.

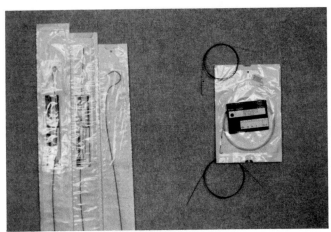

Fig. 17-17

Seldinger Technique —
catheters and guide wires

369

Special Procedure Room

The special procedure room, shown in *Figs. 17-18* and *17-19,* is equipped for all types of angiographic procedures, but with an emphasis on cranial neuroangiography. The angiographic room is usually considerably larger than a conventional radiographic room. An adjoining room or adjacent alcove is often used to house control panels, generators and physiologic monitoring equipment. A scrub area, film processor, radiograph viewing area and adequate storage facilities should be readily accessible to the procedure room. The special procedure room should be close to, but somewhat isolated from, the general radiography department. The room location should be easily accessible to the emergency department, ambulance entrance, surgery and recovery rooms.

Equipment in a Neuroangiographic Room

A modern neuroangiography suite should include: (1) biplane film changers capable of rapid simultaneous or alternating exposures, (2) changers capable of serial uniplane filming and magnification techniques, (3) automatic, mechanical contrast media injectors, (4) image-amplified television fluoroscopy that can rotate to either frontal or lateral modes, (5) appropriate generators, controls and x-ray tubes, (6) island-type table with floating top, and (7) physiologic monitoring equipment.

Additional equipment may include: (1) stereo filming capabilities, (2) linear tomography, (3) 70 or 90 mm. or larger cine′, and (4) video tape or disc recorder. The floor should be made free of any cables or wires by utilizing subfloor conduits for necessary circuitry. X-ray tubes, housings, collimators and certain other equipment can be placed on ceiling mounts and tracks to further clear the working area. Outlets for oxygen and suction should be located in the room walls.

Biplane Film Changers

The typical cerebral angiographic procedure utilizes biplane film changers in conjunction with two radiographic tubes. Each unit should be independent of the other, and the two should be easily placed at right angles to one another. This arrangement allows a series of radiographs in both the lateral position and the anteroposterior projection to be exposed with a single injection of contrast medium. Blood flow through the brain is rapid, usually passing from carotid artery to jugular vein in less than 8 seconds. Consequently, the biplane film changers must be capable of several radiographs per second, each with superb definition. There are three basic types of changers available. They include: (1) the roll film changer, (2) the cassette changer, and (3) the cut film changer. While each has advantages and disadvantages, the cut film changer, as illustrated in *Fig. 17-20,* is widely used for cerebral angiography.

The internal mechanism of the film changer moves film rapidly from the supply compartment to the exposure area intensifying screens, and finally to the receiving bin. A program selector operates the film changer during single or serial exposures, regulating film rate and the duration of each phase of the series. Therefore, the program selector controls the number of films per second as well as the total

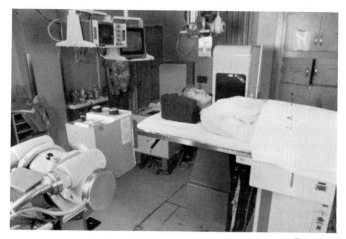

General Angiographic Room   Fig. 17-18

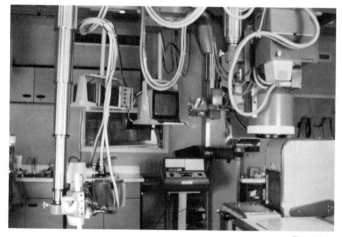

Neuroangiographic Room Equipment   Fig. 17-19

length of time that exposures are to be made. The program selector may be wired so that the contrast medium injector is synchronized with the imaging process.

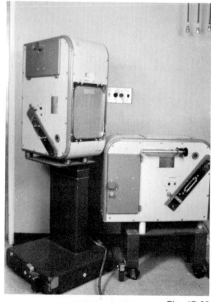

Biplane Film   Fig. 17-20
Changers

370

Automatic Contrast Medium Injector

As contrast medium is injected into the circulatory system, it is diluted by blood. The contrast material must be injected with sufficient pressure to overcome the patient's systemic arterial pressure and to maintain a bolus to minimize dilution with blood. In order to maintain the flow rates necessary for cerebral angiography, an automatic, mechanical injector must be used. The flow rate is affected by many variables, such as the viscosity of contrast medium, length and diameter of the catheter, and injection pressure. Depending on these variables and the vessel to be injected, the desired flow rate can be selected prior to injection.

A typical automatic contrast medium injector is shown in *Fig. 17-21*. Every injector has a syringe, a heating device, a high-pressure mechanism and a control panel. The syringe may be reusable or disposable. Reusable syringes must be easily disassembled for sterilization. The heating device warms and maintains the contrast medium at body temperature, reducing the viscosity of the medium. The high-pressure mechanism is usually an electromechanical device consisting of a motor drive screw that drives a piston into or out of the syringe.

Some desirable features of an automatic mechanical injector other than safety, convenience and ease of use, and reliability of flow rate settings include: (1) an obvious ready light when armed and set for injection, (2) a squirt feature for test injections, and (3) controls to preclude inadvertent injection, or excessive pressure or volume injection.

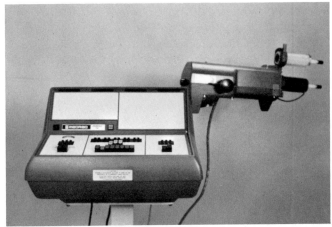

Fig. 17-21

Automatic Contrast
Media Injector

Basic Radiographic Equipment

Island Table. A basic island radiographic table and two cut film changers are shown in *Fig. 17-22*. The island-type table is necessary for femoral catheterization techniques to allow the neuroradiologist to work from either side of the patient. A four-way floating top on a central pedestal permits the changers to be placed at either end of the table and still allow room for the image intensifier. The table height should be adjustable to permit magnification techniques.

X-ray Tubes. The need to visualize smaller and smaller blood vessels during angiography, and the use of magnification techniques, have resulted in specialized x-ray tubes. These x-ray tubes provide very small, effective focal spots that are the combined result of steep angle anodes and fractional focal spots. Other modifications in the material composing the anode and focal track, as well as high-speed anode rotation, have increased the instantaneous loading capacity and the heat unit storage capabilities. The net result is an x-ray tube capable of (1) serial exposures with very high mA's and fast times and (2) superb definition production even during magnification techniques.

Collimators. Precise collimation is absolutely essential for neuroangiography. All shutters of the collimator must be in perfect alignment to prevent degradation of the image from off-focus radiation, or unwanted secondary and scatter radiation.

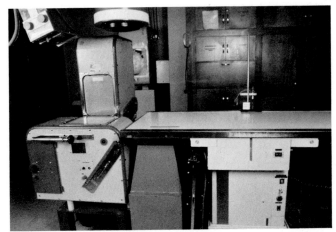

Fig. 17-22

Film Changers, Island Table
and X-ray Tubes

Sterile Supplies

Much of the cerebral angiographic procedure is carried out under aseptic conditions, and the entire exam must be carried out under clean conditions. The special procedures room and equipment must be scrupulously clean. The room should be fully stocked and prepared before the patient's arrival. All radiographic and electromechanical equipment must be checked and in working order. The appropriate sterile tray, catheters, guide wires and contrast medium must be assembled.

Basic Sterile Tray for Seldinger Catheterization

A sterile tray, such as the one shown in *Fig. 17-23,* contains the basic equipment necessary for Seldinger catheterization of a femoral artery. Basic sterile items include: (1) hemostats, (2) control syringes with fingertip control for manual injection, (3) scalpel, (4) syringe and needle for local anesthetic, (5) medicine glasses and basins, (6) three-way stopcocks or a manifold mounting of multiple stopcocks, (7) gauze squares for skin preparation and cleansing, (8) sponge forceps, (9) draping material, towels and towel clips, (10) connecting tubing, (11) catheter to manifold adapter, and (12) gowns, gloves and, on rare occasions, caps and masks.

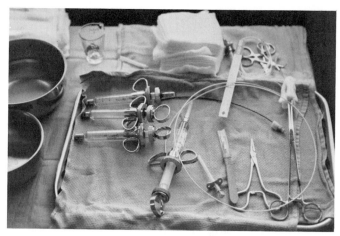

Basic Sterile Tray   Fig. 17-23

Items Added to Basic Sterile Tray

Sterile items that must be added to the basic tray are shown in *Fig. 17-24.* These include: (1) the appropriate catheter, (2) corresponding guide wire, (3) dilator and (4) arterial needle. The catheter shown in *Fig. 17-24* is a radiopaque, polyethylene tube that must be shaped at both ends by the neuroradiologist. The guide wire is a teflon-coated, safety wire with a J-shaped tip. The dilator shown is the same size as the catheter and is used whenever a non-teflon-coated catheter is used. The needle is a thin-walled needle of the Potts-Cournand design. These needles have a blunt tip with two different inserts, termed obturators. A sharp protruding obturator or a matching, blunt protruding obturator is used when needed by the neuroradiologist.

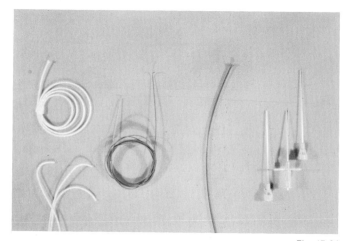

Additional Sterile Supplies   Fig. 17-24

Cerebral Angiographic Procedure

Patient Placement

After transportation to the radiology department on a stretcher, the patient is placed in the supine position on a well-padded table. A pillow or sponge support placed under areas of strain, such as the small of the back and the knees, will add to patient comfort. Even though the patient is sedated, a burning sensation will be felt on injection. Restraints may be necessary to help prevent involuntary motion during this crucial phase of the examination. Wrist and knee restraints, and possibly a compression band across the pelvis, will be helpful. The skin surface of the femoral triangle on the side to be catheterized is shaved and prepared with a germicide. Appropriate sterile drapes are then placed over the prepared area, as shown in *Fig. 17-25*.

Patient Preparation

Prior to catheterization, both femoral artery pulses should be assessed and recorded. In addition, the dorsalis pedis and posterior tibial artery pulses are evaluated and recorded bilaterally before the procedure, just prior to catheter pull-out and at the end of the procedure. Before, during and after the procedure, one member of the team should carefully note the patient's blood pressure, pulse and level of consciousness.

Reaction to the contrast medium or the premedication is a possibility and must be kept in mind. A vasovagal reaction initiated by fear may occur at any time. Genuine care and reassurance during the examination will be beneficial to all concerned.

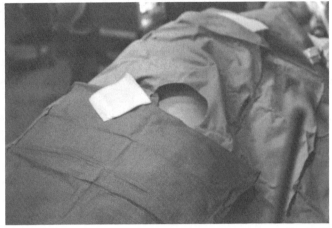

Patient Placement and Preparation Fig. 17-25

Patient Ready for the Neuroradiologist

Sterile items shown in *Fig. 17-26* are prepared for the arterial puncture by the neuroradiologist. The manifold shown on the lower part of the sterile sheet in this illustration is connected by lengths of tubing to (1) a transducer for vessel pressure readings, (2) a heparinized saline drip under pressure, and (3) an appropriate contrast medium. The syringe attached to the lower end of the manifold allows hand injection of contrast medium, while the upper end attaches to the positioned catheter.

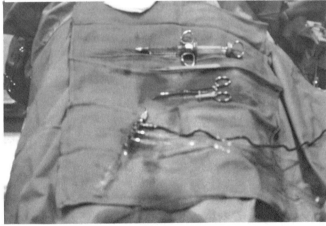

Ready for Neuroradiologist Fig. 17-26

Seldinger Catheterization Procedure

The basic Seldinger technique involves catheterization of the femoral artery. The femoral approach is versatile in that any of the four vessels supplying the brain, as well as the arch of the aorta or the external carotids, can be injected directly.

Arterial Puncture and Insertion of the Catheter. After localization and assessment of the femoral artery, the neuroradiologist punctures the femoral artery with the special arterial needle. The arterial needle is placed in the femoral artery in the left photo *(Fig. 17-27)*. The safety guide wire is advanced through the needle cannula into the femoral artery, and up to the distal aorta, if possible. The cannula is removed and the vessel puncture site is dilated with the dilator. The dilator is removed and the catheter of choice is passed over the guide wire. Finally, the guide wire is removed and the catheter is flushed and attached to a saline drip. The catheter is shown in place in the right photo of *Fig. 17-27*. At this point the catheter is advanced to the ascending aortic arch and maneuvered into the vessel chosen for study. Proposed injection sites are always tested fluoroscopically following a hand injection of contrast medium. Once it is confirmed that the catheter is correctly placed, serial radiographic filming may proceed.

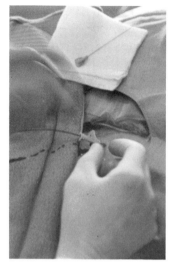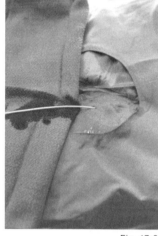

Arterial Puncture   Catheter in Place   Fig. 17-27

Positioning Routine and Examination Procedure

Scout Positioning for Internal Carotid (anterior circulation) Angiography

As soon as the patient is placed on the radiographic table, and prior to the catheterization process, scout radiographs are exposed. Scout radiographs are necessary whenever contrast medium is injected. If the primary interest is the internal carotid artery, or anterior brain circulation, an A.P. and a lateral scout are exposed. Precise positioning is essential, so care must be taken to insure that the midsagittal plane is perpendicular to the frontal changer and parallel to the lateral changer. The infraorbitomeatal line (I.O.M.L.) is placed perpendicular to the frontal changer, as shown in *Fig. 17-28*. The primary objective for the frontal projection is to superimpose the petrous ridge and the orbital plate on each side. This positioning projects the anterior and the middle cerebral arteries above the floor of the anterior fossa. A line connecting the supraorbital groove (S.O.G.) and the top of the ear attachment (T.E.A.) should be parallel to the primary beam.

The central ray is directed 2 centimeters cranial (cephalad) to this line and passes through a line connecting the two concentric points. The lateral x-ray beam is centered to the concentric point. Both beams are tightly collimated.

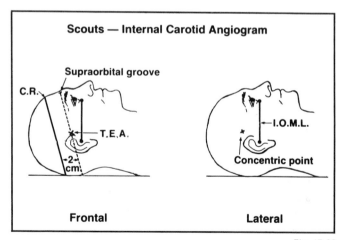

Anterior Circulation Scout   Fig. 17-28
Positioning

Scout Positioning for Vertebrobasilar (posterior circulation) Angiography

If the primary interest is the posterior circulation or vertebrobasilar system, then slightly different positioning methods are utilized. The midbrain and hindbrain must be visualized when radiographically studying the vertebrobasilar system. The frontal position utilizes a caudal angulation of approximately 30 degrees to the I.O.M.L. The central ray enters at about the hairline and exits at the level of the E.A.M. Parallax is a problem with extreme tube angles, and occasionally the neck must be hyperflexed (center illustration of *Fig. 17-29*) so that the central ray remains perpendicular to the frontal changer. This modification is especially necessary for magnification techniques. The 30-degree angle is maintained between the central ray and the I.O.M.L.

Laterally, the centering point is 2 centimeters posterior to and 1 centimeter superior to the E.A.M. Centering in this fashion corresponds to the area of the fourth ventricle.

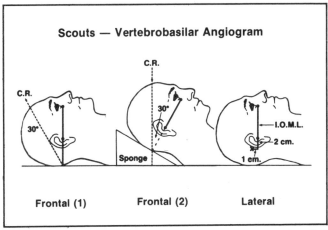

Scouts — Vertebrobasilar Angiogram

Frontal (1)   Frontal (2)   Lateral

Fig. 17-29

Posterior Circulation Scout Positioning

Position for Arch Aortography

In order to completely image the four major vessels leading to the brain, the neuroradiologist may elect to do an initial arch aortogram. Since the aorta courses posteriorly as well as to the left as it leaves the left ventricle of the heart, it is necessary to oblique the patient to open up the arch. The arch will be nearly parallel to the plane of the film, with a 30-degree right posterior oblique position or an R.P.O., as shown in *Fig. 17-30*. For this position, the left shoulder is elevated and supported with a polyurethane positioning block, and the head is turned to the lateral position.

Arch aortography allows the neuroradiologist to evaluate the major vessels for size, position, lumen status and anomalous origin. This position is rarely utilized during a three- or four-vessel angiogram, but is included as one of several possibilities.

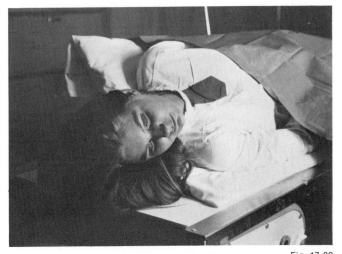

Fig. 17-30

Position (R.P.O.) for Arch Aortography

Position for Common Carotid Arteriography

A more likely beginning for a complete three- or four-vessel angiogram is two views of the neck to radiograph each common carotid artery. The position for a common carotid arteriogram is demonstrated in *Fig. 17-31*. Radiographs of the right common carotid artery in the A.P. and lateral positions are exposed to examine this artery and its bifurcation into internal and external carotid arteries. The area of bifurcation is studied carefully for occlusive disease. The left common carotid artery will be studied in a similar manner later in the examination.

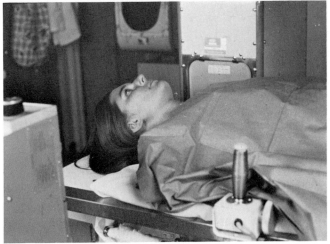

Fig. 17-31

Position for Common Carotid Arteriography

Left Common Carotid Arteriograms

An A.P. and a lateral arteriogram of the left common carotid artery are shown in *Fig. 17-32*. The catheter has been placed in the most proximal portion of the common carotid artery. The area of bifurcation is of special interest to the neuroradiologist. On the A.P. projection to the left in *Fig. 17-32*, the internal carotid artery is located more laterally than the external carotid artery. On the lateral view to the right, the internal carotid artery courses anteriorly before ascending to the base of the brain.

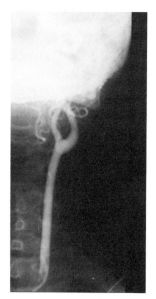
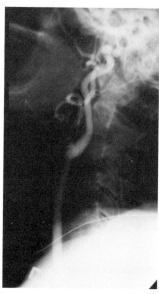

Left Common Carotid Arteriograms   Fig. 17-32

Internal Carotid Angiography

Procedure and Position for Internal Carotid Angiography

Following injection of the right or left common carotid artery, the catheter is advanced into the respective internal carotid artery. Fluoroscopic control with hand injections of contrast medium assures the neuroradiologist of correct catheter placement. The anterior cerebral circulation is studied with a sufficiently long exposure run to visualize arteries, capillaries and veins. Assuming a normal circulation time, each plane is exposed at the rate of two exposures per second for 6 to 8 seconds. Exposures usually alternate between frontal and lateral modes. Simultaneous firing of both x-ray tubes is usually not attempted due to the large amounts of cross-fogging and subsequent degradation of image quality.

Correct Positioning. Positioning for internal carotid angiography is demonstrated in *Figs. 17-33* and *17-34*. A cotton strap attached to a double-ratchet device is secured across the forehead for immobilization purposes. For the A.P. projection, the frontal x-ray tube is angled caudad so that the central ray is parallel to the line connecting the S.O.G. and T.E.A., and the central ray passes through a line connecting the two concentric points. Lateral centering is to the concentric point.

Explanation to Patient. After the patient is correctly positioned and the x-ray tubes and film changers are properly aligned, and immediately prior to injection, the neuroradiologist must explain to the patient the necessity of holding absolutely still even though a temporary burning sensation will be felt along the injection pathway. This warning cannot be minimized since, quite often, the burning sensation is intense.

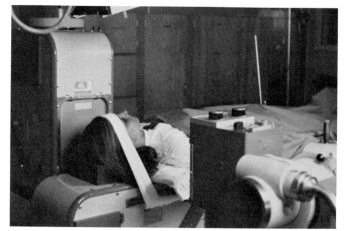

Position for Internal   Fig. 17-33
Carotid Angiography

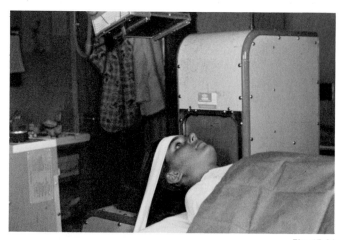

Position for Internal   Fig. 17-34
Carotid Angiography

376

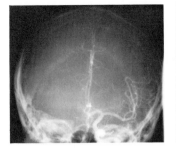
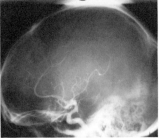

Left Internal Carotid Arteriograms

Representative radiographs of the arterial phase of a left internal carotid angiogram are shown in *Fig. 17-35*. On the frontal radiograph to the left, the floor of the anterior fossa and the petrous ridges superimpose. This allows visualization of the bifurcation of the internal carotid artery into the anterior and middle cerebral arteries.

Fig. 17-35
Left Internal Carotid Arteriograms

Magnification Radiography

Frontal Position (2X magnification)

The law of image magnification states that the width of the image is to the width of the object, as the distance of the image from the x-ray source is to the distance of the object from the x-ray source. In order to achieve 2X magnification in the frontal position, the patient's head needs to be positioned similar to the dry skull shown in *Fig. 17-36*. The center of the head is placed exactly halfway between the film and x-ray source. In 2X magnification, all anatomic structures equal to or larger than the effective focal spot size will be displayed twice their normal size on the finished radiograph.

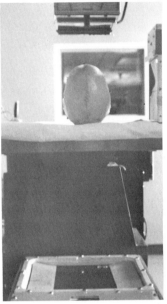

Fig. 17-36
Magnification Radiography
(frontal)

Lateral Position (2X magnification)

Head placement to achieve 2X magnification in the lateral position is shown in *Fig. 17-37*. Again, the patient's head would be placed exactly halfway between the film and the x-ray source. If the object were placed even closer to the x-ray tube, there would be greater magnification of the image. Rarely will magnification factors greater than 2X be attempted using a focus-film distance of 100 cm. Due to the size of the collimator, the head must be placed very close to the exit port of the collimator in order to achieve magnification factors greater than 2X.

Another limiting factor is the size of the film used in the automatic changer. The maximum field size of the larger changers is 35 cm. by 35 cm. Even at 2X magnification, the entire cranium barely fits on a 35 cm. by 35 cm. field.

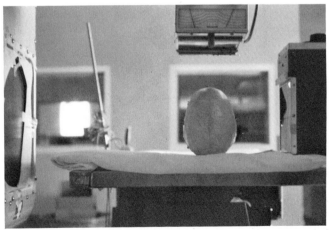

Fig. 17-37
Magnification Radiography
(lateral)

Position for Magnification Angiography of Internal Carotid Artery

Figure 17-38 demonstrates patient positioning for a magnified, internal carotid angiogram. Due to the physical limitations of this particular x-ray table in relation to the frontal film changer, a focus-film distance of less than 100 cm. is being utilized. Consequently, the frontal collimator is in close approximation with the forehead of the patient.

Air-gap Principle. A beneficial adjunct to magnification radiography is application of the air-gap principle. Whenever the image detection system is separated from the object by an appreciable distance, there is a remarkable decrease in the amount of secondary and scatter radiation that reaches the film surface. Much of the secondary and scatter radiation is directed away from the film. A large percentage of the weaker radiation emerging from the skull and directed toward the film is absorbed in the air and never reaches the film surface. The advantage offered by utilization of the air-gap principle is that a stationary grid is no longer necessary for clean-up purposes. This reduces the amount of exposure necessary and decreases the radiation exposure to the patient. In addition, both x-ray beams should be closely collimated to further reduce radiation exposure to the patient.

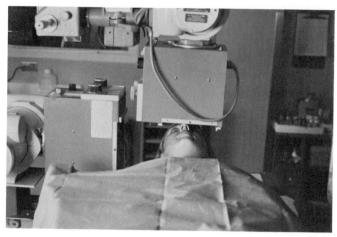

Internal Carotid Magnification   Fig. 17-38

Magnified Internal Carotid Arteriograms

Magnified radiographs of an internal carotid arteriogram are shown in *Fig. 17-39*. The frontal radiograph to the left and the lateral radiograph to the right visualize arteries much smaller than those seen on a nonmagnified study. Patient motion must be minimized during magnification techniques since any unsharpness due to voluntary or involuntary movement will be accentuated. Any motion unsharpness will be proportionately enlarged, depending on the magnification factor.

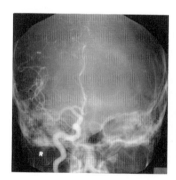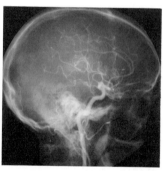

Magnified Internal
Carotid Arteriograms   Fig. 17-39

Comparison of Conventional and Magnified Carotid Arteriograms. Two lateral internal carotid arteriograms are shown for comparative purposes in *Fig. 17-40*. The routine nonmagnified study is to the left, while the 2X magnified radiograph is to the right. The phase of circulation is similar for each of these radiographs. Small arteries that cannot be delineated on the routine study are readily apparent on the magnified view.

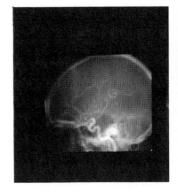
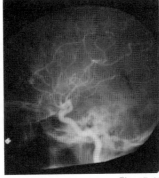

Fig. 17-40

Conventional vs. Magnified
Carotid Arteriograms

Vertebrobasilar Angiography

Position for Vertebrobasilar Angiography

Following radiographic study of the neck and anterior circulation on both sides, the posterior circulation is studied, if necessary. Usually, the left vertebral artery is catheterized first. If injection volume and pressure are adequate to visualize certain branches of the opposite vertebral artery by reflux, then the right vertebral artery is usually not injected directly. Therefore, injection of both right and left internal carotid arteries and the left vertebral artery constitute the usual **three-vessel angiogram.** If both vertebral arteries are injected, the examination is termed a **four-vessel angiogram.**

Positioning for the vertebrobasilar angiogram is similar to positioning for the internal carotid angiogram. The patient's head is immobilized, and the **I.O.M.L.** is adjusted **perpendicular** to the frontal changer. The more a patient can depress the chin, however, the better the results will be since less tube angulation is required. Frontal centering for the vertebrobasilar angiogram must include the area surrounding the fourth ventricle. Lateral centering is to the fourth ventricle, which is approximately 1 centimeter superior and 2 centimeters posterior to the E.A.M. Frontal positioning involves a modified semiaxial anteroposterior projection, maintaining a 30-degree angle between the central ray and the I.O.M.L. The central ray exits at the level of the E.A.M.

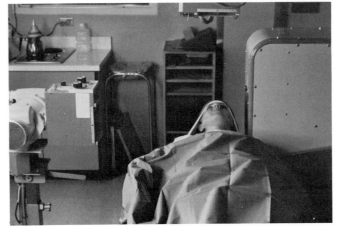

Fig. 17-41

Position for Vertebrobasilar
Angiography

Left Vertebrobasilar Arteriogram

Representative vertebrobasilar arteriograms are shown in *Fig. 17-42*. The frontal radiograph is to the left and the lateral is to the right. The frontal radiograph demonstrates a left-sided injection with adequate filling of the necessary branches of the right vertebral artery.

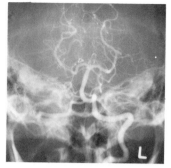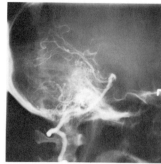

Left Vertebrobasilar
Arteriograms

Fig. 17-42

Position for Magnification Angiography of the Vertebrobasilar System

Patient position for magnification studies of the vertebrobasilar system is demonstrated in *Fig. 17-43*. The head is placed halfway between the focal spot and the film to achieve a 2X magnification. Rather than angle the x-ray tube and introduce an element of unsharpness due to parallax, the patient's head has been supported with polyurethane blocks to flex the neck so that no tube angulation is utilized. An angle of 30 degrees is maintained between the I.O.M.L. and the central ray.

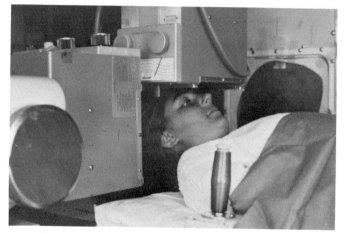

Vertebrobasilar Magnification

Fig. 17-43

Magnified Vertebrobasilar Arteriogram

Magnified vertebrobasilar arteriograms are shown in *Fig. 17-44*. The semiaxial anteroposterior projection to the left and the lateral radiograph to the right visualize a multitude of large and small arteries. Patient instructions, immobilization, close collimation and elimination of tube angulation all contribute to reduced unsharpness and, consequently, superior quality radiographs.

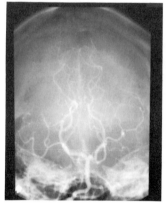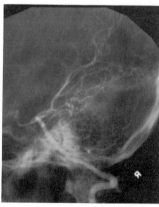

Magnified Vertebrobasilar
Arteriogram

Fig. 17-44

Aneurysm Arteriography

Special Oblique Positions

Occasionally, special oblique positions are necessary to fully evaluate aneurysms. A common site for aneurysm in the anterior circulation is near the bifurcation of the internal carotid artery into the anterior and middle cerebral arteries. The supraorbital oblique position, as shown to the left in *Fig. 17-45*, is identical to the frontal projection for the internal carotid artery, except that the head is rotated 30 degrees from the midsagittal plane.

The transorbital oblique position shown to the right utilizes a 20-degree cephalic angulation in addition to the 30-degree rotation of the head. In most cases the head is rotated 30 degrees away from the side being injected.

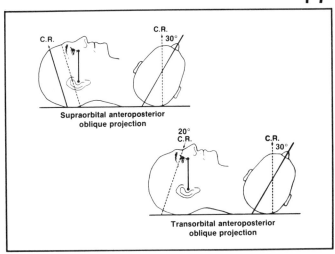

Special Oblique Positions   Fig. 17-45

Oblique Position for Internal Carotid and Branches

The position for an oblique view of the left internal carotid artery and its branches is demonstrated in *Fig. 17-46*. This illustration could represent either oblique position, depending on tube angulation. An approximate 15-degree angulation to the feet would give the supraorbital oblique position, while a 20-degree cephalic angulation would produce the transorbital position. This oblique position is usually radiographed in both frontal and lateral planes. Since only the arterial phase needs to be visualized, a run of 3 to 4 seconds is usually adequate.

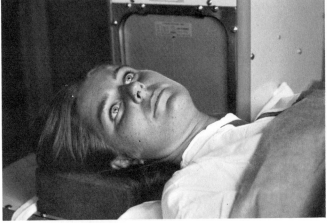

Oblique Position for Aneurysm   Fig. 17-46

Transorbital Oblique Radiography

An arteriogram utilizing the transorbital oblique position is shown in *Fig. 17-47*. A large aneurysm is evident at the bifurcation of the anterior and middle cerebral arteries.

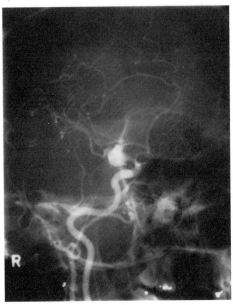

Transorbital   Fig. 17-47
Oblique Position

Photographic Subtraction

Control and Injection Radiographs

Photographic subtraction is a technique that subtracts or cancels all structures common to both a scout radiograph and an injected radiograph. In theory, this technique will produce a radiograph that shows only the opacified vessels without interference from bony structures. Both the control radiograph and the injected radiograph, as shown in *Fig. 17-48,* are obtained during the exposure series. The control radiograph is exposed immediately prior to the injection and is the first radiograph of the series. There must be no motion and no contrast medium on the control radiograph.

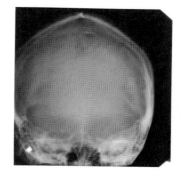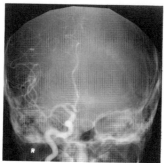

Photographic Subtraction   Fig. 17-48

Positive Mask and Subtraction Radiographs

A standard radiograph, one in which bone and opacified vessels appear white, is a negative image. The simplest method of subtraction involves first producing an exact reversal of the control radiograph. This step is accomplished in the processing room by exposing a single-emulsion film through the control radiograph. The result is a positive image, termed a positive mask or diapositive.

A composite is then made by registration. A positive mask and any radiograph in the series containing contrast medium are precisely superimposed. All bony landmarks are placed in exact register and the two radiographs are taped together. A print is made of this composite. The positive and negative radiographs tend to cancel each other, leaving a radiograph showing only the opacified blood vessels.

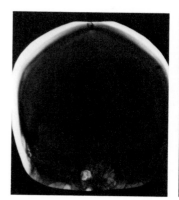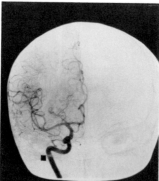

Photographic Subtraction   Fig. 17-49

Subtraction Venogram

A magnified carotid venogram and a subtraction study of the same radiograph are shown in *Fig. 17-50.* It is apparent that more diagnostic information is made available to the neuroradiologist on the subtraction study. The two techniques of (1) direct roentgen enlargement or magnification and (2) composite mask subtraction greatly enhance the more routine methods of cerebral angiography. Techniques utilized in digital angiography allow electronic subtraction of the nonessential portion of the television image.

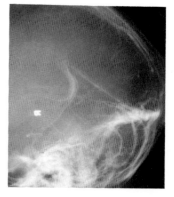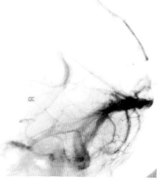

Photographic Subtraction   Fig. 17-50

CHAPTER 18

Radiographic Anatomy and Positioning Cranial Computed Tomography

Part I. Radiographic Anatomy
Cranial Computed Tomography

Computed Tomography

Computed tomography (CT) is the most dramatic advance in radiology since Roentgen's discovery of the x-ray. This imaging system substitutes radiation detectors in place of x-ray film and utilizes a computer to analyze the resultant transmission data. It is one hundred times more sensitive than any prior system.

Prior to cranial computed tomography (CCT), direct imaging methods for the cranium could visualize very little except cranial bony anatomy. Occasionally a calcified structure, often the pineal gland, would visualize. Various brain tissues, cerebrospinal-fluid-filled spaces and blood vessels merged into a homogeneous gray shadow and could not be differentiated. Therefore, invasive special procedures utilizing some type of contrast medium were required to visualize the ventricles or blood vessels. A certain degree of risk was inherent in these special examinations.

The astounding success of CCT is based on the fact that direct information concerning the structure of normal and abnormal brain tissue can be obtained without subjecting the patient to painful and potentially fatal invasive procedures. Since individual anatomic structures can be visualized on computed tomograms, a good understanding of gross and radiographic anatomy is essential. This chapter, along with Chapters 10, 16 and 17, expands the amount of cranial anatomy presented. Additionally, since CT's are viewed in sectional form, various coronal and axial sections are described in this chapter.

Central Nervous System — Brain

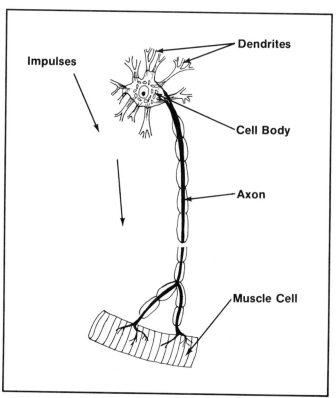

Multipolar Motoneuron

Fig. 18-1

Neurons

Neurons or nerve cells are the specialized cells of the nervous system that conduct electrical impulses. Each neuron is composed of an **axon**, a **cell body** and one or more **dendrites.** Dendrites are processes that conduct impulses toward the neuron cell body. The axon is a process leading away from the cell body. A multipolar motoneuron is shown in *Fig. 18-1*. This type of neuron is typical of the neurons conducting impulses from the spinal cord to muscle tissue. A multipolar neuron is one with several dendrites and a single axon.

Gray Matter and White Matter

The central nervous system can be divided by appearance into white matter and gray matter. White matter in the brain and spinal cord is composed of tracts, which consist of bundles of myelinated axons. Myelinated axons are those wrapped in a myelin sheath, a fatty substance having a creamy-white color. Thus, axons comprise the majority of the white matter.

The gray matter is composed mainly of neuron dendrites and cell bodies. A section of brain tissue through the cerebral hemispheres is shown in *Fig. 18-2.* At this level of the brain, gray matter forms the outer **cerebral cortex,** while the more centrally located tissue is white matter. The underlying mass of white substance is termed the **centrum semiovale.** Deep within the cerebrum, inferior to this level, is more gray matter termed the **cerebral nuclei** or basal ganglia.

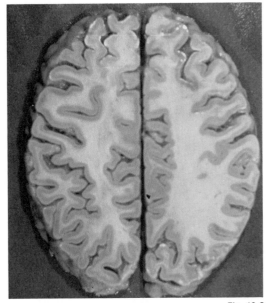

Fig. 18-2

Brain Section

Brain (midsagittal section)

The major portions of the brain are shown in midsagittal section in *Fig. 18-3.* Superiorly is the massive **right cerebral hemisphere.** Beneath the right cerebrum is the **corpus callosum,** a large commissure of white brain tissue connecting the two cerebral hemispheres. The **third** and **fourth ventricles** are midline structures filled with cerebrospinal fluid. The midbrain is directly superior to the **pons** and **medulla,** and inferior to the third ventricle. The three portions of the hindbrain are the **pons, medulla** and **cerebellum.**

Additional illustrations and descriptions of these portions of the brain are included in Chapter 16, Part I, *Radiographic Anatomy for Cerebral Pneumoencephalography.*

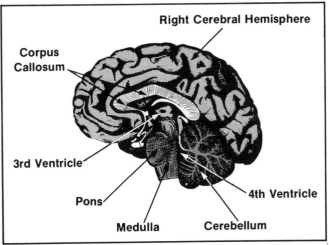

Fig. 18-3

Brain (midsagittal section)

Cerebral Nuclei

The cerebral nuclei are collections of gray matter deep within the cerebrum, as demonstrated on the cutaway drawing *(Fig. 18-4).* Four separate areas comprise the cerebral nuclei on each side. These are the (1) caudate nucleus, (2) the lentiform nucleus, composed of putamen and globus pallidus, (3) the claustrum, and (4) the amygdaloid nucleus or body. The relationship of the **brain stem** and **cerebellum** to three of the cerebral nuclei and to the **thalamus** is shown in *Fig. 18-4.* The cerebral nuclei are bilaterally symmetrical collections of gray matter located on both sides of the third ventricle.

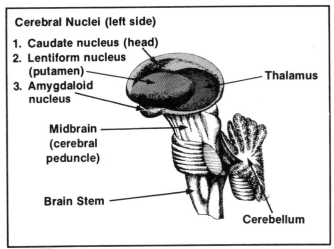

Fig. 18-4

Cerebral Nuclei

Hypothalamus

The lower border of the hypothalamus is shown in *Fig. 18-5*. Three parts of the hypothalamus labeled on this midsagittal section are the **infundibulum, posterior pituitary gland** and the **optic chiasma.** The infundibulum is a conical process projecting downward and ending in the posterior lobe of the pituitary gland. The infundibulum plus the posterior pituitary are known as the **neurohypophysis.** The optic chiasma, so named because it resembles the Greek letter X (chi), is located superior to the pituitary gland and anterior to the third ventricle.

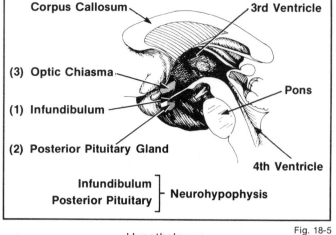

Hypothalamus

Fig. 18-5

Brain (inferior surface)

The inferior surface of the brain *(Fig. 18-6)* demonstrates the relationship of hypothalamic structures to the other parts of the brain. The **infundibulum, pituitary gland** and **optic chiasma** are shown anterior to the pons and midbrain. Extending forward from the optic chiasma are the large **optic nerves,** and extending posterolaterally are the **optic tracts.** A portion of the corpus callosum is located deep within the longitudinal fissure.

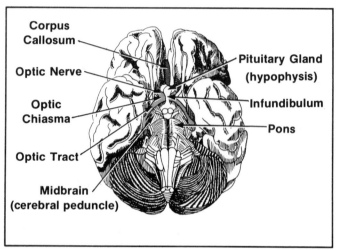

Brain (inferior surface)

Fig. 18-6

Cranial Nerves

The twelve pairs of cranial nerves are shown on the drawing of the inferior surface of the brain in *Fig. 18-7*. The pairs shown are:

1. **Olfactory Nerve**
2. **Optic Nerve**
3. Oculomotor Nerve
4. Trochlear Nerve
5. **Trigeminal Nerve**
6. Abducens Nerve
7. Facial Nerve
8. Acoustic Nerve
9. Glossopharyngeal Nerve
10. **Vagus Nerve**
11. Spinal Accessory Nerve
12. Hypoglossal Nerve

The most important of the cranial nerves are numbers 1, 2, 5 and 10. The familiar mnemonic, "On Old Olympus's Towering Tops, A Finn and German Viewed Some Hops," gives the first letter of each of the twelve pairs of cranial nerves and can be used to help remember these names.

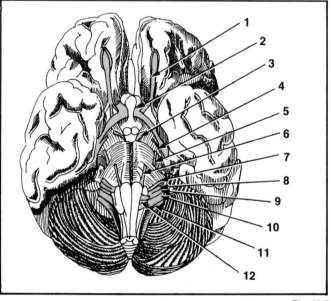

Cranial Nerves

Fig. 18-7

Cerebellum

The second largest portion of the brain, the cerebellum, occupies the major portion of the posterior cranial fossa. In the adult, the size proportion between the cerebrum and cerebellum is about eight to one. The anterior and posterior surfaces of the cerebellum are shown in *Fig. 18-8.*

The cerebellum consists of two **hemispheres** united by a narrow median strip, the **vermis,** shown on the lower drawing of the anterior surface. Toward the superior end of the anterior surface is the wide, shallow **anterior cerebellar notch.** The fourth ventricle is located within the anterior cerebellar notch, separating the pons and medulla from the cerebellum.

Inferiorly, along the posterior surface, the cerebellar hemispheres are separated by the **posterior cerebellar notch.** An extension of the dura mater, termed the falx cerebelli, is located within the posterior cerebellar notch.

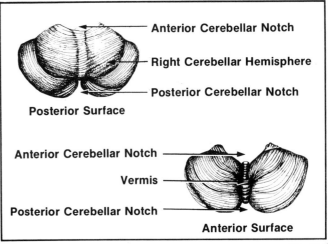

Cerebellum

Fig. 18-8

Cerebellum (midsagittal section)

A midsagittal section of the contents of the posterior fossa and, in particular, the cerebellum is shown in *Fig. 18-9.* The narrow median strip of tissue, the **vermis,** is shown in section with the left cerebellar hemisphere behind. The cerebellum is located directly posterior to the pons, medulla and fourth ventricle. Internally, both the vermis and cerebellar hemispheres exhibit an outer cortex of gray matter and an inner core of white matter. The two cerebellar hemispheres are much larger laterally than they are at the midline. The deep hollow formed at the midline on the under surface of the cerebellum is termed the **vallecula.** The cisterna magna of the subarachnoid space is located in the vallecula. To either side of the vallecula are the **cerebellar tonsils.**

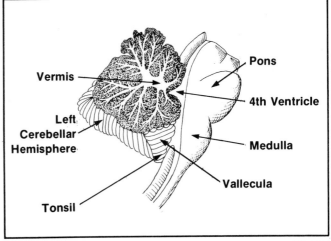

Cerebellum (midsagittal section)

Fig. 18-9

Cerebral Ventricles

The meninges are protective coverings for the brain. The subarachnoid space is located between the arachnoid layer and the pia mater. The subarachnoid space is filled with cerebrospinal fluid. The four cavities of the ventricular system of the brain are connected to the subarachnoid space and are also filled with cerebrospinal fluid. Additional information on brain coverings and spaces is included in Part I of Chapter 16.

The lateral drawing of the ventricular system in *Fig. 18-10* demonstrates the **right and left lateral ventricles,** the **third ventricle** and the **fourth ventricle.** The two lateral ventricles are located within the right and left cerebral hemispheres, while the third and fourth ventricles are midline structures.

The third ventricle lies just below the level of the bodies of the two lateral ventricles. The pineal gland is located just posterior to the third ventricle and causes a recess in the posterior part of the ventricle. The cavity of the third ventricle connects posteroinferiorly with the diamond-shaped fourth ventricle.

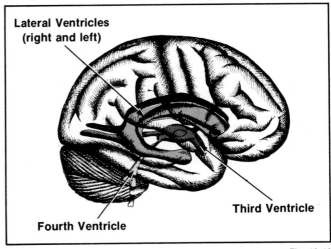

Cerebral Ventricles

Fig. 18-10

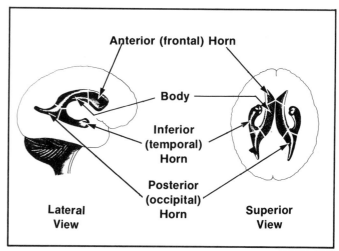

Lateral Ventricles

Each lateral ventricle is composed of four parts, a centrally located **body** and three projections or horns extending from the body. The **anterior** or **frontal horn** is toward the front and the **posterior** or **occipital horn** is toward the back. The **inferior** or **temporal horn** extends inferiorly.

Lateral Ventricles   Fig. 18-11

Subarachnoid Cisterns

The cerebrospinal-fluid-filled subarachnoid space and ventricular system are extremely important in computed tomography since these areas can be differentiated from tissue structures. Any widened areas within the subarachnoid system are termed cisterns. Only the **cisterna magna** is labeled on the drawing in *Fig. 18-12,* but the subarachnoid system has been dotted on the drawing and the locations of various other cisterns are shown with larger dots. The cisterna magna is located inferior to the cerebellar tonsils, just superior to the posterior rim of the foramen magnum and posterior to the dorsal surface of the medulla. The cisterna magna connects inferiorly to the spinal subarachnoid space, superiorly to the subarachnoid space surrounding the brain, and directly to the fourth ventricle via three foramina. Various cisterns surround the midbrain and corpus callosum.

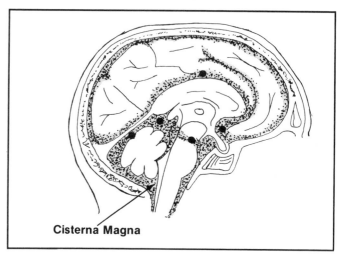

Subarachnoid Cisterns   Fig. 18-12

Other cisterns lie along the base of the brain and brain stem. The locations of these major cisterns around the base of the brain and the brain stem are shown in *Fig. 18-13*. Since the midbrain is totally surrounded by fluid-filled cisterns, this area can be well seen on a CT scan.

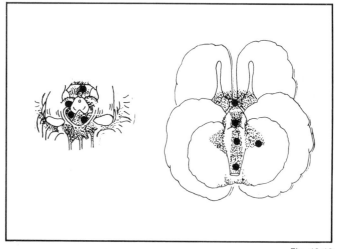

Subarachnoid Cisterns   Fig. 18-13

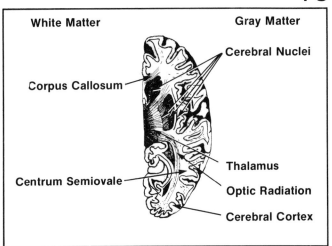

Fig. 18-14

White and Gray Matter

White Matter vs. Gray Matter

Since a cranial computed tomographic scan can differentiate between white and gray matter, a section through the cerebral nuclei provides a wealth of diagnostic information. The horizontal or axial section of the right cerebral hemisphere shown in *Fig. 18-14* demonstrates those areas that can usually be visualized. Areas of white matter include the corpus callosum and the centrum semiovale. Gray matter areas include the cerebral nuclei, the thalamus, the optic radiation and the cerebral cortex. Any portion of the cerebrospinal-fluid-filled ventricular system provides an additional density and can be readily visualized.

Orbital Cavity

The orbital cavities are often scanned as a routine part of cranial computed tomography. The orbital cavity as dissected from the front includes the **bulb** of the eye and numerous associated structures, as illustrated in *Fig. 18-15*. Orbital contents include the ocular muscles, nerves (including the large optic nerve), blood vessels, orbital fat and the lacrimal apparatus.

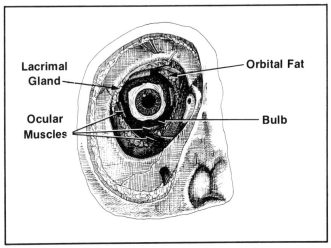

Fig. 18-15

Orbital Cavity

Orbital Cavities (superior view)

The orbital cavities are exposed from above in *Fig. 18-16* by removing the orbital plate of the frontal bone. The right orbit illustrates the normal fullness of the orbital cavity. The lacrimal gland in the upper outer quadrant, orbit fat, and ocular muscles help to fill the entire cavity. The internal carotid artery is seen entering the base of the skull. At this point, the internal carotid artery has already given off an artery that supplies the orbital contents.

The left orbital cavity, with fat and some muscles removed, illustrates the course of the **optic nerve** as it emerges from the bulb to course medially to the **optic chiasma.** Orbital tumors and foreign bodies can be readily detected through computed tomography of the orbits.

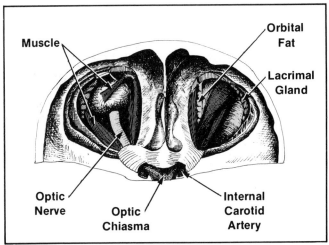

Fig. 18-16

Orbital Cavities
(superior view)

Visual Pathway

Axons leaving each eyeball travel via the **optic nerves** to the **optic chiasma.** Within the optic chiasma, some fibers cross to the opposite side and some remain on the same side, as shown in *Fig. 18-17*. After passing through the optic chiasma, the fibers form an **optic tract.** Each optic tract enters the brain and terminates in the thalamus. In the thalamus, fibers synapse with other neurons, whose axons form the **optic radiations,** which then pass to the **visual centers** in the cortex of the occipital lobes of the cerebrum. Due to the partial crossing of fibers, sight can be affected in various ways depending on the location of a lesion in the visual pathway. An example is hemianopia, which causes blindness or defective vision in only half of the visual field of each eye.

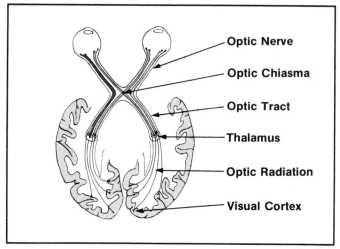

Visual Pathway

Fig. 18-17

Sectional Anatomy of the Brain

Coronal Sections

Coronal Section 1

Cranial computed tomography displays thin, cross-sectional, gray-scale images of cranial structures. Understanding this type of radiographic information requires a good understanding of cranial anatomy displayed in sectional form.

Beginning with *Fig. 18-18,* seven coronal or frontal sections of the cranium are shown. The first coronal section presented is the most anterior, passing through the eyeballs and frontal lobes of the cerebrum. Those structures labeled in *Fig. 18-18* are:

A. Frontal bone
B. Falx cerebri
C. Cerebral cortex
D. Centrum semiovale of the frontal lobe
E. Crista galli of the ethmoid bone
F. Ocular muscle
G. Bulb or eyeball
H. Periorbital fat

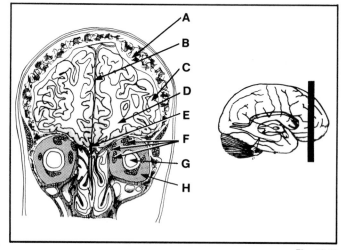

Coronal Section 1

Fig. 18-18

Coronal Section 2

Coronal section 2, shown in *Fig. 18-19,* is slightly posterior to the first coronal section. Those structures labeled are:

  A. Superior sagittal sinus
  B. Falx cerebri
  C. Centrum semiovale of the frontal lobe
  D. Corpus callosum
  E. Anterior horn of the lateral ventricle
  F. Temporal lobe
  G. Optic nerve
  H. Nasal Septum
  I. Maxillary sinus

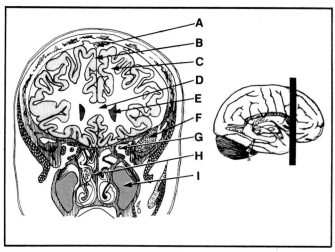

Coronal Section 2

Fig. 18-19

Coronal Section 3

Coronal section 3, shown in *Fig. 18-20,* represents a section through the pituitary gland. Those parts labeled are:
  A. Body of lateral ventricle
  B. Cerebral nuclei
  C. Pituitary gland
  D. Sphenoid sinus
  E. Greater wing of the sphenoid bone

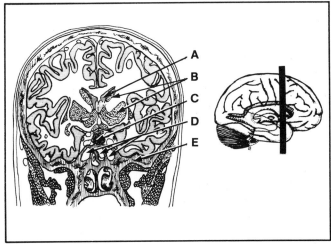

Coronal Section 3
Fig. 18-20

Coronal Section 4

The drawing in *Fig. 18-21* represents a coronal section through the main part of the thalamus. Those parts labeled are:
  A. Parietal lobe of the cerebrum
  B. Body of lateral ventricle
  C. Thalamus
  D. Inferior horn of lateral ventricle
  E. Pons
  F. Internal carotid artery
  G. Condyle of the mandible

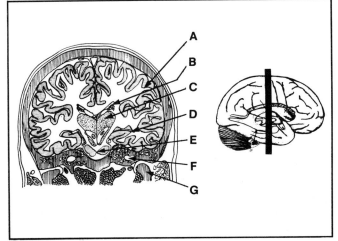

Coronal Section 4
Fig. 18-21

Coronal Section 5

The drawing in *Fig. 18-22* represents a coronal section through the posterior portion of the foramen magnum. Those labeled parts are:
  A. Superior sagittal sinus
  B. Inferior sagittal sinus
  C. Cerebellar hemisphere
  D. Midbrain
  E. Sigmoid sinus
  F. Mastoid process
  G. Medulla

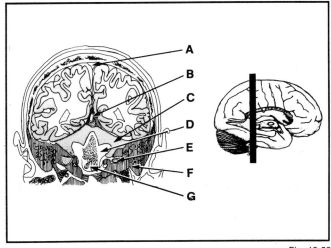

Coronal Section 5
Fig. 18-22

Coronal Section 6

The sectional drawing shown in *Fig. 18-23* depicts a section through the main substance of the cerebellum. Labeled parts are:

A. Superior sagittal sinus
B. Parietal bone
C. Falx cerebri
D. Parietal lobe of cerebrum
E. Inferior sagittal sinus
F. Sigmoid sinus
G. Cerebellar hemisphere
H. Cerebellar tonsil

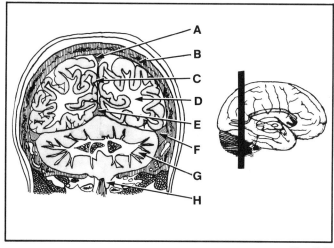

Coronal Section 6   Fig. 18-23

Coronal Section 7

The drawing in *Fig. 18-24* represents a coronal section through the confluence of the sinuses and is the most posterior of the sectional coronal slices. Labeled parts are:

A. Occipital lobe of the cerebrum
B. Occipital bone
C. Confluence of sinuses
D. Transverse sinus
E. Cerebellar hemisphere

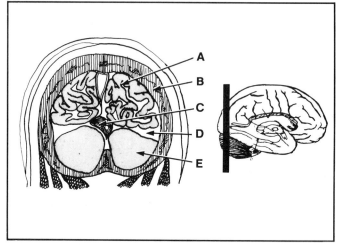

Coronal Section 7   Fig. 18-24

Axial Sections

Axial Section 1

Seven sectional drawings are now shown in axial orientation. Initial slices of the usual CCT scan are similar to the axial drawings. In computed tomography of the cranium, the patient's right is to the viewer's right. Axial section number 1, shown in *Fig. 18-25,* is the most superior of the axial sections and is termed the extreme hemispheric level. Parts labeled are:

A. Anterior portion of the superior sagittal sinus
B. Centrum semiovale (white matter of the cerebrum)
C. Falx cerebri
D. Central sulcus
E. Cerebral cortex (gray matter of cerebrum)
F. Posterior portion of superior sagittal sinus
G. Cranium

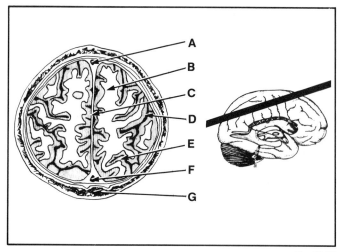

Axial Section 1   Fig. 18-25

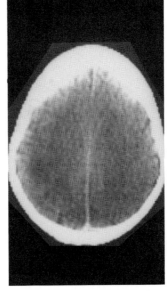

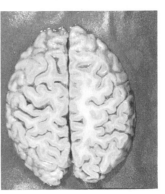

Brain Tissue and CT — Extreme Hemispheric Level

An actual slice of brain tissue and a computed tomogram corresponding to the extreme hemispheric level are shown in *Fig. 18-26.* Compare the brain tissue slice and the CT to the drawing in *Fig. 18-25.*

CT Section   Brain Tissue   Fig. 18-26

Axial Section 2

Axial section number 2 *(Fig. 18-27)* is slightly caudad to axial section number 1. This level is superior to the ventricles and is termed the high hemispheric level. The anatomy shown in axial sections 1 and 2 is similar.

A. Superior sagittal sinus

B. and C. Longitudinal fissure with the falx cerebri dipping down into the fissure.

D. White matter of the cerebrum (centrum semiovale)

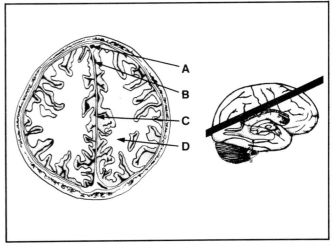

Axial Section 2   Fig. 18-27

Brain Tissue and CT — High Hemispheric Level

A photograph of an actual slice of brain tissue and a computed tomogram corresponding to the high hemispheric level are shown in *Fig. 18-28.* This photograph and radiograph are at a similar level as the drawing in *Fig. 18-27.*

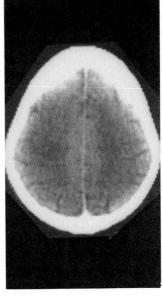

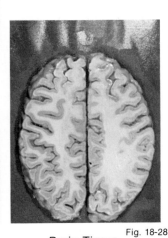

CT Section   Brain Tissue   Fig. 18-28

Axial Section 3

Progressing further toward the base of the brain, the sectional drawing in *Fig. 18-29* progresses into the lateral ventricles. Those structures labeled are:

A. Falx cerebri
B. Anterior central gyrus
C. Central sulcus
D. Posterior central gyrus

The relationship of sulci and gyri are studied carefully by the neuroradiologist since the sulci are increased in size in cases of cerebral atrophy.

E. One lateral ventricle

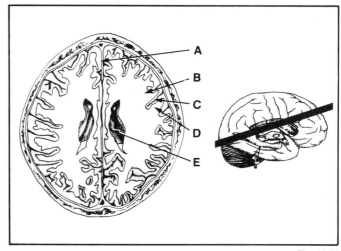

Axial Section 3   Fig. 18-29

CT — High Ventricular Level

A computed tomogram through the high ventricular level is shown in *Fig. 18-30*. Each lateral ventricle assumes a characteristic banana shape on the CCT scan at this level. The prominent cerebral sulci on this CCT scan indicate some atrophy of cerebral tissue.

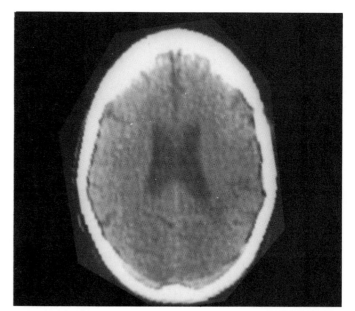

CT Section   Fig. 18-30

Axial Section 4

The drawing in *Fig. 18-31* is of the mid-ventricular level. The deep-lying cerebral nuclei are visible at this level.

A. Corpus callosum
B. Anterior horn of the right lateral ventricle
C. Cerebral nuclei
D. Thalamus
E. Third ventricle
F. Pineal gland or body
G. Corpus callosum
H. Inferior horn of the right lateral ventricle
I. Straight sinus

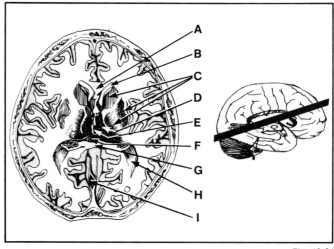

Axial Section 4   Fig. 18-31

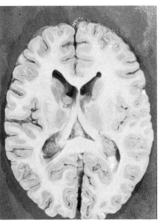
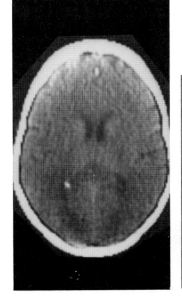

Brain Tissue and CT — Mid-ventricular Level

The photograph of brain tissue and the computed tomogram in *Fig. 18-32* are at the level of the mid-ventricles. This brain tissue slice and radiograph compare to the drawing in *Fig. 18-31*.

CT Section   Brain Tissue   Fig. 18-32

Axial Section 5

The drawing in *Fig. 18-33*, titled Axial Section 5, represents a drawing of brain tissue through the mid-third ventricle. Cerebral nuclei are visible in addition to structures of the midbrain. Those parts labeled are:

- A. Corpus callosum
- B. Anterior horn and body of the right lateral ventricle
- C. Cerebral nuclei
- D. Third ventricle
- E. Right sigmoid sinus
- F. Cerebellar hemisphere
- G. Internal occipital protuberance

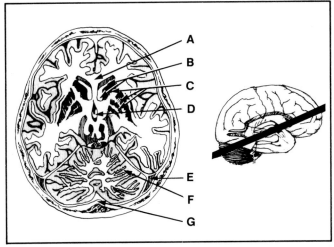

Axial Section 5   Fig. 18-33

Brain Tissue and CT — Mid-third Ventricle Level

A photograph of brain tissue and a computed tomogram through the mid-third ventricle level are shown in *Fig. 18-34*. This level corresponds to the drawing in *Fig. 18-33*.

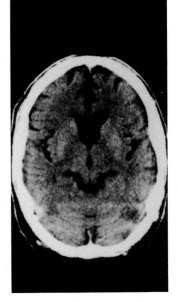
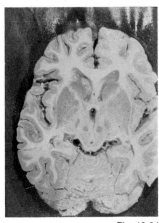

CT Section   Brain Tissue   Fig. 18-34

Axial Section 6

The drawing in *Fig. 18-35* represents the tissue plane through the sella turcica. Parts labeled are:

A. Right frontal lobe of the cerebrum
B. Pituitary gland
C. Right temporal lobe
D. Petrous pyramid
E. Pons
F. Right sagittal sinus

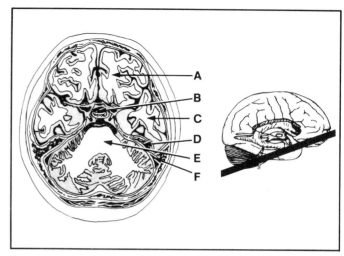

Axial Section 6

Fig. 18-35

Brain Tissue and CT — Sella Turcica Level

A photograph of actual brain tissue and a CCT scan through the level of the sella turcica are shown in *Fig. 18-36*.

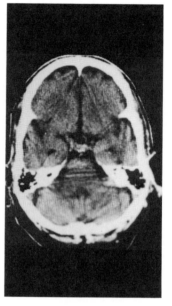
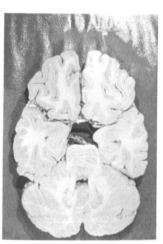

CT Section

Brain Tissue

Fig. 18-36

Axial Section 7

Axial section number 7 represents a drawing of tissue in the orbital plane. Note in *Fig. 18-37* that a different angle is used to better visualize the orbital cavities. Those structures labeled are:

A. Ocular bulb or eyeball
B. Optic nerve
C. Optic chiasma
D. Temporal lobe
E. Midbrain
F. Cerebellum
G. Occipital lobe
H. Falx cerebri
I. Superior sagittal sinus

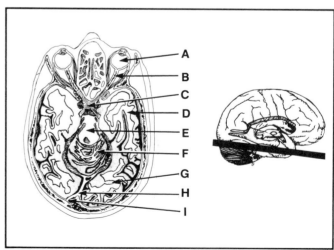

Axial Section 7

Fig. 18-37

CT — Orbital Level

A CCT scan through the orbital level is shown in *Fig. 18-38*. Compare the CT section through the orbital level with the drawing in *Fig. 18-37*. Note especially how clearly the ocular bulb and optic nerve are visualized.

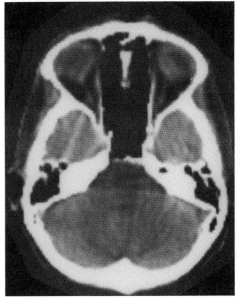

Fig. 18-38

CT Section —
Orbital Level

Part II. Basic Principles and Procedures
Cranial Computed Tomography

Cranial Computed Tomography — CCT

Definition

Cranial computed tomography refers to **radiographic examination of the cranium displayed as a thin, cross-sectional, gray-scale, tomographic image representing a computer-assisted mathematical reconstruction of numerous x-ray absorption differences of the cranial contents.**

Advantages over Conventional Radiography

Computed tomography has three distinct advantages over conventional radiography. First, three-dimensional information is presented in the form of a series of thin slices of the internal structure of the part in question. Since the x-ray beam is closely collimated to that particular slice, the resultant information is not degraded by secondary and scatter radiation from tissue outside the slice being studied. Second, the system is much more sensitive when compared to conventional radiography so that differences in soft tissue can be clearly delineated. Third, CT measures x-ray absorption of individual tissues accurately, allowing the basic nature of tissue to be studied.

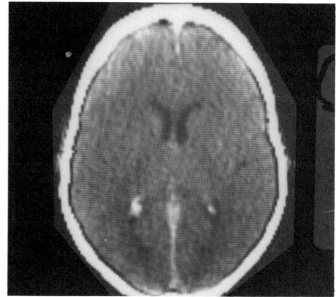

Cranial Computed
Tomogram

Fig. 18-39

Computed Tomographic System

1. Scan Unit

All computed tomographic systems consist of four major elements. One major element is the **scan unit.** The scan unit provides large amounts of information to the computer. The scan unit is usually housed in a room by itself and is the part of the computed tomographic system seen by the patient. This room is often termed the treatment room or scanner room. The scan unit consists of two parts: (1) the **patient table,** and (2) the **gantry.** The patient table or couch provides a fairly comfortable surface for the recumbent patient during the total scanning time. The gantry is a rigid support structure that encompasses the cranium within a central opening termed the **gantry aperture.** The depth to which the cranium is placed within the aperture determines the section to be studied. The gantry houses the x-ray tube or tubes and the radiation detector array.

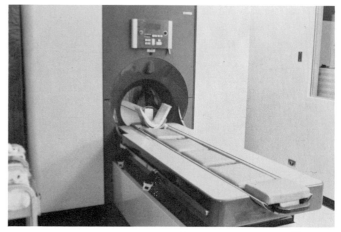

CCT Scan Unit

Fig. 18-40

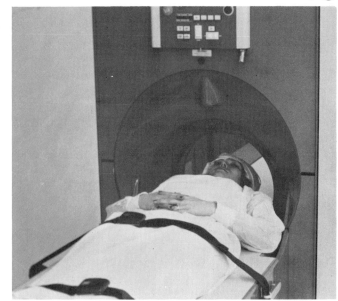

Scanning Position. The patient is shown in position in *Fig. 18-41* for the first section or scan of a CCT. The tabletop is fitted with a cradle device to allow longitudinal movement of the patient. Once the patient is immobilized and positioned for the initial scan, the patient can be moved easily into and out of the gantry aperture using the cradle device. Once the patient is in correct position and the table height is set, the concentric point of the cranium coincides with the center of the x-ray beam geometry.

CCT Scanning Position

Fig. 18-41

2. Processing Unit

A second element of any computed tomographic system is the **processing unit.** The processing unit or **computer** takes raw data and converts it into a meaningful picture form. It is the computer or processing unit that makes CT so different from conventional radiography and most other radiographic imaging modalities. Huge amounts of raw data are received directly from the scan unit by the processor. This data consists of positional, reference and calibration information, in addition to all the individual absorption readings. The transmission readings alone can amount to more than 100 thousand bits of information. This mass of information is analyzed and converted to picture form for diagnosis. Modern ingenuity and computer technology allow the scanning and image reconstruction to be performed in a matter of seconds.

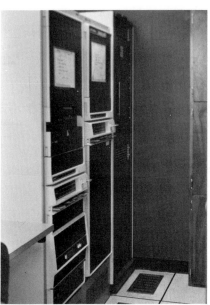

Fig. 18-42

Processing Unit
or Computer

3. Display Unit

The third major element is the **display unit** or **direct-display console.** The reconstructed image produced by the computer is made visible by the display unit. Most systems project the picture on a gray-scale television screen. Various techniques are available to make the picture more easily interpreted. For example, portions of the picture can be enlarged, the contrast scale can be manipulated, and subtractions can be made to allow complete image analysis.

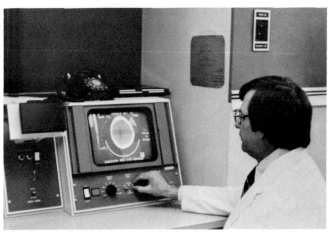

Fig. 18-43

Display Unit

Operator Console. The operator console is a part of the display unit and is located in the same room. Once the patient is properly positioned, all the necessary controls to proceed through each examination are located at the operator console. The radiographer communicates with the computer through a keyboard. The operator console speeds the scanning procedure and minimizes errors by talking the operator through each step of the procedure. Several variables can be manipulated by the radiographer at the operator console under direction by the neuroradiologist.

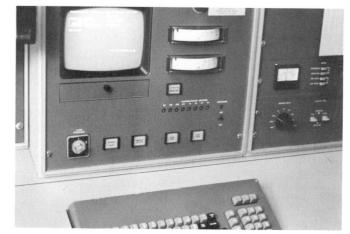

Operator Console

Fig. 18-44

4. Storage System

The fourth and final major element of all computed tomographic systems is a **storage system,** allowing individual computed tomograms to be viewed or reviewed at any time following the actual scan. Various types of storage are utilized, depending on the length of time the information must be held. Immediate storage is provided by the main memory of the computer system. Information is stored on a disc that holds a relatively small number of pictures. Immediate access is necessary to allow scans to be viewed while the patient is still on the table. When full sets of scans are completed on several patients, the information is usually transferred to medium- or long-term storage. The usual medium-term storage device is the floppy disc. For long-term storage, the information is placed on magnetic tape, as shown in *Fig. 18-45.*

Each of these storage devices — main memory, floppy disc and magnetic tape — store the complete picture information. When this information is retrieved, the image can be manipulated if necessary. Other forms of archival storage include radiographic or Polaroid film. These film methods only store what is seen on the display console.

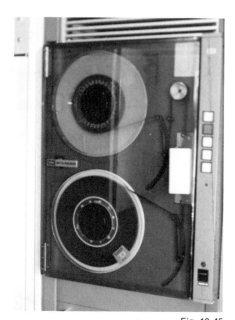

Fig. 18-45

Computer
Long-term Storage

400

Basic Principles of Computed Tomography

Basic Principle

The basic principle of computed tomography is that **the internal structure of any three-dimensional subject can be reconstructed from many different projections or views of that subject. This necessitates the collection of large amounts of data in order to reconstruct an accurate picture of the original structure.**

X-ray Transmission and Collection of Data

At least 180 different projections are required to obtain a diagnostically useful radiograph. This fact is demonstrated by assuming that the patient anatomy in question is a mass of homogeneous tissue with an air-filled cross in the center, as shown in *Fig. 18-46*. Several narrow beams of x-rays are directed through the section of tissue from right to left. All of the photons that pass through the tissue slice are collected on the left side of this "blockhead" illustration. Due to the shape and configuration of the air-filled cross, more x-rays pass through the center of the slice than pass through either the top or the bottom. By plotting the intensity of radiation collected along the left side of the section, a profile of the emergent radiation is formed. If the x-ray beam were directed through the tissue at one-degree intervals until 180 readings were made, 180 different profiles would be formed. Collecting this large amount of transmission data for processing by the computer is the function of the scan unit.

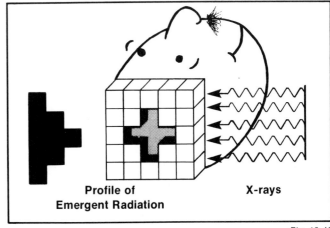

Fig. 18-46

One Profile of Emergent Radiation

Scanner Principles

Since the introduction of clinical CCT scanning in 1972, data gathering has progressed through four generations. The first generation scanners required about 4½ minutes to gather enough information per slice of tissue. Each subsequent generation of scanner has decreased the amount of scan time necessary to gather the required volume of data. Fourth generation scanners require only 2 to 10 seconds per scan.

Fourth Generation Scanner

Fourth generation scanners possess a ring of 600 or more detectors, completely surrounding the patient in a full circle within the gantry. A single x-ray tube rotates through a 360-degree arc during data collection. Throughout the continuous rotary motion, short bursts of radiation are provided by a pulsed, rotating-anode x-ray tube.

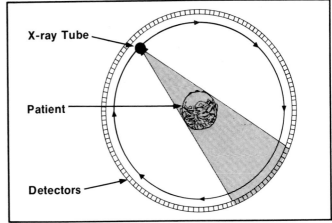

Fig. 18-47

Fourth Generation Scanner

Source and Detector Collimation

In CCT, very close collimation is necessary to limit the radiation beam to the area of interest. The x-ray beam is actually collimated on both sides of the patient's head. The source collimator is located very close to the x-ray tube, and a detector collimator is located close to each detector in the detector array. The actual **thickness of the tomographic slice is controlled by the source collimator** and ranges from 1 to several millimeters. The detector collimators limit the amount of scatter radiation picked up by the detectors. Since each section is very thin, little secondary and scatter radiation escapes to neighboring tissue. The location of the two collimators is shown diagrammatically in *Fig. 18-48.* The width and length of each individual transmission of radiation is limited by the collimators.

Volume Element (Voxel). After many transmissions of x-ray data, the reconstructed anatomy appears to be composed of a large number of tiny, elongated blocks. Each of the tiny blocks shown in the drawing of the "blockhead" represents a volume of tissue as defined by the opening in the source collimator. In CT language, each block is termed a **volume element,** which is shortened to **voxel.** Any CT slice is composed of a large number of voxels.

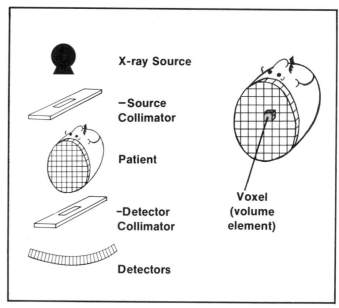

Fig. 18-48

Collimation and Volume
Element (Voxel)

Principles of Image Reconstruction

The large amounts of data accumulated by the scan unit must be processed by the computer to provide a meaningful picture form. A simplified method of image reconstruction is shown in *Figs. 18-49* through *18-53* to demonstrate the principle utilized by computed tomography. The actual methods of reconstruction are much more complex and extensive than shown, but the basic principle is the same.

Exposure and Information Profile

Our subject is the "blockhead" with an air-filled cross located within a mass of homogeneous tissue. The total tissue volume of the slice in question is divided into a 5 x 5 system of **25 voxels,** as shown in Step A of *Fig. 18-49*. Step B of this illustration shows two beams of **x-radiation** directed through the slice of tissue in question. One beam is directed from right to left, while the second beam is directed from top to bottom. The collected data produces two **profiles** of information, as shown in Step C.

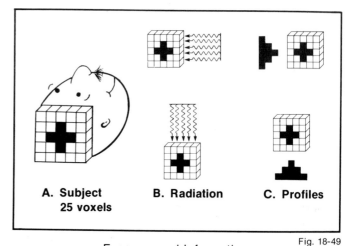

**A. Subject
25 voxels**   **B. Radiation**   **C. Profiles**

Fig. 18-49

Exposure and Information
Profile

Attenuation

Radiation is attenuated or absorbed more readily by the tissue surrounding the cross than by the air in the cross. Assume that each voxel of tissue absorbs one unit of radiation, and each air-filled voxel absorbs no radiation. This is represented in Step D of *Fig. 18-50* by assigning the **number 1 to each tissue voxel** and **0 (zero) to each air-filled voxel.** Therefore, the two drawings in Step D represent relative attenuation values in very simplified form.

The next step, as shown by the two illustrations in Step E, is to **add the numbers in the direction of the two beams of radiation.** Each beam of radiation passes through a total of five voxels. The maximum number of 5 occurs along each border of the cross where the x-rays pass through five tissue voxels. Addition of numbers in the central portion of the cross results in the number 2 since only two voxels represent tissue in that direction. Addition of each row of numbers results in two profiles of radiation represented by the numbers, as shown in Step E of this illustration.

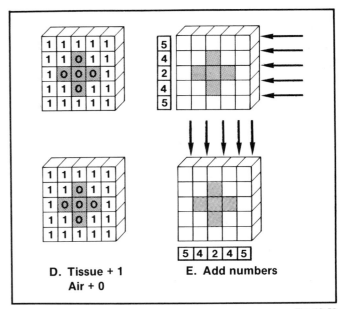

D. Tissue + 1
Air + 0

E. Add numbers

Attenuation

Fig. 18-50

Summation

The next step involves combining the two numerical profiles into one, as shown in Step F. This is done by adding the numbers in each of the two directions. Therefore, the upper right voxel in Step F is represented by the number 10 since the transmission readings were 5 in each of the two directions. The sum for the lower voxel is 6, since 4 was obtained in one direction and 2 in the other direction. The numerical composite, shown on the right in Step G, is the sum of the numbers comprising each profile. This addition process is essentially what the computer does with the large mass of transmission data accumulated by the scan unit.

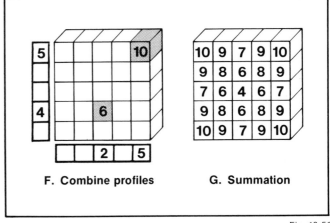

F. Combine profiles

G. Summation

Summation

Fig. 18-51

Picture Reconstruction

The large amount of numerical data obtained by summation must now be transformed into a picture. This is done by assigning various shades of gray, black or white to various numbers. As shown in Step H of this illustration, the number 4 is assigned white and the number 10 is black. Any numbers between 4 and 10 are assigned darker and darker shades of gray, as shown in the table to the right in *Fig. 18-52*. A projection of this reconstruction as an image looks like the gray-scale drawing in Step H.

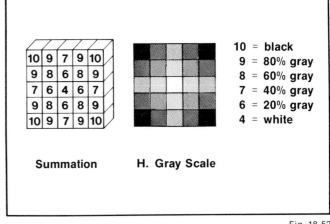

10	= black
9	= 80% gray
8	= 60% gray
7	= 40% gray
6	= 20% gray
4	= white

Summation   **H. Gray Scale**

Picture Reconstruction

Fig. 18-52

Image Manipulation

Finally, the gray-scale image shown in Step H can be manipulated to give a more accurate reconstruction of the original image. Increasing the contrast or, in effect, removing the gray from the image results in a black and white image, shown in Step I of *Fig. 18-53*. This image results if any number equaling 6 or less is assigned white, and any number 7 or larger is assigned black. Basically, this describes cranial computed tomography. The internal structure of any three-dimensional structure can be reconstructed from many different projections of that subject.

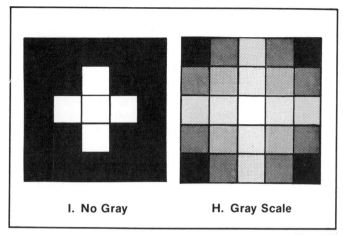

I. No Gray   **H. Gray Scale**

Image Manipulation   Fig. 18-53

Computed Tomographic Image

Degree of Attenuation of Each Voxel (Differential Absorption)

A computed tomographic image is shown in *Fig. 18-54*. Each voxel in the tissue slice is assigned a number proportional to the degree of x-ray attenuation of the entire chunk of tissue or voxel. Attenuation or differential absorption is defined as the reduction in the intensity of the x-ray beam as the beam passes through matter. X-ray photons are removed from the incident beam through absorption or scattering as a result of interaction with individual atoms or molecules comprising the matter. Many photons pass through the matter in question without any type of interaction.

Many variables affect the degree of attenuation. Variables include the energy of the x-ray beam, as well as the density, effective atomic number and number of electrons per gram of the subject matter. Generally, production of diagnostic images in radiology and in computed tomography depend entirely on the differential absorption or attenuation between adjacent tissues.

Converting Three-dimensional Voxels to Two-dimensional Pixels

Once the degree of attenuation of each voxel is determined, each three-dimensional tissue slice is projected on the television screen as a two-dimensional image. This **two-dimensional image** is termed the **display matrix** and is composed of tiny picture elements termed **pixels.** Each voxel is represented on the television screen as a pixel. The number of individual elements or pixels comprising the display matrix is determined by the manufacturer and may range from a fairly coarse matrix of 80 x 80 pixels to a very fine matrix of 512 x 512 pixels.

Computed Gray Scale

After the CT computer (through thousands of separate mathematical equations) determines a relative linear attenuation coefficient for each pixel in the display matrix, the values are then converted to another numerical scale involving CT numbers. Shades of gray are then assigned to the CT numbers. The end result is a gray-scale, computed tomographic image, as shown in *Fig. 18-54*.

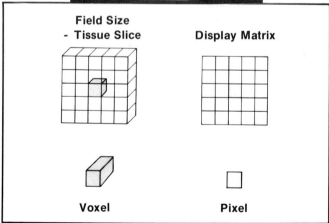

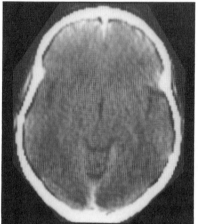

**Field Size
- Tissue Slice**   **Display Matrix**

Voxel   **Pixel**

Computed Tomographic Image   Fig. 18-54

Cranial Computed Tomography Procedure

Purpose

The primary purpose of cranial computed tomography is to provide accurate diagnostic information, significantly improving the management of the patient. The ideal result is a definitive diagnosis that does not require collaborative tests for verification. CCT, in many instances, does provide this high degree of reliability. Acute trauma to the head, for example, may result in epidural or subdural hematoma formation. This type of lesion can be quickly, accurately and unequivocally diagnosed by CCT.

Indications

Virtually any suspected disease process involving the brain is an indication for cranial computed tomography. In the short time since the first patient was scanned on a prototype CCT unit in 1972, neuroradiologic emphasis has greatly changed. CCT has virtually eliminated the need for cerebral pneumography and echoencephalography. Furthermore, a substantial decrease in the number of cerebral angiograms and radionuclide brain scans has resulted. Some of the more common indications for cranial computed tomography include suspected brain neoplasms or masses, brain metastases, intracranial hemorrhage, aneurysm, abscess, brain atrophy, posttraumatic abnormalities such as epidural and subdural hematomas, and acquired or congenital abnormalities.

Contraindications

Contraindications to cranial computed tomography are few. About 50 percent of all CCT's do not require contrast enhancement; consequently, these examinations are noninvasive. If the patient can be transported to the CT treatment room, the examination can be performed. With some very ill or massively injured patients, the transfer from patient room to treatment room and the transfer from patient bed to CT patient table may be the most hazardous part of the examination. For the other half of all CCT's that require contrast enhancement, injection of an iodinated contrast medium is necessary. A very small percentage of persons may react adversely to an injection of iodinated contrast medium. A careful history must be taken prior to such an injection. Should the patient's history indicate a possible severe reaction, the patient's physician may choose to medicate prior to the examination or cancel the contrast-enhanced portion of the study. Except for the patient with an actual history of severe reaction to iodinated contrast medium, and the nontransportable patient, there are no real contraindications to cranial computed tomography.

Patient Preparation

There is usually no patient preparation for a CCT. Unpleasant side effects such as nausea and/or vomiting may occur whenever iodinated contrast medium is introduced into the human circulatory system. For the contrast-enhanced examination, it is prudent to examine the patient with an empty stomach to prevent complications associated with premature gastric emptying. Patient preparation may be necessary for the uncooperative type of individual. Patient motion during the scan is a serious impairment to the diagnostic CCT, so some cooperation is essential. Many circumstances may render the patient less cooperative than usual. Brain lesions may affect the patient in bizarre ways, depending on the location and amount of brain tissue involved. Events prior to an acute head injury may include ingestion or inhalation of a variety of substances that may also alter normal behavior. Therefore, should sedation or anesthesia be necessary to allow scan completion without unwanted patient motion, appropriate medication must be administered by medical personnel. Preparation for resuscitative measures, including endotracheal tube placement capabilities, are mandatory for the sedated patient.

Contrast Media

The contrast media utilized for cranial computed tomography are identical to those used for excretory urography. These iodinated contrast media are usually administered as a bolus injection, but may be introduced via an intravenous infusion.

Complications

True anaphylactoid reaction to currently used iodinated contrast media is rare, but possible minor or major reactions must be foremost in the minds of radiology staff members whenever such injections are necessary. Complications arising from such injections are treated according to a well-established departmental protocol. Postprocedure care includes careful observation since delayed reactions to contrast media are possible, although most reactions will occur within the first 5 minutes following injection if they are going to happen.

Scanner Room Preparation

Room preparation for a CCT is fairly simple. Basically, three steps need to be taken. First, the scanner or treatment room should be clean and tidy. All patients, as they are brought into the scanner room, should be made to feel that they are the first patient to utilize the equipment. Second, assemble any patient support items necessary. If oxygen, suction or IV pole are necessary, these should be provided. If the patient must be ventilated during examination or anesthetized prior to the procedure, the appropriate personnel must be assembled.

Finally, the operator console, direct display console and computer must be activated. The computer must be instructed via the typewriter to prepare for the appropriate procedure. If the examination is to be a contrast-enhanced procedure, then it is necessary to prepare for injection or infusion in the standard, sterile manner.

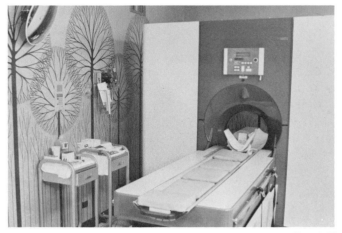

Room Preparation   Fig. 18-55

Cranial Computed Tomography Positioning

Routine positioning for cranial computed tomography is shown in *Fig. 18-56*. **The neck is flexed until a line 25 degrees to the I.O.M.L. is parallel to the x-ray beam.** This positioning requires that the chin be depressed. An exact 25-degree angle is not absolutely necessary since both sides are seen on the finished reconstruction. More important is placement of the head so that no rotation and no tilt are detected on the scan. The basic principles of skull positioning used in conventional radiography apply equally to computed tomography, with one major exception. In CCT, the **section of interest is placed parallel to the x-ray beam** rather than perpendicular to it. With accurate positioning, interested physicians can examine bilateral symmetry in the normal scan and asymmetry in the abnormal reconstruction.

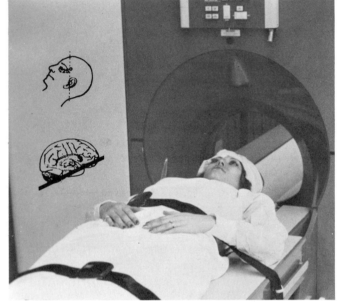

Routine CCT Positioning   Fig. 18-56

Alternate Positioning Method. An alternate positioning method for routine cranial scanning is to use **a line connecting the S.O.G.** (supraorbital groove) **and the T.E.A.** (top of ear attachment). By placing this line parallel to the x-ray beam, similar results can be obtained when compared to the 25 degree to the I.O.M.L. method. Positioning the head in this position allows most of the cerebellum to be visualized on the same slice as the area of the sella turcica.

Procedure for Complete CCT

The procedure for a complete CCT scan may vary from facility to facility, but usually the initial sequence is six to ten scans. These six to ten scans cover the entire brain from base to vertex, in up to 13 millimeter sections. Depending on the scan unit in use, the sections may be thinner, such as 5, 8 or 10 millimeters. The initial sequence is usually performed without contrast enhancement. Should enhancement be indicated, as determined by the provisional diagnosis and/or departmental routine, a second sequence is then performed. The same brain sections are again examined; but, for the second series, contrast medium is injected or infused.

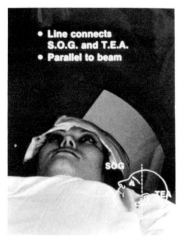

• Line connects S.O.G. and T.E.A.
• Parallel to beam

Alternate   Fig. 18-57
Positioning

CCT Scan

One of the axial sections in the cranial computed tomographic series is shown in *Fig. 18-58.* No rotation or tilt is detected on the section. The bilateral symmetry of the brain and cranial structures is demonstrated on this radiograph.

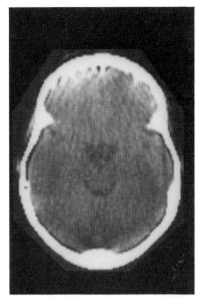

Fig. 18-58

CCT Scan
(axial section)

Orbital Scan Positioning

One variation to the basic CCT routine is orbital scanning. Some routines call for the automatic inclusion of approximately three sections through the orbits, utilizing a slightly different head position. The patient is shown in position for orbital scanning in *Fig. 18-59.* The head is in a neutral position so that the **radiation beam parallels the I.O.M. line.** An alternative line used for the same result is one connecting the midlateral orbital margin and the T.E.A. This line is parallel to the I.O.M.L.

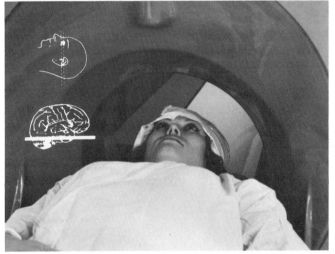

Orbital Scan Positioning

Fig. 18-59

Orbital Scan

The radiograph in *Fig. 18-60* is an orbital scan utilizing the neutral head position. This radiograph clearly shows the orbital cavities, including the ocular bulbs and optic nerves.

Other positioning angles may be utilized to meet different needs. Certain scanners allow different positions to be assumed, including the basilar position for coronal sections. Certain units allow reconstruction of coronal sections based on axial section data stored in the computer.

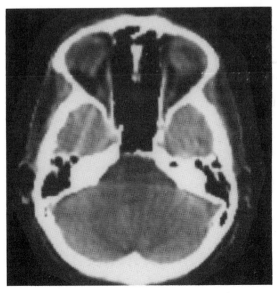

Fig. 18-60

Orbital Scan

Contrast Enhancement

The brain is well supplied with blood vessels that supply oxygen and nutrients. Oxygen must be in constant supply since total oxygen deprivation for the short time of 4 minutes can lead to permanent brain cell damage. Similarly, glucose must be continually available since carbohydrate storage in the brain is limited. Glucose, oxygen and certain ions pass readily from the circulatory blood into extracellular fluid, then into brain cells. Other substances found in the blood normally enter brain cells quite slowly. Still others, such as proteins, most antibiotics and contrast media, will not pass at all from the normal cranial capillary system into brain cells. The brain is different from other tissues in that there is a natural barrier to the passage of certain substances. This natural phenomenon is termed the "blood-brain barrier." Contrast medium appearing outside the normal vascular system is an indication that something is wrong. In *Fig. 18-61,* a normal cranial computed tomograph is shown to the left, while the same level is shown to the right with contrast enhancement. Both are normal, without any disruption of the blood-brain barrier.

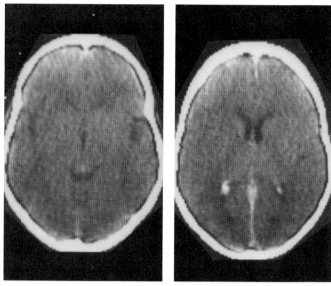

Contrast-enhanced CCT   Fig. 18-61

Positive CCT (Glioma)

An example of a positive CCT is shown in *Fig. 18-62.* This particular lesion is a glioma. To the left is the noncontrast tomogram and to the right is the contrast-enhanced version of the same slice. Contrast enhancement is necessary for all suspected neoplasia due to possible breakdown of the normal blood-brain barrier.

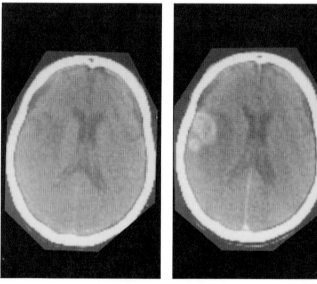

Positive CCT (Glioma)   Fig. 18-62

Subdural Hematoma and Hydrocephaly

Two additional positive examples of cranial computed tomograms are illustrated in *Fig. 18-63.* To the left is an example of large bilateral, frontal, subdural hematomas of at least three weeks' duration. This type of lesion, whether acute or chronic, can be diagnosed without contrast enhancement. To the right is an example of hydrocephalus. Note the enlarged ventricles and how well they visualize on the CCT.

With well-maintained and properly functioning equipment, computed tomography of the head is not a difficult examination for the radiographer to perform, or for the neuroradiologist to interpret. CCT is an exciting, diagnostic, radiographic tool and is proving invaluable to the diagnosis of cranial disease.

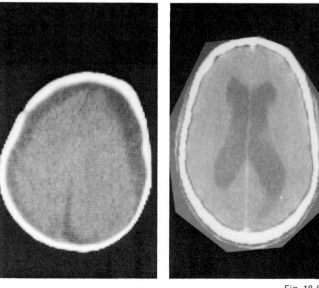

Positive CCT's   Fig. 18-63

CHAPTER 19
Radiographic Anatomy and Positioning of the
Upper Gastrointestinal System

Part I. Radiographic Anatomy
Upper Gastrointestinal System

Digestive System

The digestive system includes the entire **alimentary canal** and several **accessory organs.** The alimentary canal begins at the **mouth,** continues as the **pharynx, esophagus, stomach** and **small intestine,** and ends as the **large intestine,** which terminates as the **anus.** Accessory organs of digestion include the **teeth, salivary glands, pancreas, liver** and **gallbladder.**

The digestive system performs three primary functions. The first function is the **intake** of water, vitamins and minerals, plus the **intake** and **digestion** of food. Food is ingested in the form of carbohydrates, lipids and proteins. These complex food groups must be broken down or digested so that absorption can take place. The second primary function of the digestive system is to **absorb** digested food particles, along with water, vitamins and essential elements from the alimentary canal into the blood or lymphatic capillaries. The third function is to **eliminate** any unused material in the form of solid waste products.

Common radiographic procedures involving the upper gastrointestinal system are presented in this chapter. Common radiographic procedures are those examinations performed routinely in large and small radiology departments, as well as in certain clinics and physician's offices. All common radiographic examinations involve the **administration** of a **contrast medium.**

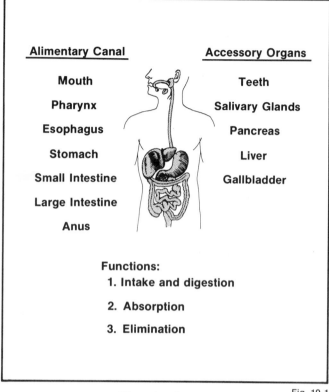

Digestive System   Fig. 19-1

Common Radiographic Procedures

(Contrast media are administered)

1. Esophagram or Barium Swallow
   - Study of pharynx and esophagus

2. Upper Gastrointestinal Series (U.G.I.) (Upper G.I.)
   - Study of distal esophagus, stomach and duodenum

A radiographic examination specifically of the pharynx and esophagus is termed an **esophagram** or **barium swallow.** The procedure designed to study the distal esophagus, stomach and duodenum in one examination is termed an **upper gastrointestinal series.** Alternative designations for upper gastrointestinal series include U.G.I., upper, G.I. or, most commonly, **upper G.I.** One radiograph from an upper G.I. series is shown in *Fig. 19-2.* Barium sulfate mixed with water is the contrast medium of choice for the entire alimentary canal. It is the white material within the stomach and duodenum on this radiograph.

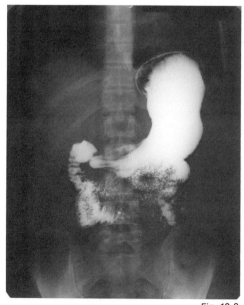

Fig. 19-2

P.A. - Upper G.I. Series

Mouth (Oral Cavity or Buccal Cavity)

The alimentary canal is a continuous hollow tube, beginning with the mouth. The **mouth** may also be referred to as the **oral cavity** or **buccal cavity.** The mouth and surrounding structures are visualized in midsagittal section in *Fig. 19-3.*

The main cavity of the mouth is bounded in front and on the sides by the inner surfaces of the **upper** and **lower teeth.** The roof of the mouth is formed by the **hard** and **soft palates,** while the main part of the floor is formed by the **tongue.** The mouth or oral cavity connects posteriorly with the **pharynx.**

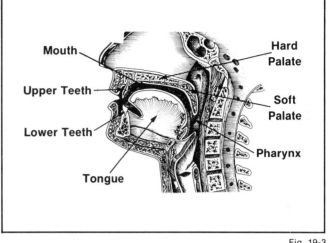

Mouth (Oral Cavity or Buccal Cavity)   Fig. 19-3

Accessory Organs in the Mouth

Accessory organs of digestion associated with the mouth are the **teeth** and the **salivary glands.** The teeth and tongue cooperate in chewing movements to reduce the size of food particles and to mix food with saliva. These chewing movements, termed **mastication,** initiate the mechanical part of digestion. The salivary glands are three pairs of glands that secrete saliva into the mouth. Saliva is over 99 percent water. Between 1000 and 1500 milliliters are secreted daily by the salivary glands. Saliva dissolves foods so that they can be tasted and so that digestion can begin. Mucous lubricates food being chewed so that the food can form into a ball or bolus for swallowing. The act of swallowing is termed **deglutition.**

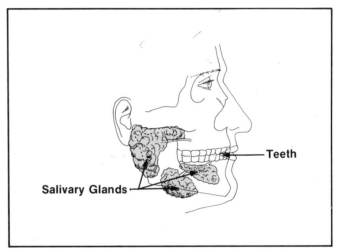

Accessory Organs in the Mouth   Fig. 19-4

Pharynx

The alimentary canal continues as the pharynx posterior to the mouth. The **pharynx** is about 12.5 centimeters long, and is that part of the digestive tube found behind the nasal cavities, mouth and larynx. A coronal section of the pharynx, seen from the posterior, is shown in *Fig. 19-5.* The three parts of the pharynx are named according to their location. The **nasopharynx** is behind the **nasal septum** and nasal cavities, and above the level of the soft palate. The **oropharynx** is directly behind the oral cavity proper. The oropharynx extends from the **soft palate** to the **epiglottis.** The epiglottis is a membrane-covered cartilage that flops down to cover the opening of the larynx during swallowing.

The third portion of the pharynx is termed the **laryngopharynx** or **hypopharynx.** The laryngopharynx extends from the level of the epiglottis to the level of the lower border of the cricoid cartilage, where it continues as the **esophagus.** In *Fig. 19-5,* the **trachea** is seen anterior to the esophagus.

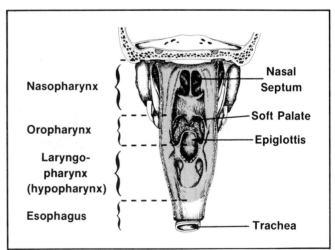

Pharynx   Fig. 19-5

Cavities Communicating with the Pharynx

The surface drawing in *Fig. 19-6* illustrates that there are seven cavities communicating with the three portions of the pharynx. The two **nasal cavities** and the two **tympanic cavities** connect to the **nasopharynx.** The tympanic cavities of the middle ears connect to the nasopharynx via the auditory or Eustachian tubes. The **mouth** connects posteriorly to the **oropharynx.** Inferiorly, the **laryngopharynx** connects to both the **larynx** and the **esophagus.**

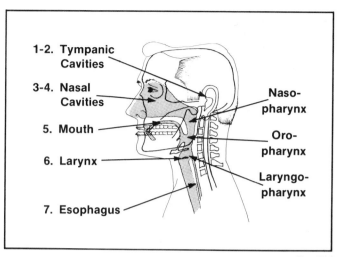

Pharynx

Fig. 19-6

Deglutition (Swallowing)

It is most important that food and fluid travel from the oral cavity directly to the esophagus during the act of swallowing or deglutition. During swallowing, the soft palate closes off the nasopharynx to prevent swallowed substances from regurgitating into the nose. The tongue prevents the material from re-entering the mouth.

During swallowing, the epiglottis is depressed to cover the laryngeal opening like a lid. In addition, the actual opening to the larynx is tightly closed by folds of tissue on either side of the epiglottis. These actions combine to prevent food and fluid from going down the "wrong pipe." Also, respiration is inhibited during most of deglutition to help prevent swallowed substances from entering the trachea and lungs. Occasionally, bits of material pass into the larynx and trachea during swallowing. A forceful episode of reflex coughing is usually necessary to reject these offensive intruders.

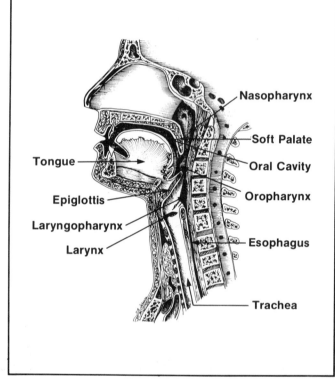

Pharynx

Fig. 19-7

Esophagus

The **esophagus** or gullet is a muscular canal, about 25 centimeters long, extending from the inferior **pharynx** to the stomach. The esophagus begins posterior to the level of the lower border of the **cricoid cartilage** of the **larynx,** which is at the level of the **sixth cervical vertebra** (C-6). The esophagus terminates at its connection to the stomach, at the level of the **eleventh thoracic vertebra** (T-11).

In *Fig. 19-8,* one can see that the esophagus is located posterior to the larynx and trachea. The spatial relationship of the esophagus to both the trachea and the thoracic vertebrae is a very important relationship to remember. The esophagus is both posterior to the trachea, and just anterior to the cervical and thoracic vertebral bodies.

The descending thoracic aorta is between the distal esophagus and the lower thoracic spine. The **heart,** within its **pericardial sac,** is immediately posterior to the **sternum,** anterior to the esophagus, and superior to the **diaphragm.**

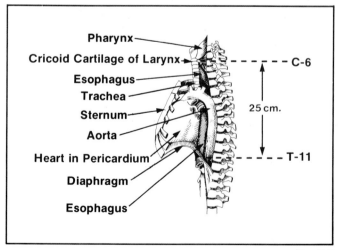

Esophagus

Fig. 19-8

The **esophagus** is essentially vertical as it descends to the stomach. This swallowing tube is the narrowest part of the entire alimentary canal. The esophagus is most constricted, first, at its upper end where it enters the thorax, and, second, where it passes through the diaphragm at the esophageal hiatus or opening. The esophagus pierces the diaphragm at the level of **T-10.** Just before passing through the diaphragm, the esophagus presents a distinct dilatation.

As the esophagus descends within the posterior mediastinum, two indentations are present, as shown in *Fig. 19-9.* One indentation occurs at the **aortic arch,** and the second is found where the esophagus crosses the **left bronchus.** The lower portion of the esophagus lies close to the posterior aspects of the **heart.**

Diaphragm Openings

The **esophagus** passes through the **diaphragm** slightly to the left and somewhat posterior to the midpoint of the diaphragm. The drawing on the left in *Fig. 19-10* represents the inferior surface of the diaphragm and indicates the relative positions of the **esophagus, inferior vena cava** and **aorta.** The drawing on the right shows the short abdominal portion of the esophagus. The **abdominal segment of the esophagus,** termed the **cardiac antrum,** measures between 1 and 2 centimeters. The cardiac antrum curves sharply to the left after passing through the diaphragm to attach to the stomach.

The opening between the esophagus and the stomach is termed the cardiac orifice. Cardiac is an adjective denoting a relationship to the heart, therefore the cardiac antrum and the cardiac orifice are located near the heart. The junction of the stomach and the esophagus is normally securely attached to the diaphragm, so the upper stomach tends to follow the respiratory movements of the diaphragm.

Swallowing

The **esophagus** contains a well-developed muscular layer composed of both longitudinal and circular fibers. Unlike the trachea, the esophagus is a collapsible tube that only opens when swallowing occurs. The process of deglutition continues in the esophagus after originating in the mouth and pharynx. Fluids tend to pass from the mouth and pharynx to the stomach primarily by gravity. A bolus of solid material tends to pass both by gravity and by peristalsis. Peristalsis is a series of muscular contractions propelling solid and semisolid materials through the tubular alimentary canal. The bolus of barium sulfate, seen in the esophagus in *Fig. 19-11,* is descending to the stomach both by gravity and by peristalsis.

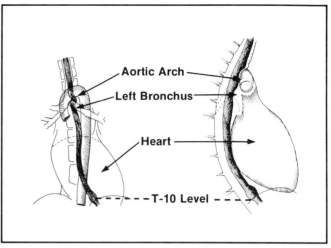

Esophagus   Fig. 19-9

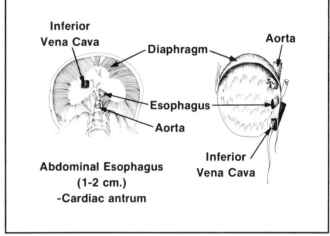

Esophagus and Diaphragm   Fig. 19-10

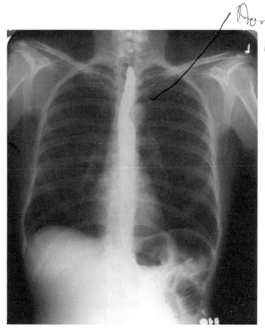

Esophagram   Fig. 19-11

Stomach

The **stomach,** located between the **esophagus** and the **small intestine,** is the most dilated portion of the alimentary canal. When empty, the stomach tends to collapse. When the stomach must serve as a reservoir for swallowed food and fluid, it is remarkably expandable. At times, the stomach may stretch almost to the point of rupture.

Synonyms for stomach are the Latin word *ventriculus,* meaning "little belly," and the Greek word *gaster,* meaning "stomach." *Gastro* is a common combining form denoting stomach. Since the shape and position of the stomach are highly variable, the average shape and location will be utilized in the following illustrations, with variations to follow later in this chapter.

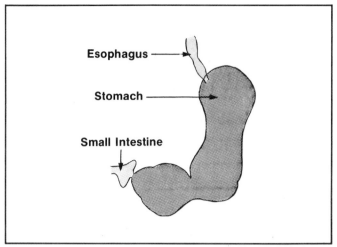

Stomach   Fig. 19-12

Stomach Openings and Lesser Curvature

The **cardiac orifice,** the aperture or opening between the esophagus and the stomach, is guarded by circular sphincter muscles. In a similar fashion, the orifice leaving the distal stomach is termed the **pyloric orifice** or **pylorus.** The pyloric sphincter is a thickened muscular ring that relaxes periodically during digestion to allow stomach or gastric contents to move into the first part of the small intestine.

The lesser curvature forms a concave border as it extends between the cardiac and pyloric openings on the right side of the stomach. An obvious notch, termed the **incisura angularis** or **angular notch,** is located along the lesser curvature, closer to the pyloric orifice than to the cardiac orifice. This notch divides the stomach inferior to the cardiac orifice into a small right portion and a large left portion.

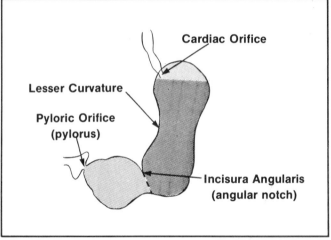

Stomach   Fig. 19-13

Stomach Subdivisions

The stomach is composed of three main subdivisions: (1) the **fundus,** (2) the **body** or **corpus,** and (3) the **pyloric portion.** The fundus is that ballooned portion lying to the left of and superior to the cardiac orifice. The upper portion of the stomach, including the cardiac antrum of the esophagus, is relatively fixed to the diaphragm and tends to move with motion of the diaphragm. In the upright or erect position, the fundus is usually filled by a bubble of swallowed air.

Left of the incisura angularis (the patient's left) and inferior to the fundus is the large portion of the stomach called the body or corpus. The smaller terminal portion of the stomach to the right of the incisura angularis is the pyloric portion of the stomach, which terminates at the pyloric valve or pylorus.

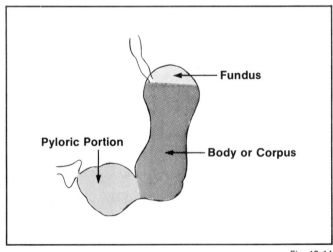

Stomach   Fig. 19-14

Greater Curvature and Rugae

The **greater curvature** extends along the left border of the stomach from the **cardiac orifice** to the **pylorus.** This greater curvature is four to five times longer than the lesser curvature and is convex rather than concave. The notch found at the junction of the esophagus and the greater curvature is termed the **incisura cardiaca** or **cardiac notch.**

When the stomach is empty, the internal lining is thrown into numerous longitudinal folds termed **rugae.** A gastric canal, formed by rugae along the lesser curvature, is believed to funnel fluids directly to the pylorus.

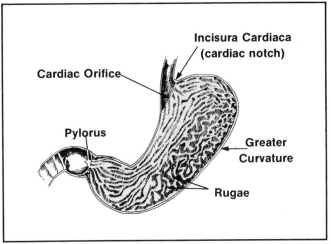

Stomach   Fig. 19-15

Stomach Position

The illustration in *Fig. 19-16* shows the typical orientation of an average, empty stomach. The frontal view is to the left and the lateral view is to the right. The **fundus,** in addition to being the most superior portion of the stomach, is located posterior to the **body** of the stomach. The body can be seen to curve downward and forward from the fundus. The **pyloric portion** is directed toward the posterior. The **pylorus** or pyloric valve and the first part of the small bowel are very near the posterior abdominal wall.

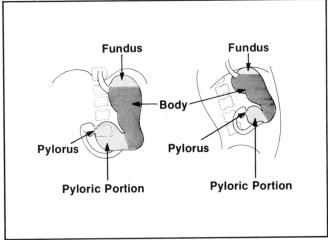

Average Empty Stomach Orientation   Fig. 19-16

Air-Barium Distribution in Stomach

If an individual were to swallow some barium sulfate and water mixture, along with some air, the position of the person's body would determine where the barium and the air would go. The illustration in *Fig. 19-17* shows air as black and the barium sulfate mixture as white. The drawing on the left depicts the stomach of a person who is **standing.** In the erect position, air will rise to fill the fundus, while barium will descend by gravity to fill the pyloric portion of the stomach.

The middle drawing shows the stomach of a person in a **prone** position. Since the fundus is more posterior than the lower body of the stomach, air will be found primarily in the fundus, while barium will gravitate to the lower body and the pyloric portion of the stomach.

The drawing on the right depicts the stomach of a person in a **supine** position. In a supine position, barium will travel to the fundus, while air will locate toward the distal end of the stomach. When studying radiographs of a stomach containing both air and barium sulfate, one can determine the patient's position by the relative locations of air versus barium.

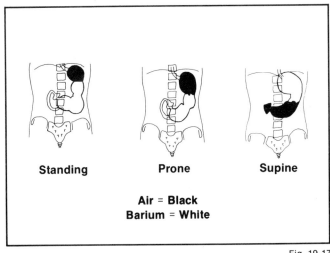

Air-Barium Distribution in the Stomach   Fig. 19-17

Duodenum

The first portion of the small intestine is the **duodenum.** Since the duodenum is examined radiographically during the routine upper G.I. series, the duodenum will be studied in Chapter 19, while the remainder of the small bowel will be studied in Chapter 20. The duodenum is about 25 centimeters long, and is the shortest, widest and most fixed portion of the small bowel.

The drawing in *Fig. 19-18* demonstrates that the C-shaped duodenum is closely related to the **head of the pancreas.** The head of the pancreas, nestled in the C-loop of the duodenum, has been affectionately labeled the "romance of the abdomen" by certain authors.

The duodenum is shaped like a letter C and consists of four parts. The **superior portion** begins at the **pylorus.** The first part of the superior portion is termed the duodenal bulb or cap. It is shaped somewhat like an arrowhead. The duodenal bulb is easily located during barium studies of the upper G.I. tract and must be carefully studied since this area is a common site of ulcer disease.

The second part of the duodenum is the **descending portion,** the longest segment. The descending portion of the duodenum receives both the common bile duct and the main pancreatic duct.

The third part of the duodenum is the **horizontal portion.** This horizontal portion curves back to the left to join the final segment, termed the **ascending portion.** The junction of the duodenum with the rest of the small bowel is relatively fixed and is held in place by the **ligament of Treitz.**

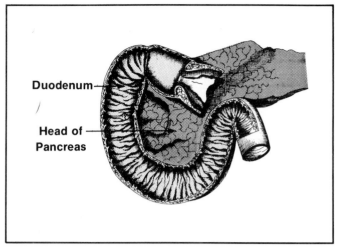

Duodenum   Fig. 19-18

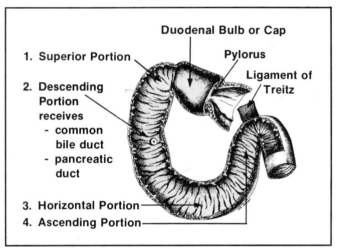

Duodenum   Fig. 19-19

Digestion

Mechanical Digestion

Digestion can be divided into a mechanical process and a chemical component. Mechanical digestion includes all movements of the G.I. tract, beginning in the mouth with chewing or mastication, and continuing in the mouth, pharynx and esophagus with swallowing or deglutition. Peristaltic activity can be detected in the lower esophagus as well as in the remainder of the alimentary canal.

The stomach, acting as a reservoir for food and fluid, also acts as a large mixing bowl. Peristalsis tends to move the gastric contents toward the pyloric valve, but this valve opens selectively. If it is closed, the stomach contents are churned or mixed with saliva and other stomach fluids into a semifluid mass termed chyme. When the valve opens, small amounts of chyme are passed into the duodenum by stomach peristalsis. Gastric emptying is a fairly slow process, taking one to four hours to totally empty after an average meal.

The small intestine continues mechanical digestion with a churning motion within segments of the small bowel. This churning or mixing activity is termed rhythmic segmentation. Rhythmic segmentation tends to thoroughly mix food and digestive juices, and to bring the digested food into contact with the intestinal lining or mucosa to facilitate absorption. Peristalsis is again present to propel intestinal contents along the alimentary canal.

Mouth (Teeth and Tongue)	Mastication (Chewing) Deglutition (Swallowing)
Pharynx	Deglutition
Esophagus	Deglutition Peristalsis (waves of muscular contraction)
Stomach	Mixing (chyme) Peristalsis
Small Intestine	Rhythmic Segmentation (Churning) Peristalsis

Summary of Mechanical Digestion   Fig. 19-20

Chemical Digestion

Chemical digestion includes all of the chemical changes that food undergoes as it travels through the alimentary canal. Six different classes of substances are ingested: (1) carbohydrates or complex sugars, (2) proteins, (3) lipids or fats, (4) vitamins, (5) minerals and (6) water. Only the carbohydrates, proteins and lipids need to be chemically digested in order to be absorbed. Vitamins, minerals and water are used in the form in which the body ingests them.

Chemical digestion is speeded up by various enzymes. Enzymes are biological catalysts found in the various digestive juices. The various enzymes are organic compounds, frequently proteins, which accelerate chemical changes in other substances without actually appearing in the final products of the reaction.

Carbohydrate digestion of starches is begun in the mouth and stomach, and is completed in the small intestine. The end products of digestion of these complex sugars are simple sugars. Protein digestion is begun in the stomach and is completed in the small intestine. The end products of protein digestion are amino acids. Lipid or fat digestion essentially takes place only in the small bowel, although small amounts of the enzyme necessary for fat digestion are found in the stomach.

Bile, manufactured by the liver and stored in the gallbladder, is discharged into the duodenum to assist in the breakdown of lipids. Bile contains no enzymes, but it does serve to emulsify fats. During emulsification, large fat droplets are broken down to small fat droplets. Appropriate enzymes can more easily catalyze smaller fat droplets. The end products of fat or lipid digestion are fatty acids and glycerol.

Most absorption of digestive end products takes place in the small intestine. Simple sugars, amino acids, fatty acids and glycerol are absorbed into the bloodstream or the lymphatic system through the lining of the small intestine. Limited absorption takes place in the stomach and may include some water, alcohol and certain drugs. Any residues of digestion or any unabsorbed digestive products are eliminated from the large bowel as a component of feces.

Substances Ingested and Digested

1) Carbohydrates (complex sugars) ⟶ (⟶) Simple Sugars

2) Proteins ⟶ Amino Acids

3) Lipids (fats) ⟶ Fatty Acids and Glycerol

Substances Ingested but NOT Digested

4) Vitamins

5) Minerals

6) Water

Enzymes
- biological catalysts

Bile
- emulsifies fats

Summary of Chemical Digestion

Fig. 19-21

Primary Functions of the Digestive System

In summary, three primary functions of the digestive system are accomplished within the alimentary canal. First, ingestion and/or digestion takes place in the mouth, pharynx, esophagus, stomach and small intestine. Second, digestive end products along with water, vitamins and minerals are absorbed by the small intestine and, to a much lesser degree, by the stomach, and are transported into the circulatory system. Third, unused or unnecessary solid material is eliminated by the large intestine.

1) **Ingestion and/or Digestion**
   (Mouth, Pharynx, Esophagus, Stomach and Small Intestine)

2) **Absorption**
   (Small Intestine and Stomach)

3) **Elimination**
   (Large Intestine)

Fig. 19-22
Primary Functions of the Digestive System

Bodily Habitus

The general form or shape of the body is termed bodily habitus. There are four general classes of bodily habitus: (1) **hypersthenic,** (2) **sthenic,** (3) **hyposthenic,** and (4) **asthenic.** The hypersthenic type of body build is the massive type, representing about 5 percent of the total population. The average body type is the sthenic designation, describing about half or 50 percent of all individuals. The word sthenic actually means active or strong. Slightly more slender than the sthenic type is the hyposthenic habitus, representing about 35 percent of the total population. The very slender type is the asthenic category which comprises about 10 percent of all subjects.

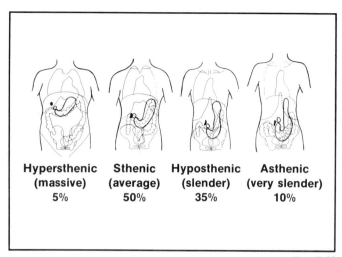

Bodily Habitus

Fig. 19-23

Hypersthenic vs. Asthenic

The two extremes of bodily habitus are the hypersthenic and the asthenic builds. The **hypersthenic** type designates the **massive body build,** with the chest and abdomen being very broad and deep from front to back. The lungs are short and wide, and the diaphragm is quite high. The heart is short and wide, and lies in a transverse axis. The transverse colon is quite high, and the entire large bowel extends the periphery of the abdominal cavity. The gallbladder is higher and more to the right compared to the average position. The gallbladder is almost transverse and lies well away from the midline. The stomach is also very high and assumes a transverse position.

The opposite extreme is the **extremely slender build** or **asthenic** type. This individual is often very frail and has poor muscle tone. In the asthenic bodily habitus, the chest cavity is narrow, shallow and quite long, so that the diaphragm lies very low. The heart is long and slender. The large intestine folds on itself, and is found very low and toward the midline. The gallbladder and stomach are both low, vertical and near the midline. The abdominal cavity is shallow, with its greatest capacity in the pelvic region.

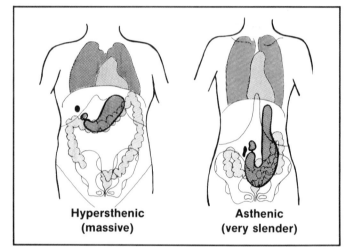

Hypersthenic vs. Asthenic

Fig. 19-24

Sthenic vs. Hyposthenic

The **average body build** is the **sthenic** type, which is a more slender version of the hypersthenic classification. The stomach is more J-shaped and is located lower than in the massive body type. The gallbladder is less transverse and lies midway between the lateral abdominal wall and the midline. The large bowel lies mainly within the abdominal cavity. The splenic flexure is often quite high, resting under the left hemidiaphragm.

The **hyposthenic** type is considered to be a modification of the more slender asthenic build. The stomach is elongated, J-shaped and extends to the iliac crest or below. The gallbladder is lower and more toward the midline compared to the sthenic type of build. The large bowel is located lower than in the average habitus, but the splenic flexure may still be found high in the upper left quadrant.

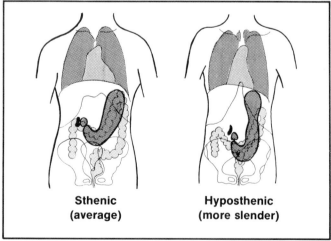

Sthenic vs. Hyposthenic

Fig. 19-25

Variations in Bodily Habitus

Bodily habitus determines the relative size, shape, position, muscular tone and motility of all organs. The two organs most dramatically affected by bodily habitus are the stomach and gallbladder. Many radiographic examinations are done daily on these two organs. It is necessary to assess the bodily habitus of each patient requiring radiographs of these two organs. The assessment requires a knowledge of bodily habitus and an ability to judge the relative position of the stomach and gallbladder from among the wide variations present in the general public.

In addition to bodily habitus, other factors affecting the position of the stomach include posture, stomach contents and respiration. Posture refers to the relative position of the body. Depending on whether one is upright, supine, prone, on one side, or in the Trendelenburg position, the position of various organs, especially the stomach, will change. Whether the stomach is empty, full or in some phase of digestion will affect stomach position.

Finally, since the upper stomach is attached to the diaphragm, whether one is in full inspiration or expiration, or somewhere in between will affect the cephalic extent of the stomach. As a radiographer, correct localization of all borders of the stomach and other organs will come with sufficient positioning practice.

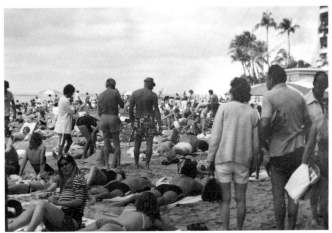

Fig. 19-26

Variable Bodily Habitus

Part II. Radiographic Positioning
Upper Gastrointestinal System

Radiography of the Alimentary Canal

Similarities of Radiographic Examinations of the Entire Alimentary Canal

Radiographic examinations of the entire alimentary canal are similar in three general aspects. **First,** since most parts of the G.I. tract are comparable in density to those tissues surrounding them, some type of **contrast medium** must be added to visualize these structures. Ordinarily, the only parts of the alimentary canal that can be seen on plain radiographs are the fundus of the stomach (in the upright position) due to the gastric air bubble, and parts of the large intestine due to pockets of gas and collections of fecal matter.

Most of the alimentary canal simply blends in with the surrounding structures and cannot be visualized without the use of contrast media. This fact is illustrated in *Fig. 19-27* by comparing a plain abdominal radiograph to an upper G.I. series radiograph using barium sulfate as a contrast medium.

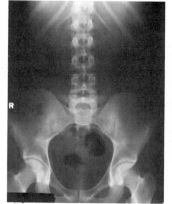
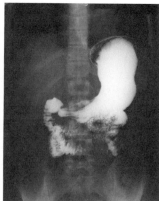

Use of Contrast Medium   Fig. 19-27

A **second** similarity is that the initial stage of each radiographic examination of the alimentary canal is carried out utilizing **fluoroscopy.** Fluoroscopy allows the interested physician to (1) observe the G.I. tract in motion, (2) produce radiographs during the course of the examination, and (3) determine the most appropriate course of action to take for the complete radiographic examination. To be able to view organs in motion and to isolate anatomical structures is absolutely essential for radiographic examination of the upper G.I. tract. The structures in this area assume a wide variety of shapes and sizes depending on the bodily habitus of the individual involved.

In addition, the functional activity of the alimentary canal exhibits a wide range of differences that are considered within normal limits. In addition to these variations, a large number of abnormal conditions exist, making it important that these organs be viewed directly by fluoroscopy.

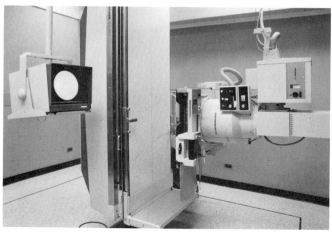

Fluoroscopy Room   Fig. 19-28

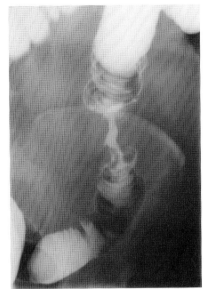

Large Intestine   Fig. 19-29
Carcinoma

A **third** similarity is that **radiographs are produced during and after the fluoroscopic examination** of any part of the alimentary canal to provide a permanent record of the normal or abnormal findings. A positive radiograph from a barium enema is shown in *Fig. 19-29*. This particular radiograph illustrates a carcinoma involving a segment of the large intestine.

Contrast Media

Radiolucent and radiopaque contrast media are utilized to render the G.I. tract visible radiographically. **Radiolucent** or **negative contrast media** include swallowed **air** and the normally present **gas bubble** in the stomach. Other gas forming concoctions may be administered if additional radiolucency is required.

The most common **positive** or **radiopaque contrast medium** used to visualize the gastrointestinal system is **barium sulfate, (BaSO₄).** As illustrated in *Fig. 19-30,* barium sulfate is a powdered, chalklike substance. The powdered barium sulfate is mixed with water prior to ingestion by the patient. This particular compound, which is a salt of barium, is relatively inert because of its extreme insolubility in water and other aqueous solutions, such as acids. All other salts of barium tend to be toxic or poisonous to the human system. Therefore, the barium sulfate used in radiology departments must be chemically pure.

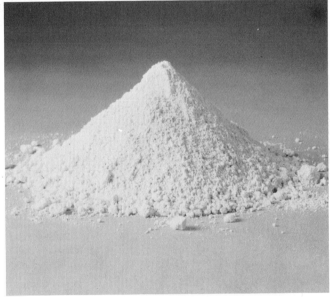

Barium Sulfate $(BaSO_4)$ Fig. 19-30

A mixture of barium sulfate and water forms a **suspension,** not a solution. In order to be a solution, the molecules of the substance added to water must actually dissolve in the water. In a suspension, such as barium sulfate and water, the particles suspended in the water tend to settle out when allowed to sit for a period of time.

The radiograph shown in *Fig. 19-31* is of several cups of barium that were mixed with a ratio by volume of one part water to one part barium sulfate and then allowed to sit for 24 hours. Since different brands of barium sulfate were used, some cups exhibit more settling out than others. When the barium sulfate and water are mixed before they are actually needed, each cup must be well stirred before actual use.

Many special barium sulfate preparations are available commercially. Most of these preparations contain finely divided barium sulfate in a special suspending agent, so these preparations tend to resist settling out and, therefore, stay in suspension longer. Each of these suspensions must be well mixed before use, however. Various brands have different smells and different flavors, such as chocolate, chocolate malt, vanilla, lemon, lime or strawberry.

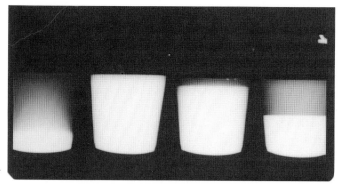

Cups of Barium (24 hrs.)　　Fig. 19-31

Thin Barium

Barium sulfate may be prepared or purchased in a relatively thin or thick mixture. The **thin barium sulfate** and water mixture, as illustrated in *Fig. 19-32,* contains one part $BaSO_4$ to one part of water. Thin barium is the consistency of cream and is used to study the entire G.I. tract.

The motility, or speed with which barium sulfate passes through the G.I. tract, depends on the suspending medium and additives, the temperature and the consistency of the preparation, as well as upon the general condition of the patient and his G.I. tract. It is most important to mix the preparation exactly, according to radiologist preferences and departmental protocol. When the mixture is cold, the chalky taste is much less objectionable. Every radiographer should sample a plain barium sulfate and water mixture, as well as various special preparations.

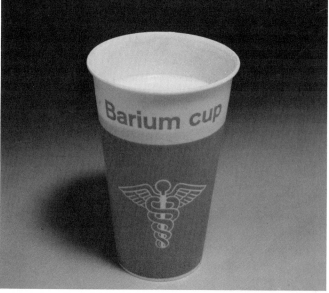

Barium Sulfate and Water Mixture　　Fig. 19-32

Thick Barium

Thick barium contains three or four parts of $BaSO_4$ to one part of water and should be the consistency of cooked cereal. Thick barium is well suited for use in the esophagus since it will descend slowly and will tend to coat the mucosal lining.

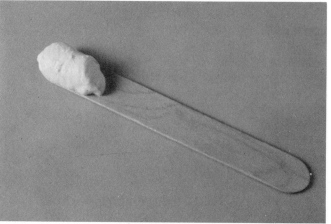

Thick Barium Sulfate Mixture　　Fig. 19-33

Contraindications to Barium Sulfate

Occasionally, barium sulfate mixtures are contraindicated. If there is any chance that the mixture might escape into the peritoneal cavity, such as through a perforated viscus, or if surgery is anticipated following the radiographic procedure, then **water-soluble**, iodinated contrast media are used. Preparations of this type, such as Gastrografin® or Oral Hypaque ®, can be easily removed by aspiration before or during surgery. Should any of this water-soluble material escape into the peritoneal cavity, the body can readily absorb it. Barium sulfate, on the other hand, will not be absorbed and must be removed by the surgeon whenever it is found outside the alimentary canal. One drawback to the water-soluble materials is their bitter taste. Although these iodinated contrast media are sometimes mixed with carbonated soft drinks to mask the taste, they are often used "as is" or diluted with water. The patient should be forewarned that the taste may be slightly bitter.

One of the normal functions of the large intestine is the absorption of water. Any barium sulfate mixture remaining in the large intestine after either an upper G.I. series or a barium enema may become hardened and somewhat solidified in the large bowel, and consequently be difficult to evacuate. Certain patients may require a laxative after these examinations to help remove the barium sulfate. If laxatives are contraindicated, the patient should force fluids or use mineral oil until stools are free from all traces of white.

Radiography — Fluorography Equipment

General Fluoroscopy Unit

A conventional combination radiography-fluorography (R/F) unit is illustrated in *Fig. 19-35*. The modern general purpose fluoroscopy room is equipped with a variety of electronic devices. These include an **image intensifier** and **spot film device** which move as the table is tilted up or down. The electronically enhanced image can be viewed either with a **mirror optical system** or with a **television monitor.** This room utilizes the television monitor system. The television system is much more versatile and more widely accepted than the mirror system. Since these television systems are always closed-circuit systems, monitors can be placed outside the fluoro room for simultaneous viewing during the examination.

During fluoroscopy, the viewer is able to position a part so that the anatomy in question can be best seen by isolating it from objectionable overlying shadows. The fluoroscopic unit is equipped with a spot film device to permanently record optimum images. Cassettes of various sizes can be moved into position to permit a conventional, phototimed radiographic exposure. When fluoroscopy is being performed, these cassettes are in a lead-protected park position.

Many fluoroscopic systems utilize a **spot film camera** in addition to the direct filming methods related to the spot film device. This particular fluoroscopic unit is equipped with a 105 mm. spot film camera in addition to a conventional spot film device. The spot film cameras are similar to movie cameras, but the framing frequency is slower and the film size is larger. Framing can be adjusted from a single exposure to 6 or 12 frames per second. The principal advantage of spot film cameras over direct filming methods is much less radiation exposure to the patient.

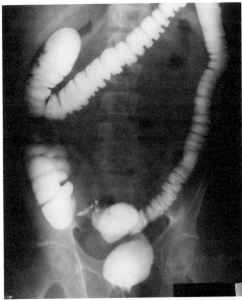

Barium Enema   Fig. 19-34

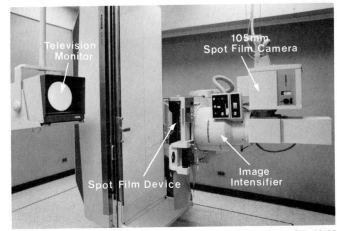

General Fluoroscopy Room   Fig. 19-35

Image Intensification

Conventional early fluoroscopy had two serious limitations:
(1) the image was statistically inferior and (2) the amount
of light given off prevented the use of daylight or cone vision.
In the early 1950's, the invention of the **image intensifier**
revolutionized fluoroscopy. The image intensifier utilizes
the radiation that passes through the patient and enhances
the resultant image by electronically making this image
much brighter. The modern image intensifier produces an
image at least 1,000 times brighter than the older fluoroscopy
screen techniques, and, in some cases, as much as 6,000
times brighter. The image produced through image intensi-
fication is bright enough to be seen with cone vision. The
room lights are dimmed and the fluoroscopic examination
is carried out in a comfortably illuminated room.

In *Fig. 19-36,* the image intensifier is located above the
tabletop, while the x-ray tube is located beneath the tabletop.

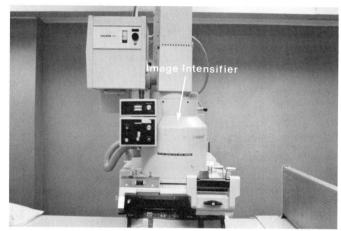

Image Intensifier   Fig. 19-36

Esophagram (Barium Swallow)

An esophagram or barium swallow is the common radiographic examination of the pharynx and esophagus, utilizing
a radiopaque contrast medium. The purpose of an esophagram is to radiographically study the form and function of
the swallowing portion of the upper gastrointestinal system,
as well as to detect abnormal anatomy, impaired swallowing
mechanics and even congenital anomalies.

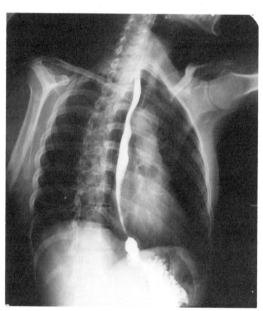

Esophagram - R.A.O.   Fig. 19-37

Patient Preparation

Radiographic examination of any part of the alimentary
canal requires that the portion of the tract to be studied be
empty. Since the esophagus is empty most of the time,
there is no patient preparation for an esophagram unless
an upper G.I. series is to follow. When combined with an
upper G.I., or if the primary interest is the lower esophagus,
preparation for the U.G.I. takes precedence.

For an esophagram only, all clothing and anything metallic
between the mouth and the waist should be removed and
the patient should wear a hospital gown. Prior to the fluoroscopic procedure, a pertinent history should be taken and
the examination should be carefully explained to the patient.

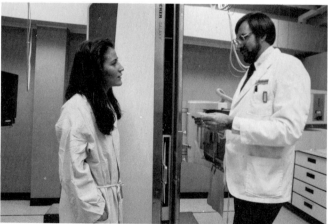

Patient Preparation   Fig. 19-38

Room Preparation

The first part of an esophagram involves fluoroscopy with a positive contrast medium. The examination room should be clean and tidy, and appropriately stocked before the patient is escorted to the room. The appropriate amount and type of contrast medium should be ready. Esophagrams utilize both thin and thick barium. Additional items useful in the detection of a radiolucent foreign body are: (1) cotton balls soaked in thin barium, (2) barium pills or gelatin capsules filled with $BaSO_4$, and (3) marshmallows followed by thin barium. The control panel should be set for fluoroscopy with the appropriate technical factors selected. The fluoroscopy timer should be set for its maximum, usually five minutes. The spot film mechanism should be in proper working order and a supply of spot film cassettes should be handy. The appropriate number and size of conventional cassettes should be provided. The spot film camera should be loaded and in working condition.

Since the esophagram begins with the table in the vertical position, the footboard should be in place and tested for security. Lead aprons and lead gloves should be provided for the radiologist, as well as lead aprons for all other personnel to be in the room. Proper radiation protection methods must be observed at all times during fluoroscopy. In most fluoroscopy units, the Bucky tray must be positioned at the foot end of the table. Appropriately place the radiation foot switch and provide the radiologist a stool, except where the examination is controlled from a remote area. Tissues, towels, emesis basins, spoons, drinking straws and a waste receptacle should be readily accessible.

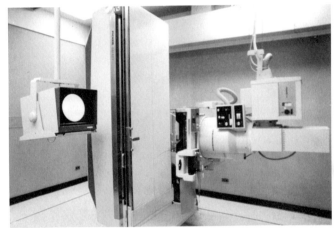

Room Preparation

Fig. 19-39

General Routine Procedure

With the room prepared and the patient ready, the patient and radiologist are introduced, and the patient's history and the reason for the exam are discussed. The fluoroscopic examination usually begins with a general survey of the patient's chest, including heart, lungs and diaphragm, and the abdomen.

During fluoroscopy, the radiographer's duties, in general, are to follow the radiologist's instructions, to assist the patient as needed and to expedite the procedure in any manner possible. Since the examination is begun in the upright or erect position, a cup of thin barium is placed in the patient's left hand close to his left shoulder. He is then instructed to follow the radiologist's instructions concerning how much to drink and when. The radiologist will observe the flow of barium with the fluoroscope. Deglutition of thin barium is observed with the patient in various frontal and oblique positions. Similar positions may be utilized while the patient swallows thick barium. The use of thick barium allows better visualization of mucosal patterns and any lesion within the esophagus. The type of barium mixture to be used will be determined by the radiologist, however.

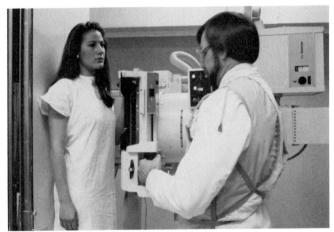

Fluoroscopy

Fig. 19-40

After the upright studies, horizontal and Trendelenburg positions with thick and thin barium may follow. A patient is shown in the **Trendelenburg position** with a cup of thin barium in *Fig. 19-41*. The pharynx and cervical esophagus are usually studied fluoroscopically with spot films, while the main portion of the esophagus down to the stomach is studied both with fluoroscopy and with overhead radiographs. Radiographs using a spot film device or the spot film camera are exposed to document any abnormalities or suspicious areas.

Other possibilities during fluoroscopy include: (1) various breathing exercises, (2) the water test, and (3) the toe-touch test. Fluoroscopy is often a highly variable exercise depending on the patient, the problem and the radiologist. The various breathing exercises are all designed to increase both the intrathoracic and intra-abdominal pressures. The most common breathing exercise is the **Valsalva maneuver.** The patient is asked to take in a deep breath and, while holding the breath in, to bear down as though trying to move the bowels. This maneuver forces air against the closed glottis. A **modified Valsalva maneuver** is accomplished by having the patient pinch off his nose, close his mouth and try to blow his nose. The cheeks should expand outward as though the patient were blowing up a balloon. A **Mueller maneuver** is performed by having the patient exhale and then try to inhale against a closed glottis.

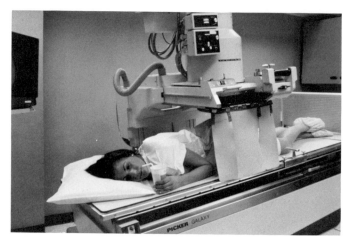

Trendelenburg Postion   Fig. 19-41

Water Test. The water test is done with the patient supine and turned up slightly on his left side. This slight L.P.O. position will fill the fundus with barium. The patient is asked to swallow a mouthful of water through a straw. Under fluoroscopy, the radiologist closely observes the esophagogastric junction. A positive water test occurs when large amounts of barium regurgitate into the esophagus from the stomach.

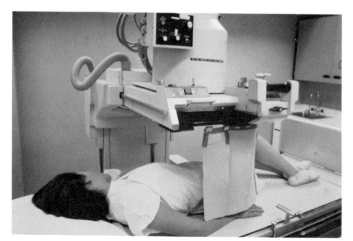

Water Test   Fig. 19-42

426

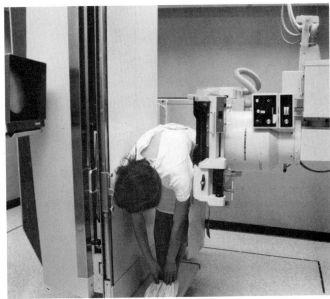

Fig. 19-43

Toe-touch Maneuver

Toe-touch Maneuver. The toe-touch maneuver is also performed to study possible regurgitation into the esophagus from the stomach. Under fluoroscopy, the cardiac orifice is observed as the patient bends over and touches his toes. Esophageal reflux and hiatal hernias are sometimes demonstrated using the toe-touch maneuver.

Post Fluoroscopy Imaging

Following the fluoroscopy portion of the esophagram, radiographs are obtained of the entire barium-filled esophagus. General positioning is similar to chest radiography. The area from the lower neck to the diaphragm must be visualized, requiring centering at the level of T-5 or T-6.

One to three spoonfuls of thick barium are fed to the patient before each exposure. The final spoonful is held in the patient's mouth until just before the exposure. The exposure is made after the bolus has been swallowed. It is usually unnecessary to have the patient stop breathing since respiration is suspended for approximately two seconds after deglutition. The patient may be examined in either the recumbent or upright position. The thick barium will not descend as rapidly when the patient is lying down, and more complete filling of the esophagus will be accomplished.

Three positions or projections are considered routine for an esophagram or barium swallow. These include: (1) **R.A.O.,** (2) **P.A. or A.P.,** and (3) **left lateral.** Left lateral positioning is accomplished with the arms clasped above the head in the usual left lateral chest position.

Variations of the routine lateral are sometimes required. These variations include (1) the retrosternal lateral position and (2) the soft tissue lateral position. The retrosternal lateral position, with the arms on the hips and the shoulders rotated well backwards, allows better visualization of the upper esophagus. When a foreign body is suspected high in the respiratory or digestive tracts, a soft tissue lateral is often the initial radiograph. Positioning is similar to an upright lateral of the cervical spine, although technical factors are adjusted so that 10 kVp less are used. Opaque foreign bodies and some nonopaque foreign bodies can be demonstrated with this position.

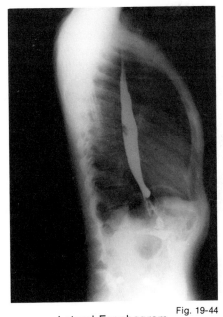

Fig. 19-44

Lateral Esophagram

Cardiac Series

The cardiac series is a radiographic examination very similar to the esophagram. The cardiac series consists of **four radiographs,** each exposed with the esophagus well filled with a thick barium sulfate mixture. Fluoroscopy is not done prior to these four overhead radiographs. Since the cardiac series is used to study heart size and configuration, each of these radiographs is performed utilizing a 72 in. (183 cm.) F.F.D.

The four radiographs in a cardiac series are: (1) a **P.A.**, (2) a **left lateral**, (3) a **45° right anterior oblique**, and (4) a **60° left anterior oblique.** The difference in degrees of obliquity for these two obliques is important to remember. This difference is due to the position of the heart, which is to the left of the midline. Each oblique attempts to place the barium-filled esophagus between the heart shadow and the thoracic vertebrae. In order to fill the esophagus adequately, three spoonfuls of thick barium should be ingested prior to each exposure.

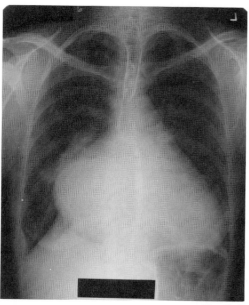

Fig. 19-45

Cardiac Series, P.A.

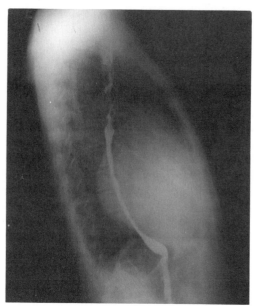

Fig. 19-46

Cardiac Series, Left Lateral

The P.A. from a cardiac series *(Fig. 19-45)* and the left lateral *(Fig. 19-46)* illustrate a massively enlarged heart. This patient suffered from rheumatic fever as a young person. Rheumatic fever attacks and damages the valves of the heart so that the myocardium or heart muscle has to work extra hard to pump adequate blood through the arteries. Whenever individual fibers of a muscle overwork, the result is an enlargement of the entire muscle, termed hypertrophy. These radiographs are an excellent demonstration of cardiac hypertrophy.

Upper Gastrointestinal Series

Radiographic examination of the distal esophagus, stomach and duodenum is termed an upper G.I. series. The purpose of the upper G.I. series is to study radiographically the form and function of the esophagus, stomach and duodenum, as well as to detect abnormal anatomical and functional conditions.

Some of the more common abnormalities seen in this portion of the G.I. tract are peptic ulcers, which include gastric and duodenal ulcers, hiatal hernias, acute or chronic gastritis, carcinomas and benign lesions such as polyps or diverticulae.

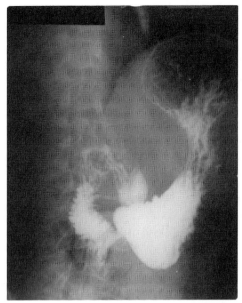

Fig. 19-47

Upper G.I. Series

Patient Preparation

The goal of patient preparation for an upper G.I. series is for the patient to arrive in the radiology department with a completely empty stomach. For an examination scheduled in the morning hours, the patient should have nothing by mouth from midnight until time for the examination. Food and fluids should be withheld for at least eight hours prior to the exam. The patient is also instructed not to smoke cigarettes or chew gum during the N.P.O. period. These activities tend to increase gastric secretions and salivation.

The upper G.I. series is often a time-consuming procedure so the patient should be forewarned of the time the examination may take when the appointment is made. This is especially true if the U.G.I. is to be followed by a small bowel series. The importance of an empty stomach should also be stressed when the appointment is made so that the patient will arrive properly prepared both physically and psychologically.

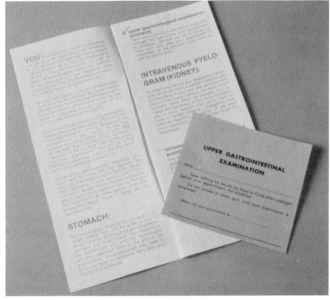

Fig. 19-48

Patient Preparation

Room Preparation

Responsibilities of the radiographer prior to the patient's arrival include setting up the room for fluoroscopy. Room set-up for a U.G.I. series is very similar to that for an esophagram. The thin barium sulfate mixture is the usual contrast medium necessary for an upper G.I. series. On occasion, thick barium may be used in addition to some type of gas-forming preparation. On rare occasions, water-soluble contrast media will be used in preference to the barium sulfate mixture.

The fluoroscopy table is raised to the vertical position, although with some very ill patients the exam must be started with the table horizontal. The room should be clean and tidy, and the control panel should be set for fluoroscopy. The spot film mechanism and the spot film camera should be properly loaded and in working condition. All cassettes for the entire exam should be provided. Lead aprons and lead gloves should be provided for the radiologists, as well as lead aprons for all other personnel in the room. Any other equipment to be utilized during the examination should be readily accessible.

Prior to introduction of the patient and the radiologist, the examination procedure should be carefully explained to the patient and the patient's history should be obtained.

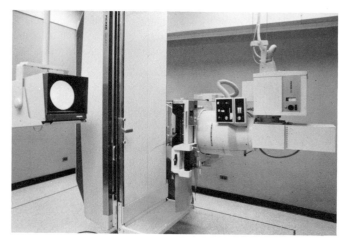

Room Preparation   Fig. 19-49

General Routine Procedure

General duties during fluoroscopy for an upper G.I. series are similar to those for an esophagram. The radiographer should follow the radiologist's instructions, assist the patient as needed and expedite the procedure in any manner possible. The fluoroscopic routine followed by radiologists varies greatly. The general routine of each physician may also vary since each patient and each examination is different. The fluoroscopy routine is usually begun with the patient in the upright position, as illustrated in *Fig. 19-50*. A wide variety of table moves, patient moves and special maneuvers follows until fluoroscopy is complete.

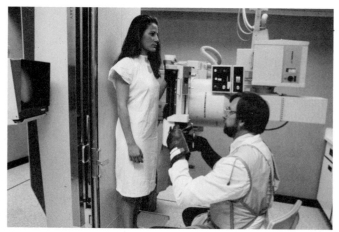

Fluoroscopy   Fig. 19-50

Since a large number of position changes are made during the fluoroscopic examination, the radiographer must help the patient with the barium cup, provide a pillow when the patient is lying down and keep the patient adequately covered at all times. The barium cup should be held by the patient in the left hand near the left shoulder whenever he is upright. The cup must be taken from the patient when the table is tilted up or down.

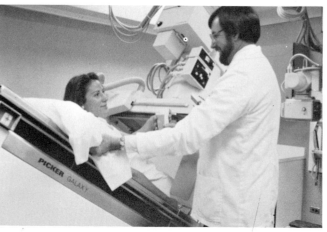

Table Moves   Fig. 19-51

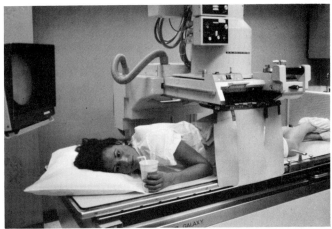

Various patient moves combined with table moves are made during the fluoroscopic procedure. The right anterior oblique position, illustrated in *Fig. 19-52,* allows barium to migrate toward the pyloric portion or distal stomach, while any air in the stomach will shift toward the fundus.

Patient Moves   Fig. 19-52

Post Fluoroscopy Routines

Following fluoroscopy, certain routine positions or projections are obtained to further document any tentative diagnosis concluded fluoroscopically. These overhead radiographs must be obtained immediately following fluoroscopy, before too much of the barium meal has passed into the jejunum.

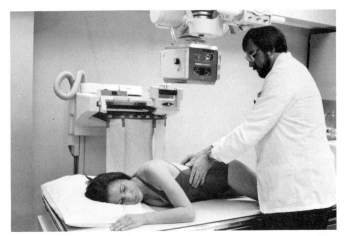

R.A.O. Positioning   Fig. 19-53

Basic and Optional Projections/Positions

Certain basic and optional positions or projections of the esophagus, stomach and duodenum are described and demonstrated on the following pages.

Esophagram. Three positions or projections are considered routine for an esophagram or barium swallow. These include: (1) **R.A.O.,** (2) **P.A. or A.P.,** and (3) **left lateral.** The right anterior oblique is the best single position since the barium-filled esophagus is well demonstrated between the thoracic vertebrae and heart shadow. Variations of the routine left lateral are sometimes required depending on what portion of the patient's anatomy must be best visualized. The retrosternal lateral position removes the shoulders from the area of the esophagus, allowing better visualization of the upper esophagus. When a foreign body is suspected high in the respiratory or digestive tracts, a soft tissue lateral is often the initial radiograph.

Esophagram
  (Barium Swallow)
Basic
- R.A.O. (35 to 40°)
- P.A. or A.P.
- Left Lateral
Optional
- Retrosternal Lateral
- Soft Tissue Lateral

Cardiac Series. The four positions or projections of the cardiac series are considered routine. These include: (1) the **R.A.O. with a 45° obliquity,** (2) the **L.A.O. with a 60° rotation,** (3) the **left lateral,** and (4) the **P.A.** These radiographs are usually taken in this order to insure optimal filling of the esophagus during the P.A. projection.

> **Cardiac Series**
> Basic
> * P.A.
> * Left Lateral
> * R.A.O. (45°)
> * L.A.O. (60°)

Upper G.I. Series. The four most common positions or projections following fluoroscopy during an upper G.I. series are: (1) **the recumbent right anterior oblique position** (R.A.O.), (2) **the recumbent posteroanterior projection** (P.A.), (3) **the recumbent right lateral position** and (4) **the recumbent left posterior oblique position** (L.P.O.). These four positions or projections are listed in order of clinical usefulness. While the routine of each radiologist or other clinical specialist may vary, the R.A.O. and P.A. are considered a minimum series. The routine may include other positions in addition to these four.

Five of the more common optional possibilities following an upper G.I. series include: (1) the upright P.A., (2) the upright left lateral, (3) the recumbent A.P., (4) the recumbent A.P. in the Trendelenburg position, and (5) the recumbent P.A. with a 35 to 45° cephalic angulation of the x-ray beam. The upright P.A. could be compared to the recumbent P.A. to document gastric mobility. The **right** lateral must always be taken when the patient is recumbent to insure filling of the duodenal bulb and distal stomach. The left lateral projection can be taken while the patient is upright, since not only will the distal stomach be barium filled, but also the stomach will be closer to the film. The closer an object is to the film, the better will be the radiographic definition.

The recumbent A.P. can be compared to the P.A. since air and barium will migrate to opposite ends of the stomach. The A.P. Trendelenburg may be utilized to visualize a hiatal hernia, while the angled P.A. is especially helpful to better visualize the hypersthenic type of stomach.

> **Upper G.I. Series**
> Basic
> * R.A.O.
> * P.A.
> * Right Lateral
> * L.P.O.
> Optional
> * P.A. - Upright
> * Left Lateral - Upright
> * A.P.
> * A.P. - Trendelenburg
> * P.A. - Cephalic Angulation

Esophagram
Basic
- **R.A.O.**
- P.A. or A.P.
- Left Lateral

Optional
- Retrosternal Lateral
- Soft Tissue Lateral

Esophagram (Barium Swallow)
• Right Anterior Oblique Position

Film Size:
14 x 17 in. (35 x 43 cm.)

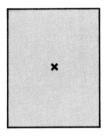

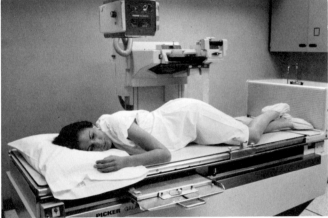

R.A.O. — Recumbent   Fig. 19-54

Bucky:
- Moving or stationary grid.

Patient Position:
- Semiprone or upright with body rotated **35 to 40°.**

Part Position:
- Right anterior body against film holder or table.
- Right arm down; left arm up.
- Flex left knee.

Central Ray:
- C.R. perpendicular to film holder.
- Center to thorax at T-5 to T-6 level.
- 40 in. (102 cm.) or 72 in. (183 cm.) F.F.D.

NOTE: • One to three spoonfuls of thick barium ingested before exposure. • Expose after last bolus is swallowed.

Structures Best Shown:
Esophagus between vertebral column and heart shadow.

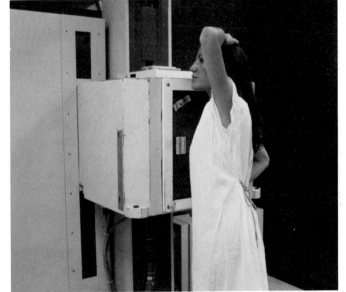

R.A.O. — Upright   Fig. 19-55

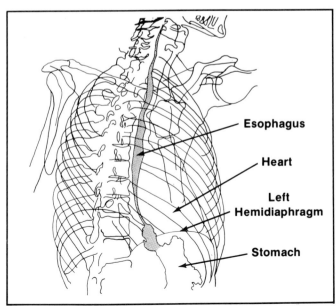

Esophagus

Heart

Left
Hemidiaphragm

Stomach

Fig. 19-57

R.A.O.

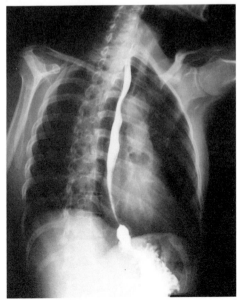

R.A.O.   Fig. 19-56

Esophagram
Basic
- R.A.O.
- **P.A. or A.P.**
- Left Lateral
Optional
- Retrosternal Lateral
- Soft Tissue Lateral

Esophagram (Barium Swallow)

- **Posteroanterior Projection**
- **Anteroposterior Projection**

Film Size:

14 x 17 in. (35 x 43 cm.)

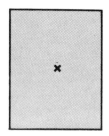

Bucky:

- Moving or stationary grid.

Patient Position:

- Upright with anterior chest against film holder, or supine.
- Midsagittal plane centered to midline of table and/or film.

Part Position:

- True P.A.
- If upright, rotate shoulders against film holder.

Central Ray:

- C.R. perpendicular to film holder.
- Center to thorax at T-5 to T-6 level.
- 40 in. (102 cm.) or 72 in. (183 cm.) F.F.D.

NOTE: • One to three spoonfuls of thick barium ingested before each exposure. • Increase mAs by 50% over P.A. chest exposure since thoracic vertebrae will superimpose esophagus.

Structures Best Shown:

Esophagus.

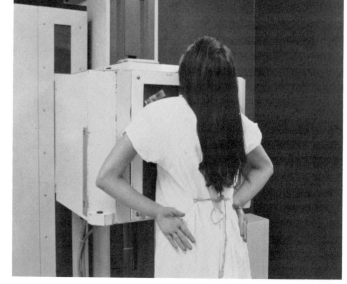

P.A. Upright   Fig. 19-58

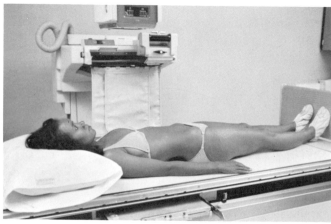

A.P. Recumbent   Fig. 19-59

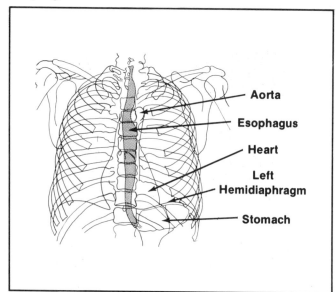

Fig. 19-61

- Aorta
- Esophagus
- Heart
- Left Hemidiaphragm
- Stomach

P.A.

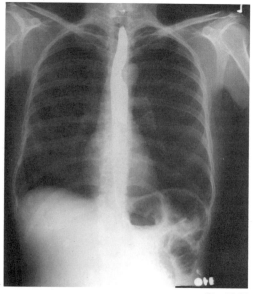

P.A.   Fig. 19-60

Esophagram
Basic
- R.A.O.
- P.A. or A.P.
- **Left Lateral**
Optional
- Retrosternal Lateral
- Soft Tissue Lateral

Esophagram (Barium Swallow)

• Left Lateral Position

Film Size:
14 x 17 in. (35 x 43 cm.)

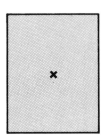

Bucky:
- Moving or stationary grid.

Patient Position:
- Upright with left side against film holder, or left lateral recumbent.

Part Position:
- True lateral; no rotation.
- Arms up.

Central Ray:
- C.R. perpendicular to film holder.
- Center to thorax at T-5 to T-6 level.
- 40 in. (102 cm.) or 72 in. (183 cm.) F.F.D.

NOTE: • One to three spoonfuls of thick barium ingested before exposure.

Structures Best Shown:
Esophagus between vertebral column and heart shadow.

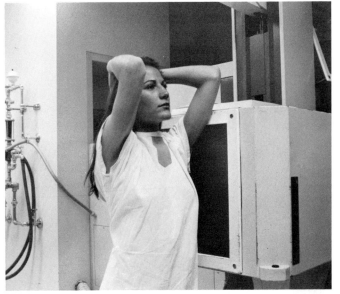

Left Lateral - Upright   Fig. 19-62

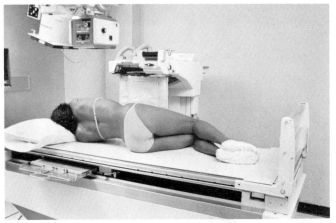

Left Lateral - Recumbent   Fig. 19-63

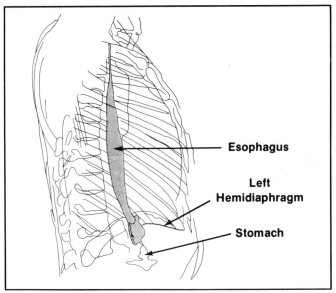

Esophagus

Left
Hemidiaphragm

Stomach

Fig. 19-65
Left Lateral

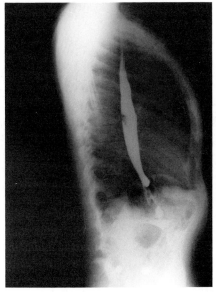

Left Lateral   Fig. 19-64

Esophagram
Basic
- R.A.O.
- P.A. or A.P.
- Left Lateral

Optional
- **Retrosternal Lateral**
- **Soft Tissue Lateral**

Esophagram (Barium Swallow)

• Retrosternal Lateral Position
• Soft Tissue Lateral

Film Size:

Retrosternal Lateral
14 x 17 in. (35 x 43 cm.)

Soft Tissue Lateral
10 x 12 in. (24 x 30 cm.)

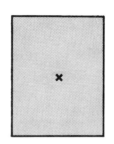
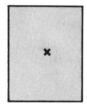

Bucky or Non-Bucky:
- Grid or Screen.

Patient Position:
- Lateral upright.

Part Position:

Retrosternal Lateral
- Same as lateral esophagram, except hands are placed on hips, and both arms and shoulders rotated backward.

Soft Tissue Lateral
- Sitting with shoulders depressed and chin elevated. Similar to lateral cervical spine.

Central Ray:

Retrosternal Lateral
- Center to thorax at T-5 to T-6 level, with C.R. perpendiclar to film holder.

Soft Tissue Lateral
- Center to laryngeal prominence, with C.R. perpendicular to film holder.

NOTE: • Soft tissue lateral is excellent for foreign body visualization.

Structures Best Shown:

Retrosternal Lateral — upper esophagus.

Soft Tissue Lateral — laryngopharynx, larynx, upper esophagus and upper trachea.

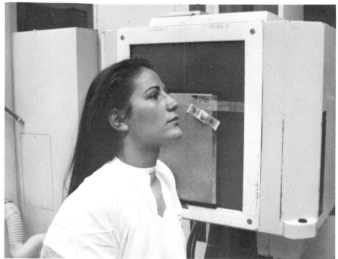

Retrosternal Lateral   Fig. 19-66

Soft Tissue Lateral   Fig. 19-67

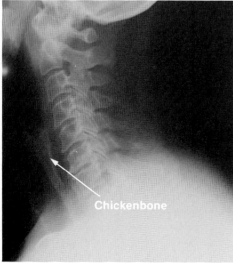

Fig. 19-69   Soft Tissue Lateral
(Positive - Chickenbone)

Chickenbone

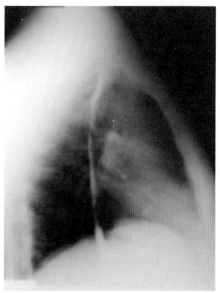

Retrosternal   Fig. 19-68
Lateral

Cardiac Series
Basic
- **P.A.**
- **Left Lateral**
- R.A.O. (45°)
- L.A.O. (60°)

Cardiac Series
- **Posteroanterior Projection**
- **Left Lateral Position**

Film Size:
14 x 17 in. (35 x 43 cm.)

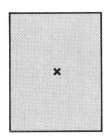

Bucky:
- Moving or stationary grid.

Patient Position

P.A.
- **Upright** with anterior chest against film holder.
- Shoulders rotated forward.
- Backs of hands on hips.

L.Lat.
- **Upright** with left side against film holder.
- Arms up.

Part Position:
- True P.A. or lateral with NO rotation.

Central Ray:
- C.R. perpendicular to film holder.
- Center to thorax at T-6 level.
- 72 in. (183 cm.) F.F.D.

NOTE: • One to three spoonfuls of thick barium ingested before each exposure. • Increase mAs by 50% over P.A. chest exposure.

Structures Best Shown:
Heart and aortic arch and their relationship to lungs and mediastinal structures, including barium-filled esophagus.

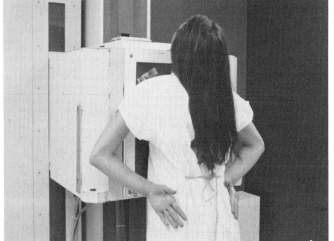

P.A.   Fig. 19-70

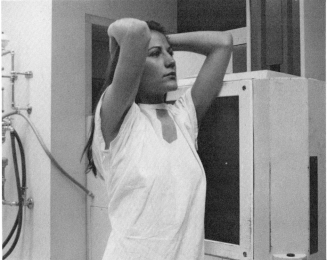

Left Lateral   Fig. 19-71

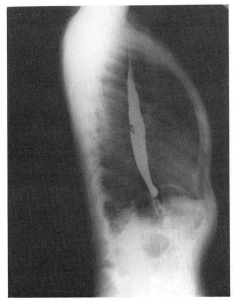

Fig. 19-73   Left Lateral

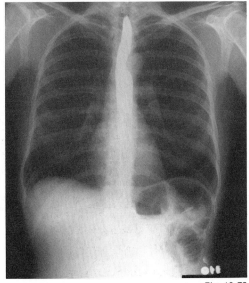

P.A.   Fig. 19-72

Cardiac Series

<table>
<tr><td>
Cardiac Series
Basic
• P.A.
• Left Lateral
• **R.A.O.** (45°)
• **L.A.O.** (60°)
</td></tr>
</table>

Cardiac Series

• **Right Anterior Oblique Position**
• **Left Anterior Oblique Position**

Film Size:

14 x 17 in. (35 x 43 cm.)

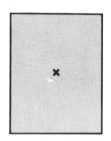

Bucky:
- Moving or stationary grid.

Patient Position:
- Upright with anterior chest against film holder.

Part Position

R.A.O.
- Right anterior chest against film holder with body rotated **45°**.
- Right arm down; left arm up.

L.A.O.
- Left anterior chest against film holder with body rotated **60°**.
- Left arm down; right arm up.

Central Ray:
- C.R. perpendicular to film holder.
- Center to thorax at T-6 level.
- 72 in. (183 cm.) F.F.D.

NOTE: • One to three spoonfuls of thick barium ingested before each exposure. • Heart should be shown between vertebral column and barium-filled esophagus.

Structures Best Shown:
Heart and aortic arch and their relationship to lungs and mediastinal structures, including barium-filled esophagus.

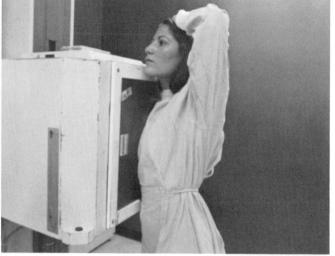

R.A.O. (45°)   Fig. 19-74

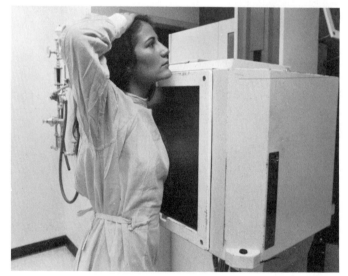

L.A.O. (60°)   Fig. 19-75

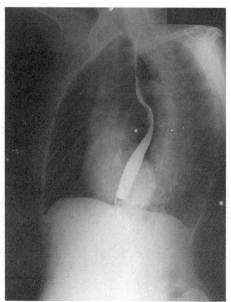

Fig. 19-77   L.A.O.

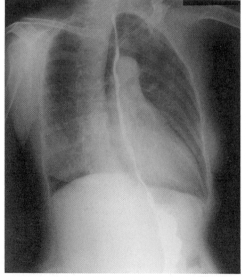

R.A.O.   Fig. 19-76

Upper G.I. Series
Basic
- **R.A.O.**
- P.A.
- Right Lateral
- L.P.O.

Upper G.I. Series
• Right Anterior Oblique Position

Film Size:
    10 x 12 in. (24 x 30 cm.)

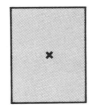

Bucky:
- Moving or stationary grid.

Patient Position:
- Recumbent with right anterior trunk against table.
- Right arm down; left arm up.

Part Position:
- Body usually rotated 45°.
- Longitudinal plane halfway between vertebral spinous processes and lateral margin of body should coincide to center of film.

Central Ray:
- C.R. perpendicular to film holder.
- Center to level of duodenal bulb or **L-2.**
- 40 in. (102 cm.) F.F.D.

NOTE: • Body rotation and exact centering depends on bodily habitus. • Iliac crest and vertebral column should be visible on radiograph. • Closely collimate and expose on expiration.

Structures Best Shown:
Stomach and duodenum with barium in distal stomach and duodenal bulb.

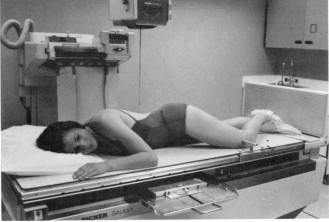

R.A.O.   Fig. 19-78

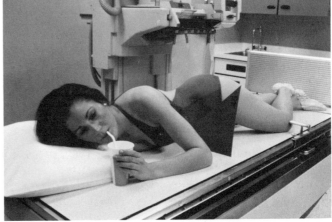

R.A.O.   Fig. 19-79

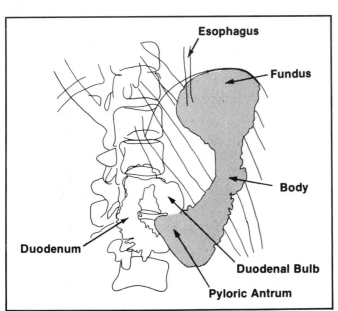

Fig. 19-81

R.A.O.

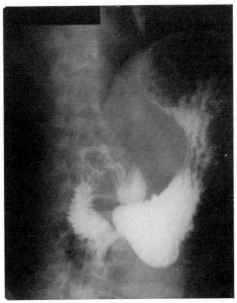

R.A.O.   Fig. 19-80

Upper G.I. Series
Basic
• R.A.O.
• **P.A.**
• Right Lateral
• L.P.O.

Upper G.I. Series

• Posteroanterior Projection

Film Size:

    14 x 17 in. (35 x 43 cm.)

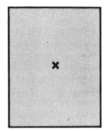

Bucky:

- Moving or stationary grid.

Patient Position:

- Prone with arms up.

Part Position:

- No body rotation.
- Midsagittal plane centered to midline of film and/or table.

Central Ray:

- C.R. perpendicular to film holder.
- Center to level of duodenal bulb or **L-2.**
- 40 in. (102 cm.) F.F.D.

NOTE: • ¾ of radiograph should be above iliac crest.
• Collimate and expose on expiration.

Structures Best Shown:

Distal esophagus, stomach and duodenum, with barium in distal stomach and duodenal bulb.

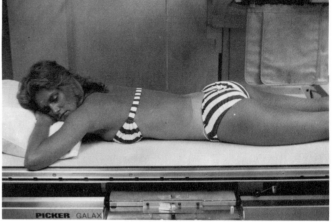

P.A.   Fig. 19-82

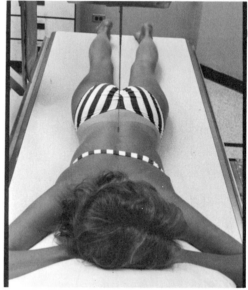

P.A.   Fig. 19-83

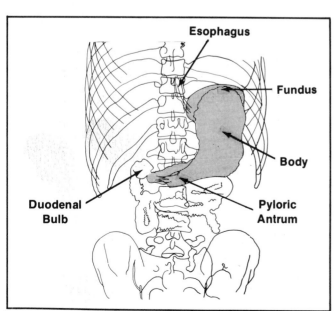

Fig. 19-85   P.A.

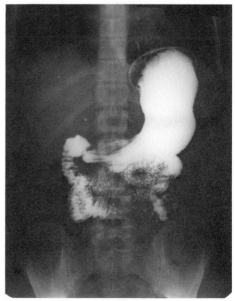

P.A.   Fig. 19-84

Upper G.I. Series
Basic
• R.A.O.
• P.A.
• **Right Lateral**
• L.P.O.

Film Size:
    10 x 12 in. (24 x 30 cm.)

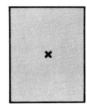

Bucky:
- Moving or stationary grid.

Patient Position:
- Right lateral recumbent.
- Knees flexed; arms up.

Part Position:
- True lateral; no rotation.
- Longitudinal plane halfway between anterior margin of vertebral bodies and anterior abdomen should coincide to center of film.

Central Ray:
- C.R. perpendicular to film holder.
- Center to duodenal bulb or **L-1.**
- May place bottom of cassette at iliac crest.
- 40 in. (102 cm.) F.F.D.

NOTE: • Stomach is located higher in this position; therefore, center one vertebral body more cephalic than on P.A. or R.A.O. • Vertebral bodies should be visible on radiograph for reference purposes. • Closely collimate and expose on expiration.

Structures Best Shown:
Stomach and duodenum, with barium in distal stomach and duodenum.

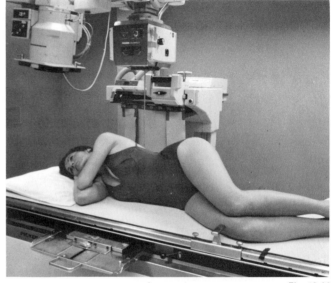

Right Lateral   Fig. 19-86

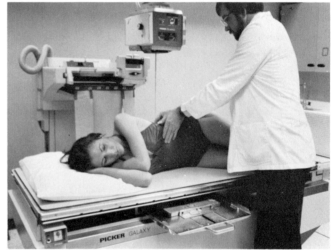

Right Lateral   Fig. 19-87

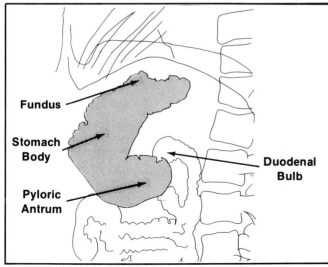

Fig. 19-89

Right Lateral

Fundus

Stomach Body

Pyloric Antrum

Duodenal Bulb

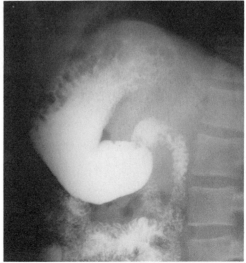

Right Lateral   Fig. 19-88

Upper G.I. Series
Basic
- R.A.O.
- P.A.
- Right Lateral
- **L.P.O.**

Upper G.I. Series
• Left Posterior Oblique Position

Film Size:
10 x 12 in. (24 x 30 cm.)

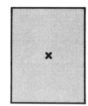

Bucky:
- Moving or stationary grid.

Patient Position:
- Recumbent with left posterior trunk against table.
- Left arm down; right arm up.

Part Position:
- Body usually rotated **45°**.
- Longitudinal plane halfway between vertebral spinous processes and lateral margin of body should coincide with center of film.

Central Ray:
- C.R. perpendicular to film holder.
- Center to level of duodenal bulb or **L-1.**
- 40 in. (102 cm.) F.F.D.

NOTE: • Stomach is located higher in this position; therefore, center one vertebral body more cephalic than on P.A. or R.A.O. • Closely collimate and expose on expiration.

Structures Best Shown:
Stomach and duodenum, with barium in fundus, and air plus barium in distal stomach and duodenum.

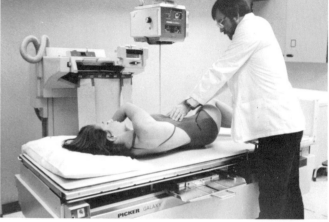

L.P.O.   Fig. 19-90

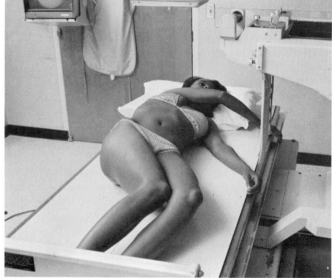

L.P.O.   Fig. 19-91

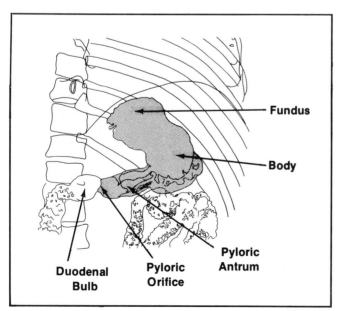

Fig. 19-93

L.P.O.

Labels: **Fundus**, **Body**, **Pyloric Antrum**, **Pyloric Orifice**, **Duodenal Bulb**

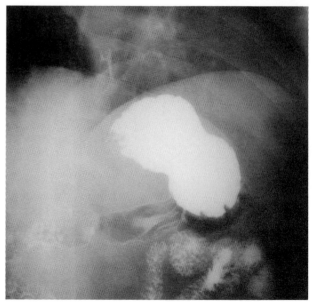

L.P.O.   Fig. 19-92

442

Upper G.I. Series

• Upright Posteroanterior Projection
• Upright Left Lateral Position

Film Size:
14 x 17 in. (35 x 43 cm.)

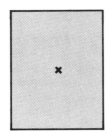

Bucky:
- Moving or stationary grid.

Patient Position:
P.A.
- Upright with thorax against film holder; arms to sides.
L. Lat.
- Upright with left side against film holder; arms up.

Part Position:
- True frontal or lateral position; no rotation.
- Midline of body coincides with midline of film and/or table.

Central Ray:
- C.R. perpendicular to film holder.
- Center to level of duodenal bulb or **L-3 to L-4.**
- 40 in. (102 cm.) F.F.D.

NOTE: • Stomach is much lower when patient is upright.
• Collimate and expose on expiration.

Structures Best Shown:
Stomach and duodenum, with barium in distal stomach and duodenum.

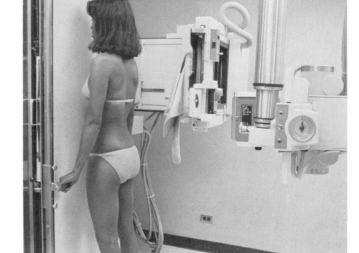

P.A. - Upright

Fig. 19-94

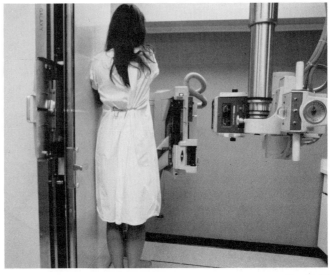

Left Lateral - Upright

Fig. 19-95

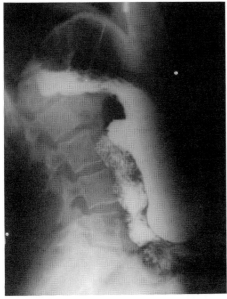

Fig. 19-97
Left Lateral - Upright

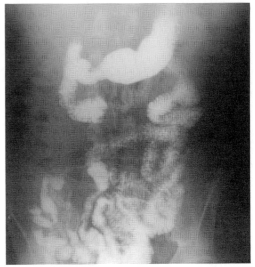

Fig. 19-96

P.A. - Upright

Upper G.I. Series
Optional
- P.A. (Upright)
- Left Lateral (Upright)
- **A.P.**
- **A.P. - Trendelenburg**
- P.A. - Cephalic Angulation

Upper G.I. Series
- **Anteroposterior Projection**
- **Trendelenburg Anteroposterior Projection**

Film Size:
> 14 x 17 in. (35 x 43 cm.)
> **or**
> 10 x 12 in. (24 x 30 cm.)

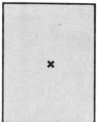

Bucky:
- Moving or stationary grid.

Patient Position:
- Supine with arms down.

Part Position:
- Midsagittal plane coincides with center of film and/or table.

Central Ray:
- C.R. perpendicular to film holder.
- Center to level of duodenal bulb or **L-1.**
- 40 in. (102 cm.) F.F.D.

NOTE: • Stomach is high within abdomen in these positions. • Expose on expiration.

Structures Best Shown:
Stomach and duodenum, with barium in fundus, and air plus barium in distal stomach and duodenum. These positions are helpful in demonstration of hiatal hernia.

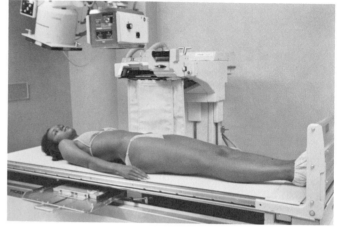

A.P.   Fig. 19-98

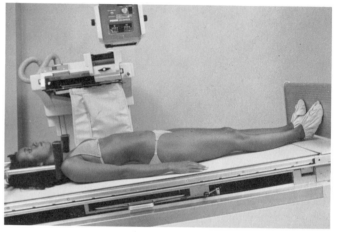

A.P. - Trendelenburg   Fig. 19-99

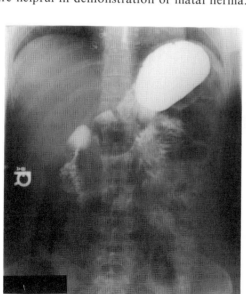

Fig. 19-101

A.P. - Trendelenburg

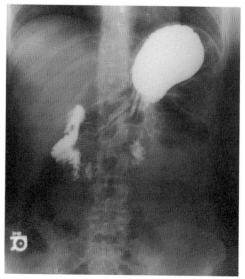

A.P.   Fig. 19-100

Upper G.I. Series

• Posteroanterior Projection with Cephalic Angulation

Film Size:
14 x 17 in. (35 x 43 cm.)

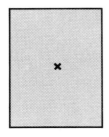

Bucky:
- Moving or stationary grid.

Patient Position:
- Prone with arms up.

Part Position:
- No body rotation.
- Midsagittal plane centered to midline of film and/or table.

Central Ray:
- Center to duodenal bulb or L-2, with cephalic angulation of **35** to **45°**.
- 40 in. (102 cm.) F.F.D.

NOTE: • Used to "open up" the high transverse stomach and project this type of stomach in the shape of a "J".

Structures Best Shown:
Stomach and duodenum, with barium in distal stomach and duodenum. Demonstrates greater and lesser curvatures, pyloric antrum and duodenal bulb.

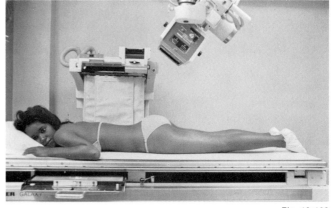

P.A. - Cephalic Angulation   Fig. 19-102

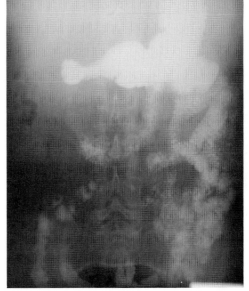

P.A. -   Fig. 19-103
Cephalic Angulation

CHAPTER 20

Radiographic Anatomy and Positioning of the Lower Gastrointestinal System

Part I.   Radiographic Anatomy
Lower Gastrointestinal System

Digestive System

The alimentary canal of the digestive system continues beyond the stomach as the **small intestine.** If the entire small bowel were removed from the body at autopsy, separated from its mesenteric attachment, uncoiled and stretched out, it would average 7 meters or 23 feet in length. During life, with good muscle tone, the actual length of the small intestine is shorter, measuring between 4.5 and 5.5 meters or 15 to 18 feet. Tremendous individual variation does exist, however. In one series of one hundred autopsies, the small bowel varied in length from 15 to 31 feet.

The **large intestine** begins in the lower right quadrant near its connection with the small intestine. The large intestine extends around the periphery of the abdominal cavity to end at the **anus.** The large intestine is about 1.5 meters or 5 feet long.

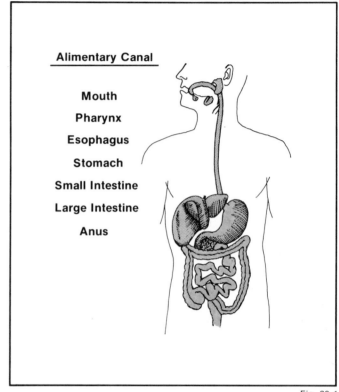

Alimentary Canal

Mouth

Pharynx

Esophagus

Stomach

Small Intestine

Large Intestine

Anus

Digestive System

Fig. 20-1

Common Radiographic Procedures

Common radiographic procedures involving the lower gastrointestinal system are presented in this chapter. All common radiographic examinations of the lower gastrointestinal system involve administration of a contrast medium.

Common Radiographic Procedures
(Contrast media are administered)

1. Small Bowel Series (S.B.S.)
   - Study of small intestine

2. Barium Enema (B.E.) (Lower G.I. Series) (Colon)
   - Study of large intestine

Radiographic examination specifically of the small intestine is termed a **small bowel series** or S.B.S. This examination is often combined with an upper G.I. series and, under these conditions, may be termed a small bowel follow-through.

The radiographic procedure designed to study the large intestine is most commonly termed a **barium enema.** Alternate designations include B.E., lower G.I. series or colon. An example of a barium enema radiograph is shown in *Fig. 20-2.*

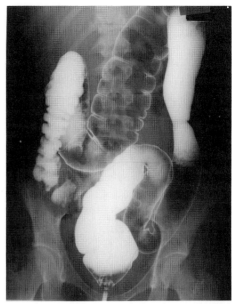

A.P. — Barium Enema   Fig. 20-2

Small Intestine

The small intestine is located primarily in the central portion of the abdominal cavity. Beginning at the pyloric valve of the stomach, the three parts of the small bowel, in order, are **duodenum, jejunum** and **ileum.** The duodenum or first part of the small intestine is the shortest, widest and most fixed portion of the small bowel. Since the jejunum and ileum are much longer than the duodenum, and since the duodenum is posteriorly located, the many loops of small bowel shown in *Fig. 20-3* are jejunum and ileum. A detailed study of the C-shaped duodenum is presented in Chapter 19.

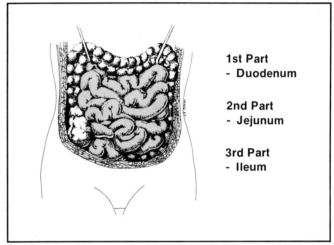

**1st Part
- Duodenum**

**2nd Part
- Jejunum**

**3rd Part
- Ileum**

Small Intestine   Fig. 20-3

Duodenum

The **duodenum** measures a fairly constant 10 inches (25 centimeters) in length and is much shorter than the other two sections of the small intestine. The usual position of the duodenum is outlined with small x's in *Fig. 20-4.*

Jejunum

The **jejunum** is located primarily to the left of midline in the upper and lower quadrants of the abdomen, making up about **two-fifths** of the small bowel remaining after the duodenum. The normal region of the jejunum is illustrated by the light gray portion of *Fig. 20-4.*

Ileum

The **ileum** is located primarily in the midabdomen and pelvis. Approximately **three-fifths** of the small bowel remaining after the duodenum is ileum. The usual area of the ileum is illustrated in *Fig. 20-4* by the dark gray area. The terminal ileum ascends from the pelvis to join the large intestine at the ileocecal valve.

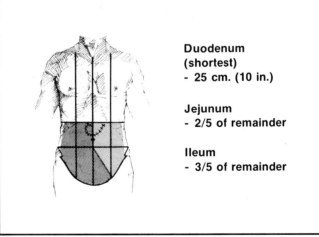

**Duodenum
(shortest)
- 25 cm. (10 in.)**

**Jejunum
- 2/5 of remainder**

**Ileum
- 3/5 of remainder**

Small Intestine   Fig. 20-4

Section Differences

The various sections of small intestine can be identified radiographically by their location and appearance. The C-shaped **duodenum** is fairly fixed in position. The proximal duodenum with its **bulb** or **cap** is unique and can be easily recognized on radiographs of the duodenum. The internal lining of the descending duodenum is thrown into circular folds. The circular folds continue throughout the remainder of the duodenum and are found in the jejunum as well. Radiographically, when the distal duodenum and the **jejunum** contain air, and especially when the bowel is distended, the internal lining of the duodenum and jejunum resemble a **coiled spring** or a stack of silver dollars. When it contains barium, the appearance is described as **feathery.**

While there is no abrupt end to the circular folds, the **ileum** tends not to have these indentations. Consequently, the internal lining of the ileum as it appears on a radiograph is **smoother** and does not have the feathery appearance. A final observable difference in the three sections of small intestine is that the internal diameter gets progressively smaller from duodenum to ileum.

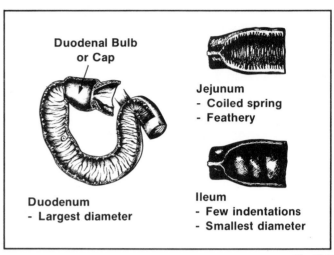

Small Intestine

Fig. 20-5

Radiographs

Two radiographs illustrating differences in the various portions of the small intestine are shown in *Fig. 20-6*. The small bowel radiograph to the left demonstrates the visible difference between the jejunum and the ileum. In the patient's left upper abdomen is seen a feathery-appearing small bowel. This feathery appearance is characteristic of the **jejunum.** Lower in the midabdomen, loops of ileum are shown. The **ileum** appears more like a small pipe than does the duodenum or jejunum. The terminal ileum connects to the large bowel at the **ileocecal valve** in the lower right quadrant.

The radiograph on the right demonstrates the coiled spring appearance of the proximal small bowel. This patient has a small bowel obstruction so the more proximal jejunum is markedly expanded with air.

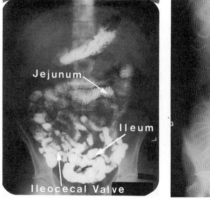

Small Intestine Radiographs

Fig. 20-6

Large Intestine

The large intestine begins in the lower right quadrant near the **ileocecal valve.** That portion of the large intestine inferior to the ileocecal valve is a saclike area termed the **cecum.** The appendix is a relatively long, narrow, blind tube that communicates with the cecum.

The vertical portion of the large intestine superior to the cecum is the **ascending colon,** which continues as the **transverse colon** after the **hepatic flexure.** The **descending colon** continues from the transverse colon after another sharp bend termed the **splenic flexure.** The descending colon continues as the S-shaped **sigmoid colon** in the lower left quadrant. The final segment of the large bowel is the **rectum.** The distal rectum contains the anal canal which ends at the **anus.**

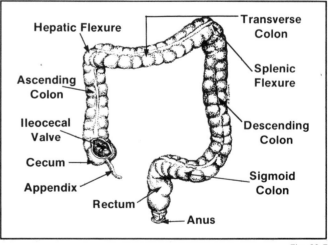

Large Intestine

Fig. 20-7

Large Intestine vs. Colon

Large intestine and colon are **NOT** synonyms, although many persons use these terms interchangeably. According to *Gray's Anatomy,* the **colon** consists of four parts and does not include the cecum and rectum. The four parts of the colon are (1) the **ascending colon,** (2) the **transverse colon,** (3) the **descending colon,** and (4) the **sigmoid colon.** The cecum and rectum are considered part of the large intestine, but are not part of the colon.

Alternate names for certain parts of the large bowel are given in *Fig. 20-8.* **Colic valve** is a second name for the more common ileocecal valve. The more common appendix may be referred to as the **vermiform process.** The hepatic flexure may be referred to as the **right colic flexure,** while the splenic flexure may be called the **left colic flexure.** The distal portion of the descending colon is sometimes called the **iliac colon,** while the sigmoid colon may be termed the **pelvic colon.**

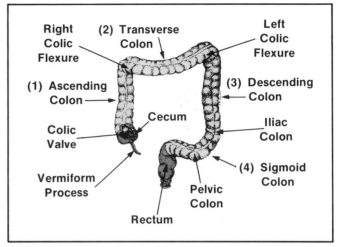

Colon

Fig. 20-8

Cecum

The **cecum** is a large, blind pouch located below the level of the ileocecal valve. The cecum, with its attached **appendix,** is the most proximal portion of the large bowel. The internal appearance of the cecum and **terminal ileum** is shown in *Fig. 20-9.* The most distal part of the ileum ascends from the depths of the pelvis to join the cecum at the **ileocecal valve.** The ileocecal valve consists of two lips that extend toward the large bowel.

The ileocecal valve acts as a sphincter to prevent the contents of the ileum from passing too quickly into the cecum. A second function of the ileocecal valve is to prevent reflux, or a backward flow of large intestine contents, into the ileum. The ileocecal valve does only a fair job of preventing reflux since some barium can almost always be refluxed into the terminal ileum when a barium enema is done. The cecum is the widest portion of the large intestine and is fairly free to move about in the lower right quadrant.

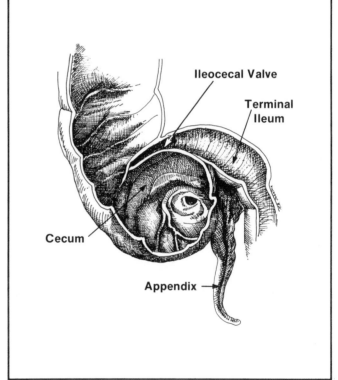

Cecum

Fig. 20-9

451

Appendix

The **appendix** or **vermiform process** is a long, narrow, worm-shaped tube extending from the cecum. The term, vermiform, in fact, means wormlike. The appendix is usually attached to the posteromedial aspect of the cecum and commonly extends toward the pelvis. It may pass back of the ileum, however, or even lie posterior to the cecum. Since the appendix has a blind ending, infectious agents may enter an appendix that does not or cannot empty itself. The result is appendicitis. An inflamed appendix may require surgical removal, termed an appendectomy, before the diseased structure ruptures and causes peritonitis. Peritonitis is inflammation of the lining of the abdomen. Occasionally, fecal matter or barium sulfate from a G.I. tract study may fill the appendix and remain there indefinitely.

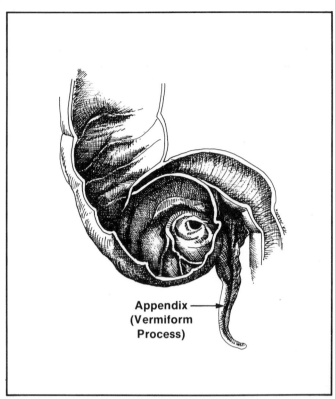

Appendix (Vermiform Process)

Appendix   Fig. 20-10

Colon

The four parts of the colon are smaller in diameter than is the **cecum.** The **transverse colon** is the longest part of the colon and possesses considerable up and down movement. It normally loops downward beyond the hepatic flexure as it passes to the left along the anterior surface of the abdominal cavity. Since the liver is such a large, solid organ, the hepatic flexure usually lies lower in the abdomen than does the splenic flexure which lies beneath the inferior pole of the spleen.

The sigmoid colon normally lies in the pelvis, but does possess a wide freedom of motion. The sigmoid colon and the cecum are the two parts of the large intestine that possess the widest freedom of motion. The sigmoid colon finally passes posteriorly and inferiorly along the curve of the sacrum to continue as the **rectum.**

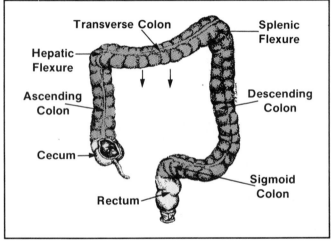

Transverse Colon — Splenic Flexure — Hepatic Flexure — Ascending Colon — Descending Colon — Cecum — Rectum — Sigmoid Colon

Colon   Fig. 20-11

Rectum

The **rectum** extends from the sigmoid colon to the **anus.** The rectum begins at the level of S-3 and is about 12 centimeters long. The final 3 centimeters of rectum are constricted to form the **anal canal.** The anal canal terminates as an opening to the exterior, the anus. The rectum closely follows the sacrococcygeal curve as demonstrated in *Fig. 20-12.*

The **rectal ampulla** is a dilated portion of the rectum located anterior to the coccyx. The initial direction of the rectum along the **sacrum** is down and back; however, in the region of the rectal ampulla, the direction changes to down and forward. A second abrupt change in direction occurs in the region of the anal canal, which is directed downward and backward. Therefore, the rectum presents **two anteroposterior curves.** This fact must be remembered when a rectal tube or enema tip is inserted into the lower G.I. tract.

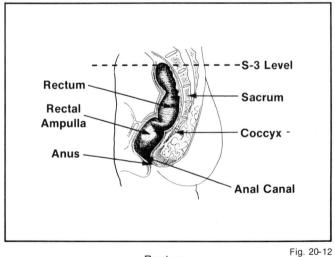

Rectum — Rectal Ampulla — Anus — S-3 Level — Sacrum — Coccyx — Anal Canal

Rectum   Fig. 20-12

452

Intestine Differences

Certain characteristics readily differentiate the large intestine from the small intestine. Although the internal diameter of the large intestine is usually greater than the diameter of the small bowel, two other distinguishing characteristics are radiographically apparent. The longitudinal muscle fibers of the large bowel form three **bands of muscle** which tend to pull the large intestine into pouches. Each of these pouches or sacculations is termed a **haustrum,** so one primary identifying characteristic of the large bowel is the presence of haustra.

Another key to differentiation is the relative positions of the two structures. The **large intestine** extends around the **periphery** of the abdominal cavity, while the **small intestine** is more **centrally** located.

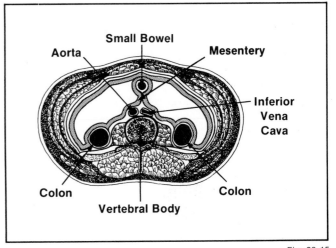

Intestine Differences   Fig. 20-13

Abdominal Cavity

Peritoneum

The abdominal cavity contains many organs. Not only does this largest of all cavities contain the major portion of the gastrointestinal system and its accessory organs, but it also contains certain organs of the endocrine, circulatory and urogenital systems. Most of these structures, as well as the wall of the abdominal cavity in which they are contained, are covered to varying degrees by an extensive serous membrane termed the **peritoneum.** In fact, the total surface area of peritoneum is about equal to the total surface area of the skin covering the entire body.

A simplified transverse section of the abdominal cavity is shown in *Fig. 20-14*. Peritoneum adhering to the cavity wall is termed **parietal peritoneum,** while that portion covering an organ is termed **visceral peritoneum.** The parietal and visceral layers form one continuous sheet. Inside this peritoneal lining is a cavity, the **peritoneal cavity,** which is mainly filled with various organs. If all the loops of bowel and the other organs of the abdominal cavity were drawn in, there would be very little actual space left in the peritoneal cavity.

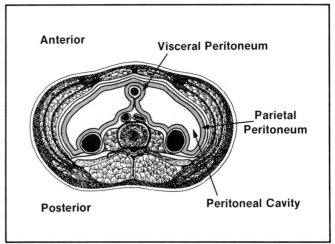

Abdominal Cavity   Fig. 20-14
(cross section)

Mesentery

The simplified cross section of the abdominal cavity illustrated in *Fig. 20-15* demonstrates three important facts. First, there is a double fold of peritoneum extending anteriorly from the region in front of the vertebral body at this level. This double fold of peritoneum completely envelops a loop of small bowel. The specific term for a double fold of peritoneum connecting the posterior abdominal wall to an organ is **mesentery.** Second, a layer of parietal peritoneum partially covers certain organs. At this level, both the ascending colon and the descending colon are partially covered. Third, some structures, such as the aorta and inferior vena cava, are located completely behind or posterior to the parietal peritoneum. Organs or other structures located behind the peritoneum are termed **retroperitoneal structures.**

Abdominal Cavity   Fig. 20-15
(cross section)

Greater Sac vs. Lesser Sac

The midsagittal sectional drawing of an adult female, *Fig. 20-16*, shows peritoneum partially or completely covering various abdominal organs, as well as lining the abdominal cavity itself. The major portion of the peritoneal cavity, shown in dark gray, is termed the **greater sac.** A smaller portion of the peritoneal cavity located posterior to the stomach is termed the **lesser sac.** In *Fig. 20-16,* **mesentery** is seen connecting a loop of small bowel (ileum) to the posterior abdominal wall. Mesentery also connects the transverse colon to the posterior abdominal wall. This specific double fold of peritoneum is termed the **transverse mesocolon.**

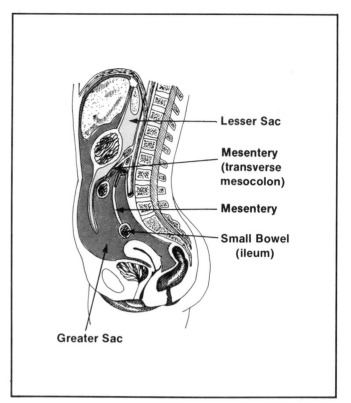

Fig. 20-16

Abdominal Cavity
(midsagittal section)

Omentum

A different type of double fold of peritoneum, termed **omentum,** is shown in *Fig. 20-17.* Omentum is a term applied to a double fold of peritoneum extending from the stomach to another organ. The **lesser omentum** extends superiorly from the stomach to portions of the liver. The **greater omentum** connects the transverse colon to the stomach inferiorly. The greater omentum extends down over the small bowel to form an apron along the anterior abdominal wall.

Note that certain structures such as the rectum, bladder and uterus lie beneath the parietal peritoneum within the true pelvis.

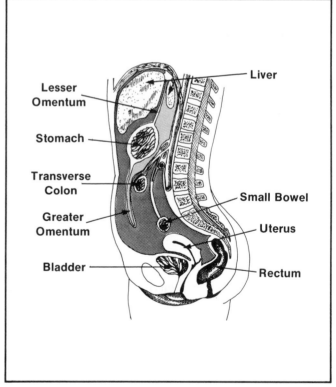

Fig. 20-17

Abdominal Cavity
(midsagittal section)

Greater Omentum

The drawing on the left in *Fig. 20-18* demonstrates the abdominal cavity with the anterior abdominal wall, muscles and peritoneum removed. The first structure encountered beneath the peritoneum is the **greater omentum.** Varying amounts of fat are deposited in the greater omentum, which serves as a layer of insulation between the abdominal cavity and the exterior. A portion of the greater omentum has been omitted from this drawing to reveal the organs beneath.

The drawing on the right in *Fig. 20-18* illustrates the apron-like construction of the greater omentum. The bottom edge of the greater omentum could be lifted, as shown, to expose the small bowel beneath and to show the connection between the greater omentum and the transverse colon. The **transverse mesocolon** is seen connecting the transverse colon to the posterior abdominal wall.

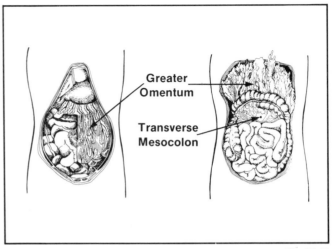

Greater Omentum   Fig. 20-18

Retroperitoneal and Pelvic Organs

Figure 20-19 illustrates the abdominal cavity after removal of all structures either partially or completely covered by visceral peritoneum. Organs that have been removed are the liver, gallbladder, spleen, stomach, jejunum, ileum, cecum and the entire colon. The remaining organs are considered **retroperitoneal** or **pelvic,** that is, those structures lying entirely behind or under the parietal peritoneum.

Retroperitoneal Organs. Structures that are retroperitoneal are the **kidneys** and **ureters, adrenal glands, pancreas, duodenum** and the **large blood vessels.** Two structures very often confused and erroneously thought to be located within the abdominal cavity are the **pancreas** and **duodenum.** These two structures are retroperitoneal.

Pelvic Organs. Located beneath the peritoneum in the **true pelvis** are the **rectum, urinary bladder** and **reproductive organs.**

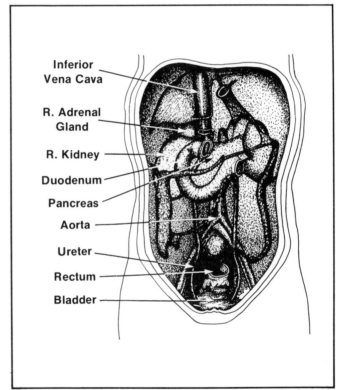

Retroperitoneal and Pelvic Organs   Fig. 20-19

Abdominopelvic Cavity (from left side)

The relative locations of various abdominal organs, as seen from the **left side,** are shown in *Fig. 20-20.* The **stomach** lies just inferior to the diaphragm, with its **fundus** much more posterior than the **body.** The **spleen** of the circulatory system nestles against the stomach and against the posterior abdominal wall. The spleen is ordinarily protected by the lower posterior rib cage.

The **transverse colon** lies underneath the greater omentum. The transverse colon is far anterior in the abdominal cavity, while its continuation, the **descending colon,** lies against the posterior abdominal wall. The S-shaped **sigmoid colon** first extends toward the anterior, then loops back posteriorly to continue as the rectum.

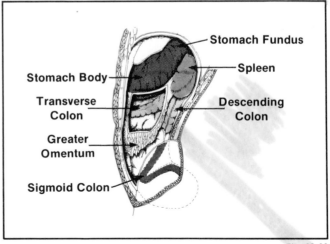

Abdominopelvic Cavity
(left side)   Fig. 20-20

Abdominopelvic Cavity (from right side)

The **abdominopelvic cavity** as seen from the **right side** is shown in *Fig. 20-21*. The large **liver** occupies most of the upper abdominal cavity on this side. Lying beneath the liver, but anterior to the midaxillary line, is the **gallbladder**. The right **kidney,** right **adrenal gland, duodenum** and **head of the pancreas** are retroperitoneal structures.

The **transverse colon** is far anterior compared to the **cecum** which lies against the posterior abdominal wall. The worm-like **appendix** extends inferiorly from the **cecum.** The cecum and appendix lie below the level of the **iliac crest.** The relative positions of various abdominal organs, both side to side and front to back, are important for the radiographer to know.

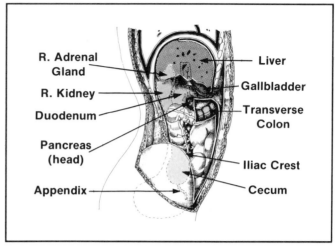

Abdominopelvic Cavity
(right side)

Fig. 20-21

Relative Locations of Air and Barium in Stomach and Intestine

The simplified drawing in *Fig. 20-22* represents the stomach and large bowel in both the **prone** and **supine positions.** If the stomach and large intestine were to contain both **air** and **barium sulfate,** the air would tend to rise and the barium would tend to sink due to gravity. The displacement and ultimate location of air is shown as dark gray. When a person is supine, air rises to fill those structures that are most anterior, which are the transverse colon, sigmoid colon, and the body and distal end of the stomach. The barium sinks to fill primarily the fundus of the stomach, the duodenal portion of the small bowel, and both the ascending and descending portions of the colon and the rectum.

When a patient is prone, barium and air reverse positions. The drawing on the right illustrates the prone position, hence, air has risen to fill the rectum, ascending colon, descending colon, fundus and duodenal bulb. This spatial relationship is important both during fluoroscopy and during radiography when performing the barium enema or stomach examinations.

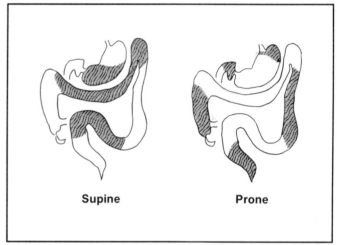

Supine   **Prone**

Barium versus Air

Fig. 20-22

Supine Barium
fundus
Duodenum
Ascending Colon
Descending Colon
Rectum

456

Mechanical Digestion

Small Intestine. Mechanical digestion throughout the length of the small bowel consists of (1) **peristalsis** to propel intestinal contents along the digestive tract, and (2) **rhythmic segmentation** to thoroughly mix digested food and facilitate absorption.

Large Intestine. In the large intestine, mechanical digestion continues with (1) **peristalsis,** (2) **haustral churning,** (3) **mass peristalsis** and (4) **defecation.** Mass peristalsis tends to move the entire large bowel contents into the sigmoid colon and rectum, usually happening once every 24 hours. Defecation is a so-called bowel movement or emptying of the rectum.

Small Intestine	Peristalsis Rhythmic segmentation
Large Intestine	Peristalsis Haustral churning Mass peristalsis Defecation

Mechanical Digestion

Fig. 20-23

Digestive Functions of the Intestines

Three primary digestive functions accomplished largely by the small and large intestines are **digestion, absorption** and **elimination.** Most digestion and absorption take place within the small bowel, while any unused or unnecessary material is eliminated by the large bowel. Certain necessary substances are also absorbed from the large bowel.

Large Intestine. The primary function of the large intestine is the elimination of feces. Feces consist normally of 40 percent water and 60 percent solid matter, such as food residues, digestive secretions and bacteria. Other specific functions of the large bowel are absorption of water, absorption of inorganic salt, and absorption of vitamins **K** and **D** in addition to certain amino acids. These vitamins and amino acids are produced by a large collection of naturally occurring microorganisms found in the large intestine.

1) Digestion
   (small intestine)

2) Absorption
   (small intestine)

3) Elimination
   (large intestine)

Lower Digestive System Functions

Fig. 20-24

Part II. Radiographic Positioning
Lower Gastrointestinal System

Lower Gastrointestinal System

The plain abdominal radiograph shown in *Fig. 20-25* is of a healthy, ambulatory adult. The many meters of small intestine are not visible in the central portion of the abdomen. In the normal, ambulatory adult, any collection of gas in the small intestine is considered abnormal. Without any gas present, the small bowel simply blends in with other soft tissue structures and cannot be visualized.

Due to variable amounts of gas and fecal matter normally present in the large intestine, this structure is grossly, but inadequately, visualized on the plain radiograph. Therefore, radiographic examination of the alimentary canal distal to the stomach and duodenum requires the introduction of contrast media for diagnostic visualization.

Small Bowel Series

Radiographic examination specifically of the small intestine is termed a **small bowel series,** or S.B.S. The upper G.I. series and small bowel series are often combined. Under these circumstances, the small bowel portion of the exam may be termed a small bowel follow-through.

Purpose. The purpose of the small bowel series is to study radiographically the form and function of the three parts of the small intestine, as well as to detect any abnormal conditions.

Common Abnormalities. Common abnormalities seen in the small intestine are (1) enteritis, often involving the stomach as well, thus gastroenteritis; (2) neoplasms, including benign lesions and, rarely, carcinomas; (3) various malabsorption syndromes and (4) ileus, which means obstruction. Two types of obstruction are seen. First is the adynamic or paralytic ileus that results when the bowel does not propel its contents forward properly. In this type of ileus, the intestine slows or ceases normal function, due usually to an infection in neighboring structures, such as peritonitis or appendicitis. A second type is the mechanical ileus that results from a blockage caused by adhesions, strictures, hernias or other mechanical problems.

Contraindications. There are few strict contraindications to contrast media studies of the intestinal tract. Presurgical patients and patients suspected of having a perforated, hollow viscus should **not** receive barium sulfate. The water-soluble, iodinated media should be used instead. Barium sulfate by mouth is contraindicated in patients with a possible large bowel obstruction. An obstructed large bowel should first be ruled out with an acute abdominal series and a barium enema.

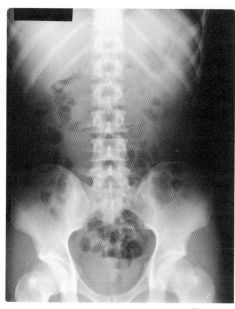

Fig. 20-25

Plain
Abdominal Radiograph

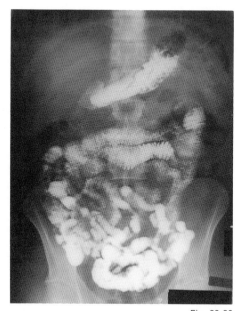

Fig. 20-26

Small Bowel
Radiograph

458

Small Intestine Radiographic Examinations

Five methods are used to study the small intestine radiographically. These are listed in order of the most common to the least common. Of the five methods used to study the small intestine, the combination upper G.I. — small bowel is the most often used. Next are the small bowel only series and the accelerated methods. Seldom used are the small bowel enemas, and the retrograde small bowel or reflux method.

1. Upper G.I. — Small Bowel Combination

For the upper G.I. — small bowel combination, a routine upper G.I. series is done first. After the routine stomach study, progress of the barium is followed through the entire small bowel. During a routine upper G.I. series, the patient should have ingested one full cup or 8 ounces of barium sulfate mixture. For any small bowel examination, the exact time that the patient initially ingested barium should be noted because timing for sequential radiographs is based on the first ingestion of barium.

After completion of fluoroscopy and routine radiography of the stomach, the patient is given one additional cup of barium to ingest. The second cup of barium may be difficult for the patient to down since that amount of barium is a lot to swallow. Thirty minutes after the initial barium ingestion, a P.A. radiograph of the proximal small bowel is obtained. This first radiograph of the small bowel series (marked "30 minutes") is usually obtained about 15 minutes after completion of the U.G.I. series.

Radiographs are obtained at specific intervals throughout the small bowel series until the barium sulfate column passes through the ileocecal valve and progresses into the ascending colon. For the first 2 hours in the small bowel series, radiographs are usually obtained at half-hour intervals. If it becomes necessary to continue the examination beyond the 2-hour time frame, then radiographs are usually obtained every hour until barium passes through the ileocecal valve.

Inspection of Radiographs. As soon as each radiograph in the small bowel series is processed, it should be inspected by the radiologist. The physician may wish to examine any suspicious area under the fluoroscope or request additional radiographs. The region of the terminal ileum and ileocecal valve is usually studied fluoroscopically. Spot filming of the terminal ileum usually indicates completion of the examination. The patient shown in *Fig. 20-27* is in position under the compression cone, which may be utilized to spread out loops of ileum to better visualize the ileocecal valve. The radiologist may request delayed imaging in order to follow the barium through the entire large bowel. A barium meal given by mouth usually reaches the rectum in 24 hours.

Small Intestine Studies

1. U.G.I. — small bowel combination
2. Small bowel only series
3. Accelerated small bowel series
4. Small bowel enema
5. Retrograde small bowel or reflux method

SUMMARY OF PROCEDURE

1. Upper G.I. — Small Bowel Combination

Procedure:

- Routine U.G.I. first
- Note time patient ingested first cup (8 oz.) of barium
- Ingest second cup of barium
- 30-minute P.A. radiograph (center high for proximal S.B.)
- Half-hour interval radiographs, centered to iliac crest, until barium reaches large bowel (usually 2 hrs.)
- One-hour interval radiographs, if more time is needed after two hours

Optional:

- Fluoroscopy and spot filming of ileocecal valve and terminal ileum (compression cone may be used)

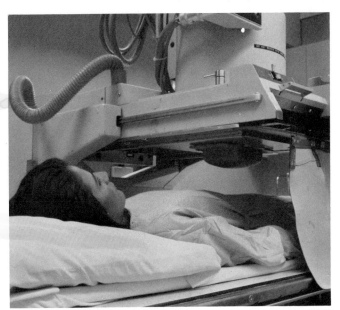

Fig. 20-27

Compression Cone

2. Small Bowel Only Series

The second possibility for study of the small intestine is the small bowel only series. For every contrast medium examination, including the small bowel series, a plain radiograph should be obtained before introduction of the contrast medium. If a routine abdomen was not obtained previously, it would be the first radiograph of any series depicting the small bowel. For the small bowel only series, 2 cups of barium are ingested by the patient. One-half hour later the first radiograph of the series is obtained with high centering to include the diaphragm. From this point on, the exam is exactly like the follow-up series of the U.G.I. Half-hour radiographs are taken for 2 hours, with one-hour radiographs thereafter, until barium is well into the ascending colon. In the routine small bowel series, regular barium sulfate ordinarily reaches the large intestine within 2 or 3 hours.

3. Accelerated Small Bowel Series

The accelerated small bowel series is done if normal gastric and intestinal motility is **not** a prime reason for performing the examination. If there is a need to see the entire small bowel as quickly as possible, then a different barium recipe or examination approach is needed. Three methods are commonly used to accelerate the normal transit time to less than one hour. The first method uses normal saline, rather than water, when mixing the barium sulfate suspension. Additionally, the mixture should be well chilled before use. A second method calls for the usual chilled barium and water mixture with 10 milliliters of Gastrografin® added. Finally, various drugs may be injected into the patient to increase peristaltic activity of the small bowel and thus increase motility. Each of these methods causes acceleration of the barium meal.

The special barium sulfate mixture is ingested after a plain scout radiograph. Half-hour interval radiographs are obtained until barium sulfate reaches the large intestine.

4. Small Bowel Enema

The fourth method of small bowel examination is termed the small bowel enema. This method requires passage of the long tube through the nose, esophagus and stomach, and into the small intestine. When the end of the tube reaches the part of the small bowel to be studied radiographically, barium is injected into the opposite end of the tube. The injection is usually made under fluoroscopic control, then radiographs are exposed every half hour until the exam is terminated by the radiologist.

SUMMARY OF PROCEDURE

2. Small Bowel Only Series

Procedure:

- Plain abdomen radiograph
- 2 cups of barium ingested (note time)
- 30-minute radiograph (center high)
- Half-hour interval radiographs until barium reaches large bowel (usually 2 hrs.)
- One-hour interval radiographs, if more time is needed

SUMMARY OF PROCEDURE

3. Accelerated Small Bowel Series

Three methods:

1 - Saline used rather than water, when mixing barium
2 - 10 ml. of Gastrografin® added to regular barium.
3 - Various drugs injected into patient

Procedure:

- Plain abdominal radiograph
- Barium ingested
- Half-hour interval radiographs until barium reaches large bowel (usually 1 hr. or less)

SUMMARY OF PROCEDURE

4. Small Bowel Enema

Procedure:

- Tube inserted through nose into small bowel
- Barium injected into tube (under fluoroscopic control)
- Radiographs taken at 30-minute intervals until the exam is terminated

---

5. Retrograde Small Bowel or Reflux Method

The final method of small bowel study is termed the retrograde small bowel or reflux method. As the name suggests, the small bowel is filled retrograde (reverse direction of normal flow) through the rectum and large intestine. When large amounts of barium followed by normal saline are given via barium enema, some of the barium will reflux into the small intestine. After the small bowel is filled, the patient is allowed to evacuate the large intestine contents. Radiographs and fluoroscopic spots are then made of the small bowel. The small bowel enema and the retrograde small bowel are the least commonly used techniques to study the small intestine.

5. Retrograde Small Bowel or Reflux Method

Procedure:

- Enema tip inserted into rectum

- Large intestine filled with barium followed by normal saline

- Barium allowed to reflux into the small bowel until it is filled

- Large intestine contents evacuated

- Small bowel fluoroscoped and radiographed

Patient Preparation

Patient preparation for a small bowel series is identical to that for an upper G.I. series. In fact, the most common method of small bowel study is a combination of the two examinations into one long examination with the small bowel series following the U.G.I. series. The goal of patient preparation for either the upper G.I. series or the small bowel series is an empty stomach. Food and fluid must be withheld for at least 8 hours prior to these exams. In addition, the patient should not smoke cigarettes or chew gum during the N.P.O. period.

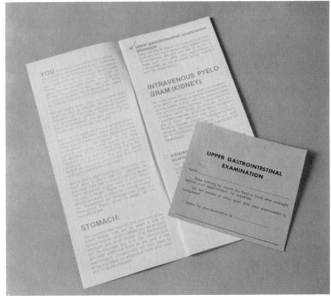

Patient Preparation

Fig. 20-28

Radiographic Room Preparation

Radiographic room preparation depends on the type of small bowel series to be performed. For the upper G.I. — small bowel combination, room preparation is exactly the same as for an upper G.I. series. One additional full cup (8 ounces) of barium sulfate mixture is needed. Initial radiographs for both the small bowel only series and the accelerated small bowel series can be made in any general radiographic room, unless the radiologist wishes to fluoroscope the patient's abdomen prior to ingestion of the barium sulfate mixture. Most of the sequentially timed radiographs in any small bowel series are performed in a general radiographic room.

For the small bowel enema, a general fluoroscopic room is necessary since a nasogastric tube must be advanced to the proximal small bowel. Since the retrograde small bowel or reflux method begins as a barium enema, a general fluoroscopic room is necessary and room preparation for a barium enema is required. In *Fig. 20-29,* a patient is shown in position for the initial 30-minute radiograph in any small bowel series. The room being used in this case is a general radiographic/fluorographic room.

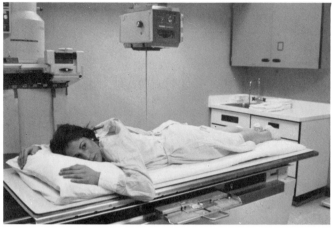

Room Preparation   Fig. 20-29

Method of Imaging

Imaging for any overhead radiograph during a small bowel series is done on 14 x 17 in. (35 x 43 cm.) film in order to visualize as much of the small intestine as possible. Spot filming of selected portions of the small bowel is done on smaller sized film. The prone position is usually used during a small bowel series, unless the patient is unable to assume that position. For the 30-minute radiograph, the film is placed high enough to include the diaphragm on the finished radiograph. This requires longitudinal centering to the duodenal bulb and side-to-side centering to the midsagittal plane. Approximately three-fourths of the film should extend above the iliac crest. Since most of the barium will be in the stomach and proximal small bowel, a high kVp technique should be utilized on this initial radiograph.

All radiographs after the initial 30-minute one will be centered to the iliac crest. For the one-hour and later radiographs, medium kilovoltage techniques may be used since barium is spread through more of the alimentary canal and not concentrated in the stomach. Spot filming of the terminal ileum usually completes the examination.

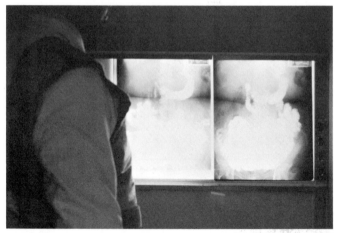

Small Bowel Imaging   Fig. 20-30

462

Barium Enema (B.E.) (Lower G.I. Series)

Specific radiographic examination of the large intestine is most commonly termed a barium enema. Alternate designations include B.E. and lower G.I. series.

Purpose

The purpose of the barium enema is to study radiographically the form and function of the lower gastrointestinal system, as well as to detect any abnormal conditions.

Common Abnormalities

There are a wide variety of indications for contrast media studies of the entire G.I. tract. These range from life-threatening emergencies to vague abdominal complaints. Many new patients receive both upper and lower G.I. examinations as part of a gastrointestinal system workup.

Some of the more common abnormalities encountered in the lower G.I. system are: (1) colitis, one specific kind being idiopathic ulcerative colitis; (2) diverticulosis and, if infected, diverticulitis; (3) neoplasms such as benign adenomas and polyps, as well as carcinomas; (4) volvulus; (5) intussusception and (6) appendicitis. Carcinoma of the large bowel and its effects are a leading cause of death in both males and females. The lesion often encircles a small section of the bowel. The radiographic appearance leads to the descriptive terms apple core lesion or napkin ring lesion.

A double-contrast barium enema, as shown in *Fig. 20-31,* must be used to demonstrate small growths, such as polyps, within the large bowel.

Volvulus is a twisting of a portion of the intestine on its own mesentery. Blood supply to the twisted portion is compromised, leading to obstruction and necrosis or localized death of tissue. While a volvulus may be found in portions of the jejunum or ileum, the most common sites are in the cecum and sigmoid colon, due to their increased mobility. Intussusception is the telescoping of one part of the bowel into the next part. Again, obstruction and necrosis may follow if the problem is not corrected.

While the water-soluble iodinated agents are useful under certain conditions, these media must be used with caution in elderly persons, young patients and any patient who is dehydrated. These media tend to reverse the normal flow of water. They tend to draw water into the bowel, rather than to allow water to be reabsorbed into the circulatory system.

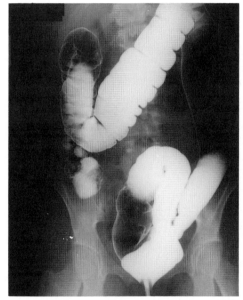

Fig. 20-31
Barium Enema Radiograph
(double-contrast)

Large Bowel Radiographic Examination
(1) Single-contrast Barium Enema
(2) Double-contrast Barium Enema

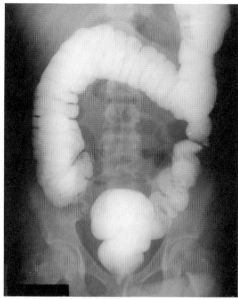

Single-contrast Barium Enema

The single-contrast barium enema utilizes only a positive contrast medium. In most cases the contrast material is barium sulfate in a thin mixture. Occasionally, the contrast medium will have to be a water-soluble contrast material. If the patient is to be taken to surgery following the B.E., then a water-soluble contrast medium must be used. An example of a single-contrast barium enema utilizing barium sulfate as the contrast medium is shown in *Fig. 20-32*.

Fig. 20-32

Single-contrast
Barium Enema

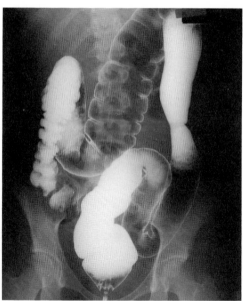

Double-contrast Barium Enema

The double-contrast barium enema utilizes both barium sulfate and air or, in some cases, barium sulfate and carbon dioxide. An example of a double-contrast barium enema utilizing barium sulfate and air is shown in *Fig. 20-33*.

Fig. 20-33

Double-contrast
Barium Enema

Patient Preparation

Preparation of the patient for a barium enema is more involved than is preparation for the stomach and small bowel. The final objective, however, is the same. The section of alimentary canal to be examined must be empty. Thorough cleansing of the entire large bowel is of paramount importance to the satisfactory contrast medium study of the large intestine.

Contraindications to Cathartics. Certain conditions contraindicate the use of very effective cathartics or purgatives needed to thoroughly cleanse the large bowel. These exceptions are (1) gross bleeding, (2) severe diarrhea, (3) obstruction and (4) inflammatory lesions such as appendicitis. A cathartic or purgative is a substance that produces frequent, soft or liquid bowel movements. These substances increase peristalsis in the large bowel, and occasionally in the small bowel as well, by irritating the sensory nerve endings in the intestinal mucosa. This increased peristalsis dramatically accelerates intestinal contents through the digestive system.

Two Classes of Cathartics. Two different classes of cathartics may be prescribed. First are the irritant cathartics such as castor oil, and second are the saline cathartics such as magnesium citrate or magnesium sulfate. For best results, bowel cleansing procedures should be specified on patient instruction sheets for both inpatients and outpatients. One should be completely familiar with the type of preparation used in each radiology department. The importance of a clean bowel for a barium enema, and especially for a double-contrast barium enema, cannot be overstated because any retained fecal matter may obscure the normal anatomy or give false diagnostic information.

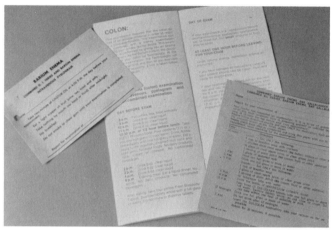

Patient Preparation

Fig. 20-34

Radiographic Room Preparation

The radiographic room should be prepared in advance of the patient's arrival. The fluoroscopic room and examination table should be clean and tidy for each and every patient. The control panel should be set for fluoroscopy with the appropriate technical factors selected. The fluoroscopy timer should be set at its maximum, usually 5 minutes. The spot film mechanism should be in proper working order and a supply of spot film cassettes should be handy. The appropriate number and size of conventional cassettes should be provided. Protective lead aprons and lead gloves should be provided for the radiologist, as well as lead aprons for all other personnel to be in the room. The fluoroscopic table should be placed in the horizontal position, with waterproof backing or disposable pads placed on the tabletop. Waterproof protection is essential in case of premature evacuation of the enema.

The footboard is not necessary for the B.E. and should be removed. The Bucky tray must be positioned at the foot end of the table if the fluoroscopy x-ray tube is located beneath the tabletop. Place the radiation foot switch appropriately for the radiologist or prepare the remote control area. Tissues, towels, replacement linen, bedpan, extra gowns, a room air freshener and a waste receptacle should be readily available. Prepare the appropriate contrast medium or media, container, tubing and enema tip. A proper lubricant should be provided for the enema tip. The type of barium sulfate used and the concentration of the mixture varies considerably depending on radiologist preferences and the type of examination to be performed.

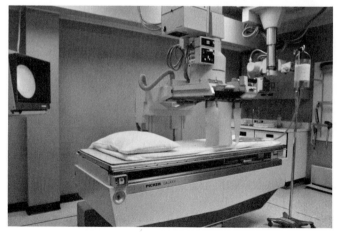

Room Preparation

Fig. 20-35

Closed System vs. Open System

Two different systems are used to administer the barium sulfate or barium sulfate and air combination during the barium enema. These are termed (1) the closed system and (2) the open system. These systems are shown in *Fig. 20-36*. The closed system consists of a one-time-use plastic bag with its own connective tubing. Using this system, the $BaSO_4$ is mixed within the bag to the desired concentration. Air or CO_2 can be added to the plastic bag. After the examination, much of the barium can be drained back into the bag by lowering the system below tabletop level. The entire bag and tubing are disposed of after a single use.

The open system consists of a plastic or stainless steel can and associated tubing, with a hemostat or another type of volume control clamp. A Y-connector and air insufflator are added for the double-contrast B.E. If reflux from the bowel into this open system contaminates the apparatus, a method for thoroughly cleansing and sterilizing the container and tubing is essential. This open system cannot be lowered like the plastic bags since the entire system would then be contaminated. Each of these systems should hold at least 2 liters of barium sulfate mixture.

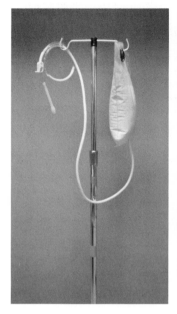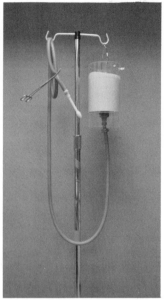

Fig. 20-36

Enema Containers

Closed System   Open System

Enema Tips and Rectal Tubes

Various types and sizes of enema tips or rectal tubes are available. The soft plastic disposable tips are most commonly used. Rectal retention catheters are used on those patients who have a relaxed anal sphincter or who, for any reason, cannot retain the enema. These retention tips may be reusable or disposable. Rectal retention catheters consist of a double lumen tube with a thin rubber balloon at the distal end. This balloon can be carefully inflated with air to assist the patient in retaining the barium enema. These retention catheters should be **fully inflated only with fluoroscopic guidance by the radiologist.**

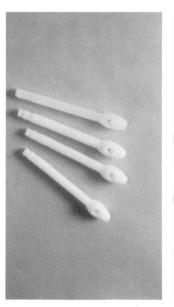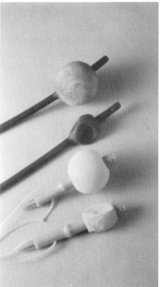

Fig. 20-37

Enema Tips and Rectal Tubes

General Routine Procedure

A barium enema patient is examined in an appropriate hospital gown. A cotton gown with the opening and ties in the back is preferable. Never use the type of gown that must be pulled over the patient's head to remove. Sometimes the gown will become soiled during the examination. The outpatient is instructed to remove all clothing, including shoes and socks or hose. Disposable slippers should be provided in case some barium is lost on the way to the restroom.

After the fluoroscopic room is completely prepared and the contrast medium is ready, the patient is escorted to the examination room. Prior to insertion of the enema tip, a pertinent history should be taken and the examination should be carefully explained. Since complete cooperation is essential, and since this examination can be somewhat embarrassing, every effort should be made to reassure the patient at every stage of the exam. Any previous radiographs should be available for the radiologist. The patient is placed in the Sims' position prior to insertion of the enema tip.

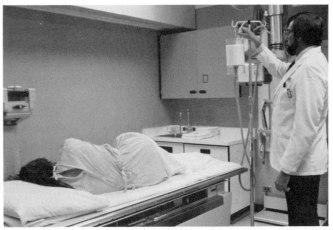

Routine Procedure

Fig. 20-38

Sims' Position

The Sims' position is shown in *Fig. 20-39*. The patient is asked to roll onto the left side and to lean well forward. The right leg is flexed at the knee and hip, and is placed in front of the left leg. The left knee is comfortably flexed. The Sims' position relaxes the abdominal muscles and decreases pressure within the abdomen.

During the procedure, each phase of the rectal tube insertion must be explained. Prior to rectal tube insertion, the barium sulfate solution should be well mixed. Before insertion, a little of the barium mixture should be run into a waste receptacle to insure that no air remains in the tubing or enema tip.

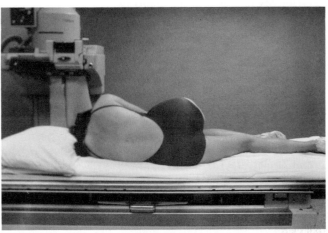

Sims' Position

Fig. 20-39

Rectal Tube

Figure 20-40 shows a rectal retention catheter ready for insertion. The radiographer wears a rectal glove and enfolds the enema tip in several sheets of paper toweling. The rectal tube is well lubricated with a water-soluble lubricant. If the radiologist has given approval to use the retention catheter, the distal end of the catheter should be made as small as possible by squeezing out all of the air and clamping the air insertion tube. Retention tips must be especially well lubricated since the end to be inserted will be irregular in shape and larger than the straight tip.

Before the examination, the patient should be instructed to (1) keep the anal sphincter tightly contracted against the rectal tube to hold it in position and prevent leakage, (2) relax the abdominal muscles to prevent increased intra-abdominal pressure and (3) concentrate on breathing by mouth to reduce spasms and cramping. The patient must be assured that barium flow will be stopped during cramping.

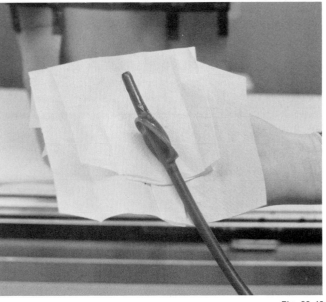

Rectal Tube

Fig. 20-40

Rectal Tube Insertion

To insert the rectal tube, adjust the opening in the back of the patient's gown to expose only the anal region. The rest of the patient should be well covered when inserting the rectal tube. Protect the patient's modesty in any way you can during the barium enema examination. The right buttock should be raised to open the gluteal fold and expose the anus. The patient should take in a few deep breaths prior to actual insertion of the rectal tube. Since the abdominal muscles relax on expiration, the tip should be inserted during the exhalation phase of respiration. Since the rectum and anal canal present a double curvature, the tube is first inserted in a forward direction approximately 3 to 5 centimeters. This initial insertion should be aimed toward the umbilicus. After the initial insertion, the rectal tube is directed superiorly and slightly anteriorly to follow the normal curvature of the rectum. The total insertion of the tube should not exceed 10 to 12 centimeters to avoid possible injury to the wall of the rectum. The rectal tube may be taped in place at this point.

After insertion of the rectal tube, the patient is rolled into position for the fluoroscopy portion of the examination. This position is usually supine, but may be prone depending on the preference of the radiologist. If the retention tube is necessary, most departments allow the radiographer to instill one or two squirts of air into the balloon end. The bulb should be filled to its maximum, however, only under fluoroscopic control.

Fluoroscopy Routine

During barium enema fluoroscopy, the general duties of the radiographer are to follow the radiologist's instructions, to assist the patient as needed and to expedite the procedure in any way possible. The radiographer must also control the flow of barium and/or air, and change fluoro spot cassettes. The flow of barium will be started and stopped several times during the B.E. Each time the radiologist asks that the flow be started, the radiographer should say "barium on" after the clamp or hemostat is released. Each time the radiologist requests that the flow be stopped, the radiographer should say "barium off" after the tubing is clamped.

The radiologist is summoned to the radiographic room when all room and patient preparations are completed. Following introduction of the physician and patient, the patient's history and the reason for the examination are discussed.

Many changes in patient position are made during fluoroscopy. These positional changes are made to better visualize superimposed sections of bowel, as well as to aid in advancement of the barium column. Areas of the large intestine best studied by positional changes include the rectosigmoid area, the two flexures and the cecal area. The radiographer may need to assist the patient with positional moves, and make sure that the tubing is not kinked or accidentally pulled out during the examination.

The fluoroscopic procedure begins with a general survey of the patient's abdomen and chest. If the retention type catheter is required, the air balloon is inflated under fluoroscopic

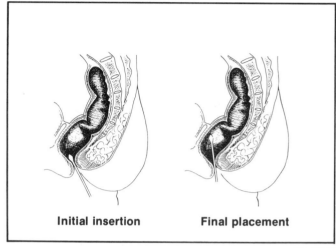

Initial insertion   **Final placement**

Rectal Tube Insertion

Fig. 20-41

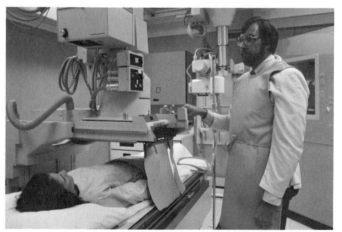

Fluoroscopy

Fig. 20-42

control at this point. Various spot radiographs are obtained of selected portions of the large intestine as the barium column proceeds in retrograde fashion from rectum to cecum. At the end of the fluoroscopic procedure, a little barium is refluxed through the ileocecal valve and fluoro spots are obtained of that area. Moderate discomfort is usually experienced when the large bowel is totally filled, so the examination must be concluded as rapidly as possible. Routine overhead radiographs are obtained with the bowel filled.

Method of Imaging

After fluoroscopy and before the patient is allowed to empty the large bowel, one or more radiographs of the filled bowel should be obtained. The standard enema tip is usually removed prior to these radiographs since this may make it easier to hold in the enema. The retention catheter, however, is obviously not removed until one wants the large bowel to empty.

In *Fig. 20-43,* a model is shown in the most common position for a routine barium enema. This is the P.A. projection with a full-sized cassette centered to the iliac crest. The film and cassette should be centered to include the rectal ampulla on the bottom of the finished radiograph. This positioning will usually include the entire large intestine with the exception of the splenic flexure. It is acceptable to cut off the splenic flexure on the radiographs since the radiologist previously obtained a spot film of each flexure. Other positions or projections may be obtained prior to evacuation of the barium. These radiographs must be obtained as rapidly as possible since the patient may have difficulty retaining the barium.

Once the routine pre-evacuation radiographs and any supplemental radiographs have been obtained, the patient is allowed to expel the barium. For the patient who has had the enema tip removed, a quick trip to a nearby restroom is necessary. For the patient who cannot make such a trip, a bedpan should be provided. For the patient who is still hooked up to a closed system, simply lowering the plastic bag to floor level and allowing most of the barium to drain back into the bag is helpful. For the patient with a retention catheter in place, the catheter must be clamped, first, and then unhooked from the enema tubing and container. Once the patient is safely on a bedpan or commode, air is released from the bulb and the catheter is removed. After most of the barium has been expelled, a postevacuation radiograph is obtained. The postevac radiograph is usually taken prone, but on occasion it is taken supine.

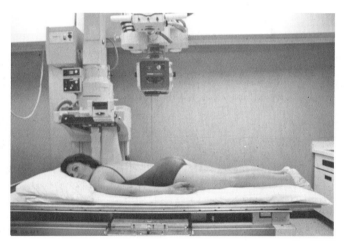

Post Fluoroscopy Radiography

Fig. 20-43

Double-contrast Barium Enema

Radiographic and fluoroscopic procedures for a double-contrast barium enema are somewhat different in that both air and barium must be introduced into the large bowel. An absolutely clean large bowel is essential to the double-contrast study, and a much thicker barium mixture is required. Although exact ratios depend on the commercial preparations utilized, the ratio approaches a one-to-one mix so that the final product is like heavy cream.

One preferred method of coating the bowel is to utilize a two-step procedure with either the open or closed systems. Initially, the thick barium is allowed to fill the left side of the bowel. Air is then instilled into the bowel, pushing the barium column through to the right side. The patient is then allowed to evacuate as much of the barium as possible. The second step consists of inflating the bowel with a large amount of air. These steps are carried out under fluoroscopic control since the air column cannot be allowed to get in front of the barium column. Spot radiographs are obtained to document any suspicious area. The patient may be asked to rotate several times to distribute the barium and air better. Routine positioning for a double-contrast barium enema includes at least four positions or projections and, in many cases, more than four. In addition, the radiologist may specify that the overhead radiographs be done in a particular order. A radiograph with a patient in one of the routine positions, the right lateral decubitus, is shown in *Fig. 20-44.*

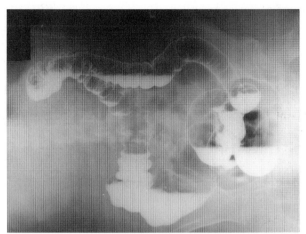

Double-contrast
B.E. Radiograph

Fig. 20-44

Basic and Optional Projections/Positions

Certain basic and optional projections or positions of the small and large intestine are demonstrated and described on the following pages. The radiologist and radiographer must closely coordinate their efforts during both the small bowel series and the barium enema. A great deal of individual variation exists among radiologists. The routine or basic positions or projections listed may vary from hospital to hospital. The radiographic routine for the barium enema, in particular, must be thoroughly understood by the radiographer in advance of the examination since any radiographs needed must be obtained as rapidly as possible.

Small Bowel Series
Basic
- P.A.

Barium Enema
Basic
- P.A.
- R.A.O.
- L.A.O.
- P.A. - Postevacuation

Barium Enema
Optional
- L. or R. Lateral
- A.P. Butterfly
- L.P.O. Butterfly
- P.A. Butterfly
- R.A.O. Butterfly
- Chassard - Lapine'

B.E. - Double-contrast
Basic
- P.A.
- A.P.
- R. Lat. Decub.
- L. Lat. Decub.

<table>
<tr><td>

Small Bowel Series
Basic
● **P.A.**

</td></tr>
</table>

Small Bowel Series

● **Posteroanterior Projection**

Film Size:
 14 x 17 in. (35 x 43 cm.)

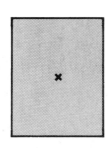

Bucky:
- Moving or stationary grid.

Patient Position:
- Prone (supine, if necessary).
- Midsagittal plane of body centered to midline of table and/or film.
- Legs extended with support under ankles.
- Arms up beside head.

Part Position:
- Trunk of body, including pelvis, comfortable and not rotated.

Central Ray:
(1) Half-hour — Center to duodenal bulb or transpyloric plane (¾ of film above crest).
(2) Hourly — Center to iliac crest.
- C.R. perpendicular to film holder.
- 40 in. (102 cm.) F.F.D.

NOTE: ● Half-hour radiograph includes entire stomach (use high kVp). ● Hourly radiographs include small intestine (use medium kVp). ● The total series includes half-hour radiographs through 2 hours, then hourly until barium is well into cecum. ● Timing begins with first ingestion of barium.

Structures Best Shown:
Contrast-filled small intestine.

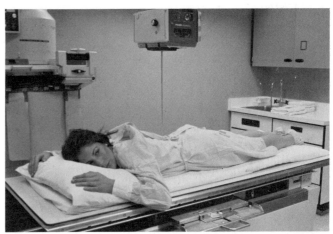

P.A. (half-hour)   Fig. 20-45

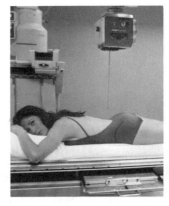 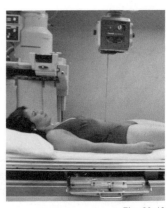

Prone Position   Supine Position   Fig. 20-46
                        (if necessary)

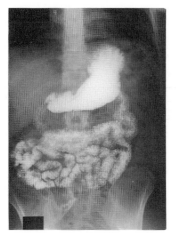

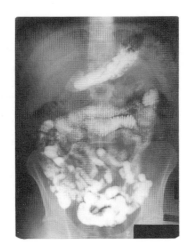

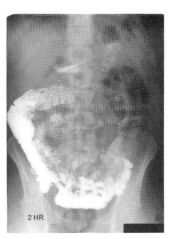

S.B.S. (½ hour)   S.B.S. (1 hour)   S.B.S. (2 hours) Fig. 20-47

Barium Enema (Single-contrast)

• Posteroanterior Projection

Film Size:
    14 x 17 in. (35 x 43 cm.)

Bucky:
- Moving or stationary grid.

Patient Position:
- Prone.
- Midsagittal plane of body centered to midline of table and/or film.
- Legs extended with support under ankles.
- Arms elevated.

Part Position:
- Trunk of body, including pelvis, comfortable and not rotated.

Central Ray:
- C.R. perpendicular to film holder.
- Center to level of iliac crest and midsagittal plane.
- 40 in. (102 cm.) F.F.D.

NOTE: • Proceed as rapidly as possible. • Include rectal ampulla on radiograph (splenic flexure may not be visible). • Standard enema tip is removed before overhead radiographs. • A.P. projection may be added. • Use high kVp.

Structures Best Shown:
Entire large intestine with exception of splenic flexure.

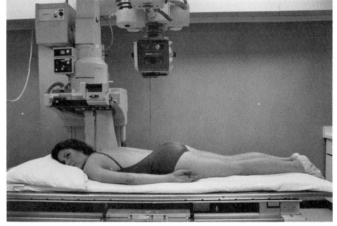

P.A.   Fig. 20-48

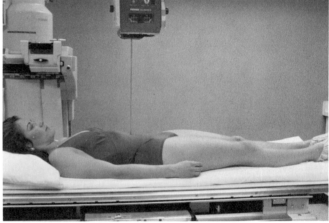

A.P. (sometimes added)   Fig. 20-49

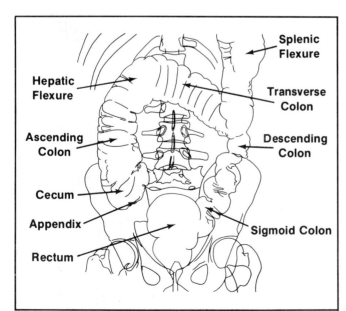

Splenic Flexure

Hepatic Flexure

Transverse Colon

Ascending Colon

Descending Colon

Cecum

Appendix

Sigmoid Colon

Rectum

Fig. 20-51   P.A.

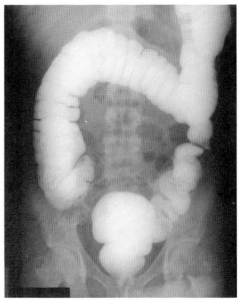

P.A.   Fig. 20-50

Barium Enema
Basic
- P.A.
- **R.A.O.**
- L.A.O.
- P.A. - Postevacuation

Barium Enema
(Single-contrast)

- **Right Anterior Oblique Position**
- **Left Anterior Oblique Position**

Film Size:

    14 x 17 in. (35 x 43 cm.)

Bucky:
- Moving or stationary grid.

Patient Position:
- Semiprone; body rotated 45°.

Part Position:

R.A.O.
- Right arm down; left arm up.
- Flex left knee; rest on right anterior body.
- Check posterior pelvis and trunk for 45° rotation.

L.A.O.
- Left arm down; right arm up.
- Flex right knee; rest on left anterior body.
- Check anterior pelvis and trunk for 45° rotation.

Central Ray:
- C.R. perpendicular to film holder.
- Center to iliac crest.
- 40 in. (102 cm.) F.F.D.

NOTE: • Obliques may show portions of bowel that are superimposed and not clearly visible on P.A. • Proceed as rapidly as possible. • Use high kVp.

Structures Best Shown:
Large intestine. L.A.O. best shows left half of large bowel and R.A.O. best shows right half and sigmoid colon.

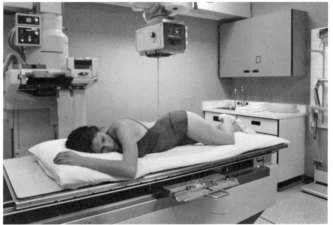

R.A.O.   Fig. 20-52

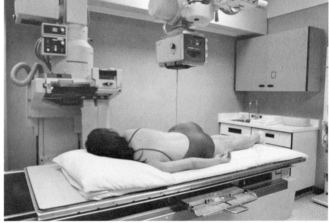

L.A.O.   Fig. 20-53

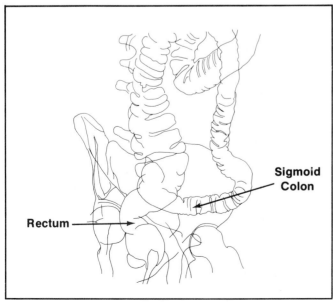

Fig. 20-55

R.A.O.

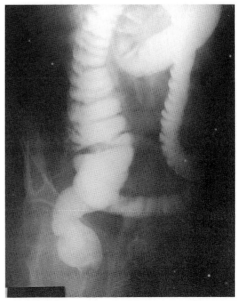

R.A.O.   Fig. 20-54

Barium Enema
Basic
- P.A.
- R.A.O.
- L.A.O.
- **P.A. - Postevacuation**

Barium Enema
(Single-contrast)

● Posteroanterior Projection
Postevacuation

Film Size:
 14 x 17 in. (35 x 43 cm.)

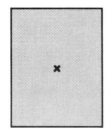

Bucky:
- Moving or stationary grid.

Patient Position:
- Prone (supine, if necessary).

Part Position:
- Midsagittal plane of body centered to midline of table and/or film.
- Legs extended; arms elevated.
- Trunk of body, including pelvis, comfortable and not rotated.

Central Ray:
- C.R. perpendicular to film holder.
- Center to iliac crest.
- 40 in. (102 cm.) F.F.D.

NOTE: ● Include rectal ampulla. ● Use medium kVp.

Structures Best Shown:
Large intestine, especially mucosal pattern.

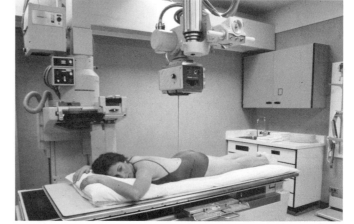

P.A. Postevacuation
Fig. 20-56

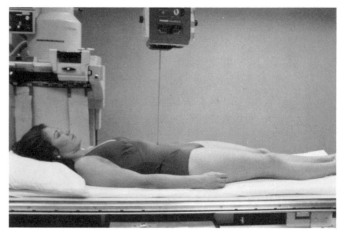

A.P. (if necessary)
Fig. 20-57

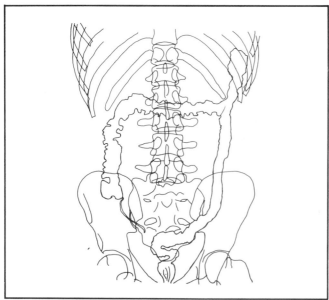

Fig. 20-59

P.A. Postevacuation

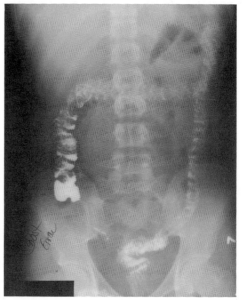

P.A. Postevacuation
Fig. 20-58

Barium Enema
Optional
- **L. or R. Lateral**
- A.P. Butterfly
- L.P.O. Butterfly
- P.A. Butterfly
- R.A.O. Butterfly
- Chassard — Lapiné

Barium Enema
- **Left Lateral Position**
- **Right Lateral Position**

Film Size:
10 x 12 in. (24 x 30 cm.)

Bucky:
- Moving or stationary grid.

Patient Position:
- Lateral recumbent position.

Part Position:
- Insure that pelvis is in true lateral position.
- Knees flexed; arms elevated.

Central Ray:
- C.R. perpendicular to film holder.
- C.R. 5 cm. posterior to midaxillary plane and 5 cm. superior to upper symphysis pubis.
- 40 in. (102 cm.) F.F.D.

NOTE: • Best position for unobstructed view of rectum.
• Use high kVp.

Structures Best Shown:
Rectum.

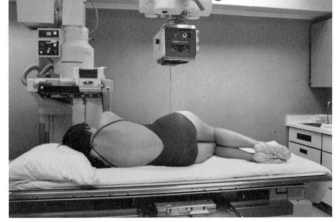

Left Lateral of Rectum   Fig. 20-60

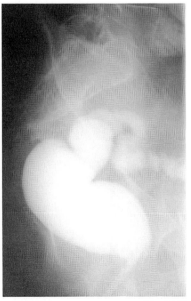

Right Lateral of Rectum   Fig. 20-61

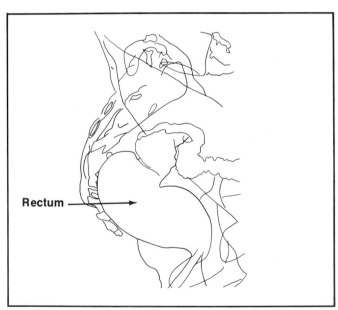

Rectum →

Fig. 20-63
Left Lateral of Rectum

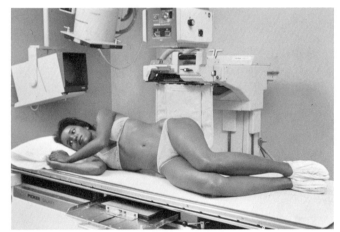

Left Lateral of Rectum   Fig. 20-62

Barium Enema
- ## Tube Angled Anteroposterior Projection
  - ### - Butterfly Position
- ## Tube Angled Left Posterior Oblique Position
  - ### - Butterfly Position

Film Size:
14 x 17 in. (35 x 43 cm.)

Bucky:
- Moving or stationary grid.

Patient Position:
- Supine or semisupine.

Part Position:

A.P.
- Insure no rotation.

L.P.O.
- Oblique patient 30 to 35° toward left side.

Central Ray:
- Angle cephalad 30 to 35°.
- 40 in. (102 cm.) F.F.D.

A.P.
- Center to A.S.I.S.

L.P.O.
- C.R. passes through point 5 cm. medial to right A.S.I.S.

NOTE: • Tube angulation and/or body rotation unravels sigmoid colon.

Structures Best Shown:
Rectosigmoid portion of large intestine.

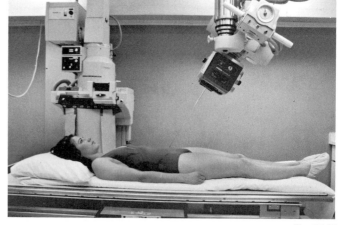

A.P. Butterfly   Fig. 20-64

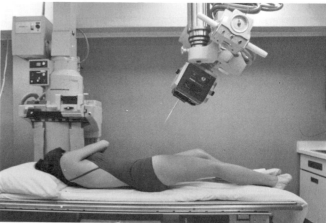

L.P.O. Butterfly   Fig. 20-65

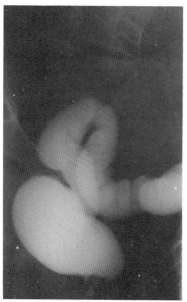

Fig. 20-67
L.P.O. Butterfly

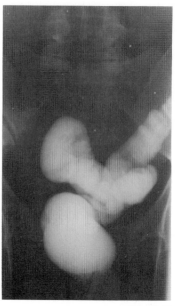

A.P. Butterfly   Fig. 20-66

Barium Enema
Optional
- L. or R. Lateral
- A.P. Butterfly
- L.P.O. Butterfly
- **P.A. Butterfly**
- **R.A.O. Butterfly**
- Chassard — Lapine'

Barium Enema

- **Tube Angled Posteroanterior Projection**
  - **Butterfly Position**
- **Tube Angled Right Anterior Oblique Position**
  - **Butterfly Position**

Film Size:

14 x 17 in. (35 x 43 cm.)

Bucky:

- Moving or stationary grid.

Patient Position:

- Prone or semiprone.

Part Position:

P.A.

- Insure no rotation.

R.A.O.

- Oblique patient 30 to 35° toward right side.

Central Ray:

- Angle caudad 30 to 35°.
- 40 in. (102 cm.) F.F.D.

P.A.

- Center to A.S.I.S.

R.A.O.

- C.R. passes through point 5 cm. medial to right A.S.I.S.

NOTE: • Tube angulation and/or body rotation unravels sigmoid colon.

Structures Best Shown:

Rectosigmoid portion of large intestine.

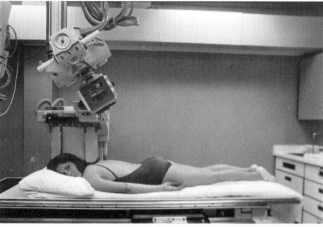

P.A. Butterfly   Fig. 20-68

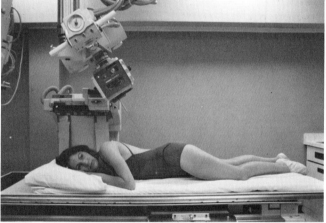

R.A.O. Butterfly   Fig. 20-69

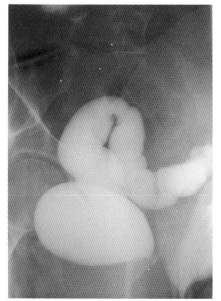

Fig. 20-71

R.A.O. Butterfly

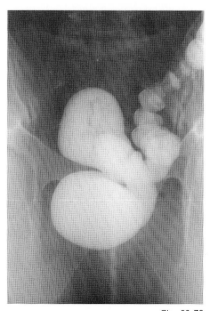

P.A. Butterfly   Fig. 20-70

Barium Enema
Optional
- L. or R. Lateral
- A.P. Butterfly
- L.P.O. Butterfly
- P.A. Butterfly
- R.A.O. Butterfly
- **Chassard — Lapine'**

Barium Enema
- **Chassard — Lapine' Axial Position**
  - Squat Shot or Bucket Shot

Film Size:
14 x 17 in. (35 x 43 cm.)
Lengthwise to table.

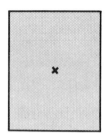

Bucky:
- Moving or stationary grid.

Patient Position:
- Patient seated on side of table, leaning well forward.

Part Position:
- Patient should lean forward as far as possible and grasp ankles.
- Sit well back on table.
- Abduct thighs to help patient lean farther forward.

Central Ray:
- C.R. perpendicular to film holder and through line passing between greater trochanters.
- 40 in. (102 cm.) F.F.D.

NOTE: • Can only be attempted on patients with excellent sphincter control (may otherwise be done after evacuation).

Structures Best Shown:
Rectosigmoid portion of large intestine.

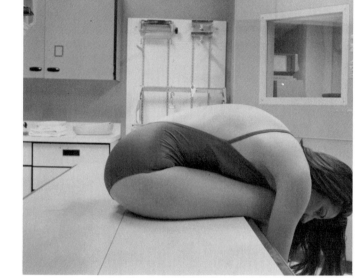

Chassard — Lapine' Axial Position
Fig. 20-72

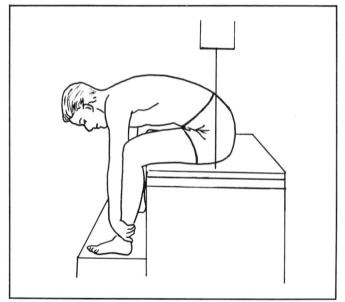

Chassard — Lapine' Axial Position
Fig. 20-73

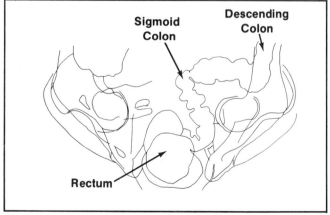

Fig. 20-75

Axial Position

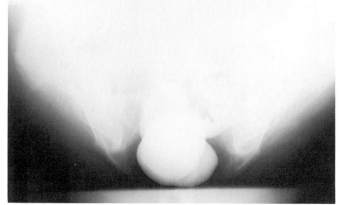

Axial Position
Fig. 20-74

B.E. - Double-contrast
Basic
- **P.A.**
- **A.P.**
- R. Lat. Decub.
- L. Lat. Decub.

Barium Enema (Double-contrast)

- **Posteroanterior Projection**
- **Anteroposterior Projection**

Film Size:

14 x 17 in. (35 x 43 cm.)

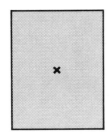

Bucky:
- Moving or stationary grid.

Patient Position:
- Prone or supine.

Part Position:
- No body rotation.
- Arms and legs comfortable.

Central Ray:
- Center to iliac crest, perpendicular to film holder.
- 40 in. (102 cm.) F.F.D.

NOTE: • Proceed as rapidly as possible. • Use medium kVp. • Table may or may not be tilted down 10 to 15°. • Rectal tube should not be removed. • Include all of rectal ampulla.

Structures Best Shown:
Large intestine. Internal growths such as polyps are especially well shown.

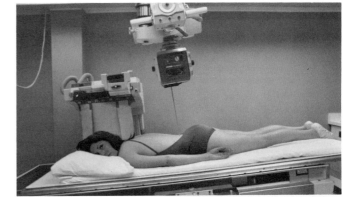

P.A. with table tilt   Fig. 20-76

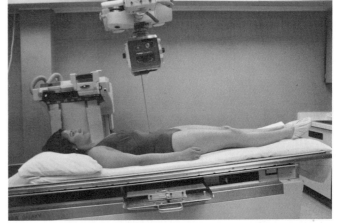

A.P. with table tilt   Fig. 20-77

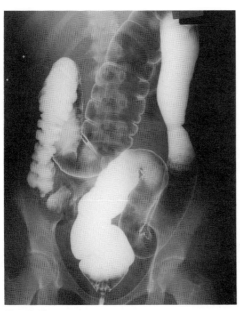

Fig. 20-79   A.P.

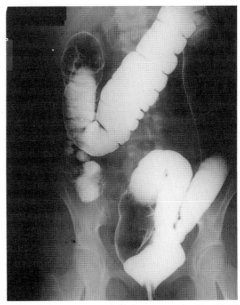

P.A.   Fig. 20-78

B.E. — Double-contrast
Basic
- P.A.
- A.P.
- R. Lat. Decub.
- L. Lat. Decub.

Barium Enema
(Double-contrast)

- **Right Lateral Decubitus**
- **Left Lateral Decubitus**

Film Size:

14 x 17 in. (35 x 43 cm.)
Lengthwise to patient.

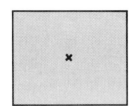

Bucky:
- Moving or stationary grid.

Patient Position:
- Patient in lateral recumbent position.
- Knees flexed, one on top of other.
- Arms up near head.

Part Position:
- Trunk of body, including pelvis, not rotated.

Central Ray:
- C.R. perpendicular to film holder.
- Center to iliac crest and midsagittal plane.
- 40 in. (102 cm.) F.F.D.

NOTE: • Table or grid cassette vertical. • A.P. projection may be more comfortable for patient. • Use medium kVp. • Rectal tube should not be removed. • Include all of rectal ampulla.

Structures Best Shown:
Large intestine, especially polyps.

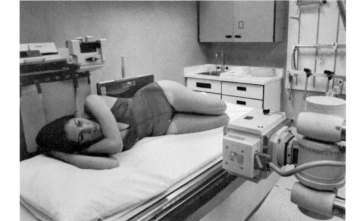

Right Lat. Decub.   Fig. 20-80

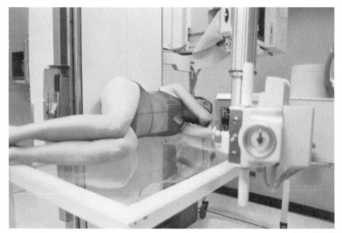

Left Lat. Decub.   Fig. 20-81

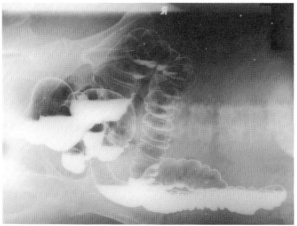

Fig. 20-83   Left Lat. Decub.

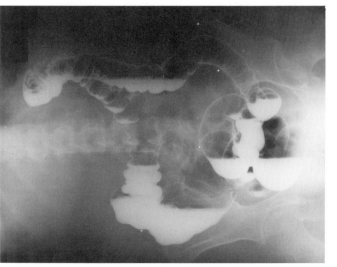

Right Lat. Decub.   Fig. 20-82

CHAPTER 21

Radiographic Anatomy and Positioning of the Gallbladder and Urinary System

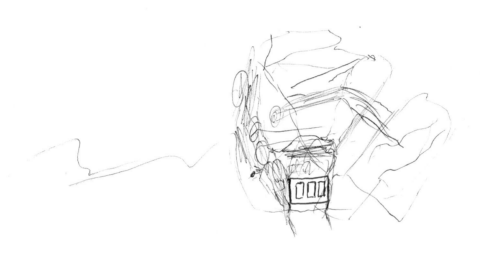

Part I. Radiographic Anatomy
Gallbladder and Biliary Ducts

Liver, Gallbladder and Biliary Ducts

Liver

Radiographic examination of the biliary system involves studying the manufacture, transport and storage of bile. Bile is manufactured by the liver, transported by the various ducts and stored in the gallbladder. In order to understand radiographic examination of the biliary system, one should understand the basic anatomy and physiology of the liver, gallbladder and connecting ducts. The liver is the largest solid organ in the human body and occupies most of the upper right quadrant. As viewed from the front in *Fig. 21-1*, the liver is triangular in shape. The upper border is the widest part of the liver and is convex to conform to the inferior surface of the **right hemidiaphragm.** The right border of the liver is its greatest vertical dimension and, in the average person, extends to slightly below the lateral portion of the tenth rib. The liver is fairly well protected by the lower right rib cage. Since the liver is highly vascular and easily lacerated, protection by the ribs is very necessary.

Gallbladder. The distal end of the **gallbladder** extends slightly below the anterior, inferior margin of the liver. The rest of the gallbladder lies along the inferior surface of the liver.

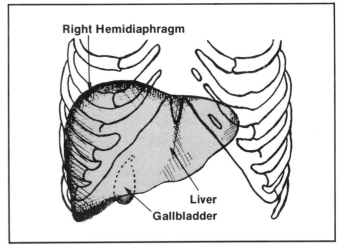

Liver and Gallbladder

Fig. 21-1

Lobes of the Liver. The liver is incompletely divided into two major lobes and two minor lobes. As viewed from the front in *Fig. 21-2*, only the two major lobes can be seen. A much larger **right lobe** is separated from the smaller **left lobe** by the **falciform ligament.** The two minor lobes can be seen only when viewing the visceral or inferior surface of the liver.

Function. The liver is an extremely complex organ and is one absolutely essential to life. The liver performs over 100 different functions, but the one function most applicable to radiographic study is the production of bile. Bile contains various waste products such as bile salts, cholesterol and bile pigments, primarily bilirubin. A major function of bile is to aid in the digestion of fats by emulsifying lipid material.

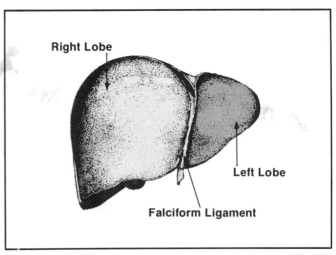

Liver

Fig. 21-2

Gallbladder and Extrahepatic Biliary Ducts

The gallbladder and the biliary ducts located outside of the gallbladder are shown in *Fig. 21-3*. Bile is formed in small lobules of the liver and travels by small ducts to either the **right** or **left hepatic duct.** The right and left hepatic ducts join to continue as the **common hepatic duct.** Bile is either carried to the **gallbladder** via the **cystic duct** for temporary storage or poured directly into the **duodenum** by way of the **common bile duct.**

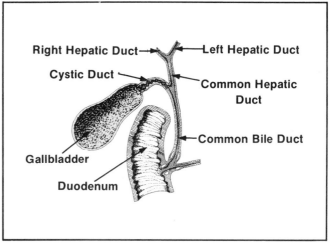

Fig. 21-3

Gallbladder and
Extrahepatic Biliary Ducts

Gallbladder and Cystic Duct

The gallbladder and cystic duct are shown in *Fig. 21-4*. The gallbladder (G.B.) is a pear-shaped sac composed of three parts — **fundus, body** and **neck.** The fundus is the distal end and the broadest part of the gallbladder. The main section of the gallbladder is termed the body. The narrow proximal end is termed the neck, which continues as the **cystic duct.** The cystic duct is 3 to 4 centimeters long, containing several membranous folds along its length. These folds are termed the **spiral valve,** which functions to prevent distension or collapse of the cystic duct. The normal gallbladder is from 7 to 10 centimeters long, about 3 centimeters wide and normally holds 30 to 40 cc's of bile.

Functions of the Gallbladder. The three primary functions of the gallbladder are to store and concentrate bile, and to contract when stimulated. First, if bile is not needed for digestive purposes, it is stored for future use in the gallbladder. Second, bile is concentrated within the gallbladder because the gallbladder normally absorbs water and salts from the stored bile. In the abnormal situation, if too much water is absorbed or if the bilirubin, calcium or cholesterol becomes too concentrated, gallstones (choleliths) may form in the gallbladder. As a third function, the gallbladder normally contracts when foods such as fats or fatty acids are in the duodenum. These foods stimulate the duodenal mucosa to secrete the hormone cholecystokinin-pancreozymin (CCK-PZ). Increased levels of CCK-PZ in the blood cause the gallbladder to contract and the terminal opening of the common bile duct to relax. In addition, CCK-PZ causes increased exocrine activity by the pancreas.

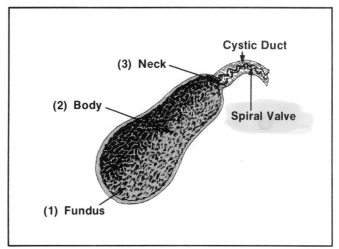

Fig. 21-4

Gallbladder and Cystic Duct

Common Bile Duct

The common hepatic duct draining the liver joins with the cystic duct of the gallbladder to form the **common bile duct** (ductus choledochus). The common bile duct averages about 7.5 centimeters in length and has an internal diameter about the size of a drinking straw. The common bile duct descends behind the superior portion of the duodenum and the head of the pancreas to enter the second or **descending portion** of the **duodenum.**

The end of the common bile duct is closely associated with the end of the **main duct** of the **pancreas,** as shown in *Fig. 21-5.* In the majority of individuals, these two ducts empty into the duodenum via one opening. Near this terminal opening, the duct walls contain circular muscle fiber, termed the **sphincter of Oddi.** The sphincter of Oddi relaxes when there are increased levels of CCK-PZ in the bloodstream. The presence of this ring of muscle causes a protrusion into the lumen of the duodenum. This protrusion is termed the **duodenal papilla** or papilla of Vater.

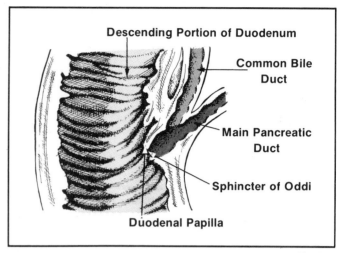

Common Bile Duct   Fig. 21-5

Gallbladder Location

The simplified lateral drawing in *Fig. 21-6* illustrates the arrangement of the **liver, gallbladder** and **biliary ducts** as seen from the right side. The gallbladder is anterior to the midaxillary plane, while the duct system is about midway between the front and the back. This spatial relationship influences optimal positioning of either the gallbladder or the biliary ducts. If it were necessary to place the gallbladder as close to the film surface as possible, the prone position would be much better than the supine position. If the primary purpose is to drain the gallbladder into the duct system, the patient would be placed supine to assist this drainage.

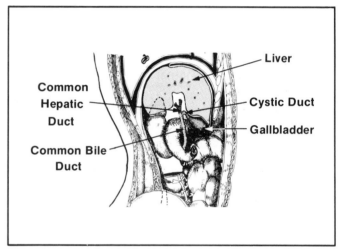

Gallbladder and Biliary Ducts   Fig. 21-6

Gallbladder Location Variation

The usual position of the gallbladder varies according to the body build of the patient. In the average body build, which includes the **sthenic** and **hyposthenic** types, the gallbladder is usually located halfway between the xiphoid tip and the lower lateral rib margin.

In the **hypersthenic** bodily habitus, the gallbladder is usually located higher and more to the right than average. In the **asthenic** bodily habitus, the gallbladder is much lower and more toward the vertebral column than average.

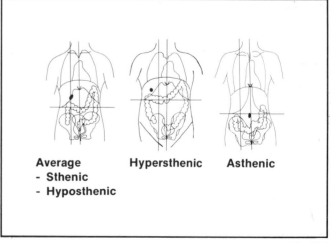

Gallbladder Variation   Fig. 21-7

Part II. Radiographic Positioning
Gallbladder and Biliary Ducts

Gallbladder and Biliary Duct Radiography

Since the liver is such a large, solid organ, it can be easily located in the upper right quadrant on abdominal radiographs. The gallbladder and biliary ducts, however, blend in with other abdominal soft tissues and in most cases cannot be visualized without the addition of contrast media. The radiograph shown in *Fig. 21-8* illustrates one exception to this general rule. The location of this patient's gallbladder can be inferred by the calcium-containing gallstones or choleliths. About 15 percent of all gallstones contain enough calcium to be visualized on a plain abdominal radiograph.

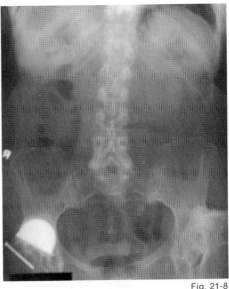

Fig. 21-8

Calcium Gallstones

Cholecystography

Radiographic examination specifically of the gallbladder is termed **cholecystography**. *Chole-* is a prefix denoting a relationship to bile. *Cysto-* means sac or bladder. Therefore, chole combined with cysto literally translates as bile sac or gallbladder.

Oral Cholecystography

The most common way to get contrast media into the biliary system is orally or by mouth. Most cholecystography is accomplished following ingestion of four to six tablets or capsules during the evening preceding the examination. These oral contrast media for visualization of the gallbladder are termed cholecystopaques.

Purpose. The purpose of the oral cholecystogram is to study radiographically the anatomy and function of the biliary system. The oral cholecystogram tests (1) the functional ability of the liver to remove the orally administered contrast medium from the bloodstream and to excrete it along with the bile, (2) the patency and condition of the biliary ducts and (3) the concentrating and contracting ability of the gallbladder.

Common Abnormalities. A variety of abnormal conditions may be demonstrated during oral cholecystography. The most common abnormality diagnosed by the cholecystogram is the presence of gallstones in the gallbladder or in the duct system. The contrast medium assists in the detection of these biliary calculi or choleliths. Other abnormalities that can be detected during oral cholecystography are neoplasms, biliary stenosis, developmental anomalies and lesions of the head of the pancreas.

Contraindications. Contraindications to cholecystography are few, but do include: (1) advanced hepatorenal disease, especially those with renal impairment; (2) active gastrointestinal disease such as vomiting or diarrhea, which would prevent absorption of the oral contrast medium and (3) hypersensitivity to iodine-containing compounds.

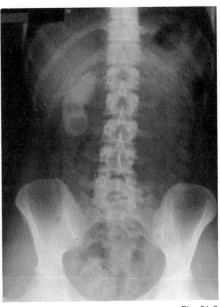

Fig. 21-9

Oral Cholecystogram

Patient Preparation

Patient preparation for the oral cholecystogram blends nicely with preparations for an upper G.I. series, so these exams are usually scheduled on the same morning. If the patient has been on a fat-free diet, he should eat some fats for one or two days before the gallbladder examination. Ingestion of fats causes the gallbladder to contract. By making sure that the gallbladder has emptied prior to the administration of contrast medium, chances are increased that the newly formed bile, with contrast medium added, will be stored in the gallbladder. Laxatives are to be avoided during the 24-hour period before the exam. The evening meal before the examination should be a light one and should not contain any fats or fried foods. When combined with an upper G.I., the patient must be N.P.O. for at least eight hours, and must refrain from chewing gum or smoking until after the exams.

Depending on the contrast medium used, either four or six tablets or capsules are taken after the evening meal, but before 9 p.m. The usual cholecystopaques are most effective taken 10 to 12 hours before the exam. No breakfast is permitted and the patient reports to radiology in the early a.m. The exact patient prep and contrast medium utilized will vary from hospital to hospital.

When the patient arrives in the radiology department for oral cholecystography, all clothing should be removed from the chest and abdomen, and the patient should put on a hospital gown. Before the scout radiograph, the patient must be questioned about taking the contrast medium. The patient should **first** be asked how many pills were taken and at what time. It may be necessary to have the patient describe the capsules or tablets to confirm that they were the correct ones. **Second,** the patient should be questioned regarding any reaction from the pills. Nausea followed by vomiting would prevent adequate absorption, as would active diarrhea. Any anaphylactoid or hypersensitivity reactions should be noted. **Third,** it should be determined that the patient has not had breakfast. **Fourth,** make sure that the patient still has a gallbladder. On those rare occasions when the patient has already had the gallbladder surgically removed, there is no need to do the cholecystogram.

Cholecystogram Scout

After appropriate questioning, a scout radiograph is taken on a full-sized film. The scout radiograph is made with the patient prone, as shown in *Fig. 21-12.* Since iodine is the major radiation-absorbing component of the contrast medium, a kilovoltage near 70 should be used. The scout radiograph must be checked to determine the presence or absence of an opacified gallbladder.

If the gallbladder shadow is present, the radiographer should determine (1) its exact location, (2) if there is overlap by intestine or bone, (3) if there is sufficient concentration for additional imaging and (4) if the exposure factors were optimal. If the gallbladder did not opacify adequately for imaging, the patient needs to be questioned again in detail about his preparation and, especially, about

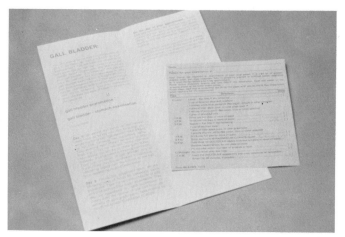

Patient Preparation Fig. 21-10

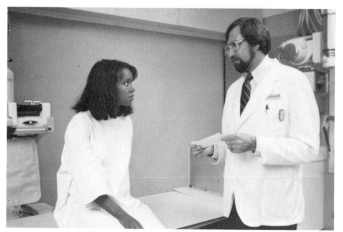

Patient Interview Fig. 21-11

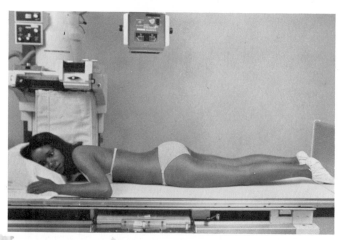

Cholecystogram Scout Fig. 21-12

his diet for the past 24 hours. Nonvisualization on the first day may result in a two-day study with a second dose of contrast medium or, perhaps, a trip to the ultrasound department for cholecystosonography.

General Routine Procedures

One or more positions may be utilized if the gallbladder visualizes adequately on the scout radiograph. At least one position or projection utilizing a horizontal beam is essential. A wide range in both the location and the pathology of the gallbladder make cholecystography an individual examination. The right lateral decubitus position, as shown in *Fig. 21-13*, or the upright position is utilized to stratify or layer out gallstones. This is the reason for at least one horizontal beam radiograph. Depending on the density of the stones in relation to the specific gravity of bile, stones may sink, rise or layer out in these two positions. Additionally, these positions allow the gallbladder to assume a different position in the abdomen and, perhaps, allow better visualization.

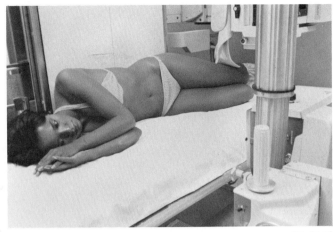

Radiography   Fig. 21-13

Method of Imaging

Many radiologists request fluoroscopy and spot films of the gallbladder in the upright position in addition to a variety of conventional radiographs. Spot filming allows use of compression and small positional changes to optimally visualize the gallbladder. A model is shown in position for upright fluoroscopy of the gallbladder in *Fig. 21-14*. If an upper G.I. series is scheduled in addition to the oral cholecystogram, the patient would then be in position for ingestion of barium.

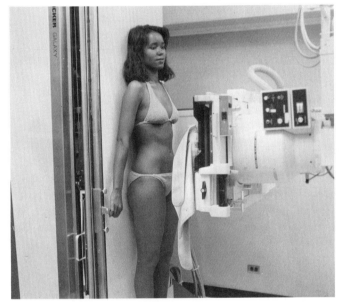

Fig. 21-14

Fluoroscopy

Cholecystogogue Usage

Occasionally, after adequate imaging of the filled gallbladder, the radiologist may wish to test the ability of the gallbladder to contract and to study the extrahepatic biliary ducts. Any agent that promotes contraction of the gallbladder is termed a **cholecystogogue.** Gallbladder contraction may be accomplished in one of two ways.

First, administration of a "fatty meal" will stimulate the duodenal mucosa to produce CCK-PZ which, in turn, will cause the gallbladder to contract. Commercially available fatty meal substitutes are administered for this purpose. The patient is placed in an R.P.O. position after the fatty meal *(Fig. 21-15)* so that the gallbladder can best drain. Radiographs are obtained in the same R.P.O. position every 15 minutes until satisfactory visualization of the duct system is obtained.

The second method for gallbladder stimulation and contraction is much faster and more direct. Either cholecystokinin-pancreozymin or a synthetic substitute is injected into the patient's venous system. This usually causes contraction of the gallbladder in five to ten minutes.

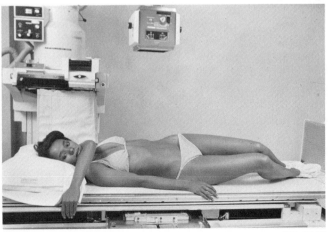

Gallbladder Drainage Position   Fig. 21-15
(R.P.O.)

Cholangiography

Intravenous Cholangiography

Intravenous cholangiography is radiographic examination of the biliary ducts following injection of an iodinated contrast medium.

Purpose. Intravenous cholangiography (I.V.C.) may be ordered to visualize the duct system in patients who previously have had their gallbladders removed. Additionally, the I.V.C. may be helpful in visualizing the ducts and, perhaps, gallbladders of patients who have had nonvisualization of the gallbladder following one or two days of orally administered contrast medium, or who cannot retain the oral contrast medium long enough for absorption due to vomiting or diarrhea. The position most often utilized for the entire series of an I.V.C. is a 15-to 30-degree right posterior oblique, as shown in *Fig. 21-16*.

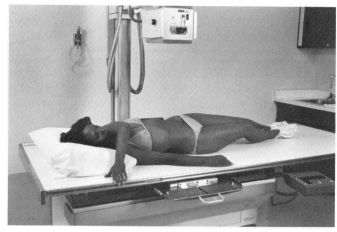

I.V. Cholangiogram   Fig. 21-16

Patient Preparation and Contrast Medium

Patient preparation ideally includes an empty stomach and a clean bowel. Occasionally an emergency I.V.C. must be done without patient preparation. The contrast medium for intravenous cholangiography is Cholografin® meglumine. The usual adult dose of Cholografin® is 100 milliliters, slowly infused over a period of 30 to 45 minutes. Infusion must be slow to lessen the likelihood of nausea and subsequent vomiting. An allergic history must be taken since this contrast medium is an iodinated, injectable type. Since hypersensitivity reaction to the contrast material is possible, a well-stocked emergency cart must be readily available.

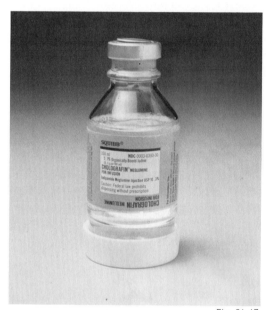

Cholografin® meglumine   Fig. 21-17

General Routine Procedure

The general procedure for an intravenous cholangiogram begins with two scout radiographs. The usual position is a 15-to 30-degree right posterior oblique. One conventional scout and one midline tomographic scout are usually obtained in this position. Once infusion of the contrast medium is begun, serial radiographs are obtained every 20 minutes until optimal visualization of the biliary ducts is obtained. Optimal visualization usually occurs 40 to 80 minutes after the start of the infusion.

Tomography is helpful during intravenous cholangiography since the contrast medium is diluted during the excretion process within the liver. Tomography may help visualize the faint ductal shadows. Once optimal visualization occurs as evidenced by the serial radiographs, tomograms are obtained. If cholecystography (visualization of the gallbladder) is desired following the cholangiography portion of the examination, radiographs at 2, 4 and 24 hours may be necessary.

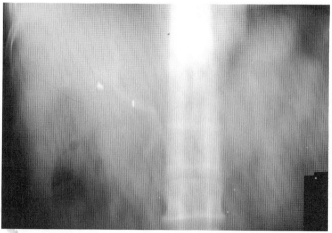

I.V.C. - Tomogram   Fig. 21-18

Percutaneous Transhepatic Cholangiography

A less common form of cholangiography involves direct injection of the ducts. **Percutaneous transhepatic cholangiography** requires puncturing the skin with a long needle. The needle is pushed through liver tissue until a duct is located. A contrast medium is then injected directly into the biliary ducts under fluoroscopic control.

Purpose. Direct injection of the biliary duct system is performed during special situations. Should the duct system be obstructed, as evidenced by a jaundiced condition, percutaneous transhepatic cholangiography may be necessary.

This examination is usually attempted only after all other methods to visualize the duct system have failed. There is a certain amount of risk during transhepatic cholangiography that the liver may hemorrhage internally or bile may escape into the peritoneal cavity.

Procedure. Percutaneous transhepatic cholangiography is performed by the radiologist under fluoroscopic control. Radiographer responsibilities are to (1) prepare the fluoroscopic suite, (2) set up the sterile tray and include the long, thin-walled needle used for the puncture, (3) arrange for patient transport, (4) provide the appropriate contrast medium which can be any of those used for excretory urography, (5) monitor the patient during the procedure, (6) change fluoro spots as necessary and (7) assist in any way possible.

Under appropriate sterile technique, the radiologist punctures the skin with the long needle and places the needle tip in an appropriate biliary duct. More than one puncture may be necessary to locate the appropriate biliary duct. After placement and injection of the contrast medium, numerous spot radiographs are exposed. Spasmolytic agents, such as glucagon, may be injected to help the sphincter of Oddi to relax.

Following fluoroscopy, conventional radiographs may be performed at the discretion of the radiologist. A postprocedure chest radiograph may be necessary to rule out a pneumothorax. Both during and after this procedure, the patient's vital signs are closely monitored to detect deterioration.

Operative or Immediate Cholangiography

Operative or immediate cholangiography is carried out during biliary tract surgery. In most hospitals, this procedure is performed in the surgical suite utilizing a high mA portable x-ray machine and grid cassettes. Prior to the patient's arrival in the surgical suite, the radiographer changes into surgical garb and makes sure that the portable unit is functional and clean. When the patient is placed on the operating table *(Fig. 21-21)*, a scout radiograph is taken.

Purpose. Operative cholangiography is done (1) to investigate the patency of the duct system, (2) to determine the functional status of the sphincter of Oddi, (3) to reveal any choleliths not previously detected and (4) to demonstrate small lesions, strictures or dilatations within the biliary ducts.

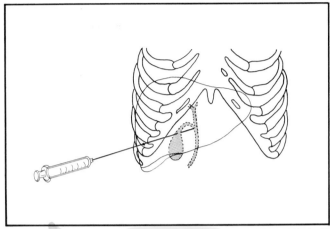

Fig. 21-19

Percutaneous Transhepatic Puncture

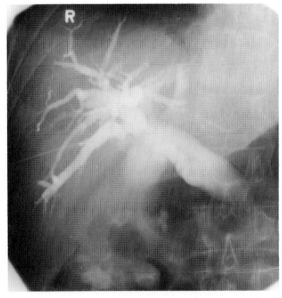

Fig. 21-20

Percutaneous Transhepatic Cholangiogram

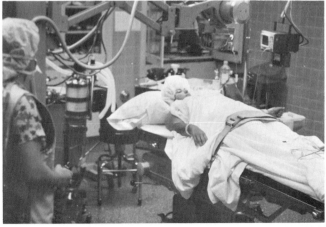

Fig. 21-21

Scout Operative Cholangiogram

Procedure. The surgeon exposes the duct system during the surgical procedure. Contrast medium is injected into the duct system before or after exploration of the biliary tract and, occasionally, after removal of the gallbladder. Radiographs are obtained following injection into a small tube placed in the common bile duct.

At least two, and preferably three, radiographs are obtained in slightly different positions. Each exposure is preceded by a fractional injection of contrast medium. The usual series consists of (1) an A.P., (2) a slight R.P.O. and (3) a slight L.P.O. The oblique positions are obtained by asking the anesthesiologist to tilt the table slightly. The grid cassette must be placed crosswise for the oblique positions to avoid objectionable grid cutoff.

Radiographs are obtained with cooperation and synchronization of the surgeon, anesthesiologist and radiographer. The surgeon must inject and then leave the exposure area. After injection, the anesthesiologist must stop patient breathing motion for the exposure. Lead aprons must be provided to those persons remaining in the exposure area.

Centering Point. The surgeon should indicate the proper centering point on the sterile sheet covering the incision or, at least, indicate appropriate landmarks such as the xiphoid tip. In *Fig. 21-22,* the surgeon has twisted the sterile drape to identify the centering point. Each fractional injection consists of 6 to 8 cc's of contrast medium. The exposure is made after the injection, after the surgeon steps back and after the anesthesiologist has stopped patient motion.

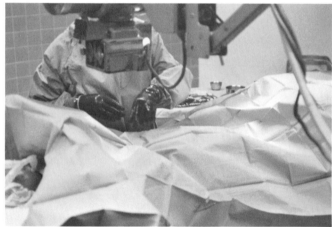

Proper Centering
Point

Fig. 21-22

T-tube, Postop or Delayed Cholangiography

T-tube cholangiography, also termed postoperative or delayed cholangiography, is usually performed about ten days after the patient's gallbladder surgery. The T-tube cholangiogram is done to assess the status of the duct system and to visualize any residual or previously undetected gallstones. A T-shaped tube (left in the common bile duct by the surgeon to provide drainage following gallbladder surgery) is injected under fluoroscopic control by the radiologist during the T-tube cholangiogram examination. Ideally, the drainage tube is clamped one day before the examination to fill the duct system with bile and prevent the accumulation of air bubbles in the duct. Bubbles in the duct system may simulate gallstones on radiographs. After duct drainage under fluoroscopic control, water-soluble iodinated contrast medium is injected fractionally and spot radiographs are exposed in various positions. Conventional or delayed radiographs may be ordered by the radiologist. Occasionally the radiologist may manipulate or remove the T-tube after consultation with the referring physician.

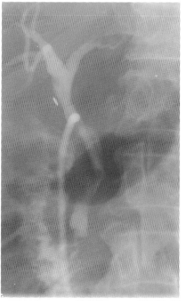

T-tube
Cholangiography

Fig. 21-23

Summary

Biliary System Radiography

In summary, **cholecystography** and **cholangiography** may be categorized by the method of contrast medium administration. Contrast medium is usually administered orally for cholecystography. For cholangiography, the biliary ducts are usually studied following intravenous infusion or direct injection of contrast medium.

Administration of Contrast Medium

(1) By mouth (oral) — cholecystography

(2) By intravenous infusion — intravenous cholangiography

(3) By direct injection of ducts
- During fluoroscopy — percutaneous transhepatic cholangiography
- During surgery — operative or immediate cholangiography
- Through indwelling drainage tube — T-tube, postop or delayed cholangiography

Basic and Optional Projections/Positions

Certain basic and optional projections or positions of the gallbladder and biliary ducts are demonstrated and described on the following pages. The radiologist and radiographer must closely coordinate their efforts during examinations of this part of the body. Individual variations exist among radiologists, and the routine or basic positions or projections listed may vary from hospital to hospital.

Oral Cholecystography
Basic
- P.A. Scout
- L.A.O.
- Right Lat. Decub.
- P.A. Upright
- A.P. Upright (Fluoro)

Oral Cholecystography
(A.F.M. or CCK-PZ)
- R.P.O.

O.R. Cholangiography
Basic
- A.P.
Optional
- R.P.O.
- L.P.O.

I.V. Cholangiography
Basic
- R.P.O.
- R.P.O. (Tomography)

Percutaneous transhepatic cholangiography and T-tube cholangiography are included as part of the basic positions or projections; however, these exams are performed by the radiologist, **NOT** the radiographer, so they are not described in the positioning section of this chapter.

Percutaneous Transhepatic Cholangiography
- Fluoro Spots
- Radiography optional

T-tube Cholangiography
- Fluoro Spots
- Radiography optional

Oral Cholecystography
• **Posteroanterior Projection** (Scout)

Film Size:

  14 x 17 in. (35 x 43 cm.)

Bucky:
- Moving or stationary grid.

Patient Position:
- Prone.
- Midsagittal plane of body centered to midline of table and/or film.
- Legs extended with support under ankles.
- Arms up beside head.

Part Position:
- Trunk of body, including pelvis, comfortable and NOT rotated.

Central Ray:
- C.R. perpendicular to film holder.
- Center to level of iliac crests and to midsagittal plane.
- 40 in. (102 cm.) F.F.D.

NOTE: • 70 kVp should be utilized. • Check scout to determine presence and location of gallbladder, adequate visualization and adequacy of exposure factors.

Structures Best Shown:
Opacified gallbladder and its relationship to bony skeleton, soft tissues and accumulations of gas.

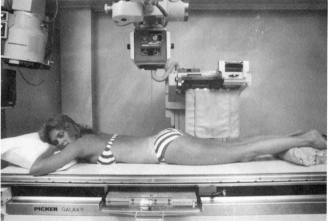
P.A. Scout   Fig. 21-24

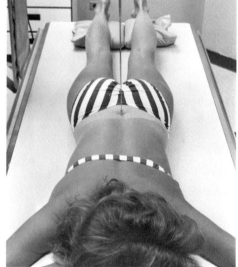
P.A. Scout   Fig. 21-25

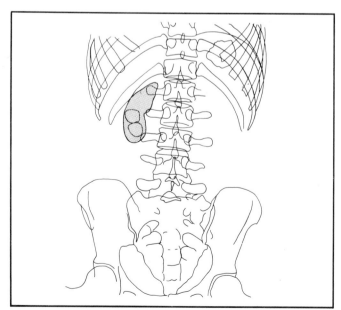
Fig. 21-27
P.A. Scout

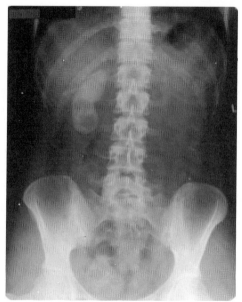
P.A. Scout   Fig. 21-26

Oral Cholecystography
Basic
• P.A. Scout
• **L.A.O.**
• **Right Lat. Decub.**
• P.A. Upright
• A.P. Upright (Fluoro)

Oral Cholecystography

• Left Anterior Oblique Position
• Right Lateral Decubitus Position

Film Size:
10 x 12 in. (24 x 30 cm.) or smaller.

Bucky:
- Moving or stationary grid.

Patient and Part Position:

L.A.O.
- From prone position, rotate into a 15 to 30° left anterior oblique.
- Right arm up; left arm down.
- Flex right knee.

Right Lat. Decub.
- Lateral recumbent.
- Knees flexed, one on top of the other.
- Arms up near head.

Central Ray:
- C.R. perpendicular to film holder.
- Center midway between spinous processes and right lateral body margin at level of the gallbladder (level of gallbladder determined from scout).
- 40 in. (102 cm.) F.F.D.

NOTE: • L.A.O. position shifts gallbladder away from vertebral column. • Decubitus position allows choleliths to stratify. • Closely collimate.

Structures Best Shown:
Opacified gallbladder.

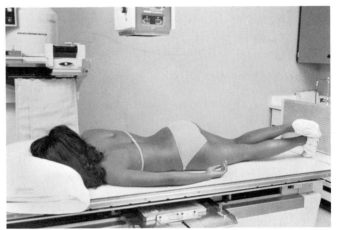

L.A.O.   Fig. 21-28

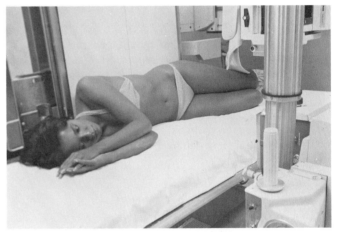

Right Lat. Decub.   Fig. 21-29

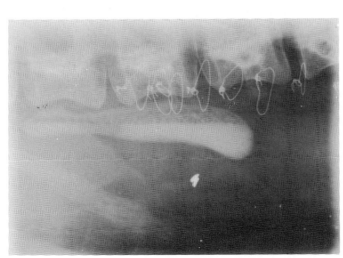

Fig. 21-31   Right Lat. Decub.

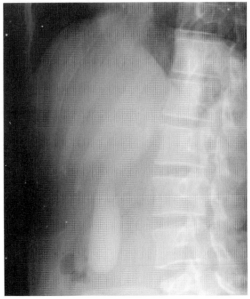

L.A.O.   Fig. 21-30

Oral Cholecystography
• **Posteroanterior — Upright**
• **Anteroposterior — Upright** (Fluoro)

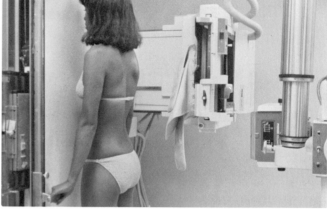

P.A. Upright   Fig. 21-32

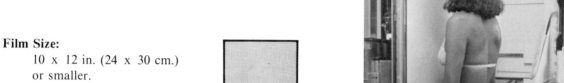

Film Size:

   10 x 12 in. (24 x 30 cm.) or smaller.

Bucky:
- Moving or stationary grid.

Patient and Part Position:

P.A.
- Upright, facing table or film holder.

A.P.
- Upright with back against table or film holder.

Central Ray:
- C.R. perpendicular to film holder.
- Center midway between midsagittal plane and right lateral body margin at level of gallbladder. Gallbladder will be 1 to 2 in. (2.5 to 5 cm.) more inferior than on the scout.
- 40 in. (102 cm.) F.F.D. (may be less for fluoro).

NOTE: • Upright positions allow choleliths to stratify. • Closely collimate. • Change centering for extremes of body build.

Structures Best Shown:
Opacified gallbladder.

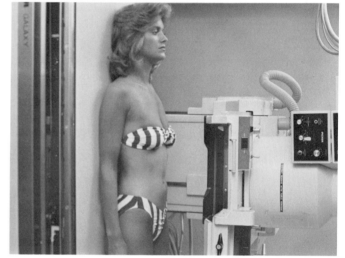

A.P. Upright (Fluoro)   Fig. 21-33

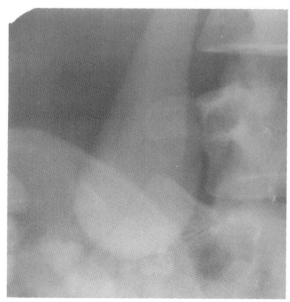

Fig. 21-35
A.P. Upright (Fluoro)

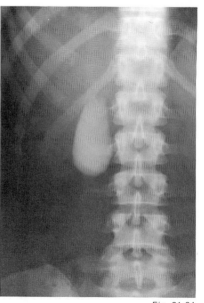

Fig. 21-34
P.A. Upright

Oral Cholecystography (A.F.M. or CCK-PZ) Basic • R.P.O.

Oral Cholecystography

• **Right Posterior Oblique Position**
A.F.M. (After Fatty Meal) **or**
CCK-PZ (Post CCK-PZ Injection)

Film Size:
10 x 12 in. (24 x 30 cm.)
or smaller.

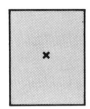

Bucky:
- Moving or stationary grid.

Patient and Part Position:
- From supine position, rotate into a 15 to 30° right posterior oblique.
- Support hip and shoulder.

Central Ray:
- C.R. perpendicular to film holder.
- Center midway between spinous processes and right lateral body margin at the level of the gallbladder. Gallbladder level is determined from scout, although the G.B. may be slightly more superior than when prone.
- 40 in. (102 cm.) F.F.D.

NOTE: • R.P.O. position allows better drainage since gallbladder is now superior to ducts. • Closely collimate.

Structures Best Shown:
Contraction of opacified gallbladder allows visualization of cystic duct and common bile duct.

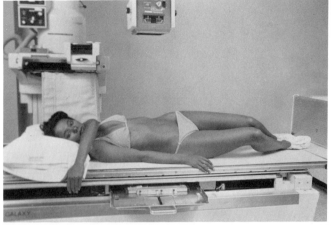

R.P.O.   Fig. 21-36

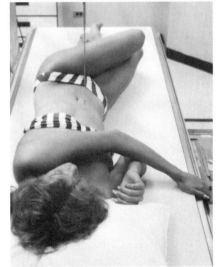

R.P.O.   Fig. 21-37

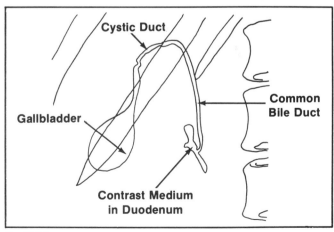

Fig. 21-39
R.P.O. (A.F.M.)

Cystic Duct

Common
Bile Duct

Gallbladder

Contrast Medium
in Duodenum

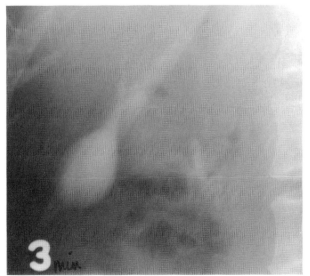

R.P.O. (A.F.M.)   Fig. 21-38

| I.V. Cholangiography
Basic
• R.P.O.
• R.P.O. Tomo |

Intravenous Cholangiography

• Right Posterior Oblique Position
• R.P.O. (Tomography)

21
Gallbladder
and
Biliary Ducts

Film Size:

    10 x 12 in. (24 x 30 cm.)

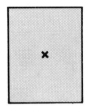

Bucky:

- Moving or stationary grid.

Patient and Part Position:

- From supine position, rotate into a 15 to 30° right posterior oblique position.
- Support hip and shoulder.

Central Ray:

- C.R. perpendicular to film holder.
- Center midway between spinous processes and right lateral body margin at level halfway between lower rib margin and xiphoid process.
- 40 in. (102 cm.) F.F.D.

NOTE: • R.P.O. position allows better biliary duct drainage. • Tomography is usually necessary to optimally visualize the faintly visible biliary ducts. • Closely collimate.

Structures Best Shown:

Common bile duct. Cystic duct, common hepatic duct and gallbladder may visualize.

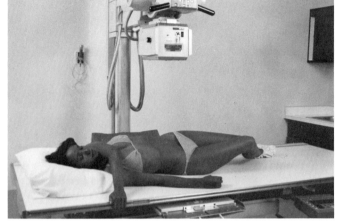

R.P.O.

Fig. 21-40

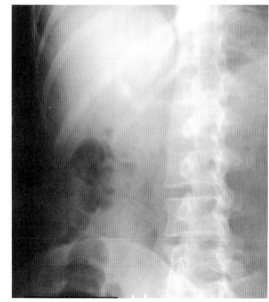

R.P.O.

Fig. 21-41

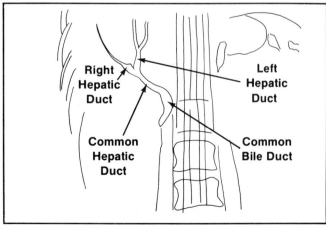

Fig. 21-43

R.P.O. Tomogram

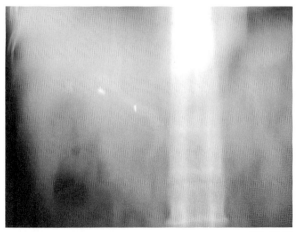

R.P.O. Tomogram

Fig. 21-42

Operative Cholangiography
• Anteroposterior Projection

O.R. Cholangiography
Basic
• **A.P.**
Optional
• R.P.O.
• L.P.O.

Film Size:
   10 x 12 in. (24 x 30 cm.)

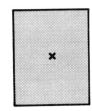

Bucky:
- Stationary grid.

Patient and Part Position:
- Supine.
- Table is tilted slightly for each oblique.

Central Ray:
- Center halfway between right lower rib margin and xiphoid tip, or to where surgeon indicates.
- 40 in. (102 cm.) F.F.D.

NOTE: • Place grid cassette crosswise for obliques to avoid grid cutoff. • Each exposure done after surgeon injects and anesthesiologist stops patient motion. • Closely collimate.

Structures Best Shown:
Biliary duct system, drainage into duodenum and any retained gallstones.

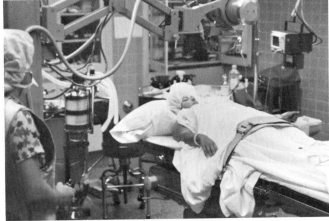

Scout A.P.

Fig. 21-44

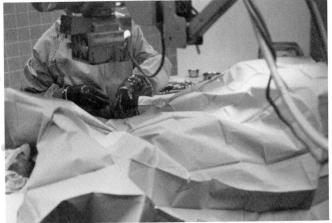

A.P. (Centering point)

Fig. 21-45

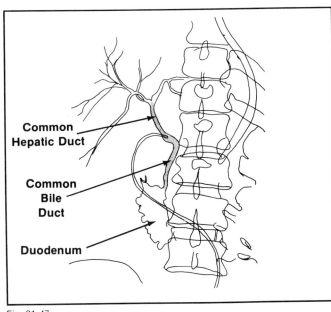

Common Hepatic Duct

Common Bile Duct

Duodenum

Fig. 21-47

A.P.

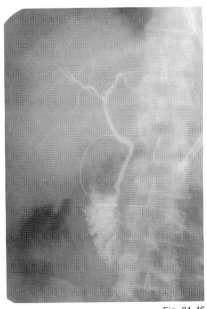

A.P.

Fig. 21-46

Part III. Radiographic Anatomy
Urinary System

Kidneys, Ureters, Bladder and Urethra

Urinary System

Radiographic examinations of the urinary system are among the most common contrast medium procedures performed in radiology departments. The urinary system consists of two **kidneys,** two **ureters,** one **urinary bladder** and one **urethra.** The two kidneys are glandular organs lying in the retroperitoneal space. These two bean-shaped organs lie on either side of the vertebral column in the most posterior part of the abdominal cavity. Near the upper part of each kidney is an adrenal gland. These important glands of the endocrine system are located in the fatty capsule surrounding each kidney. Each kidney connects to the single urinary bladder by its own ureter. Waste material, in the form of urine, travels from the kidneys to the bladder via these two narrow tubes, termed ureters. The saclike urinary bladder serves as a reservoir to store urine until it can be eliminated from the body via the urethra.

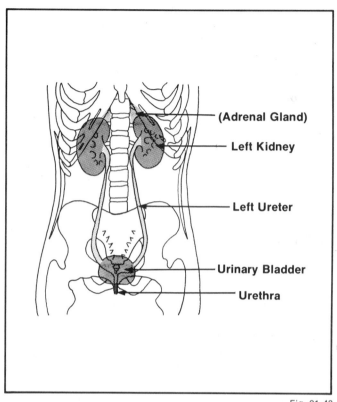

Urinary System   Fig. 21-48

Kidneys. The various organs of the urinary system and their relationship to the bony skeleton are shown from the left side in *Fig. 21-49.* The posteriorly placed **kidneys** lie on either side of the vertebral column in the upper abdomen. The lower rib cage forms a protective enclosure for the kidneys.

Ureters. Most of each **ureter** lies anterior to its respective kidney. The ureters follow the natural curve of the vertebral column. Each ureter initially curves forward following the lumbar lordotic curvature and then curves backward upon entering the pelvis. After passing into the pelvis, each ureter follows the sacrococcygeal curve before entering the posterolateral aspect of the bladder.

Urethra. The **urethra** connects the bladder to the exterior. The urethra exits from the body inferior to the symphysis pubis.

The entire urinary system is either posterior to or below the peritoneum. The kidneys and ureters are retroperitoneal structures, while the bladder and urethra are infraperitoneal structures.

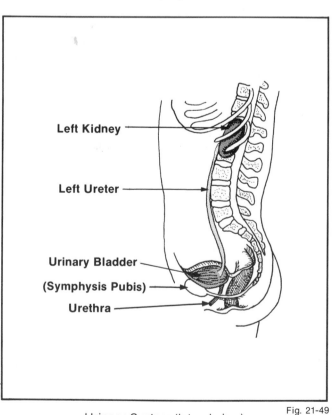

Urinary System (lateral view)   Fig. 21-49

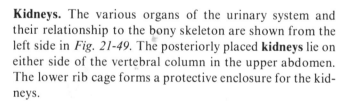

498

Kidneys

Each kidney is fairly small, weighing about 150 grams. Despite their small size, at least one functional kidney is absolutely essential for normal well-being. Failure of both kidneys, unless corrected, means inevitable death. The average measurements of each kidney are about 11 centimeters long, about 6 centimeters wide and about 3 centimeters thick. Large quantities of blood pass through the kidneys daily. Large **renal blood vessels** enter and leave the medial aspect of each kidney. One **ureter** also leaves each kidney medially near the location of the large renal blood vessels. Each kidney is arbitrarily divided into an upper part and a lower part, termed the **upper pole** and the **lower pole.**

Functions

The primary function of the urinary system is the production of urine and its elimination from the body. During production of urine, the kidneys (1) remove nitrogenous wastes, (2) regulate water levels in the body and (3) regulate acid-base balance and electrolyte levels of the blood. Nitrogenous waste products such as urea and creatinine are formed during the normal metabolism of proteins. Build-up of these nitrogenous wastes in the blood results in the clinical condition termed uremia.

Urine Production

The average water intake for humans during each 24-hour period is about 2.5 liters. This water comes from ingested liquids and foods, and from the end products of metabolism. These 2.5 liters of water eventually end up in the bloodstream. Vast quantities of blood are filtered every 24 hours. More than one liter of blood flows through the kidneys every minute of the day, which results in about 180 liters of filtrate being removed from the blood every 24 hours. Over 99 percent of this filtrate is reabsorbed by the kidneys and returned to the bloodstream. During the reabsorption process, the blood pH and amounts of various electrolytes such as sodium, potassium and chloride are regulated.

From the large amount of blood flowing through the kidneys daily, about 1.5 liters or 1,500 cc's of urine are formed. This is an average amount that varies greatly depending on fluid intake, amount of perspiration and other factors.

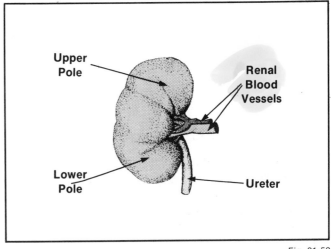

Kidney

Fig. 21-50

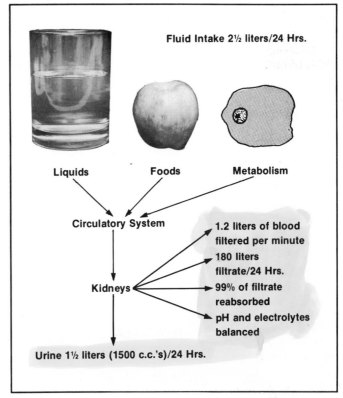

Urine Production

Fig. 21-51

Renal Blood Vessels

Large blood vessels are needed to handle the vast quantities of blood flowing through the kidneys daily. About 25 percent of the blood pumped out of the heart with each beat passes through the kidneys. Arterial blood is received by the kidneys directly from the **abdominal aorta** via the left and right renal arteries. Each **renal artery** branches and rebranches until a vast capillary network is formed in each kidney.

Since most of the blood volume entering the kidneys is returned to the circulatory system, the **renal veins** must also be large vessels. The renal veins connect directly to the large **inferior vena cava** to return to the right side of the heart. Along the medial border of each kidney is a centrally located, longitudinal fissure termed the **hilum.** The hilum serves to transmit the renal artery and renal vein, lymphatics, nerves and the **ureter.** The Latin designation for kidney is *ren,* and *renal* is a common adjective referring to kidney.

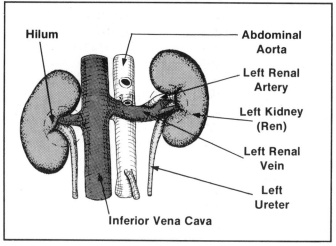

Renal Blood Vessels

Fig. 21-52

Macroscopic Structure

The macroscopic internal structure of the kidney is shown in *Fig. 21-53.* Directly under the **fibrous capsule** surrounding each kidney is the **cortex,** forming the peripheral or outer portion of the kidney substance. The internal structure termed the **medulla** is composed of from 8 to 18 conical masses termed **renal pyramids.** The cortex periodically dips into the internal medullary substance. The renal pyramids are primarily a collection of tubules.

Each renal pyramid ends in a **minor calyx.** There are from 4 to 13 minor calyces which unite to form 2 to 3 **major calyces.** The major calyces unite to form the **renal pelvis.** Each expanded renal pelvis continues as the **ureter.** Thus, urine formed in the microscopic or nephron portion of the kidney finally reaches the ureter by passing through the various collecting tubules, to a minor calyx, to a major calyx and then to the renal pelvis.

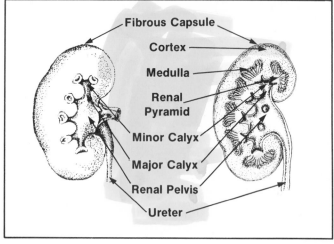

Renal Structure

Fig. 21-53

Microscopic Structure

The structural and functional unit of the kidney is the microscopic **nephron.** There are over one million nephrons in each kidney. One such nephron is shown in *Fig. 21-54.* Small arteries in the kidney substance form tiny capillary tufts, termed **glomeruli.** Blood is initially filtered through the many glomeruli. Each glomerulus is surrounded by a **Bowman's capsule,** which is the proximal portion of each nephron. The glomerular filtrate travels from the Bowman's capsule to a **proximal convoluted tubule,** to the **loop of Henle,** to a **distal convoluted tubule,** to a **collecting tubule** and, finally, into a **minor calyx.** The filtrate is termed urine by the time it reaches the minor calyx. Between glomeruli and minor calyces, over 99 percent of the filtrate is reabsorbed into the kidney's venous system. Microscopically, the glomeruli and Bowman's capsules of the many nephrons are located within the cortex of the kidney. The various tubules are located primarily within the medulla. The renal pyramids within the medulla are primarily a collection of tubules.

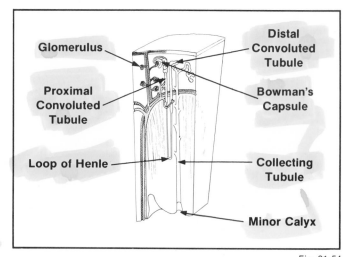

Microscopic Structure (Nephron)

Fig. 21-54

Kidney Orientation

The usual orientation of the kidneys in the supine individual is shown in *Fig. 21-55*. The large muscles on either side of the vertebral column cause the kidneys to form an angle of about 20 degrees with the midsagittal plane. These large muscles include the two **psoas major muscles.** These muscle masses get larger as they progress inferiorly from the upper lumbar vertebrae. This gradual enlargement causes the upper pole of each kidney to be closer to the midline than its lower pole.

These large posterior abdominal muscles also cause the kidneys to rotate backward within the retroperitoneal space. As a result, the medial border of each kidney is more anterior than is the lateral border of each kidney. The kidneys are located fairly close to the posterior aspect of the **diaphragm.** Since the kidneys are only loosely attached within the retroperitoneal space, they will move up and down with breathing movements of the diaphragm.

A transverse section through the level of L-2 is shown in *Fig. 21-56*. This visual illustrates the usual amount of backward rotation of the kidneys. The normal kidney rotation of about 30 degrees is due to the midline location of the vertebral column and the large muscles on either side. When posterior oblique positions are utilized during radiographic studies of the urinary system, each kidney, in turn, is placed parallel to the film plane. The body is rotated about 30 degrees in each direction to place one kidney, and then the other, parallel to the film plane. An L.P.O. will position the right kidney parallel to the film, and an R.P.O. will position the left kidney parallel.

Each kidney is surrounded by a mass of fatty tissue termed the **adipose capsule** or **perirenal fat.** It is the presence of these fatty capsules around the kidneys that permits radiographic visualization of the kidneys on plain abdominal radiographs. There is sufficient density difference between fat and muscle to visualize the outline of each kidney on a technically satisfactory, abdominal radiograph.

Normal Kidney Location

Most abdominal radiographs, including urograms, are performed on expiration with the patient supine. The combined effect of these two factors allows the kidneys to lie fairly high in the abdominal cavity. Under these conditions, the kidneys normally lie halfway between the **xiphoid tip** and the **iliac crest.** The left kidney normally lies about 1 centimeter more superior than does the right one. The presence of the liver on the right side tends to push the right kidney slightly caudad. The top of the left kidney is usually at the level of the **T-11 — T-12 interspace.** The bottom of the right kidney is most often level with the upper part of **L-3.** Each renal pelvis is usually near or slightly below the **transpyloric plane.**

Kidney Movement. Since the kidneys are only loosely attached within their fatty capsule, they tend to move up and down with movements of the diaphragm and with position changes. When one inhales deeply or stands upright, the kidneys normally drop about one lumbar vertebra or 5 centimeters. If the kidneys tend to drop more than one lumbar vertebra, a condition termed nephroptosis is said to exist. Any excessive downward displacement of the kidneys is termed nephroptosis. With some very thin patients, in particular, the kidneys may drop dramatically and end up within the pelvis.

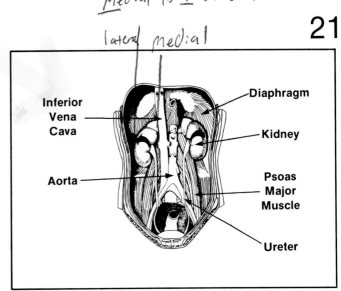

Kidney Orientation

Fig. 21-55

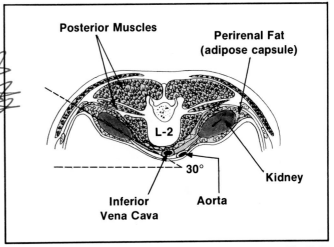

Kidney Orientation
(cross section, top view)

Fig. 21-56

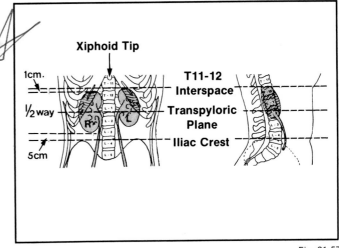

Normal Kidney Location

Fig. 21-57

Ureters

The ureters convey urine from the kidneys to the urinary bladder. Slow peristaltic waves force urine down the ureters. The renal pelvis leaves each kidney at the hilum to become the **ureter.** The ureters vary in length from 28 to 34 centimeters, with the right one being slightly shorter than is the left. As the ureters pass caudad, they lie on the anterior surface of each psoas major muscle. Continuing to follow the curvature of the vertebral column, the ureters eventually enter the posterolateral portion of each side of the **urinary bladder.**

Prior to any pelvic surgery, the exact course of the ureters should be determined radiographically. The ureters are very narrow tubes and closely resemble surrounding tissue, therefore care must be exercised during surgery to leave the ureters intact. This is especially true during hysterectomies since the ureters are located close to the uterus.

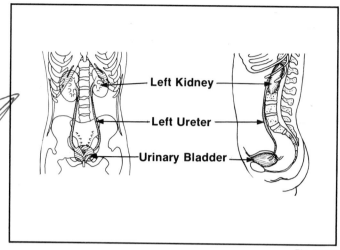

Ureters   Fig. 21-58

Ureter Size and Points of Constriction

The ureters vary in diameter from 1 millimeter to almost 1 centimeter. Normally, there are three constricted points along the course of each ureter. Should a kidney stone attempt to pass from kidney to bladder, it would have trouble passing these three spots. The first point is the **ureteropelvic junction,** the second is near the **brim of the pelvis** where the iliac blood vessels cross, and the third is where the ureter joins the bladder. This third narrow spot is termed the **ureterovesical junction** or U.V. junction. Most kidney stones passing down the ureter tend to hang up at the U.V. junction, but once the stone passes this point it will have little trouble passing through the bladder and urethra to the exterior.

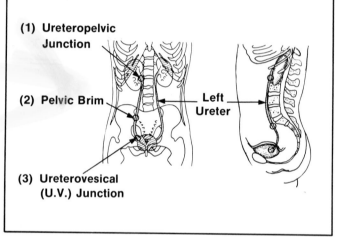

(1) Ureteropelvic Junction

(2) Pelvic Brim

(3) Ureterovesical (U.V.) Junction

Left Ureter

Ureters   Fig. 21-59

Urinary Bladder

The urinary bladder or vesica urinaria is a musculomembranous sac that serves as a reservoir for urine. The empty bladder is somewhat flattened and only assumes the more oval shape when partially or fully distended. Basically, the bladder consists of two parts. The first is a triangular portion along the inner, posterior surface, termed the **trigone.** The second part is the smooth muscle of the bladder wall. The trigone, shaded in *Fig. 21-60*, is the muscular area formed by the entrance of the two **ureters** from behind and the exit site of the **urethra.** The trigone is firmly attached to the floor of the pelvis. As the bladder fills, it is the top of the bladder that expands upward and forward toward the abdominal cavity.

The gland surrounding the proximal urethra in *Fig. 21-60* is the **prostate gland.** Only males possess a prostate gland so this drawing represents a male bladder, although the internal structure of the bladder in both sexes is similar.

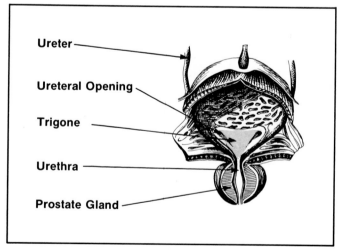

Ureter

Ureteral Opening

Trigone

Urethra

Prostate Gland

Urinary Bladder   Fig. 21-60

Bladder Functions

The **bladder** functions as a reservoir for urine and, aided by the urethra, it expels urine from the body. There is normally some urine in the bladder at all times, but as the amount reaches 250 milliliters there is a desire to void. The act of voiding is termed urination or micturition. Normally, urination is under voluntary control and the desire to void may pass if the bladder cannot be emptied right away. The total capacity of the bladder varies from 350 milliliters to 500 milliliters. As the bladder becomes fuller and fuller, the desire to void becomes more and more urgent. If the internal bladder pressure rises too high, involuntary urination will occur. Involuntary urination, whether due to excessive pressure or to organic problems, is termed incontinence.

Size and Position of the Bladder. The size, position and functional status of the bladder depends somewhat on surrounding organs and on how full the bladder is. When the rectum contains fecal matter, the bladder is pushed up and forward. A term pregnancy, as shown in *Fig. 21-61,* exerts tremendous pressure on the bladder.

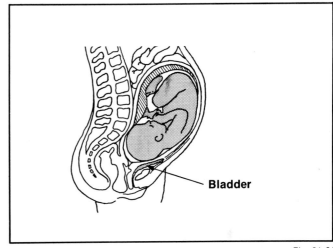

Term Pregnancy

Fig. 21-61

Male Pelvic Organs

The male pelvic organs are shown in midsagittal section in *Fig. 21-62.* When the **urinary bladder** is empty, most of the bladder lies directly posterior to the upper margin of the symphysis pubis. As the bladder distends, as it would during a cystogram or radiographic study of the bladder, more and more of the bladder will lie above the level of the symphysis pubis.

The male **urethra** extends from the internal urethral orifice to the external urethral orifice at the end of the penis. The urethra extends through the **prostate gland** and through the length of the penis. The male urethra averages 17.5 to 20 centimeters in length and serves two functions. Not only does the male urethra serve as the distal portion of the urinary tract, helping to eliminate urine stored in the bladder, but it also is the terminal portion of the reproductive system, serving as a passageway for semen.

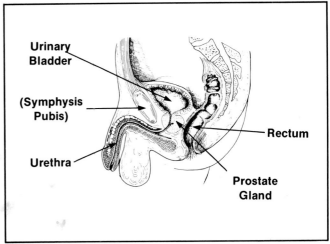

Male Pelvic Organs

Fig. 21-62

Female Pelvic Organs

The female pelvic organs are shown in midsagittal section in *Fig. 21-63*. The **urinary bladder** lies behind or above the upper margin of the symphysis pubis, depending on the amount of bladder distension. The female **urethra** is a narrow canal, about 4 centimeters long, extending from the internal urethral orifice to the external urethral orifice. The single function of the female urethra is the passage of urine to the exterior. There is a close relationship between the urethra and bladder, and the **uterus** and **vagina.** The urethra is imbedded in the anterior wall of the vagina. The spatial relationship of the three external openings becomes important during certain radiographic procedures. The anal opening is most posterior, the urethral opening is most anterior, and the vaginal opening is in between.

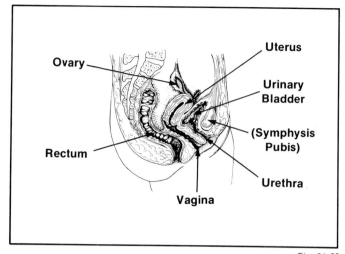

Female Pelvic Organs

Fig. 21-63

Part IV. Radiographic Positioning
Urinary System

Kidney, Ureter, Bladder and Urethra Radiography

The plain abdominal radiograph or K.U.B. shown in *Fig. 21-64* demonstrates very little of the urinary system. The gross outlines of the kidneys are demonstrated due to the fatty capsule surrounding the kidneys. In addition, the generalized gray area in the pelvis represents the urine-filled, urinary bladder. The rest of the urinary system blends in with the other soft tissue structures of the abdominal cavity. Contrast media must be utilized to visualize the internal, fluid-filled portion of the urinary system radiographically.

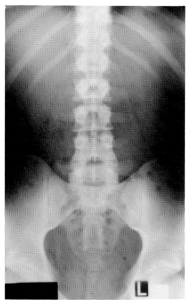

Fig. 21-64

Abdominal
Radiograph

Urography

Radiographic examination of the urinary system, in general, is termed urography. *Uro* is a prefix denoting a relationship to urine or to the urinary tract. The contrast media utilized to visualize the urinary tract are introduced into the human system in one of two ways. First, the contrast medium may be introduced into the bloodstream. This process is most often accomplished by intravenous injection. The second requires some form of catheterization so that the contrast medium can be delivered directly into the structure to be studied radiographically. Radiographic examinations of the urinary system utilizing these two methods of contrast delivery are discussed in the remainder of this chapter. An excretory urogram following intravenous injection of a contrast medium is shown in *Fig. 21-65*.

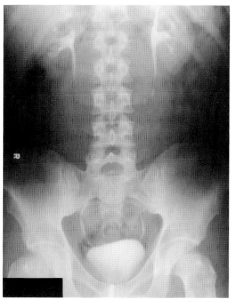

Fig. 21-65

Excretory Urogram

505

Contrast Media

Various contrast media are used to visualize the different parts of the urinary system radiographically. Various brands of contrast media are available for use in urography. The basic molecule for each of the different types of urographic contrast media is the triiodobenzoic acid molecule, which contains three organically bound iodine atoms per molecule. This basic iodine-containing molecule is found in those contrast media that are injected directly into the bloodstream, as well as in those media that are delivered directly into a hollow structure via catheterization.

Complications may follow administration of any contrast medium, but the majority of side effects and reactions occur following an intravascular injection. Since most studies of the kidneys require an intravenous injection, complications should be expected. Adverse reactions to contrast media cannot be predicted. Both the radiologist and the radiographer must be prepared for a reaction whenever contrast medium is injected.

General Procedure. Prior to any contrast medium injection, one should (1) prepare the patient psychologically, (2) obtain a careful and pertinent patient history, (3) select the correct contrast medium and prepare it for injection and (4) make sure a properly stocked emergency cart is readily available. Radiographic examinations requiring intravascular injections are likely to cause patient anxiety. One can reduce this anxiety by preparing for the exam in a confident, professional manner and by explaining the procedure to the patient in understandable terms.

Common Side Effects. Two common side effects following an intravenous injection of iodinated contrast media are a temporary hot flash and a metallic taste in the mouth. Both the hot flash, particularly in the face, and the metallic taste in the mouth usually pass quickly. Discussion of these possible effects and careful explanation of the examination will help to reduce patient anxiety and help to prepare the patient psychologically.

Patient History. A careful patient history may serve to alert the medical team to a possible reaction. Patients with a history of allergy are more likely to experience adverse reactions to contrast media than those who have no allergies. Questions to ask the patient should include: (1) Are you allergic to anything? (2) Have you ever had hay fever, asthma or hives? (3) Are you allergic to any drugs or medications? (4) Are you allergic to iodine? (5) Are you allergic to seafood or shellfish? (6) Are you allergic to other foods? and (7) Have you ever had an x-ray examination that required an injection into an artery or vein? A positive response to any of these questions will alert the injection team to an increased probability of reaction.

If the patient is a female, then a menstrual history must be obtained. Irradiation of an early pregnancy is one of the most hazardous situations in diagnostic radiography. Any x-ray examination of the abdomen of a potentially pregnant female should be governed by the "ten-day rule." X-ray examinations such as the X.U., which include the pelvis and

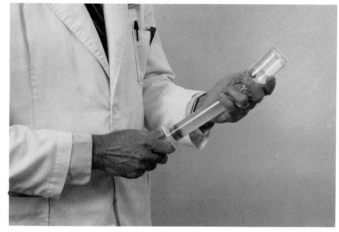

Contrast Medium
for Injection

Fig. 21-66

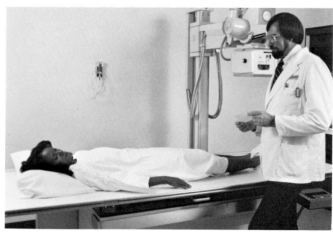

Discussion of History

Fig. 21-67

506

uterus in the primary beam, should never be done on pregnant females unless absolutely necessary. Any female of child-bearing age should have such radiographic procedures only during the 10-day period after the start of menstruation. This is the only time when pregnancy can be ruled out with any certainty. Abdominal radiographs of a known pregnancy should be delayed at least until the third trimester, if done at all.

Selection and Preparation of Contrast Media. Selection and preparation of the correct contrast medium are important steps prior to injection. Since labels on various media containers are similar, one should always read the label three times. In addition, the empty container should be shown to the radiologist or other person making the actual injection. Whenever contrast medium is withdrawn into a syringe, be certain to maintain sterility of the medium, the syringe and the needle.

Preparation for Possible Reaction. Since contrast medium reaction is possible and unpredictable, a fully stocked emergency cart must be readily available whenever an intravenous injection is made. In addition to emergency drugs, the cart should contain cardiopulmonary resuscitation equipment, portable oxygen, suction and blood pressure apparatus, and possibly a defibrillator and monitor.

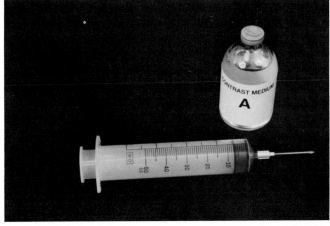

Possible Adverse Reactions   Fig. 21-68

Reactions to Contrast Media

Most reactions to contrast media occur rapidly if they are going to happen, but, on occasion, a delayed reaction may occur. Reactions to contrast media can be classed as **mild, moderate** or **severe.** Mild reactions are usually self-limiting and require no medication for relief of symptoms. A moderate reaction is one that requires treatment for both the symptoms and the comfort of the patient. Any reaction that produces life-threatening symptoms requiring vigorous, active treatment is classed as a severe reaction. Any reaction, regardless of how minor it may seem, deserves careful observation. Mild reactions sometimes signal a more serious reaction to follow. The patient should never be left alone following an intravenous injection. As the necessary radiographs are produced, observe the patient and question the patient regarding any changes. The radiologist or other responsible physician should remain within immediate reach for five minutes following an injection, and within easy reach for one hour thereafter. The physician must be summoned immediately for any moderate or severe reaction.

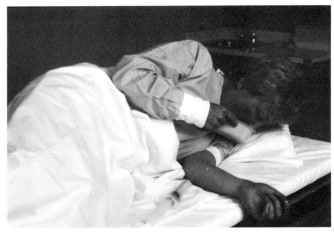

Mild Reaction   Fig. 21-69

Mild Reactions. The majority of reactions to contrast media are mild, usually requiring no treatment other than support and verbal reassurance. Mild reactions such as nausea and vomiting are fairly common. One should not forewarn the patient of their possible occurrence, however. Sometimes the power of suggestion is enough to bring on this type of reaction. Have an emesis basin handy in case of vomiting and a cold towel for the forehead in case of nausea. Take care that the patient does not vomit while supine. Either sit the patient up or turn the patient onto the left side, as shown in *Fig. 21-69*.

Other mild reactions include hives or urticaria, itching and sneezing. These reactions cause some concern because they may signal a more severe response.

Mild reactions may also occur at the injection site, particularly if some of the contrast medium leaks out of the vein into the surrounding tissue. Such leakage is termed extravasation. Pain, burning or numbness may result when extravasation occurs. A warm towel over the injection site may speed absorption of the contrast material. Another mild reaction is a response to fear termed the vasovagal response. Sometimes the sight of a needle or the sensation of a needle stick may trigger a vasovagal reaction. Symptoms include a sensation of weakness or dizziness, sweating and the feeling that precedes fainting. Explanation of the procedure and a confident injection team often deter this type of reaction. The patient's blood pressure should be taken during a vasovagal reaction since a marked drop in pressure indicates a more serious reaction.

Moderate Reactions. Moderate reactions require administration of some type of medication while the patient is still in radiology. Moderate reactions include excessive urticaria, tachycardia or rapid heartbeat, giant hives and excessive vomiting. These symptoms usually respond rapidly and completely to the appropriate medication.

Severe Reactions. Severe reactions are life-threatening and require immediate, intensive treatment. Very low blood pressure, cardiac or respiratory arrest, loss of consciousness, convulsions, laryngeal edema, cyanosis, difficulty in breathing and profound shock are examples of severe reactions. Delayed or inappropriate treatment for any of these symptoms or conditions could result in the patient's death. If a moderate or severe reaction is suspected, get help and summon the physician immediately.

Mild Reactions
- Reaction Examples
  - Nausea and vomiting
  - Hives (urticaria)
  - Itching
  - Sneezing
  - Burning or numbness at injection site (with extravasation)
  - Vasovagal response (fear) — weakness, dizziness, sweating, feeling of passing out

Moderate Reactions
- Require medication
- Reaction Examples
  - Excessive urticaria
  - Giant hives
  - Tachycardia (rapid heartbeat)
  - Excessive vomiting

Severe Reactions
- Life-threatening — require **immediate** treatment
- Reaction Examples
  - Very low blood pressure
  - Cardiac or respiratory arrest
  - Loss of consciousness
  - Convulsions
  - Laryngeal edema
  - Cyanosis
  - Difficulty in breathing
  - Profound shock

Excretory Urography (X.U.)

The excretory urogram or X.U. is the most common radiographic examination of the urinary system. This examination is often referred to as an I.V.P. or intravenous pyelogram. *Pyelo* refers only to the renal pelvis, however, and since the X.U. normally visualizes more anatomy than just the renal pelvis, the term I.V.P. should not be used. The excretory urogram visualizes the minor and major calyces, renal pelves, ureters and urinary bladder following an intravenous injection of contrast medium.

The X.U. is a true functional test since the contrast medium molecules are rapidly removed from the bloodstream and are excreted completely by the normal kidney.

Purpose. The purpose of an excretory urogram is to visualize the collecting portion of the urinary system and to assess the functional ability of the kidneys. An example of an excretory urogram is shown in *Fig. 21-70.*

Common Indications. The excretory urogram is one of the most common contrast media examinations performed in the radiology department, and there are a wide variety of conditions that lead to requests for excretion urography. Some of the more common indications for an X.U. are (1) abdominal or pelvic mass, (2) renal or ureteral calculus, (3) kidney trauma, (4) flank pain, (5) hematuria or blood in the urine, (6) preop pelvic surgery, (7) renal failure, (8) hypertension and (9) urinary tract infections. Although there are other indications for the X.U., these are the primary ones.

Contraindications. Present-day contrast media are relatively safe so there are few strict contraindications to excretory urography. One such contraindication is anuria, an absence of urine excretion. Another contraindication is a known severe sensitivity to the particular contrast medium to be used. The highly sensitive patient may need to be examined using some other imaging modality, or may need to be premedicated prior to the X.U. High risk patient conditions include the following: (1) multiple myeloma, (2) diabetes, (3) severe hepatic or renal disease, (4) congestive heart failure, (5) pheochromocytoma and (6) sickle cell anemia. Dehydration increases risk for the patient with multiple myeloma (bone marrow cancer) or the patient with severe renal impairment. These patients must be well hydrated for an X.U.

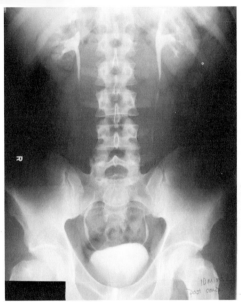

Fig. 21-70

Excretory Urogram

Patient Preparation

Patient preparation for both the excretory urogram and the barium enema are similar. The intestinal tract should be free of gas and solid fecal matter for both exams. If both exams are to be performed on the same patient, they are usually done on the same day. The X.U. is done first with the B.E. to follow.

Preparation for an excretory urogram usually consists of a light evening meal, a bowel-cleansing cathartic, enemas until clear in the a.m., and a light breakfast. Children usually receive no bowel preparation at all for an X.U., and adults requiring an emergency study are usually done "as is." Many preparation variations do exist, however. Some physicians feel that the patient should be dehydrated for an X.U., withholding all fluids for eight hours prior to the exam. Dehydration results in slower and more concentrated excretion of the contrast medium. The current trend is toward normal hydration, however, coupled with an injection of 50 to 60 cc's of contrast material. This amount of contrast material is considered a "double dose" and results in a higher concentration of contrast medium in the circulatory system.

Prior to the excretory urogram, all clothing except shoes and socks should be removed and replaced with a short-sleeved hospital gown. The opening and ties should be in the back. Always make certain that the patient scheduled for this examination or any other radiographic procedure is the correct patient. Double check the inpatient identification band and verify the outpatient with appropriate questions. The patient should void just prior to the examination for two reasons: (1) a bladder that is too full could rupture, especially if compression is applied early in the exam, and (2) urine already present in the bladder dilutes the contrast medium accumulating there.

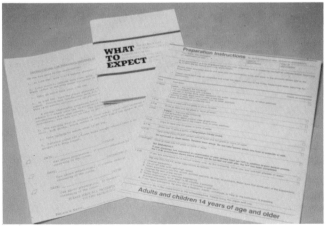

Fig. 21-71

Patient Preparation

Radiographic Room Preparation

Equipment needed for excretory urography, in addition to a suitable radiographic room, are: (1) correct type and amount of contrast medium drawn up in an appropriate syringe, (2) the empty container of contrast medium to show the physician or assistant doing the injection, (3) a selection of sterile needles to include a 19-gauge butterfly needle and tubing, (4) alcohol sponges or wipes, (5) tourniquet and (6) towel or sponge to support the elbow. Items also needed are (7) male gonadal shield, (8) emesis basin, (9) lead numbers, minute marker, and R and L markers, (10) emergency cart handy, (11) epinephrine or adrenalin ready for emergency injection, (12) ureteric compression device and (13) a cold towel for the forehead or a warm towel for the injection site, if necessary. These items should be assembled and ready before the patient is escorted to the radiographic room. Be certain that the room is clean and tidy for each and every patient, and make sure that the patient has voided prior to placing the patient on the radiographic table.

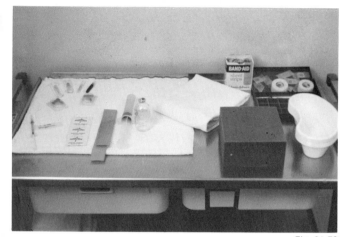

Excretory Urography
Equipment

Fig. 21-72

X.U. Scout Radiograph

A scout radiograph is necessary since contrast medium is to be utilized. With iodine-containing contrast media the optimal kVp is 70, so the scout and series should be performed at this kilovoltage level. The model is shown in position for the scout radiograph in *Fig. 21-73*. The scout for an excretory urogram is similar to a plain abdominal radiograph. A large-sized film is used so that the kidneys, ureters and bladder can be included on the resultant radiograph. The midsagittal plane of the patient should be centered to the midline of the film. Center to the iliac crest and make sure that the symphysis pubis will be shown on the bottom of the radiograph.

The knees should be flexed to (1) reduce the lumbar lordosis, (2) place the kidneys closer to the film and (3) put the kidneys more parallel to the plane of the film. In most cases, the exposure is made on full expiration with breathing stopped. Suspended inspiration is sometimes used, however, to move the kidneys lower in the abdominal cavity.

While the scout radiograph is being processed, complete the necessary preinjection questioning of the patient and carefully explain the examination procedure. Depending on the patient's current problem, one of several possible radiographic routines will be followed after injection. The scout radiograph must be checked by the radiologist to identify and locate abnormal calcifications, to identify any unusual shadows that may be on or under the patient, to identify unsuspected aortic aneurysm or other abdominal mass, and to determine adequacy of patient preparation.

The radiographer should check the scout to be sure that the technical factors were optimum and that there was no patient motion. Check to see that the upper poles of both kidneys are both visualized and that the upper border of the symphysis pubis is on the radiograph. Knowing exactly where the kidneys are is necessary since well-collimated radiographs of the kidneys may be ordered early in the examination. By making sure that the symphysis pubis is just on the bottom of the radiograph, one should be able to include kidneys, ureters and bladder on the full-sized radiographs.

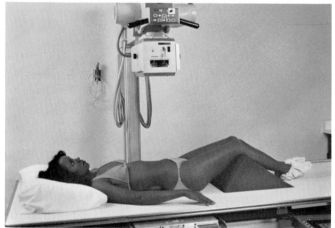

X.U. Scout

Fig. 21-73

Trendelenburg X.U. Scout. Some departmental routines require that the scout and early series radiographs be taken in the Trendelenburg position, as shown in *Fig. 21-74*. The head end of the table is tilted down 15 degrees. The patient will feel more secure if the shoulder support is utilized. The purpose of the Trendelenburg position is to enhance filling of the pelvicalyceal system. The contrast medium in the urine will tend to stay in the kidneys longer in this position since the kidneys will be much lower than the ureters.

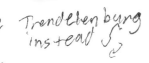
e Trendelenburg instead ς

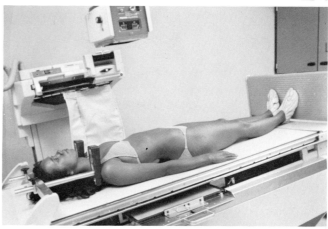

Trendelenburg X.U. Scout   Fig. 21-74

Ureteric Compression. A second method utilized to enhance filling of the pelvicalyceal system is ureteric compression. One such compression device is shown in position on the model in *Fig. 21-75*. The belt is placed around the waist with inflatable balloons over the lower abdomen. When properly applied, pressure will be placed over the ureters at the brim of the pelvis, retaining contrast medium in the kidneys longer. Compression should not be used on patients with (1) possible ureteral stones, (2) abdominal mass, (3) aortic aneurysm, (4) recent abdominal surgery, (5) severe abdominal pain or (6) acute abdominal trauma.

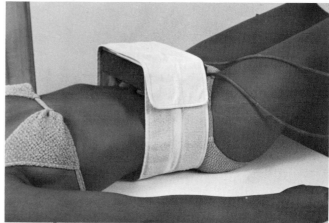

Ureteric Compression   Fig. 21-75

General Routine Procedure

After the scout radiograph is checked and all other preparations are complete, the radiologist or his designate makes the injection. The patient's history and any other pertinent information are discussed prior to the injection. Depending largely on regional standards of practice, the radiologist may utilize a "test dose" prior to the full injection. The test dose consists of a small amount of contrast medium being slowly injected into the patient. For a period of one minute, the radiologist watches the patient for any adverse reaction. When satisfied that the test dose is not causing a reaction, the full injection is completed. Since the test dose is known to have little value in predicting hypersensitivity or allergic reactions, it is currently used primarily for medicolegal purposes.

When the full injection is made, one should note the exact starting time and the length of the injection. Timing for the entire series is based on the start of the injection, not on the end of it. The injection usually takes between 30 seconds and one minute to complete. As the examination proceeds, carefully observe the patient and question the patient regarding any physical changes.

After the full injection of contrast medium, radiographs are taken at specific time intervals, depending on depart-

Xuratory urogram

mental protocol, the patient's particular problem and evaluation of each radiograph by the radiologist. For instance, a basic routine for an X.U. might be supine radiographs at one minute, five minutes and 15 minutes, both posterior obliques at 20 minutes, and either an upright or prone post-voiding radiograph to complete the series. Many variations in routine do exist, however, and the radiologist may order specific positions at any time during the usual series.

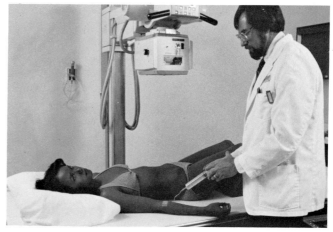

X.U. Injection   Fig. 21-76

Nephrogram. Radiographs taken very early in the series are termed **nephrograms.** The renal parenchyma or functional portion of the kidney consists of many thousands of nephrons. Since individual nephrons are microscopic, the nephron phase is a blush of the entire kidney substance. This blush results from contrast medium throughout the many nephrons, but not into the collecting tubules as yet. The usual nephrogram is obtained with a radiograph at one minute after the start of injection. Ureteric compression, if used, tends to prolong the nephron phase to as long as five minutes in the normal kidney. Since the primary interest in nephrography is the two kidneys, centering and film size should be confined to the kidneys. Center halfway between the iliac crest and the xiphoid process unless a better centering point is determined after viewing the scout radiograph. The model in *Fig. 21-77* is shown in correct position for a one-minute nephrogram. Timing is critical on this radiograph so be certain that the exposure is made exactly 60 seconds after the start of the injection. The table, film and control panel must be in readiness even before the injection is begun since the injection will sometimes take nearly 60 seconds to complete.

Hypertensive X.U. One special type of excretory urogram is the hypertensive X.U. This examination is done on patients with high blood pressure to determine if the kidneys are the cause of the hypertension. During the hypertensive X.U., several early radiographs are obtained. The hypertensive series will include, at least, one-, two- and three-minute radiographs, with the possibility of additional radiographs every 30 seconds. Timing is extremely important during a hypertensive X.U. so these radiographs must be taken at the exact times after the start of injection. Occasionally, tomography of the kidneys during the nephrogram phase may be ordered.

After the very early radiographs in a standard X.U., imaging is done on full-sized film to include the kidneys, ureters and bladder. Any supine radiographs are done exactly as described for the scout.

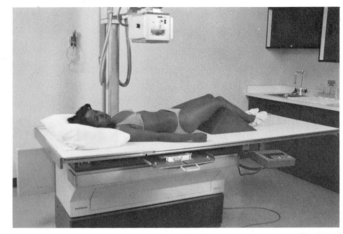

Nephrogram

Fig. 21-77

Postrelease or Spill Procedure (Ureteric Compression). A postrelease or spill radiograph may be requested when ureteric compression is used. This is a full-sized radiograph taken immediately after releasing the compression. Explain to the patient what will be done, then release the air pressure as illustrated in *Fig. 21-78*. After removing the apparatus, immediately make the exposure. The spill radiograph or any other delayed imaging is usually done in the supine position.

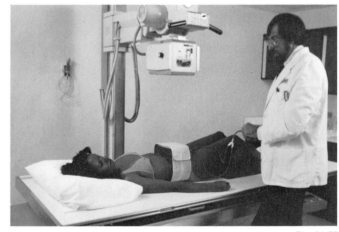

Postrelease or Spill Procedure

Fig. 21-78

Series Completion. Near the end of the series when the entire collecting system from kidney to bladder is well opacified, both posterior obliques are often taken. A body rotation of 30 degrees is utilized. This amount of rotation will place the kidney farthest from the film parallel to the film plane. Thus, in the L.P.O. position, the right kidney will be placed nearly parallel to the film plane. The full-sized film is used and centering is to the iliac crest.

At the completion of the usual X.U. series, a postvoid radiograph is often obtained in either the prone or the upright position. By emptying the bladder, small abnormalities of the bladder may be detected on the postvoid radiograph. The upright position, as shown in *Fig. 21-79*, will demonstrate any unusual movement of the kidneys.

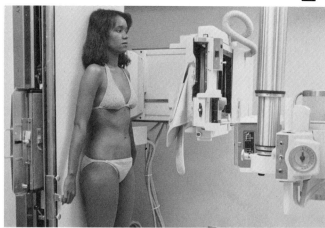

Postvoid Upright Position   Fig. 21-79

Summary of Excretory Urography (X.U.) Procedure

- **Scout radiograph taken**
  (may require Trendelenburg position or ureteric compression routine)
- **Patient's history taken**
- **Injection of contrast medium**
  (may include test dose)
  - Time noted at beginning of injection
  - Radiographs taken

    Possible Routine
- 1 min. supine
  (nephrogram, center to kidneys)
- 5 min. supine
- 15 min. supine
- 20 min. L.P.O. and R.P.O.
- Erect or prone postvoid

Retrograde Urography

Retrograde urography is a nonfunctional examination of the urinary system during which contrast medium is introduced directly into the pelvicalyceal system via catheterization by a urologist during a minor surgical procedure. Retrograde urography is nonfunctional since the patient's normal physiologic processes are not involved in the procedure.

Surgery personnel place the patient on the combination cystoscopic-radiographic table, usually located in the surgery department. The patient is placed in the modified lithotomy position, which requires that the legs be placed in stirrups as illustrated in *Fig. 21-80*. The patient is usually either sedated or anesthetized for this examination. The urologist inserts a cystoscope through the urethra into the bladder. After examining the inside of the bladder, the urologist inserts ureteral catheters into one or both ureters. Ideally, the tip of each ureteral catheter is placed at the level of the renal pelvis.

After catheterization, a scout radiograph is exposed. The scout radiograph allows the radiographer to check technique and positioning, and allows the urologist to check catheter placement. The second radiograph in the usual retrograde urographic series is a pyelogram. The urologist injects 3 to 5 cc's of any of the urographic contrast media directly into the renal pelvis of one or both kidneys. Respiration is suspended immediately after injection, and the exposure is made.

The third and final radiograph in the usual series is a ureterogram. The head end of the table may be elevated for this final radiograph. The urologist withdraws the catheters and simultaneously injects contrast material into one or both ureters. The urologist indicates when to make the exposure. This examination is used to directly visualize the internal structures of one or both kidneys and ureters.

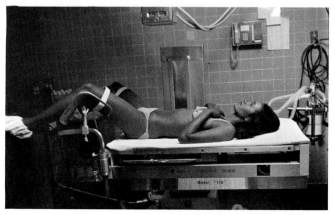

Retrograde Urography   Fig. 21-80
Scout Position

Cystography

Cystography is another nonfunctional urinary system examination. Cystography is a radiographic examination of the urinary bladder following instillation of an iodinated contrast medium via a urethral catheter. There is no patient preparation for this examination, although the patient should empty the bladder prior to catheterization. After routine bladder catheterization under aseptic conditions, the bladder is drained of any residual urine. The bladder is then filled with dilute contrast medium as illustrated in *Fig. 21-81*. The contrast material is allowed to flow in by gravity only, using an asepto syringe. One should never get in a hurry and attempt to inject the contrast medium under pressure. Bladders have been ruptured through the use of unnecessary pressure.

After the bladder is filled, which may require 150 to 500 cc's, either fluorographic spot radiographs are taken by the radiologist or various overhead positions are exposed by the radiographer. Routine positioning for a cystogram includes an A.P. with a 15-degree caudal angle and both posterior obliques. An optional position is the true lateral which may or may not be included in the routine due to the large gonadal radiation exposure necessary. The caudal angulation of 15 degrees with the legs extended for the A.P.

projection will help to project the symphysis pubis below the filled bladder. A steeper oblique is used to visualize the bladder during cystography than is used to visualize the kidneys during excretory urography. Cystogram obliques are usually 45 to 60 degrees depending on the radiologist's preference. The steep oblique allows the posterolateral aspect of the bladder and the location of the ureterovesical junction to be examined radiographically.

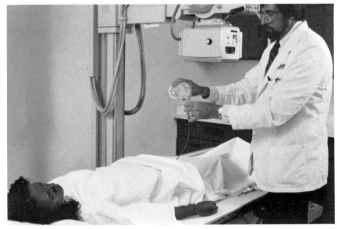

Fig. 21-81

Cystography —
instilling contrast medium

Voiding Cystourethrography

Voiding radiographs may be taken after the routine cystogram. When combined in this manner, the examination would be termed a cystourethrogram or voiding cystourethrogram (V.C.U.). The voiding phase of the examination is best done utilizing fluoroscopic control and a spot film camera. The procedure is sometimes done with the patient supine, although the upright position makes it easier to void. The key to a good voiding study is to gently remove the catheter from the bladder and urethra. First remove any liquid from the balloon portion of the catheter, if this type of catheter was used, and ever so gently remove the catheter. The urethra can be traumatized if care is not exercised. The female is usually examined in the A.P. or slight oblique position, as shown on the radiograph in *Fig. 21-82*. The male is best examined in a 30-degree right posterior oblique position. An adequate receptacle or absorbent padding must be provided for the patient. After voiding is complete and adequate imaging is obtained, a postvoiding A.P. may be requested.

Bead-chain Cystogram

A special type of voiding cystourethrogram is performed on females with a diagnosis of stress incontinence or involuntary loss of urine. This examination is termed the bead-chain cystogram and is done to determine the anatomical relationship of the bladder and the urethra. Four radiographs are taken in the usual bead-chain cystogram. Two upright A.P.'s and two upright laterals are taken. First, the physician inserts a flexible, metallic bead chain into the bladder. The distal end rests on the floor of the bladder,

while the proximal end is taped to the patient's thigh. A catheter is then introduced and about 60 cc's of contrast medium are instilled in the bladder. After removing the catheter and standing the patient up, an A.P. and lateral are exposed while the patient is relaxed. A second set of radiographs is taken while the patient bears down or strains. A towel placed between the thighs will help the patient apply full pressure on straining. She may fear involuntary urination, otherwise.

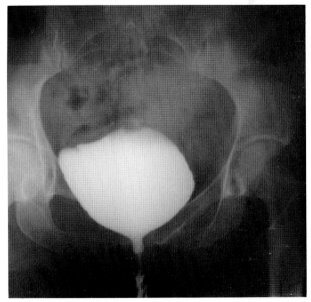

Fig. 21-82

Female Voiding
Cystourethrogram

Retrograde Urography

A retrograde urethrogram is sometimes performed on the male patient to demonstrate the full length of the urethra. Contrast medium is injected into the distal urethra until the entire urethra is filled in retrograde fashion. Injection of contrast material is sometimes facilitated by a special device termed a Brodney clamp, which is attached to the distal penis. A 30-degree right posterior oblique is the position of choice, and centering is to the symphysis pubis. The tip of the syringe is inserted into the distal urethra and the injection is made. Ample contrast medium is used to fill the entire urethra and exposures are made. An R.P.O. retrograde urethrogram on a male patient is shown in *Fig. 21-83*. Ideally, the urethra is superimposed over the soft tissues of the right thigh. This prevents superimposition of any bony structures except for the lower pelvis.

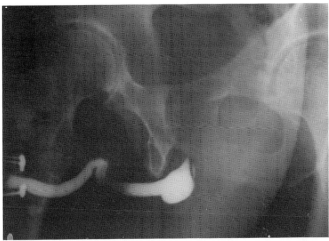

Male Retrograde
Urethrogram

Fig. 21-83

Summary

Urinary System Radiography — Urography

Urography may be categorized by the method of contrast medium administration. Contrast medium is either introduced into the circulatory system or directly into the structure to be studied.

(1) Into the bloodstream
(usually intravenous injection)
- Excretory Urography

(2) Directly into the structure to be studied
(requires catheterization)
- Retrograde Urography
- Cystography
- Voiding Cystourethrography
- Bead-chain Cystography
- Retrograde Urethrography

Basic and Optional Projections/Positions

Certain basic or optional projections or positions of the urinary system are demonstrated and described on the following pages. The radiologist and radiographer must closely coordinate their efforts during examinations of this portion of the anatomy.

Excretory Urography (X.U.)
Basic
- A.P. (Scout and Series)
- L.P.O. (30°)
- R.P.O. (30°)
- Upright A.P. - Postvoid

Optional
- A.P. - Trendelenburg
- A.P. - Ureteric Compression
- P.A. - Postvoid

Retrograde Urography
Basic
- A.P. (Scout)
- A.P. (Pyelogram)
- A.P. (Ureterogram)

Cystography
Basic
- A.P. (15° caudad)
- Both Obliques (60°)

Optional
- Lateral

Voiding Cystourethrography
Basic (Male)
- R.P.O. (30°)
Basic (Female)
- A.P.

Bead-chain Cystography
Basic
- A.P. (relaxed and straining)
- Lat. (relaxed and straining)

Retrograde Urethrography
Basic
- R.P.O. (30°)

Excretory Urography
• Anteroposterior Projection

Excretory Urography (X.U.)
Basic
- **A.P.** (Scout and Series)
- L.P.O. (30°)
- R.P.O. (30°)
- Upright A.P. - Postvoid

Optional
- A.P. - Trendelenburg
- A.P. - Ureteric Compression
- P.A. - Postvoid

Film Size:
   14 x 17 in. (35 x 43 cm.)

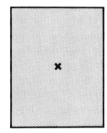

Bucky:
- Moving or stationary grid.

Patient Position:
- Supine.
- Midsagittal plane of body centered to midline of table and/or film.
- Flex knees and place support under knees.

Part Position:
- Trunk of body, including pelvis, comfortable and not rotated.
- Symphysis pubis should be on bottom of radiograph.

Central Ray:
- C.R. perpendicular to film holder.
- Center to level of iliac crests and to midsagittal plane.
- Center to kidneys for nephrogram.
- 40 in. (102 cm.) F.F.D.

NOTE: • 70 kVp should be utilized. • Suspend respiration on expiration. • Explain examination procedure and obtain patient history before injection of contrast medium. • Check scout for optimum technique and position of kidneys. • Patient voids before examination.

Structures Best Shown:
Kidneys, ureters and urinary bladder filled with contrast medium.

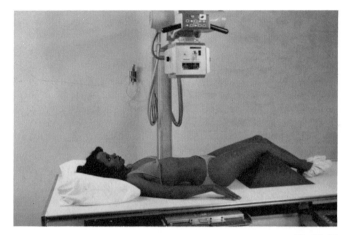

X.U. Scout and Series   Fig. 21-84

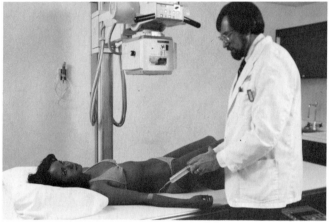

X.U. Injection   Fig. 21-85

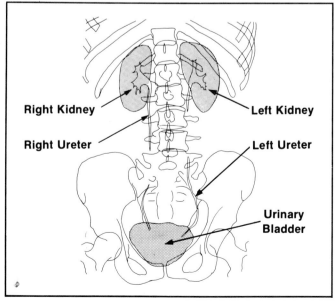

Right Kidney   **Left Kidney**

Right Ureter   **Left Ureter**

Urinary Bladder

Fig. 21-87
Urogram (15 minutes)

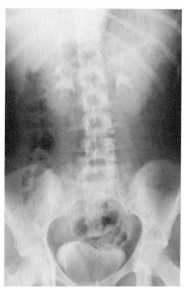

Urogram   Fig. 21-86
(15 minutes)

Excretory Urography (X.U.)
Basic
- A.P. (Scout and Series)
- **L.P.O.** (30°)
- **R.P.O.** (30°)
- Upright A.P. - Postvoid

Optional
- A.P. - Trendelenburg
- A.P. - Ureteric Compression
- P.A. - Postvoid

Excretory Urography
- **Left Posterior Oblique Position**
- **Right Posterior Oblique Position**

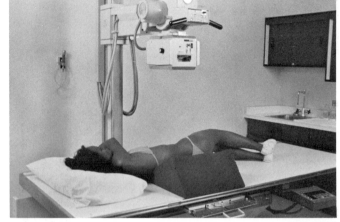

L.P.O. Position   Fig. 21-88

Film Size:
>   14 x 17 in. (35 x 43 cm.)

Bucky:
- Moving or stationary grid.

Patient and Part Position:
- Rotate body into a 30° posterior oblique for both positions.
- Plane through vertebral column should be centered to midline of table and/or film.
- Support hip and back.

Centray Ray:
- C.R. perpendicular to film holder.
- Center to level of iliac crests and to vertebral column.
- 40 in. (102 cm.) F.F.D.

NOTE: • 70 kVp should be utilized. • Suspend respiration on expiration. • 30° posterior oblique will place kidney furthest from the film parallel to plane of film.

Structures Best Shown:
Kidneys, ureters and urinary bladder filled with contrast medium. R.P.O. position best shows left kidney.

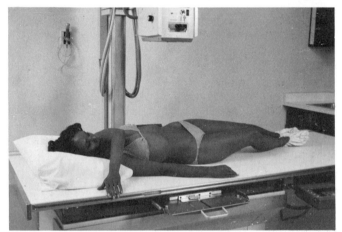

R.P.O. Position   Fig. 21-89

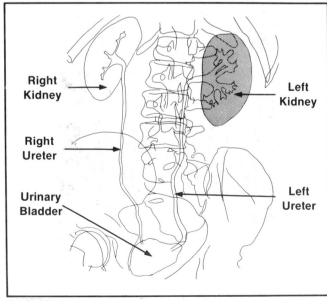

Fig. 21-91

Right Kidney

Left Kidney

Right Ureter

Left Ureter

Urinary Bladder

R.P.O.

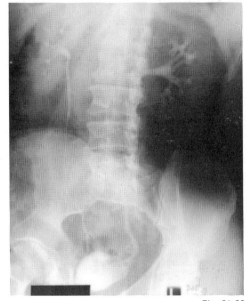

R.P.O.   Fig. 21-90

Excretory Urography (X.U.)
Basic
- A.P. (Scout and Series)
- L.P.O. (30°)
- R.P.O. (30°)
- **Upright A.P. - Postvoid**
Optional
- A.P. - Trendelenburg
- A.P. - Ureteric Compression
- **P.A. - Postvoid**

Excretory Urography
- **Upright A.P. - Postvoid**
  - **P.A. - Postvoid**

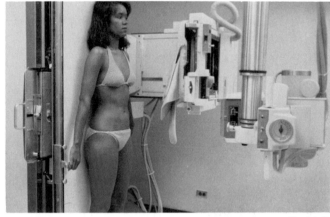
Upright A.P. (Postvoid)   Fig. 21-92

Film Size:
   14 x 17 in. (35 x 43 cm.)

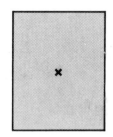

Bucky:
- Moving or stationary grid.

Patient and Part Position:

Upright A.P.
- Standing with back against table or film holder (no rotation).

P.A.
- Prone (no rotation).

Central Ray:
- C.R. perpendicular to film holder.
- Center to level of iliac crests and to midsagittal plane.
- 40 in. (102 cm.) F.F.D.

NOTE: • 70 kVp should be utilized. • Suspend respiration on expiration. • Upright radiograph will demonstrate nephroptosis, if present.

Structures Best Shown:
Kidneys (positional change) and nearly empty bladder.

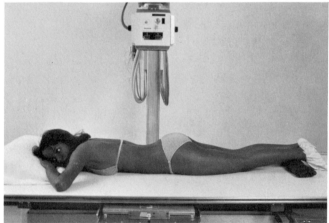
P.A. (Postvoid)   Fig. 21-93

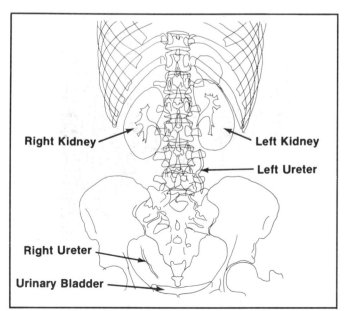

Right Kidney

Left Kidney

Left Ureter

Right Ureter

Urinary Bladder

Fig. 21-95
Upright A.P. (Postvoid)

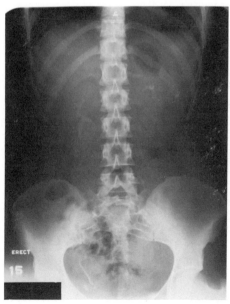
Fig. 21-94
Upright A.P. (Postvoid)

Excretory Urography
- **A.P. - Trendelenburg**
- **A.P. - Ureteric Compression**

Film Size:
14 x 17 in. (35 x 43 cm.)

Bucky:
- Moving or stationary grid.

Patient and Part Position:

A.P. - Trendelenburg
- Supine with head end of table tilted downward 15°. C.R. remains perpendicular to plane of film. Use shoulder support.

A.P. - Ureteric Compression
- Supine with compression device over lower abdomen. Compression should NOT be used with acute problems, abdominal masses or recent surgery.

Central Ray:
- C.R. perpendicular to film holder.
- Center to level of iliac crests and to midsagittal plane. Center to kidneys only if indicated.
- 40 in. (102 cm.) F.F.D.

NOTE: • Both positions enhance pelvicalyceal filling.

Structures Best Shown:
Renal pelvis and calyces.

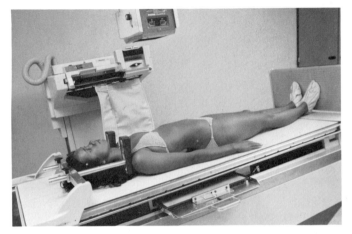

A.P. Trendelenburg   Fig. 21-96

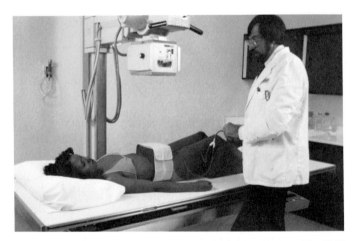

A.P. Ureteric Compression   Fig. 21-97

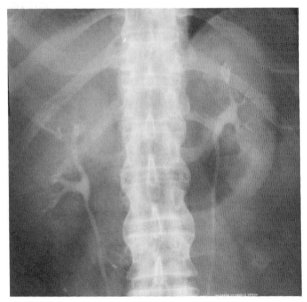

Fig. 21-99

A.P. Ureteric Compression

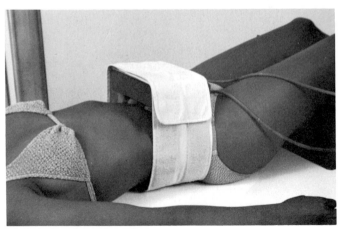

A.P. Ureteric Compression   Fig. 21-98

Retrograde Urography
Basic
- A.P. (Scout)
- A.P. (Pyelogram)
- A.P. (Ureterogram)

Retrograde Urography
• Anteroposterior Projection

Film Size:
   14 x 17 in. (35 x 43 cm.)

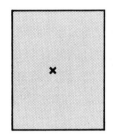

Bucky:
- Moving or stationary grid.

Patient and Part Position:
- Modified lithotomy position.

Central Ray:
- C.R. perpendicular to film holder.
- Center to level of iliac crests and to midsagittal plane.
- 40 in. (102 cm.) F.F.D.

NOTE: • Scout exposed after urologist places catheter(s).
• Pyelogram exposed after contrast medium injection into renal pelvis. • Ureterogram exposed as catheters are withdrawn. • Suspend respiration on expiration.

Structures Best Shown:
Renal pelvis, major and minor calyces, and ureters.

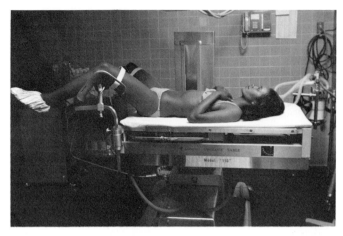

Fig. 21-100
Retrograde Urography Position

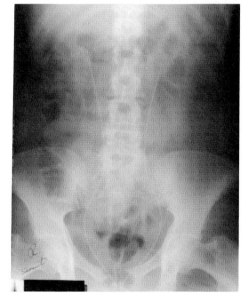

Retrograde Urogram Scout   Fig. 21-101

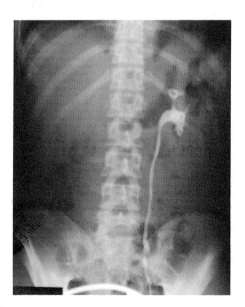

Fig. 21-103
Ureterogram — left only

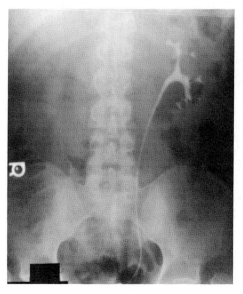

Pyelogram — left only   Fig. 21-102

Cystography
Basic
- **A.P.** (15° caudad)
- **Both Obliques** (60°)

Optional
- **Lateral**

Cystography
- **Anteroposterior Projection**
- **Posterior Oblique Positions**
- **Lateral Position**

Film Size:

    10 x 12 in. (24 x 30 cm.)

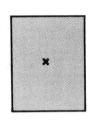

Bucky:

- Moving or stationary grid.

Patient and Part Position:

A.P.

- Supine, with legs extended.

Posterior Obliques

- 45 to 60° body rotation.

Lateral

- True lateral (no rotation).

Central Ray:

A.P.

- Center 2 in. (5 cm.) above symphysis pubis with 15° caudad tube angle.

Posterior Obliques

- Center 2 in. (5 cm.) above symphysis pubis and 2 in. (5 cm.) medial to A.S.I.S.

Lateral

- Center 2 in. (5 cm.) above and posterior to symphysis pubis.

NOTE: • Caudal angulation with the A.P. helps to project symphysis pubis inferior to bladder. • Steep obliques are used to visualize posterolateral aspect of bladder, especially U.V. junction. • Contrast medium should **never** be injected under pressure. • Lateral position optional due to large gonadal radiation dose.

Structures Best Shown:

Urinary bladder.

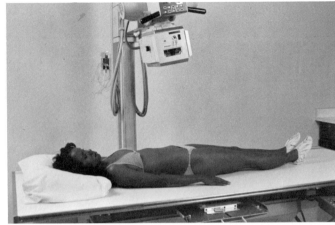

A.P. (15° caudad)   Fig. 21-104

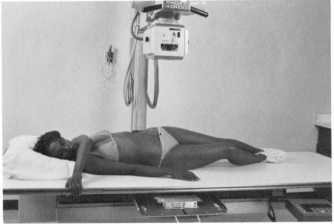

R.P.O. (60°)   Fig. 21-105

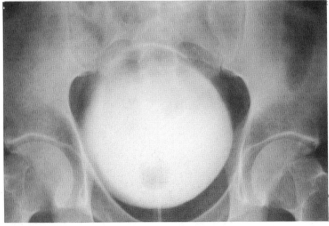

Fig. 21-107

A.P. (15° caudad)

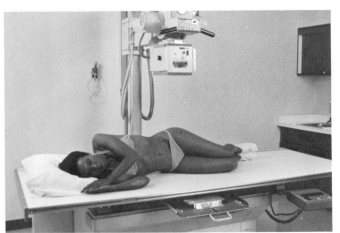

Right Lateral   Fig. 21-106

Voiding Cystourethrography
• Right Posterior Oblique (30°) - Male
• Anteroposterior - Female

<table>
<tr><td>
Voiding Cystourethrography
Basic (Male)
• R.P.O. (30°)
Basic (Female)
• A.P.
</td></tr>
</table>

Film Size:
10 x 12 in. (24 x 30 cm.)

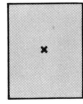

Bucky:
- Moving or stationary grid.

Patient and Part Position:

Male
- Recumbent or upright.
- Turn to 30° right posterior oblique.

Female
- Recumbent or upright.
- A.P. or slight oblique.

Central Ray:
- C.R. perpendicular to film holder.
- Center to top of symphysis pubis.
- 40 in. (102 cm.) F.F.D.

NOTE: • Male urethra should superimpose soft tissues of right thigh. • Provide adequate receptacle or absorbent padding for patient. • Best done utilizing fluoroscopic control and spot filming. • Catheter must be gently removed prior to voiding procedure.

Structures Best Shown:
Urinary bladder and urethra. Ureteral reflux may be demonstrated.

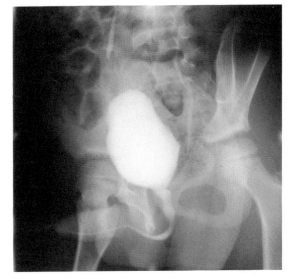
R.P.O. — Male   Fig. 21-108

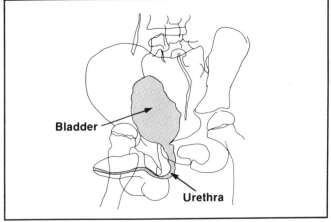
R.P.O. — Male   Fig. 21-109

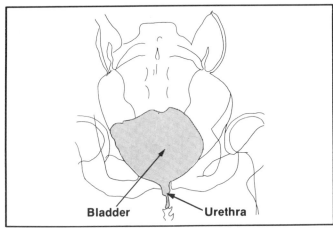
Fig. 21-111   A.P. — Female

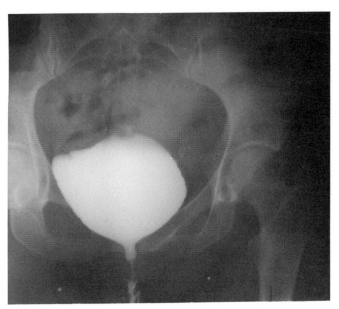
A.P. — Female   Fig. 21-110

Retrograde Urethrography
• Right Posterior Oblique (30°) Position

Film Size:
  10 x 12 in. (24 x 30 cm.)

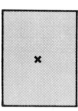

Bucky:
- Moving or stationary grid.

Patient and Part Position:
- Recumbent right posterior oblique position.
- Extend right leg so that urethra superimposes right thigh.

Central Ray:
- C.R. perpendicular to film holder.
- Center to symphysis pubis.
- 40 in. (102 cm.) F.F.D.

NOTE: • Ample contrast material must be used to fill entire length of urethra. • Device such as Brodney clamp may be used to facilitate injection.

Structures Best Shown:
Full length of male urethra.

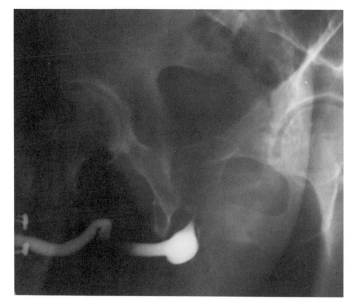

Male Retrograde Urethrogram   Fig. 21-112

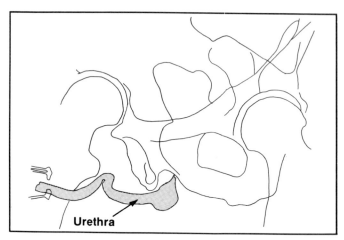

Male Retrograde Urethrogram   Fig. 21-113

CHAPTER 22
Special Radiographic Procedures

Special Radiographic Procedures

Throughout this textbook and in the audiovisual series by the same authors, all radiographic examinations and procedures are classified in three categories; **basic** or **routine examinations, common procedures** and **special procedures.**

Special neuroradiographic procedures involving the head are presented in detail in Chapters 16, 17 and 18. There are many additional special radiographic procedures with which the radiographer should be familiar. One should be aware of the name and type of all special procedures, even if one is not planning specialization in this area. These special examinations are listed and briefly described in this chapter.

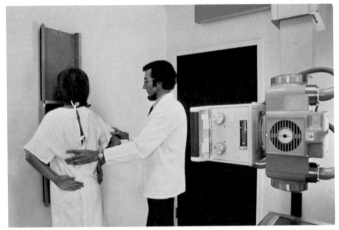

Basic (Routine) Examination,
P.A. Chest

Fig. 22-1

Basic or Routine Radiographic Examinations

Basic or routine radiographic procedures make up the majority of the caseload in the average radiology department or other medical radiographic facility. These basic or routine examinations are performed by a radiographer following an appropriate order by a physician. These examinations do not require administration of a contrast medium or the active participation of a radiologist or other physician specialist. Most basic or routine radiographic projections or positions, as well as certain optional positions or projections, are described in Chapters 2 through 15 of this text.

The most common basic or routine radiographic examination is shown in *Figs. 22-1* and *22-2.* Although the routine posteroanterior chest radiographic examination does not require instillation of a constrast medium, a natural contrast medium is utilized. Air is a negative contrast medium. The air normally found in the lungs provides a natural contrast to the other organs and structures of the chest region.

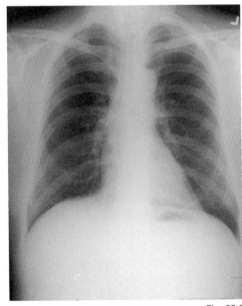

Fig. 22-2

P.A. Chest Radiograph

526

Common Radiographic Procedures

Common radiographic procedures, as described in this text, are those examinations performed in large numbers in both large and small radiology departments, as well as in certain clinics and physicians' offices. They involve the administration of some form of contrast medium. Common radiographic procedures utilizing some form of contrast medium may also involve the use of fluoroscopy or the active participation of a radiologist or other physician specialist. These contrast-medium-enhanced common radiographic procedures may comprise 20 to 30 percent of the radiology department caseload. One example of a common radiographic procedure is an esophagram, shown in *Fig. 22-3*. Common radiographic examinations involve the gastrointestinal system, the biliary system and the urinary system. These common radiographic examinations are presented in Chapters 19, 20 and 21.

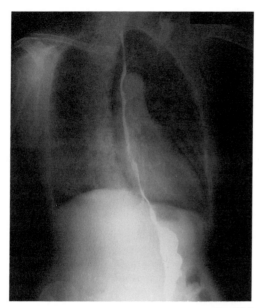

Common Examination
— Esophagram

Fig. 22-3

Special Radiographic Procedures

Special radiographic procedures are those examinations requiring specialized radiographic equipment, and specially trained radiologists and radiographers. Most special procedures require the use of a contrast medium and the services of a highly trained team of radiology personnel. An example of a special radiographic examination is the coronary arteriogram, shown in *Fig 22-4*. Three special neuroradiographic examinations involving the head are presented in Chapters 16, 17 and 18. Cranial computed tomography and cerebral angiography are among the most often performed special radiographic procedures.

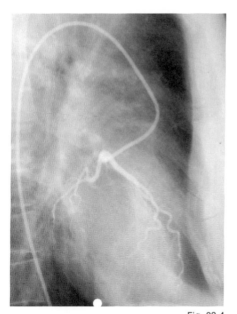

Special Examination
— Coronary Arteriogram

Fig. 22-4

Contrast Media

Radiolucent or Negative Contrast Media

Contrast media are substances that render an organ or structure more visible than is possible without the addition of a contrast medium. Contrast media added to the human body are either radiolucent or radiopaque. The addition of a radiolucent or negative contrast medium allows the passage of more x-rays than would be possible without the use of a contrast medium. Examples of negative contrast media are air, oxygen, carbon dioxide and nitrous oxide. Air added to the ventricles of the brain in pneumoencephalography allows the ventricles and subarachnoid spaces of the brain to be visualized radiographically.

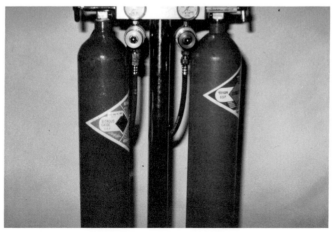

Negative Contrast Media

Fig. 22-5

Radiopaque or Positive Contrast Media

Barium Sulfate. Radiopaque or positive contrast media can cause an increase in the absorption of x-rays, producing a white image on the finished radiograph. Positive contrast agents contain elements with high atomic weights, such as iodine or barium. The most commonly used positive contrast medium is barium sulfate ($BaSO_4$). Barium sulfate is used by itself or in conjunction with a negative contrast medium in most radiographic examinations of the alimentary canal. Barium sulfate is a powdered, chalklike substance, as shown in *Fig. 22-6,* that is mixed with water prior to use. When barium sulfate and water are mixed for usage, the resultant mixture is a suspension, not a solution. Since the barium sulfate and water mixture is a suspension, the barium sulfate particles tend to settle out when allowed to sit for a period of time. Radiographic examinations of the esophagus, stomach, small intestine and large intestine, in most cases, utilize barium sulfate as the positive contrast medium.

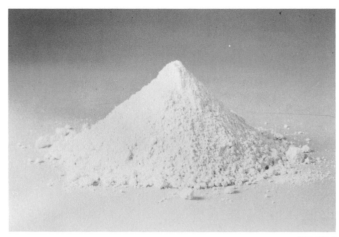

Positive Contrast Medium   Fig. 22-6

Organic Iodides and Iodized Oils. Most other radiopaque or positive contrast media utilize iodine as the radiation-absorbing component. These iodinated compounds are formulated to be soluble in water or not soluble in water. Compounds not soluble in water are the iodized oils used for lymphangiography, bronchography and some myelography. Water-soluble, organic iodides are widely used for excretory urography, angiography and intravenous cholangiography. Other organic iodides are taken orally in the form of tablets, capsules and granules for radiographic study of the gallbladder and biliary ducts.

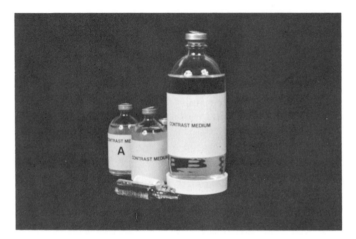

Positive Contrast Media   Fig. 22-7

Positive and Negative Contrast Media

Some radiographic examinations utilize both positive and negative contrast media. Both types of contrast media are useful in certain studies of the stomach, large intestine, joints, urinary bladder and spinal canal. A double-contrast barium enema is shown in *Fig. 22-8.* This examination utilizes the positive contrast medium, barium sulfate, and the negative contrast medium, air.

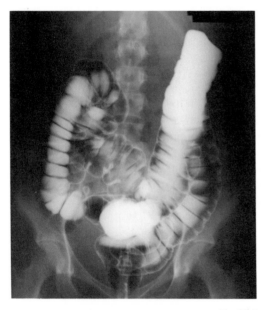

Negative and Positive   Fig. 22-8
Contrast Media

528

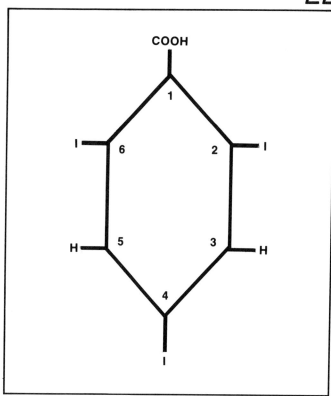

Triiodobenzoic Acid Molecule

Fig. 22-9

Water-Soluble, Injectable Contrast Media

Most water-soluble, injectable contrast media utilize the same basic molecule. This is the triiodobenzoic acid molecule, as shown in *Fig. 22-9.* This molecule has three high atomic weight iodine atoms attached to the molecule at positions 2, 4 and 6. Iodine is used extensively in radiopaque contrast media. These compounds are easily formed, do not rapidly disintegrate in the body and are readily excreted by the kidneys.

Three Most Commonly Used Triiodinated Benzoic Acid Compounds. The three main types of triiodinated benzoic acid compounds used today are the **diatrizoates,** the **iothalamates** and the **metrizoates.** These three compounds are very similar and vary only slightly at the number 3 position. The side chain at the number 5 position is identical in all three compounds. Each of these contrast medium molecules is composed of a positive portion, the cation, and a negative portion, the anion. The positive portion is either sodium or meglumine. The negative part of the molecule is one of the three salts, diatrizoate, iothalamate or metrizoate.

Desirable Properties of Injectable Contrast Media. Injectable contrast media must exhibit properties of **low toxicity, high opacity, low viscosity** and **high miscibility.** The contrast media must exhibit low toxicity so that few reactions are encountered following injection. With three iodine atoms per molecule, these contrast media exhibit a high degree of x-ray opacification. Viscosity relates to the ease or difficulty of an injection of contrast material. In special procedures requiring a quick delivery of a bolus of contrast medium, the medium selected must have a low viscosity. When the viscosity of a solution is low, rapid administration is possible. Injectable contrast media must also freely mix with the blood within the vessel being injected and, therefore, must have a high degree of miscibility.

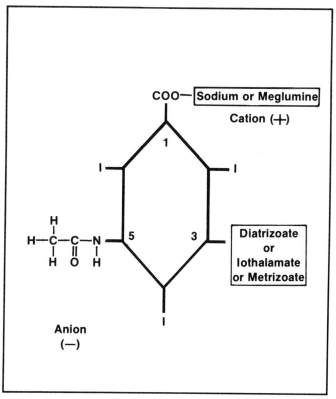

Water-soluble Injectable
Contrast Media

Fig. 22-10

Special Radiographic Examinations — Chest

Bronchography

Bronchography is radiographic examination of the lungs and bronchial trees after the bronchi have been filled with a radiopaque contrast medium. Contrast medium is usually instilled following intratracheal intubation, when a tube is passed through the nose or mouth through the glottis and into the trachea. Once the contrast medium is injected, it must be distributed throughout the bronchial tree by gravity, using many changes of body position. The patient must suppress the urge to cough until fluoroscopy spot radiographs and overhead radiographs are taken. P.A. and lateral bronchograms are shown in *Figs. 22-11* and *22-12*.

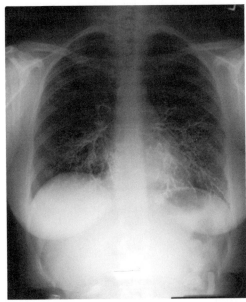

Fig. 22-11
Bronchogram — P.A.

Laryngography

Laryngography is radiographic examination of the larynx following instillation of a radiopaque contrast medium. Following anesthetization of the throat structures, and using a curved cannula, the interior of the larynx and structures above the larynx are coated with an oil-based, iodinated contrast medium. The examination is performed under fluoroscopy with permanent imaging by a spot film device or spot film camera.

Bronchial Brush Biopsy and Percutaneous Lung Biopsy

Bronchial brush biopsy or bronchial brushing is a method of obtaining cytological specimens from deep within the tissues of the lungs. Following insertion of a special catheter under fluoroscopic control, a nylon or stainless steel brush is introduced into the bronchial tree and cells are scraped from suspected areas. Percutaneous lung biopsy is also done under fluoroscopic control. A biopsy needle is introduced through the skin and into a suspected lesion within the thorax.

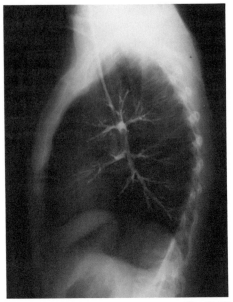

Fig. 22-12
Bronchogram — Lat.

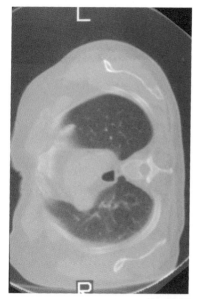

Chest C.T.   Fig. 22-13

Computed Tomography of Chest

Computed tomography of the chest is radiographic examination of any part of the thorax displayed as a thin, cross-sectional, gray-scale, tomographic image representing a computer-assisted, mathematical reconstruction of numerous x-ray absorption differences of the thoracic contents. The principles of computed tomography are described and illustrated in Chapter 18. A CT scan through the upper thorax is shown in *Fig. 22-13*.

Angiography of Thoracic Blood Vessels

Pulmonary Angiography. Pulmonary angiography is radiographic examination of the pulmonary arteries and veins following injection of a radiopaque contrast medium into the venous circulation or right heart. An example of a right pulmonary arteriogram is shown in *Fig. 22-14*.

Angiocardiography. Angiocardiography is radiographic examination of the chambers of the heart and associated great vessels following injection of an iodinated contrast medium. Angiocardiography may be done in conjunction with heart catheterization. Heart catheterizations are usually performed by a cardiologist who obtains additional information such as blood samples for analysis, direct pressure readings and other physiologic data.

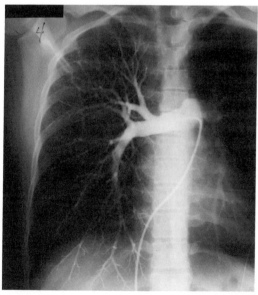

Pulmonary Arteriogram   Fig. 22-14

Thoracic Aortography. Thoracic aortography is radiographic visualization of the thoracic aorta and its branches following injection of an iodinated contrast medium. Selective thoracic angiography may follow thoracic aortography, allowing any of the smaller branches of the thoracic aorta to be located and injected. Any of the intercostal arteries, esophageal arteries or bronchial arteries may be injected.

Coronary Arteriography. Coronary arteriography is radiographic examination of the coronary arteries of the heart following manual injection of iodinated contrast medium via a catheter placed in either the left or right coronary artery. A left coronary arteriogram is shown in *Fig. 22-15*.

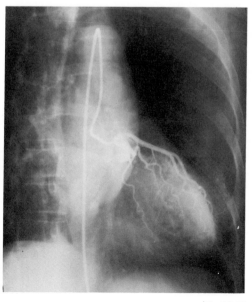

Coronary Arteriogram   Fig. 22-15

Special Radiographic Examinations — Abdomen and Pelvis

Computed Tomography of Abdomen

Computed tomography, utilizing computer-assisted reconstruction techniques, is successfully and advantageously utilized on any part of the body, including the abdomen. The abdominal contents are similar to the cranial contents in that the many soft tissue components fuse into a gray mass during conventional radiography. Utilizing computed tomography of the abdomen enables the radiologist to differentiate between various tissue structures. By using iodinated contrast media within the alimentary canal, further tissue and organ differentiation is possible. A computed tomogram of the upper abdomen utilizing contrast enhancement methods is illustrated in *Fig. 22-16.*

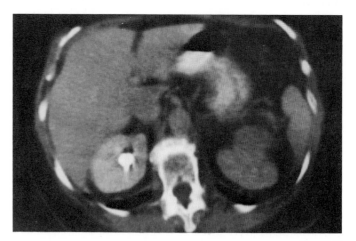

Abdomen C.T.   Fig. 22-16

Visceral Angiography

Any large organ within one of the cavities of the body, but especially the abdominal cavity, is termed a **viscus.** Any radiographic examination of the blood vessels of a viscus is termed, in general, visceral angiography.

Abdominal Aortography. Abdominal aortography is radiographic visualization of the abdominal aorta and its various branches following the injection of a water-soluble, iodinated contrast medium. The contrast medium is usually injected following catheterization of the femoral artery. Catheter placement utilizing the Seldinger technique is termed percutaneous transfemoral catheterization. A typical abdominal aortogram is shown in *Fig. 22-17.*

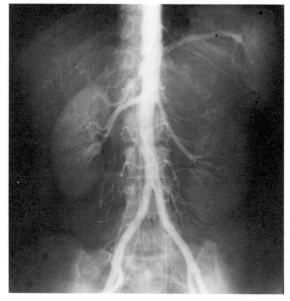

Abdominal Aortogram   Fig. 22-17

Selective Abdominal Angiography. Selective abdominal angiography is specific catheterization and radiographic visualization of any one of the major branches of the abdominal aorta. Major branches of the abdominal aorta that may be selected for specialized study are the **renal arteries,** the **celiac artery,** the **superior mesenteric artery** or the **inferior mesenteric artery.** The renal arteries supply the kidneys; the celiac artery supplies the liver, stomach and spleen; the superior mesenteric artery supplies the small intestine and the right half of the large intestine; and the inferior mesenteric artery supplies the left half of the large intestine. A selective abdominal arteriogram is shown in *Fig. 22-18.* In this example the left renal artery has been injected with contrast medium.

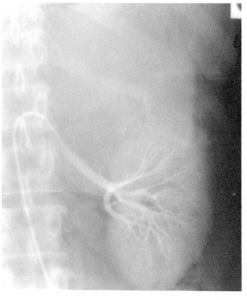

Left Renal Arteriogram   Fig. 22-18

Superselective Abdominal Angiography. Superselective abdominal angiography refers to selective catheterization and radiographic visualization of a minor branch of the abdominal aorta or a small branch from one of the major branches. Utilizing modern catheters and techniques, the radiologist angiographer can select and place the catheter tip in virtually any small blood vessel in the entire body. The radiograph shown in *Fig. 22-19* visualizes a small branch supplying the left adrenal gland area.

Interventional Radiography

Percutaneous Transluminal Angioplasty (PTA). Interventional radiography refers to several procedures offering therapeutic alternatives to surgery and other forms of treatment. Percutaneous transluminal angioplasty refers to the therapeutic use of balloons within arterial blood vessels to dilate or occlude.

Therapeutic Embolization. Therapeutic embolization deals with the use of plastic polymers to selectively block certain blood vessels. This technique is helpful in stopping gastrointestinal bleeding, and decreasing or stopping the blood supply to neoplasia.

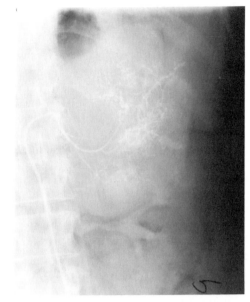

Adrenal Arteriogram   Fig. 22-19

Fistulography or Sinography

A fistula is an abnormal passage or communication, usually between two internal organs, or leading from an internal organ to the surface of the body. A sinus track is an abnormal channel permitting the escape of pus from a site of infection. Fistulography or sinography is radiographic visualization of the abnormal passage or channel to determine the extent of the track. A radiograph showing a sinus track extending from within the abdominal cavity to the anterior abdominal wall is shown in *Fig. 22-20*.

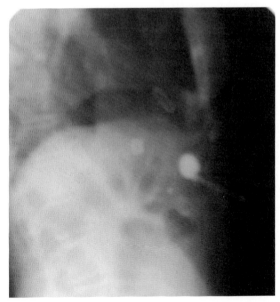

Sinus Track   Fig. 22-20

Endoscopy

Endoscopy is inspection of any cavity of the body by means of an endoscope, an instrument that allows illumination of the internal lining of an organ. Various fiberoptic endoscopes are available to examine the interior lining of the stomach, duodenum and colon. Certain fiberoptic endoscopes allow cannulation and injection of contrast medium into small ducts such as the common bile duct or pancreatic duct. The drawing in *Fig. 22-21* shows an endoscope in position to study the stomach, duodenum, common bile duct or pancreatic duct.

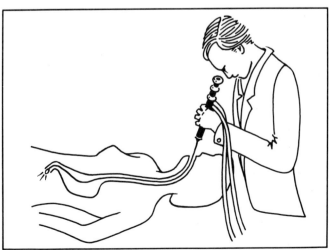

Endoscopy   Fig. 22-21

Hysterosalpingography

Hysterosalpingography is radiographic examination of the uterus and oviducts or Fallopian tubes following injection of a radiopaque contrast medium. This examination is usually performed to determine patency of the oviducts. It is important that this examination be scheduled for the seventh or eighth day following cessation of menstruation. This is the interval during which the endometrium is least congested, and more importantly, it is a few days before ovulation normally occurs, so there is no danger of irradiating a recently fertilized ovum. A hysterosalpingogram is shown in *Fig. 22-22*.

Pelvic Pneumography. Pelvic pneumography or gynography is radiographic examination of the female pelvic organs following intraperitoneal gas insufflation. By adding a negative contrast medium and allowing the gas to surround the proximal uterus, tubes and ovaries, these specific organs are visualized radiographically. In fact, by creating an artificial pneumoperitoneum, any organ within the abdominal cavity can be better visualized.

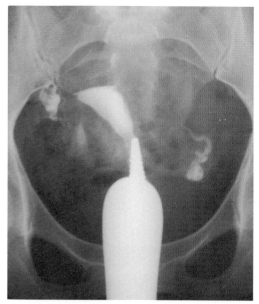

Hysterosalpingogram   Fig. 22-22

Herniography

Herniography or peritoneography is radiographic evaluation of suspected inguinal hernias following percutaneous injection of a water-soluble, positive contrast medium into the abdominal cavity. Herniography is usually performed on children possessing one known inguinal hernia in order to evaluate the clinically normal side. The radiograph is exposed in an upright position to allow the contrast medium to descend into any hernia connecting with the peritoneal cavity. A herniogram is shown in *Fig. 22-23*.

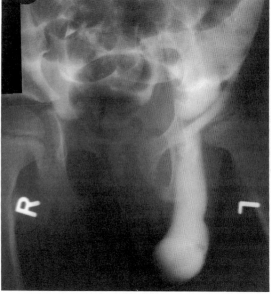

Fig. 22-23

Herniogram

Special Radiographic Examinations — Limbs or Extremities

Peripheral Arteriography

Peripheral arteriography is radiographic visualization of the arteries of either the arm or the leg. The most common examination of this type is femoral arteriography in order to study the femoral artery at its point of bifurcation in the area of the knee. The entire length of the extremity in question is usually radiographed during peripheral arteriography. The positive femoral arteriogram shown in *Fig. 22-24* demonstrates an occlusion at the point of bifurcation. Additional radiographs of the pelvis and lower leg are included in a complete examination.

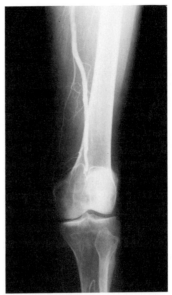

Femoral   Fig. 22-24
Arteriogram

Peripheral Venography

Peripheral venography or phlebography is radiographic examination of the veins of the arm or leg following injection of a radiopaque contrast medium. Venograms are usually performed on the veins of a leg with needle placement on the dorsum of the foot. These examinations are usually done to rule out thromboembolism. Venograms of the knee and femur areas are shown in *Fig. 22-25*.

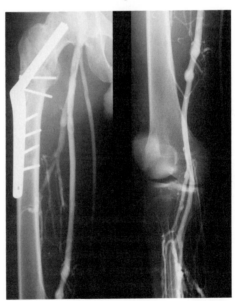

Fig. 22-25

Leg Venograms

Lymphangiography

Lymphangiography is radiographic examination of the lymph vessels following opacification by an injected, iodinated contrast medium. Lymphangiography is carried out within the first hour following injection. Lymphadenography is usually performed 24 hours later to radiographically study the lymph nodes. The peripheral lymph vessels are small and lack color, so a blue dye is injected into the subcutaneous tissues (usually between the first and second toe) about 15 minutes before the examination. The lymphatic system picks up the dye and outlines a lymph channel along the dorsum of the foot. The lymph vessel is then exposed by cutdown and is cannulated. This is one of the few examinations done in the radiology department utilizing a dye as compared to a contrast medium. Contrast media are not dyes and should not be called dyes. A pelvic lymphangiogram is shown in *Fig. 22-26*.

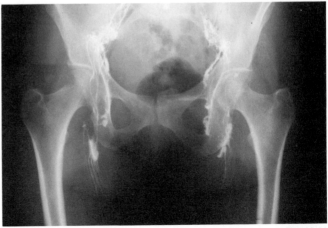

Fig. 22-26

Pelvic Lymphangiogram

Arthrography

Arthrography is radiographic examination of the soft tissue structures of joints (menisci, ligaments, articular cartilage, bursae) following injection of either a positive or a negative contrast medium into joint spaces. While arthrography may be done on any encapsulated joint (shoulder, hip, elbow, wrist, T.M.J.'s), the knee is the joint most often examined. On occasion, the joint is injected with both a negative and a positive contrast medium. A positive contrast medium arthrogram of a knee joint is shown in *Fig. 22-27*.

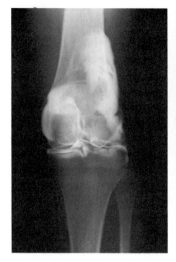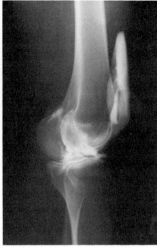

Positive Contrast Arthrogram   Fig. 22-27

Special Radiographic Examinations — Head

Tomography

Tomography is a method of radiographing a selected body plane of predetermined thickness from which unwanted shadows above and below the level of interest are reduced to a blur. In conventional radiography, a three-dimensional object (the body) is compressed to two dimensions on the finished radiograph. The negligible thickness of any radiograph in the direction of the x-ray beam results in images of a number of structures being superimposed upon one another. Conventional tomography and computed tomography eliminate unwanted images by displaying a plane of tissue on the radiograph or television screen. Most conventional tomographic units allow the patient to remain motionless while the x-ray tube and film travel in opposite directions in a prescribed manner during the exposure.

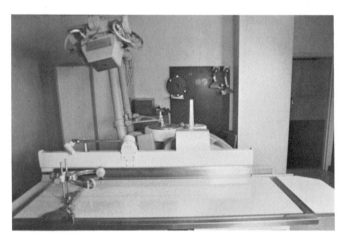

Conventional Tomographic Unit   Fig. 22-28

Those parts of the body that are very difficult to radiograph conventionally are often tomogrammed. Areas that may benefit from tomography are chest lesions, trachea, bronchi, larynx, sternum, sternoclavicular joints, odontoid process, upper thoracic spine, individual vertebrae, biliary ducts, kidneys (nephron phase of excretion), orbits, facial bones, sella turcica, sinuses, temporomandibular joints and the vertebral canal. The most common usage of conventional tomography is shown in *Fig. 22-29*. The delicate structures of the middle and inner ears lie within the dense petrous pyramid and thus benefit from body section radiography.

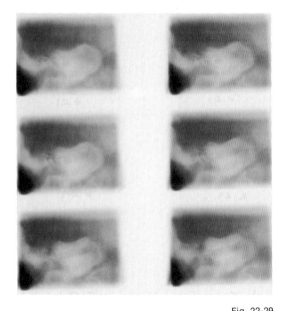

Petrous Pyramid Tomograms   Fig. 22-29

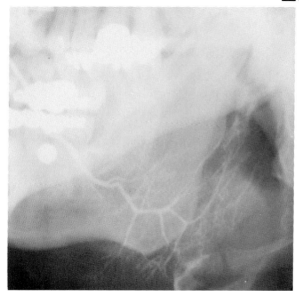

Sialography

Sialography is radiographic examination of the salivary ducts following injection of a radiopaque contrast medium. A cannula or catheter is passed into the proximal duct of the gland in question. Since there are several salivary glands in close approximation to one another, only one gland and duct can be examined at a time. After injection of an iodinated contrast medium, both the duct and the gland are visualized. An example of a sialogram is the parotid sialogram shown in *Fig. 22-30*.

Parotid Sialogram   Fig. 22-30

Digital Subtraction Angiography (DSA)

Digital radiographic systems use computers to convert impulses of the x-ray beam into numbers, and then translate them into an image on a television screen. This process permits image manipulations, storage and recall. Digital subtraction angiography is a technique of imaging arteries without visualizing the surrounding structures, as shown in *Fig. 22-31*. An image taken without a contrast medium is subtracted from one taken after material is injected. This technique is very similar to the time-consuming, film subtraction methods. By utilizing a digital computer, however, the subtraction is performed electronically and almost instantly. One of the big advantages of DSA is that arterial images can be visualized following intravenous injection. This procedure greatly decreases the risk factor for both the patient and the radiologist. An added advantage is that the examination can be done using a much lower radiation dose. Electronic radiography may someday replace film-screen radiography.

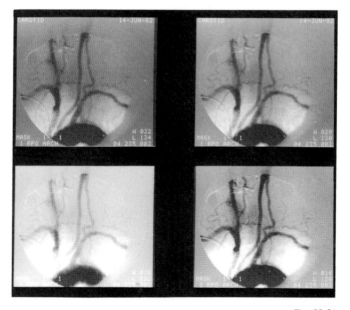

Digital Subtraction Arteriogram   Fig. 22-31

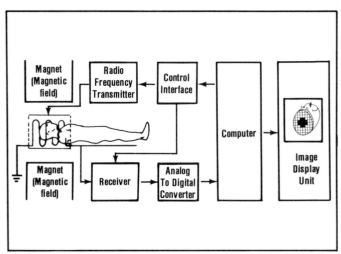

NMR Schematic   Fig. 22-32

Nuclear Magnetic Resonance (NMR)

Nuclear magnetic resonance (NMR) imaging is a new method utilized to produce a computed tomographic image similar to that produced by CT imaging and, in addition, is able to produce information concerning the chemical nature of the tissue in question. As shown in the simplified drawing in *Fig. 22-32,* the patient is placed in a strong magnetic field. A control interface and image display unit, and the gantry which houses the magnets, are shown in *Figs. 22-33* and *22-34.* (Courtesy Picker International)

Certain atomic nuclei, such as hydrogen, behave as small magnets. When these nuclei are placed in static magnetic fields, some will align themselves in the direction of the field and will rotate like a spinning top about the direction of the magnetic field. Energy is then added to these selected nuclei from a radio frequency transmitter delivering energy at just the correct phase and frequency. The specific nuclei in the tissue will absorb energy from the radio frequency transmitter only at a discrete, resonant frequency. When the radio frequency signal is removed, the excited nuclei will emit the added energy and return to their former state. Because nuclei of different elements have different resonant frequencies, the composition of the sample tissue can be determined from the energies that are given off following radio frequency transmission.

Additionally, the electrical signals can be converted to picture form and displayed as a computed section of patient anatomy. Several examples of sections produced by nuclear magnetic resonance imaging are shown in *Fig 22-35.*

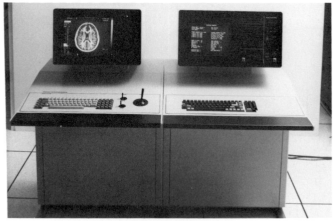

Control Interface and   Fig. 22-33
Image Display Unit

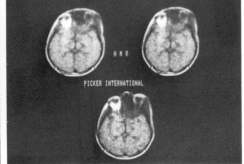

Magnet Gantry   Fig. 22-34
and Scanning Couch

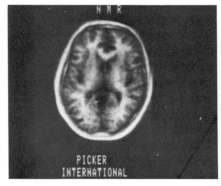

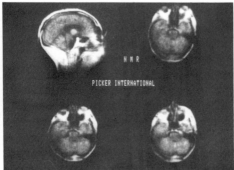

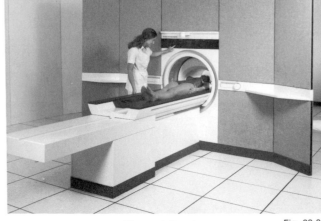

NMR Images   Fig. 22-35

Special Radiographic Examinations — Vertebral Column

Discography

Discography or nucleography is radiographic examination of individual intervertebral discs following injection of water-soluble, iodinated contrast medium into the center of the disc (nucleus pulposus). An example of a cervical discogram is shown in *Fig. 22-36*.

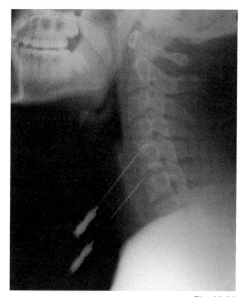

Cervical Discogram   Fig. 22-36

Myelography

Positive Contrast (Oily) Myelography. Myelography is radiographic examination of the central nervous system structures (spinal cord and spinal nerves) situated within the spinal canal following injection of a positive contrast medium. The positive contrast medium is either oil-based or water-soluble. Rarely, a negative contrast medium, air, is utilized. The contrast medium is placed within the subarachnoid space following spinal tap in the lower lumbar region or upper cervical region. An example of an oil-based cervical myelogram is shown in *Fig. 22-37*. Ideally, the oil-based contrast medium is removed following the examination since the material absorbs very, very slowly. Unless the base of the brain is to be studied, the contrast medium is not allowed to pass up onto the floor of the cranium. The neck is kept in hyperextension to prevent passage of the contrast medium past the foramen magnum.

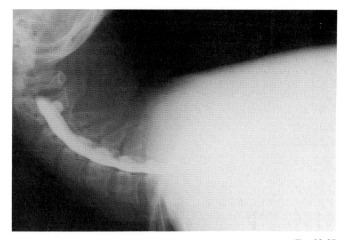

Cervical Myelogram   Fig. 22-37

Metrizamide Myelography. Myelography is also performed utilizing a water-soluble radiopaque contrast medium. Metrizamide is the basic ingredient of this contrast medium. An advantage to the use of metrizamide is that the solution need not be retrieved from the subarachnoid space. It is absorbed very rapidly into the circulatory system.

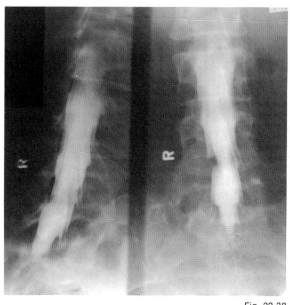

Lumbar Myelogram   Fig. 22-38

Computed Myelography. Computed myelography is computer-enhanced radiographic examination of the vertebral column, spinal cord and spinal nerves following injection of water-soluble metrizamide. In addition, nonenhanced computed tomography of the vertebral column and its contents is often performed. An example of a computed myelogram is shown in *Fig. 22-39*.

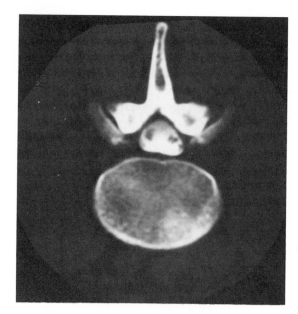

Computed Myelogram   Fig. 22-39

Epidural Venography

Epidural venography is radiographic examination of the collection of veins lining the spinal canal. This intricate plexus of veins is closely related to the intervertebral discs. This examination complements myelography in the diagnosis of intervertebral disc herniations. An example of an epidural venogram is shown in *Fig. 22-40*.

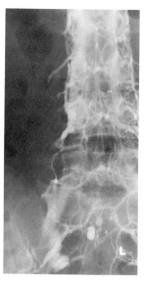

Epidural   Fig. 22-40
Venogram

Related Radiologic Imaging Modalities

Nuclear Medicine — Radionuclide Imaging

Nuclear medicine is that branch of radiology utilizing radioactive elements and compounds for both diagnosis and treatment. In nuclear medicine imaging, radioactive materials are administered to the patient. These radioactive materials will concentrate in a particular organ or system. Sensitive detectors measure the radiation, especially gamma rays, emerging from the concentrated radioactivity. Most of the radiopharmaceuticals have a short half-life, deliver a low radiation dose, emit gamma rays, are easily detected and are readily available.

Examinations commonly performed in the nuclear medicine laboratory include lung ventilation and perfusion studies, cardiac scan and flow examinations, bone scans, thyroid uptakes and scans, liver-spleen scans, brain scan and flow studies, cisternography, kidney scan and flow studies, and detection of primary and metastatic neoplasia. Certain examinations, such as lung ventilation imaging and thyroid scanning, are unique to nuclear medicine. Many other examinations complement studies performed in other parts of the radiology department.

Ultrasonography

Ultrasonography is that branch of radiology utilizing sound waves to produce signals from within the body and transform these signals to recordable images. High frequency sound waves exhibit both transmission and reflection properties as they pass through the human body. An image is formed since the sound beam reacts with each tissue interface or boundary that it encounters as it passes through the body.

Advantages and Uses of Ultrasonography. Two advantages of ultrasonography are that it is noninvasive and that it does not require the use of ionizing radiation. Since ionizing radiation is not used, multiple examinations are possible. This fact is especially important in obstetrical ultrasonography. Placental localization, fetal cephalometry, multiple or early pregnancy, and growth patterns are studied with ultrasound. Ultrasound studies of the heart, eyes, blood vessels and abdominal organs are other uses of this imaging modality. A midsagittal uterine sonogram of a term fetus is shown in *Fig. 22-42*.

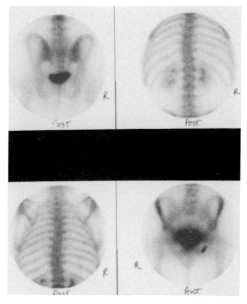

Bone Scans   Fig. 22-41

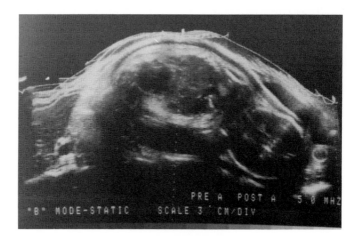

Uterine Sonogram   Fig. 22-42

Bibliography

Abrams, H., editor. Angiography, ed. 2, vol. 1. Boston: Little, Brown and Co., 1971.

Becker, R.; Wilson, J.; Gehweiler, J. The Anatomical Basis of Medical Practice, ed. 1. Baltimore: The Williams & Wilkins Co., 1971.

Clark, K.C. Positioning in Radiography, ed. 9, vols. I and II. London: Ilford Limited, William Heinemann Medical Books, Ltd., 1974.

Compere, W. Radiographic Atlas of the Temporal Bone, Book 1, ed. 1. St. Paul, Minnesota: H.M. Smyth Co., Inc., 1964.

Christensen, E.; Curry, T.; Dowdey, J. An Introduction to the Physics of Diagnostic Radiology, ed. 2. Philadelphia: Lea & Febiger, 1978.

Egan, R. Technologist Guide to Mammography, ed. 1. Baltimore: The Williams & Wilkins Co., 1968.

Etter, L. Roentgenography and Roentgenology of the Middle Ear and Mastoid Process, ed. 1. Springfield, Illinois: Charles C. Thomas, Publisher, 1965.

Gerhardt, P.; vanKaich, G. Total Body Computed Tomography, ed. 2. Stuttgart: Georg Thieme Publishers, 1979.

Gray, H. Anatomy of the Human Body, ed. 27. Philadelphia: Lea & Febiger, 1959.

Jacobi, C.; Paris, D. Textbook of Radiologic Technology, ed. 5. St. Louis: C.V. Mosby Co., 1972.

Kreel, L.; Steiner, R. Medical Imaging, ed. 1. Exeter, Great Britain: A. Wheaton & Co. Ltd., 1979.

Merrill, V. Atlas of Roentgenographic Positions and Standard Radiologic Procedures, ed. 4, vols. I, II, and III. St. Louis: C.V. Mosby Co., 1975.

Meschan, I. An Atlas of Anatomy Basic to Radiology, ed. 1. Philadelphia: Lea & Febiger, 1975.

Meschan, I. Radiographic Positioning and Related Anatomy, ed. 2. Philadelphia: W.B. Saunders Co., 1978.

New, P.; Scott, W. Computed Tomography of the Brain and Orbit, ed. 1. Baltimore: The Williams & Wilkins Co., 1975.

Norman, D.; Korobkin, M.; Newton, T., editors. Computed Tomography, ed. 1. St. Louis: C.V. Mosby Co., 1977.

Ramsey, R. Advanced Exercises in Diagnostic Radiology, #9, Computed Tomography of the Brain, ed. 1, Philadelphia: W.B. Saunders Co., 1977.

Taveras, J.; Wood, E. Diagnostic Neuroradiology, ed. 2, vol. I. Baltimore: The Williams & Wilkins Co., 1976.

Valvassori, G. Radiographic Atlas of the Temporal Bone, Book II, ed. 1. St. Paul, Minnesota: H.M. Smyth Co., Inc., 1964.

Subject Index

Book List

The following books are also available from Multi-Media Publishing, Inc.:

Radiation Protection for Student Radiographers, Mary Alice Statkiewicz-Sherer, A.S., R.T.(R), and E. Russell Ritenour, Ph.D., 277 pages, 80 illustrations, $15.95, I.S.B.N. 0-940122-10-3

Introduction to Magnetic Resonance Imaging, William R. Hendee, Ph.D., and Christopher Morgan, M.D., 215 pages, 50 illustrations, $26.95, I.S.B.N. 0-940122-13-8

Diagnostic Ultrasound For Radiographers, Patricia A. Athey, M.D., and Linda McClendon, R.T., R.D.M.S., 121 pages, 62 illustrations, $13.95, I.S.B.N. 0-940122-09-X

Textbook of Radiographic Positioning and Related Anatomy, Kenneth L. Bontrager, M.A., R.T.(R), and Barry T. Anthony, R.T.(R), 550 pages, 1,580 illustrations, $54.95, I.S.B.N. 0-940122-01-4

Radiology Management: An Introduction, Eric Bouchard, M.A., R.T.(R), 230 pages, 50 illustrations, $18.95, I.S.B.N. 0-940122-04-9

Introduction to Radiologic Technology, LaVerne T. Gurley, Ph.D., R.T.(R), FASRT, and William J. Callaway, B.A., R.T.(R) with 16 contributors, 270 pages, 66 illustrations, $16.95, I.S.B.N. 0-940122-02-2

Radiation Physics Laboratory Manual, Marianne R. Tortorici, Ed.D., R.T.(R), and Hiram M. Hunt, Ed.D., 172 pages, 60 illustrations, $12.95, I.S.B.N. 0-940122-14-6

Order from: Multi-Media Publishing, Inc.
1393 S. Inca Street
Denver, Colorado 80223
(303) 778-1404